HEALTH PROMOTION PLANNING

An Educational and Environmental Approach

HEALTH PROMOTION PLANNING
An Educational and
Environmental Approach

SECOND EDITION

Lawrence W. Green
Institute of Health Promotion Research
University of British Columbia

Marshall W. Kreuter
Health 2000

With the assistance of staff of

The Center for Health Promotion Research and Development
University of Texas Health Science Center at Houston

Center for Chronic Disease Prevention and Health Promotion
Centers for Disease Control, Public Health Service
U.S. Department of Health and Human Services

and

The Henry J. Kaiser Family Foundation

MAYFIELD PUBLISHING COMPANY

MOUNTAIN VIEW   TORONTO   LONDON

For Judith M. Ottoson and Martha F. Katz

Library of Congress Cataloging-in-Publication Data

Green, Lawrence W.
    Health promotion planning : an educational and environmental
approach / Lawrence W. Green and Marshall W. Kreuter ; with the
assistance of staff of The Center for Health Promotion Research and
Development, University of Texas Health Science Center at Houston,
Center for Chronic Disease Control and Health Promotion, Centers for
Disease Control, Public Health Service, U.S. Department of Health
and Human Services, and The Henry J. Kaiser Family Foundation. —
2nd ed.
        p.   cm.
    Includes bibliographical references and index.
    ISBN 0-87484-779-6
    1. Health promotion — United States.   2. Health education — United
States — Planning.   I. Kreuter, Marshall W.   II. Title.
RA427.8.G74   1991
613'.0973 — dc20   90-20500
                                                                          CIP

Manufactured in the United States of America
10   9   8   7   6   5   4

Mayfield Publishing Company
1240 Villa Street
Mountain View, CA 94041

Sponsoring Editor, James Bull; manuscript editor, Yvonne Howell; text designer, Diane
Beasley. The text was set in 10/12 Times Roman by Harrison Typesetting, Inc., and
printed on 50# Glatfelter Spring Forge by Thomson-Shore.

Brief Contents

Contents

4   Behavioral and Environmental Diagnosis   125

8   Applications of PRECEDE–PROCEED in
     Community Settings 261

Preface

This book and the previous edition, which was called *Health Education Planning: A Diagnostic Approach*, have been written to provide a conceptual synthesis of the roots and foundations of health education and, more recently, health promotion following a period of rapid growth and development. Before 1980, the field of action represented by health education and health promotion lacked a clear articulation of its boundaries, its methods and procedures, and the distinctions between health education and health promotion. The philosophy, intellectual roots, and systematic descriptions of health education subspecialities were well represented in textbooks, and the research foundation was growing in every direction. We proposed a single framework on which disparate new research findings could be hung, a heuristic for theorists and planners, and a practical teaching and learning tool for practitioners, professors, and students trying to make sense of the field.

For most of this century, health promotion has been relegated to the status of a philosophical ideal, subsumed under the World Health Organization's definition of health. It was seldom translated into policy — and then most often only within the confines of health education and fitness programs. In 1974, the LaLonde report, *A New Perspective on the Health of Canadians*, put the term "health promotion" on a new footing by using it with policy backing for the first time. In 1975, Public Law 94-317 gave policy support to health promotion in the United States with the Health Information and Health Promotion Act and the creation of the federal Office of Disease Prevention and Health Promotion. Since then, a wide range of government and private-sector initiatives to support a more healthful lifestyle for whole communities, and even societies, have been implemented. Major clean air initiatives and a host of local ordinances have been passed to control smoking in public places. Consumer organizations and self-help groups advocate healthful living conditions and resources to increase personal control over the factors influencing health. Increased cooperation between levels of government and between health agencies and other sectors has produced new health promotion opportunities and activities, notably in schools and worksites, but also in whole communities, states, and nations where coalitions have taken hold. Media have given increased attention to health issues, and initiatives to demand greater equity and social justice in access to health resources have been passed. However, some social equity has been lost, as well.

In the tumult of these times, when health promotion engages behavioral and social scientists, epidemiologists, physicians, nurses, political activists, physical educators, communications and marketing specialists, and others, the linchpin for health promotion is the status of health education in all its various dimensions. We place emphasis here on the single word "education," not "information," nor even "health education." Education for health empowers through the development of understanding, motivation, and skills. We emphasize not just the knowledge and skills to reduce behavioral risks, as important as they are, but also those elements that engage people more actively in their community's affairs, such as participating effectively in making health and social policy, demanding enforcement of regulations on environmental polluters, and organizing advocacy for new or revised laws and regulations. These public dimensions of health promotion require education of the electorate no less than the personal risk-reduction dimensions.

Health promotion now affords new opportunities and challenges for health practitioners as they seek to strengthen the organizational, economic, and environmental supports necessary for healthful living in modern society. We hope this book offers help to those who would accept these challenges.

Despite enormous expansion in the scope of health promotion policy and practice, responsibility for health promotion planning is still left largely to those identified as health educators. There has been no significant movement to create a new profession called health promotion, and we are not advocating such a movement with the retitling of this book. Professional training for health promotion is centered still in the departments of health education and community health of health professional schools. To varying degrees, training also occurs in the form of electives in schools of public health, medicine, nursing, dentistry, pharmacy, allied health, and physical education and recreation. Health promotion planning continues to depend on health education specialists not only because they hold many of the key positions from which to mount the expanded functions of health promotion, but also because they possess the essential combination of skills in program planning and behavioral diagnosis described in the first edition of this book. However, the field of health promotion does offer a more open invitation for people in other professions and for laypersons to take leadership roles not frequently offered by the increasingly professionalized field of health education.

Our task in this second edition has been to catch up with the rapid developments in policy, research, and practice. While maintaining the integrity of the PRECEDE planning framework that has been widely tested in various settings at the national, provincial or state, and community levels, we have expanded the model to accommodate the more comprehensive field of health promotion. Thus, the diagnostic approach now encompasses the social forces (including political, organizational, economic, and environmental) that influence lifestyle and health, as well as the more specific behavioral influences on health and the more immediate educational influences on behavior.

Within this expanded scope, we continue to emphasize an educational approach to health promotion as the essential starting point, even when the ultimate interventions must be more coercive, regulatory, or economic. Indeed, the public support and acceptance of new legislation and regulation depends on adequate preparation of the citizenry through an educational process. Many good legislative bills that would have improved the public's health have failed to pass or have been repealed because their sponsors failed to build an educated constituency for them. The continuing commitment to an educational approach to health, even within the political context of health promotion, is reflected in the new subtitle of this edition.

Our attempt here to address the essentially political dimension of health promotion is a departure from our more strictly scientific and technological approach to health education in the previous edition. We attempted then to avoid ideological traps by taking a value-free stance with respect to methods, except for one overriding principle or philosophy — that behavior change should be voluntary. We remain committed to that educational philosophy in this edition, and it remains the basis for the development of an educational diagnostic model. At the same time, we recognize that the social policy targets of health promotion sometimes call for aggressive and even coercive measures to regulate the behavior of those individuals, corporations, and government officials whose actions influence the health of others. The essential rule of thumb we suggest for justifying more coercive means of changing behavior or lifestyle is when the behavior in question is one that threatens the health or well-being of others, such as drunk driving or the promotion of unhealthful products to children. This rule runs into gray areas, of course, when the alleged threat to the well-being of others is something more remote, such as the long-term economic cost to society incurred by people who smoke or engage in other high-risk behavior today that *might* result in chronic illness or disability later. It also runs into value conflicts with constitutional protections such as the First Amendment right to free speech, which protects advertising as well as the press.

As we come to grips with more and more of these value-laden choices in health promotion, we must develop and sharpen the political understanding and skill of those who plan health promotion programs. We have put this burden particularly on Chapter 2, the quality-of-life assessment or "social diagnosis." The emphasis is on methods of assuring the active involvement of people in assessing their own needs and evaluating their own progress and programs. This is especially relevant at the local level, where values can be weighed within the context of the social culture and economy. Again, the educational perspective prevails, with the emphasis on participation and enabling people to take greater control of the decisions influencing their quality of life, but we have tried to reflect more on the political realities in carrying out this frequently neglected phase of the diagnostic process.

The original framework, which we called PRECEDE in the previous edition, remains largely intact in this edition. PRECEDE stands for "predisposing, reinforcing, and enabling constructs in educational diagnosis and evaluation." To accommodate the broader mandate of health promotion, we have superimposed an additional set of procedures which we call PROCEED for "policy, regulatory, and organizational constructs in educational and environmental development." The burden of this component of the combined model falls on what we called the administrative diagnosis in the previous edition. The administrative diagnosis is the final planning step to "precede" implementation. From there we "proceed" to promote the plan or policy, regulate the environment, and organize the resources and services, as required by the plan or policy. The promotional, regulatory, and organizational components of PROCEED take the student or practitioner beyond educational interventions to the political, managerial, and economic actions necessary to make social systems and environments more conducive to healthful lifestyles and a more complete state of physical, mental, and social well-being for all.

ACKNOWLEDGMENTS

The frameworks for planning presented in this text grew out of our combined experience in practice, research, teaching, consultation, and government service—all guided and enriched by significant teachers, colleagues, and students. PRECEDE included an amalgamation of Ronald Andersen's *Behavioral Model of Families' Use of Health Services*, Albert Bandura's Social Learning Theory, Hochbaum, Rosenstock, and Becker's Health Belief Model, Fishbein's behavioral intention mode, J. Mayone Stycos' decision model on couples' adoption of family planning methods, Kurt Lewin's force-field analysis, and Edward E. Bartlett's methods and strategies in health education. These models and our collaboration with Sigrid Deeds, David Levine, Kay Partridge, Virginia Li, and others at Johns Hopkins University in the 1970s influenced our way of thinking about health education planning, needs assessment, and evaulation.

Similarly, PROCEED was a product of the Health Field Concept of Laframboise and the LaLonde report; of our experience with Joseph Califano, Julius Richmond, James O. Mason, Michael McGinnis, Martha Katz, Donald Iverson, Lloyd Kolbe, Henry Montes, Patricia Mullen, Dennis Tolsma, and others in the U.S. federal initiative in disease prevention and health promotion, including participation in the development of the national objectives for 1990, the Model Standards for Community Preventive Health Services, and in similar processes with several state and local health agencies; of the work of Judith Ottoson, Guy

Parcel, Nell Gottlieb, Bruce and Denise Simons-Morton, and Susan Brink on implementation; of the World Health Organization's Declaration of Alma Alta and Technical Discussions of the 1983 World Health Assembly on New Policies in Health Education for Primary Health Care; of the U.S. Preventive Services Task Force; and of the Ottawa Charter for Health Promotion, which brought together the views of thirty-eight European, North American, and Western Pacific countries. We are especially grateful to Denise Simons-Morton, Susan Brink, Nell Gottlieb, Chris Lovato, Pat Mullen, Guy Parcel, and Lloyd Kolbe for help on specific chapters as noted in the footnotes.

In addition to the students, fellows, and colleagues we acknowledged in the first edition, we are indebted to the following for additional insights, helpful suggestions, and feedback from their experiences with the models: David Altman, Hans Andrianse, Jim Belloni, Robert Bertera, Bob Bolan, Arthur Brownlea, Pat Bush, Nelly Candeais, Ray Carlaw, Judy Chwalow, Helen Cleary, Bryan Cooke, Cheryl Cortines, William Cresswell, Wendy Cuneo, Lawren Daltroy, Nicole Dedobbeleer, Evelyne deLeeuw, Hein DeVries, Mark Dignan, Carole Donovan, Sharon Dorfman, Stuart Dunn, Rosemarie Erban, Michael Ericksen, Stephanie Evans, Jack Farquhar, Michael Felix, Mary Ann Fenley, Jonathan Fielding, John Fisher, Bryan Flynn, Stuart Fors, Janet Fuchs, Nell Gottlieb, Syed Jahangir Haider, Michele Hindi-Alexander, Peter Howatt, Ruby Isom, Jack Jones, Howard Kalmer, Laura Kann, Gerjo Kok, Lloyd Kolbe, Fred Kroger, Robert Lawrence, Dick Levinson, Fran Lewis, Kate Lorig, Chris Lovato, Alfred McAlister, Ken McLeroy, Donald Morisky, Charles Nelson, Gary Nelson, Ian Newman, Horace Ogden, Richard Papenfuss, Guy Parcel, David Poehler, John Raeburn, Amelie Ramirez, Marilyn Rice, Barbara Rimer, Todd Rogers, Allen Rubin, Zora Salisbury, Randy Schwartz, Bruce and Denise Simons-Morton, David Sleet, Shelagh Smith, Gene Stainbrook, Ron Stoddard, Ellen Tabak, Kathy Tiernan, Nancy Watkins, Alisa Wilson, Bente Wold, Colin Yarham, and Jane Zapka.

We are grateful also for the administrative support of the University of Texas Health Science Center, particularly Marty Lazzari, and of the Kaiser Family Foundation, particularly Beverly Wright and Carol Holt.

The final compilation of revisions produced from our collaborations in Texas, Georgia, and California was assisted by Jackie Clare Wood, Sc.D. She helped fill some last gaps. Jim Bull took over from Lansing Hays as our editor at Mayfield, providing patient encouragement and support throughout the revision process.

Lawrence W. Green, Vancouver
Marshall W. Kreuter, Atlanta

Chapter 1

Health Promotion Today and a Framework for Planning

his chapter examines the historic and epidemiologic reasons for the emergence of health promotion as the best hope of effectively combating the leading causes of death.[1] It also introduces the two components of the health promotion planning framework: (a) a diagnostic (or needs assessment) phase called **PRECEDE**, (*p*redisposing, *r*einforcing, and *e*nabling *c*onstructs in *e*ducational/ *e*nvironmental *d*iagnosis and *e*valuation) and (b) a developmental stage of health promotion planning that follows the diagnostic assessment and initiates the implementation and evaluation process. This second component is called **PROCEED** (*p*olicy, *r*egulatory, and *o*rganizational *c*onstructs in *e*ducational and *e*nvironmental *d*evelopment).

RELATION OF HEALTH PROMOTION TO HEALTH EDUCATION AND PUBLIC HEALTH

A popular notion of **health promotion**[2] is of lean and ruddy people, alone, grimly adhering to a regimen of **health-directed behavior** to reduce their risks of premature death, disease, and even aging. Important as such goal-oriented activity may be for that small minority of individuals, and much as health education can point with pride to its development in recent years, goal-oriented activity is but a small piece of the more pervasive and problematic web of the **health-related behavior** of individuals as well as families, groups, communities, and organizations. This more pervasive behavior has to do with patterns and **conditions of living** – housing, eating, playing, working, and just plain loafing – most of which lie outside the realm of the health sector and are not consciously health-directed.

1

The previous edition of this book[3] adhered to a definition of **health education** that insisted on voluntary change in behavior and hence limited its scope to conscious health-directed behavior. Health education could be shown to work most directly, effectively, and humanely when people were clearly oriented to solve a discrete and immediate behavioral or health problem of importance to them. Patient education and self-care education (in which people are motivated to cure or control a disease), immunization programs (in which people want to avoid an imminent threat), screening programs (in which people seek a specific diagnosis or reassurance), smoking cessation programs (in which people want to quit), family planning programs (in which people want to prevent or delay a pregnancy), and other highly targeted programs were advanced by the application of the framework and procedures outlined by the diagnostic approach of the previous edition.

As that book went to press in 1979, the *Surgeon General's Report on Health Promotion and Disease Prevention*[4] challenged the American public and professional health community to examine more critically our routine and usually unpremeditated health-related behaviors and the community conditions of living that account for over 50 percent of the causes of premature death and to examine the policies supporting such behaviors and living conditions. Among these, the most important were substance misuse and addiction (including tobacco and alcohol), poor diet, sedentary work and leisure, and stress-related conditions (including suicide, violence, and reckless behavior). These behavioral and **lifestyle** risk factors were estimated to account for 40–70 percent of all premature deaths, a third of all cases of acute disability, and two thirds of all cases of chronic disability. Sexual behavior was considered important in relation to teenage pregnancy and sexually transmitted diseases, but it took on much greater importance as a cause of death after the emergence of the AIDS epidemic.

CONTROVERSY CONCERNING THE SCOPE OF HEALTH PROMOTION

The complexity and value-laden character of these proposed targets of health promotion policies were shown by the language of the critiques and debates that greeted both the *Health Education Planning* book and the *Surgeon General's Report*. The controversy hinged on phrases such as individual versus social responsibility for health[5]; facilitating individual behavior change versus broader, institutional and social change approaches to health promotion[6]; behavioral versus ecological strategies[7]; healthy people versus healthy cities and healthy policies[8]; blaming the victim versus blaming the manufacturers of illness.[9]

The federal office that issued the *Surgeon General's Report* published in the same year a quasi-official definition of health promotion as "any combination of health education and related organizational, political and economic interventions designed to facilitate behavioral and environmental changes conducive to health."[10] This did not silence the critics, who continued to worry in subsequent years that the Reagan administration, which took office in 1981, would use a narrower concept of behavior and individual responsibility in its health promotion policy to justify cuts in basic health services and government programs.

At the heart of the health promotion debates and in some of the contentious phrases and ideologies, one can find both positive and pejorative uses of the word *lifestyle*. As a target for health promotion policy and programs, lifestyle is, for some people, the consciously chosen, personal behavior of individuals as it may relate to health. To others, lifestyle is a composite expression of the social and cultural circumstances that condition and constrain behavior, in addition to the personal decisions the individual might make in choosing one behavior over another.[11] Both uses of the term acknowledge that lifestyle is a more enduring (some would say habitual) *pattern* of behavior than is often connoted by the term behavior or action.

The persistence of behavior became an increasingly important dimension of health behavior as the chronic and degenerative diseases displaced acute, communicable diseases in the list of the leading causes of morbidity and mortality. Once, a single act such as getting an immunization could provide a lifetime of protection against an infectious disease; but now, a lifetime of simple, seemingly harmless acts—such as eating high-fat foods, smoking a few cigarettes each day, going to work in heavy traffic without seat belts, and driving home after a few drinks— account for most of society's disease, injury, disability, and premature death.

Although health education had been successful in public health campaigns to change single health-directed acts, many policy makers and health officials of the 1970s were not confident that health education could bring about changes in the new public health targets—the more complex, lifetime habits and the social circumstances associated with the term *lifestyle*.[12] With such elusive targets as socially embedded lifestyles, public health education could have an impact on public health only if it joined other sectors and brought multiple social forces to bear, some of which would go beyond the ethical definition of and most policy makers' understanding of health education.

There was also the question of equity and social justice.[13] As James Mason, then director of the Centers for Disease Control (CDC), now assistant secretary for health, put it a few years later:

> It is my observation that, up until now, most of the behavior changes we have promoted have involved the better-educated, upper-, and middle-class segments of our society. If health promotion is a good thing, it should be good for the whole society, not just that portion which is favorably predisposed. Unless we are able to reach all segments of the population, we will never meet the goals we have set for a national consciousness for wellness in America.[14]

Health education was drawn into the fray with the opportunity to provide leadership for an expanded public health policy of lifestyle priorities and objectives under the mantle of health promotion.[15] The previously quoted quasi-official definition of health promotion sought to position health education centrally in the new federal policies and programs. A refined and simplified version of that definition is offered here for purposes of this book: *Health promotion is the combination of educational and environmental supports for actions and conditions of living conducive to health.* The actions or behavior in question may be those of individuals, groups, or communities, of policy makers, employers, teachers, or others whose actions control or influence the determinants of health. The purpose of health promotion is to enable people to gain greater control over the determinants of their own health.[16] This control ideally resides with the individual when the determinants are ones over which he or she can exert personal control, but with some aspects of the complex lifestyle issues, especially those that affect the health of others such as drunk driving, the control that people exercise must be through community decisions and actions.[17]

COMMUNITY AS THE CENTER OF GRAVITY FOR HEALTH PROMOTION

If the first *Surgeon General's Report on Health Promotion and Disease Prevention* seemed to put too much responsibility on the individual, some of the wishful thinking of some health promotion advocates has expected too much of national policy and centralized planning.[18] If the victim-blaming implicit in policies that focused on individual behavior was unfair, the system-blaming implicit in some of the more sweeping social reform proposals offered as alternatives was unproductive. A unified middle ground must be found if health promotion is to be viable policy.[19] The value-laden, culturally and ethnically defined nature of many of the lifestyle issues such as diet make it impossible to dictate behavior uniformly from a distant central government, especially in pluralistic, democratic societies.[20] The private nature of many of these practices, such as sexual and sedentary behavior, make them inaccessible to effective surveillance and regulation. The constitutional and civil rights of citizens protect most of the behaviors, including even the right to bear arms in the United States, or the right to sexual practices among consenting adults, or freedom of speech protecting pornography and advertising of unhealthful products. The state or provincial dominion of large federation or commonwealth governments, such as those of Australia, Canada, and the United States, limit the powers of central government in favor of state or provincial rights to police power in matters of health, and most of these powers are ceded to local governments.[21]

In the final analysis, the most effective and proper center of gravity for health promotion is the community.[22] State and national governments can formulate policies, provide leadership, allocate funding, and generate data for health promotion. At the other extreme, individuals can govern their own behavior and control the determinants of their own health up to a point, and should be allowed to do so. But the decisions on priorities and strategies for *social* change affecting the more complicated lifestyle issues can best be made collectively as close as possible to the homes and workplaces of those affected. This principle assures that programs are relevant and appropriate to the people affected, and it offers greater opportunity for the people affected to be actively engaged in the planning process. The overwhelming weight of evidence from research and experience on the value of participation in learning and behavior indicates that people are more committed to initiating and upholding those changes that they helped design or adapt to their own purposes and circumstances.[23]

Community may be the town or county in sparsely populated areas or the school, worksite, or neighborhood in more populous metropolitan areas. It is, ideally, a level of collective decision making appropriate to the urgency and magnitude of the problem, the cost and technical complexity of the solutions required, the culture and traditions of shared decision making, and the sensitivity and consequences of the actions required of people after the decision is made. Once national policy settled on objectives for health promotion in countries such as Australia, Canada, Finland, the Netherlands, Sweden, and the United States, the necessity of adapting those policies to the state or provincial and community levels became inescapable.[24]

THE RENAISSANCE OF HEALTH PROMOTION

The epidemiological revolution of the nineteenth century is usually traced to the events surrounding the development of the germ theory of disease and its application in public health. But much of the actual reduction in morbidity and mortality during that century can be attributed more directly to massive changes in the lifestyles of the populations of Europe and North America.[25] These changes were brought about through the "poor laws" and social reforms in housing, food supply, and working conditions, as well as through the popularization of health through advice literature, voluntary societies, and classes on human physiology in schools.[26] The sanitary reforms of Chadwick in Great Britain and Shattuck in Massachusetts centered in large part on recommendations for the improvement of living and working conditions, not just changes in the sanitation of the physical environment. Many of these social reforms in behalf of the health of populations were characteristic of today's initiatives to ban smoking in public places, to provide fitness facilities in workplaces, and to obtain nutrition labeling on packaged foods in the name of health promotion.[27]

This broad and encompassing concept of health promotion is hardly new,[28] though its latter-day resurgence is a departure from the drift of health policy over the decades since World War II. C. E. A. Winslow, in 1920, referred to "promoting health" as "organized community effort for the . . . education of the individual in personal health, and the development of the social machinery to assure everyone a standard of living adequate for the maintenance or improvement of health."[29] The social machinery for health was turned full bore toward medical care after World War II.

THREE ERAS THAT LED TO HEALTH PROMOTION POLICY

The Era of Resource Development. The postwar years are sometimes called the era of resource development. In Europe and Japan this was a period of reconstruction in all sectors, whereas in the United States its chief product was legislation to build three types of health resources: scientific knowledge, medical facilities, and health personnel. Knowledge was developed through inauguration of the National Institutes of Health and massive investments in biomedical research. Facilities were developed through the Hill–Burton Act, mandating the building of hospitals and clinics in virtually every community. Personnel to staff these facilities came with the Health Manpower Act, renewed periodically to finance the professional training of physicians, nurses, dentists, veterinarians, and a modest number of public health and allied health personnel.

This momentous investment in health resources produced an infrastructure that was primarily biomedical rather than health in its orientation. Eventually the question arose: Are these vast resources for medical care equitably distributed?

The Era of Redistribution. In the 1960s the United States entered an era of redistribution of resources with the New Frontier initiatives, the Great Society and the War on Poverty of Presidents Kennedy and Johnson. The emphasis was on the equitable redistribution of resources, particularly with the development of neighborhood health centers and the introduction of Medicare and Medicaid in 1966. These new laws were designed to put health authority and medical purchasing power in the hands of consumers, especially the elderly and the poor.

Health education during this era was devoted largely to *increasing* the public's use of health services. Programs were designed with behavioral objectives and community organization strategies to reduce the delay in seeking medical care in response to symptoms, to increase participation in mass screening and immunization programs, and to increase attendance at well-child and family planning clinics.

The initiatives of the 1960s achieved greater equity in the distribution and use of resources. The poor now had greater access to medical services, and their rates of use of those services increased almost to the levels of the affluent.[30] But though the gap between the "haves" and the "have-nots" was significantly reduced in terms of access to medical services, morbidity and mortality indicators continued to reflect strong socioeconomic and racial disparities.[31] The nation now had to ask whether it was paying for unnecessary services rendered by physicians and hospitals eager to tap into the Medicare and Medicaid wellsprings or excessively consumed by patients uneducated to the newly accessible services.

The Era of Cost Containment. The overutilization question came as the cost of medical care was rising rapidly in many countries. Most countries were entering a period of austerity in the 1970s. In the United States, this took the form of cost-containment initiatives in government-sponsored programs, especially medical care programs. It also opened a new opportunity for health education and public health, placing disease prevention and health promotion back on the policy agenda after decades of national preoccupation with medical care resources and services.

The era of cost containment began with efforts to trim the pricing of medical care itself, but more basic solutions began to be sought on the demand side with the appointment of the President's Committee on Health Education.[32] The Committee report proposed several possibilities for the organization of federal and private-sector initiatives to control costs. These included education of the public in self-care and appropriate use of health services (primarily to *reduce* utilization) and a fundamental strengthening of health education in schools, worksites, and communities.

The Health Maintenance Organization Act of 1973 provided incentives for the medical care system to practice preventive medicine to keep patients out of expensive hospital beds. It made health education services mandatory for those health maintenance organizations (HMOs) receiving federal certification.[33] This requirement was subsequently removed, but HMOs continued to develop health education services.

The National Health Planning and Resource Development Act of 1974 specified public health education as one of the nation's health planning priorities and made it a requirement of state and regional plans.[34] Self-care education initiatives in health services research and policy gained notable prominence during this period.[35] Note that all of these initiatives of the cost-containment era were designed to *reduce* the public's use of health services, whereas in the earlier era health education's role had been to *increase* use.

FROM COST CONTAINMENT TO HEALTH PROMOTION

Cost containment gave some credence to health education as evidence came in on the effectiveness of self-care education programs in reducing unnecessary use of health services and of patient education reducing hospital days following surgery.[36] These efforts to control costs by decreasing the need for health care provided an initial policy boost for renewed interest in disease prevention and health promotion. But a second epidemiological revolution was afoot, supporting the development of health promotion policy independent of the cost-containment rationale and the medical care system.[37]

The Increase in Chronic Diseases. Around the middle of the twentieth century, chronic diseases surpassed communicable diseases as the leading causes of death in developed countries. Interest in health education and public health had waned with the decline of communicable diseases and did not immediately increase with the emergence of the chronic diseases. From the 1950s through the 1960s, health education and public health were kept alive by occasional immunization campaigns, family planning programs, work on communicable-disease control and family planning in the developing countries, and leadership in the citizen-participation component of the health planning and neighborhood health center movements of the 1960s.

The Self-Care Movement. Citizen participation was a cornerstone of the War on Poverty and health-planning initiatives.[38] At the same time, the self-care initiatives had taken the shape of a significant social movement, variously referred to as self-help, self-reliance, or self-improvement.[39] Health education and the budding health promotion movement became tools of the people seeking to take control of their own health and to control the determinants of their health, rather than tools of the establishment seeking to control people's use of health services or to gain their cooperation in managing centrally planned health programs.

Individual Participation and Responsibility. It was a short and natural step for public health to shift its emphasis from institution building and centrally planned programs to self-reliance, person-centered initiatives, and individual participation in health. The budgetary constraints on health agencies and institutions, combined with the need for behavioral change to control the chronic diseases, made the desire of the public for more personal involvement and initiative in health a welcome relief for program budgets and a tempting opportunity to shift responsibility for health from professionals and government institutions to individuals and families.[40]

Private Sector Initiatives. The rebirth of personal initiative in health was simultaneously an epidemiological necessity, a popular movement, and a budgetary convenience. In the 1970s the idea was embraced by governmental, professional, and commercial interests. Personal initiative produced consumer demand, which was followed by private sector initiative to supply commercial products and services. Self-help and dietary books were at the top of the best-seller lists more often than any other category of nonfiction. A business boom developed for vendors of health courses, self-help products, and packaged wellness programs for large employers. Private companies supported personal health initiatives with increased health insurance coverage and worksite health promotion programs for employees.[41] In response to the recommendation of the President's Committee on Health Education for private and public sector focal points, a National Center for Health Education was created in the private sector in 1973.

Independent Sector Initiatives. Coterminous with the public and private sector initiatives in health promotion have been innovations and demonstrations sponsored by voluntary health organizations and philanthropic foundations. The voluntary health associations had long maintained public health education programs and sought to influence school health curricula. The American Heart Association convened one of the first gatherings of behavioral scientists and health educators to review the state of applied social science in reducing cardiovascular risk, going beyond strictly educational approaches.[42]

The Rockefeller and Ford Foundations had a long history of supporting community development approaches to public health problems in developing countries. In the 1960s, the Ford Foundation provided much of the funding for the Population Council's mass media and community approaches to family planning in developing countries, which predated the community-based cardiovascular risk reduction projects in the United States, Finland, and Australia.[43] In 1977, The W. K. Kellogg Foundation assembled a group of "the nation's experts on health education and health behavior change to look at possible strategies for Foundation funding in promoting healthier lifestyles for all Americans."[44] The Foundation then funded over a decade a total of 81 demonstration projects covering health promotion services in worksites, schools, hospitals, universities, and communities.

In 1985, the Henry J. Kaiser Family Foundation picked up the baton with another 10-year commitment to a national health promotion program. Organizing a cofunding partnership with 13 other foundations, the Kaiser Family Foundation had provided financial support and technical assistance to more than 100 community projects by mid-1990 and had supported the development or maintenance of health promotion policy, advocacy, technical assistance, and mass-media initiatives on a national or regional scale.[45] In 1989, The Robert Wood Johnson Foundation made a $27 million commitment to community-based, comprehensive substance-abuse prevention programs.

Federal Initiatives. Canada's lead was emulated in the United States. In 1974, a Bureau of Health Education (now expanded into two divisions within the Center for Chronic Disease Prevention and Health Promotion) was created in the Centers for Disease Control. In 1976, Public Law 94-317 established an Office of Health Information and Health Promotion (now the Office of Disease Prevention and Health Promotion) in the Office of the Assistant Secretary of Health, the highest level of the U.S. Public Health Service in which health policy is made.

Concurrently, a considerable amount of new research was being sponsored by the National Institutes of Health and the National Center for Health Services Research on the efficacy and effectiveness of health promotion.[46] Data had accumulated showing that chronic diseases could be controlled through active involvement of people in their own health care, and that patient education, self-care groups, and community efforts through mass media and face-to-face communications could bring about significant changes in health behavior and reductions in risk factors.[47] Thus the pendulum had swung from institutional dominance of health resources to individual initiative and responsibility. Now there was a need for appraisal and adjustment of this balance, to find the right mix of social and individual responsibility.[48]

In 1979, the Surgeon General's Report on Health Promotion and Disease Prevention, *Healthy People*,[49] signaled America's entry into a decade of new health policy, parallel to the Canadian initiative triggered by the 1974 LaLonde Report.[50] The new era has been referred to by some as the era of health promotion or, more grandiosely, the second public health revolution. This revolution built upon the scientific foundations of the second epidemiologic revolution,[51] in which the shift from communicable diseases to chronic diseases called for new paradigms, new methods, and even new definitions of health.[52]

Global Initiatives. The turn in federal health policy, mirrored in other countries,[53] has had a parallel in World Health Organization and UNICEF policies concerning health education and health promotion. These two international agencies met in Alma-Ata, USSR, in 1978 to deliberate the future of health and to formulate a global health strategy for primary health care. The Alma-Ata Declaration designated "education concerning prevailing health problems and the methods of preventing and controlling them" as the first of eight essential elements of primary health care.[54] Community and individual participation were featured as cornerstones of the planning strategy to be followed by each country.[55] A report of the WHO Expert Committee on New Approaches to Health Education in Primary Health Care concludes that

> the WHO *Global Strategy for Health for All by the Year 2000* and the WHO Seventh General Programme of Work give to information and education for health a role more prominent that ever before . . . Health science and technology have come to a point where their contribution to the further improvement of health standards can make a real impact *only* if the people themselves become full partners in health protection and promotion . . . Too often in the past, "modern" health practices have been promoted without giving sufficient thought to their relevance to the social and cultural background of the communities concerned. An effort must be made to enable individuals and communities to play an active role in the planning and delivery of health care. To assume such a role, people need guidance and encouragement from the health care providers in ways of identifying their health problems and of finding solutions to them . . . to set targets and translate these into simple and realistic goals that can be monitored. Finally, they should realize the need to refer to the policies behind the public health programmes in setting priorities among the targets identified.[56]

OTHER ISSUES IN THE DEVELOPMENT OF HEALTH PROMOTION

The evolution just described of health policy and programs for health education and health promotion gives the impression of a pendulum swinging from heavy reliance on government and institutions to heavy reliance on individuals and families, and back. Ideological and categorical attempts to throw the responsibility more exclusively to one side or the other have met with a seemingly inescapable and inexorable cycle or teeter-totter, at least in American history, of political swings from left to right, tilting the balance of responsibility from individuals to government and back. The reality of program planning and execution is that both sides must be engaged.[57]

THE DIVISION OF RESPONSIBILITY

The methods proposed for health promotion planning in the chapters that follow are based on the assumption that the optimum mix of responsibility to be assumed by those involved — individuals, families, professionals, private or governmental organizations, and local or national agencies — must be worked out on a case-by-case basis. For each health issue or project, a determination must be made as to its urgency, its causes, its variability, and the degree to which individuals want and can exercise control over the determinants of the health problem or goal. It is essential that those directly affected have a voice in negotiating this division of responsibility. Providing an opportunity for that voice to be heard applies the principle of participation so central to learning theory and effective community organization. It also assures a link to the philosophical and ethical underpinning of the professional commitment to supporting voluntary change where possible.

The history recounted here seems to focus on the developed nations, particularly North America. Yet the global initiatives reflected by WHO and UNICEF in the primary health care approach and the Ottawa Charter make the emerging concepts of health promotion relevant to the developing nations. The case-by-case diagnosis of needs and tailoring of strategies to local circumstances, finding the right balance between personal and societal responsibility, and providing for active participation of individuals and communities in the assessment of needs and the division of responsibility all apply as much to the developing countries as to the so-called developed.[58]

If the new health promotion has shifted the locus of initiative for health and of control over its determinants from institutions and professionals to individuals and families, it did so mostly in a context of growing community and social support. Worksite health promotion expanded rapidly with notable provisions for institutional supports for employee participation.[59] Schools placed increasing emphasis on social and organizational factors in programs for the modification or development of diet and the prevention of substance abuse.[60] In most communities, new emphasis was being placed on concerns with the environment and with housing and other conditions of living that shape the lifestyle of the community.

THE LIFESTYLE CONSTRUCT

Another issue of this period of development is the use of the term *lifestyle*. Behavior is seen increasingly not as isolated acts under the autonomous control of the individual, but rather as socially conditioned, culturally embedded, economically constrained patterns of living. This growing conviction was noted most publicly in the evolution of a formal definition of health promotion by the editor of the new *American Journal of Health Promotion* between 1986, when he published the first issue of the journal,[61] and three years later when he published an amended definition, expanding on the term *lifestyle* as it appeared alone in the original definition:

> Health promotion is the science and art of helping people change their lifestyle to move toward a state of optimal health . . . . Lifestyle change can be facilitated through a combination of efforts to enhance awareness, change behavior, and create environments that support good health practices. Of the three, supportive environments will probably have the greatest impact in producing lasting changes.[62]

The lifestyle construct has its roots in anthropology, sociology, and clinical psychology, where it is used to describe patterns of behavior that have an enduring consistency and are based in some combination of cultural heritage, social relationships, geographic and socioeconomic circumstances, and personality.[63] Initially, the behavioral pattern described in the lifestyle construct was assumed to be made up of a full range of daily routines within a social fabric of family, friends, schoolmates, and workmates. Each behavior within the pattern was assumed to have some connection (and possibly a dependent relationship) with every other behavior in the lifestyle.[64] In later usage by medical sociologists and psychologists,[65] there was a search for subsets of behaviors highly correlated around health protection, health promotion, and use of health services.[66]

These features made the lifestyle construct appropriate and useful for some analyses of health-related behavior, especially those that might have a synergistic or multiplier effect on each other in producing poor health outcomes, such as smoking and consumption of high-fat foods, drinking and driving, or driving without seat belts. Unfortunately, such analyses have produced rather modest correlations among the presumably related behaviors. This leaves some doubt about the utility of the lifestyle construct in describing or explaining consistent patterns of interrelated health behavior in populations.[67]

The value of the term *lifestyle* has been further eroded by its widespread misuse in describing single acts and temporary practices. Some have gone as far as to equate lifestyle with behavior of any kind related to health. These and other criticisms of the use of the term in health promotion[68] should alert the student or practitioner to be cautious in its application and interpretation. In this book, the term is used *only* to describe a complex of related practices and behavioral patterns, in a person or group, that are maintained with some consistency over time. It includes conscious health-directed behavior as well as unconscious health-related behavior and practices that are pursued for nonhealth purposes but with health consequences or risks.

This somewhat holistic view of lifestyle as a health-related construct justifies a more holistic approach to promoting health in communities and individuals. For example, a recognition that each behavior related to health is also related to other facets of a lifestyle should make program planners and professionals more aware of the need to include in the planning process the thoughts and perspectives of those whose behavior might be expected to change (see Chapter 2). It also argues for a comprehensive approach to health promotion, with a combination of educational, organizational, economic, or other environmental supports rather than only persuasive appeals for change in each specific behavior. When a health-related behavior is seen to be embedded in a complex web of lifestyle, changing that behavior will necessarily require attention to the social norms, the cultural values, and the economic and environmental circumstances surrounding and supporting that lifestyle.[69]

Considering the complexity of lifestyle, it is prudent to stay with the terms *behavior*, *actions*, or *practices* to describe the intermediate targets of health education and health promotion. This helps in avoiding the traps of arrogance and pretentiousness that accompany practical but simplistically conceived strategies to change lifestyle. Only the most ambitious, long-term, complex health promotion programs can be expected to produce significant impact on lifestyle, and such programs are impractical for everyday health promotion planning. At the same time, this does not diminish the importance of local health education and health promotion programs, whose contribution to social and lifestyle change is vital. Helping just one person gain control over a single determinant of his or her health qualifies as health promotion in this book.

While striving to be practical and down to earth, this book does not ignore the larger tasks of social change and policy advocacy that each health professional should seek to support. As we encourage citizens to participate and become empowered advocates for the health of their communities, so too should the health professional be a part of social and policy change. But these changes require the cooperative and sustained effort of many professionals, sectors, and public constituencies. Each individual who is helped to gain control over the determinants of health in his or her own life is one more voice added to the constituencies advocating social change, a cumulative effect clearly illustrated by the development of local ordinances for smoke-free environments. Each person who successfully adapts his or her own behavior becomes a source of help, inspiration, or influence for others to make similar changes. This process has been described as the normative effect of behavior change and health promotion in groups and communities.[70]

THE PLACE OF HEALTH EDUCATION IN HEALTH PROMOTION

A third issue raised by the definition of health promotion and the recent historical trends is the central place given to health education. This chapter defined health promotion in such a way as to require health education as one of its components. Organizational, economic, or other environmental supports for action are optional, depending on which of them is needed in combination with health education. This commitment to an educational approach to health promotion is partially a matter of practical necessity and partially an outgrowth of a philosophical commitment to provide for informed consent and voluntary change *before* attempting to change social structures and systems.

In her keynote address to the Canadian Public Health Association in 1986, Dr. Ilona Kickbusch, regional officer for health promotion in the European office of the World Health Organization, related the following history:

> Health promotion emerged out of health education. There are many reasons for this. I will state just two. First: health educators became more aware of the need for positive approaches in health education—enhancing health and creating health potential rather than focusing on disease prevention. Second: it became self evident that health education could only develop its full potential if it was supported by structural measures (legal, environmental, regulatory, etc.). The issue, as formulated by Nancy Milio, was how to make healthier choices the easier choices.[71]

Finding the policy support for the organizational, economic, regulatory, and other environmental interventions necessary to accomplish the original intent of health education does not justify abandoning health education as the primary modality for democratic social and behavioral change. Health education provides the consciousness-raising, concern-arousing, action-stimulating impetus for public involvement and commitment to social reform essential to its success in a democracy. Without health education, health promotion would be a manipulative, social engineering enterprise. Health education of the public keeps the social change component of health promotion accountable to the public it is supposed to serve. Without the policy supports for social change, on the other hand, health education is often powerless to help people reach their health goals, even with successful individual change efforts.

In short, health education is aimed primarily at the voluntary actions people can take on their own, individually or collectively, as citizens looking after their own health or as decision makers looking after the health of others and the common good of the community. Health promotion encompasses health education, as defined for this book, and is aimed at the complementary social and political actions that will facilitate the necessary organizational, economic, and other environmental supports for the conversion of individual actions into health enhancements and quality of life gains:

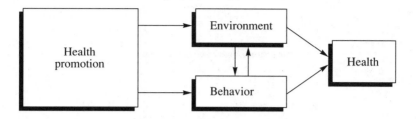

THE NOTION OF POSITIVE HEALTH

Wellness, the fourth element in the current concept of health promotion, requires some explanation: The term implies that there is more to health than the absence of disease or disability. Some people actually restrict their use of *health promotion* to refer only to the positive end of the illness–wellness continuum.[72] Nevertheless, the reduction of behavioral risk factors in individuals can be a legitimate and important task for health promotion. Recognition of this need provides considerable impetus to policy support for health promotion. In the short run, at least, reduction of health risks can be expected to accomplish greater reductions in morbidity than a focus on health enhancement in those without significant behavioral risk factors.

But it is the hope for health enhancement that captures the imagination of contemporary society. Most people who have responded personally to health promotion are interested in these kinds of promises: improved quality of life, efficient functioning, the capacity to perform at more productive and satisfying levels, and the opportunity to live out their life span with vigor and stamina. Such potential benefits also appeal to the other sectors whose support is needed for health promotion. For example, employers will sponsor worksite health promotion programs and facilities if they are assured of improved worker morale and productivity; and school administrators will support a school-based program if they are convinced that children will be able to stay awake and alert in school, perform better on standardized tests, and generally achieve better educational outcomes. In each case, the proponent of health promotion is seeking practical, situation-specific results other than the traditionally defined health outcomes. Those in other sectors have a different "bottom line," or they adopt a broader definition of health than conventional measures dictate. The cooperation of these other sectors as arenas in which health promotion can usefully operate is essential to the success of health promotion. Health practitioners and administrators seeking intersectoral cooperation from schools, churches, and private industry to extend health promotion through their channels must explicitly identify some of the other outcomes and potential benefits of health promotion.[73] Some of these other benefits are depicted in Figure 1.1 under immediate and intermediate outcomes. Schools and employers, for example, are more inclined to cooperate

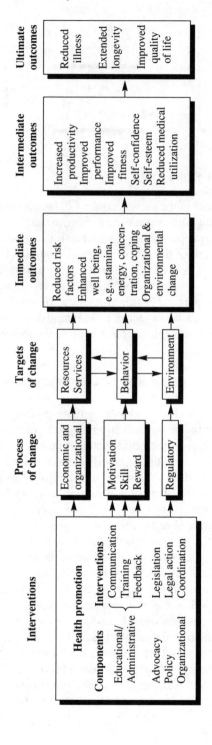

FIGURE 1.1

Approximate relationships among objects of interest to the health sector and other sectors cooperating in health promotion. [From L. W. Green, A. L. Wilson, and C. Y. Lovato, *Preventive Medicine* 15 (1986): 508–21, by permission of the publisher.]

with a health promotion program if they foresee improved stamina, energy, concentration, and productivity in their students or employees than if the only promise of the program is reduced health risk factors.

SCOPE OF HEALTH EDUCATION AND HEALTH PROMOTION

Health education is any combination of learning experiences designed to facilitate voluntary actions conducive to health. *Combination* emphasizes the importance of matching the multiple determinants of behavior with multiple learning experiences or educational interventions. *Designed* distinguishes health education from incidental learning experiences as a systematically planned activity. *Facilitate* means predispose, enable, and reinforce. *Voluntary* means without coercion and with the full understanding and acceptance of the purposes of the action. *Action* means behavioral steps taken by an individual, group, or community to achieve an intended health effect.

Health promotion was defined in the opening paragraphs of this chapter as the combination of educational and environmental supports for actions and conditions of living conducive to health. *Combination* again refers to the necessity of matching the multiple determinants of health with multiple interventions or sources of support. *Educational* refers to health education as defined in the foregoing paragraph. *Environmental* refers to the social, political, economic, organizational, policy, and regulatory circumstances bearing on the behavior or more directly on health. It is used here to refer to the dynamic social forces operating on the situation more than to the physical environment or medical services. These other environmental factors usually need to be considered in planning health promotion, but health promotion can be distinguished from the other two major components of public health by leaving the engineering of the physical environment to health protection and the management of the medical environment to preventive health services.

Living conditions permits our definition of health promotion to range beyond the strictly behavioral into the more complex web of culture, norms, and socio-economic environment associated with the broader historical meaning of *lifestyle*. This is the least well defined or researched aspect of health promotion but is the one on which perhaps the most has been written. Much of the writing about this dimension of health promotion tends to be either descriptive, as in correlational studies of the relationship of poverty and health, or exhortatory, as in polemical critiques of health promotion policies believed to be based on a victim-blaming ideology.

These definitions emphasize the scope as well as the purpose of health education and health promotion. They enable us to delineate which programs, activities, and methods may be characterized as educational or promotional. In practice, health education is usually embedded in health promotion or other programs (patient education in medical care programs, occupational health education in industrial safety and health programs, or school health education in school programs) rather than existing as autonomous, free-standing activities. Many educational components of other health programs may not even be identified as health education. Indeed, practitioners sometimes disavow any association with health education in an attempt to distinguish their efforts as more innovative, modern, technological, behavioristic, client-centered, or scientific than they perceive health education to be. Thus it happens that health education programs may not be labeled as such even when the methods employed clearly derive their philosophical, technical, and theoretical or scientific approaches from education, educational psychology, educational technology, or health education itself.

Indeed, the term *health promotion* emerged in U.S. health policy in its most recent incarnation as a last-minute substitute by Congress in 1975 for the term *health education*. As the legislative bills for a national health education act were readied to be referred to congressional committees, the term *health education* was removed in favor of *health promotion* to avoid having the bills referred to the education committees where they would have died for lack of interest or priority on health within the education field.[74] The term *health promotion* was not defined when it emerged in Public Law 94-317, The Health Information and Health Promotion Act of 1975. The Act created the Office of Health Information and Health Promotion, which had no definition of health promotion until it fashioned an operational definition in 1979. This definition, much like the one just given, was expressly designed to seize the larger terrain of organizational and political interventions, which enlightened health educators had always presumed were their responsibilities but which others usually assumed were beyond the scope of health education.[75]

The most extensive exercise in delineating the elements of health education came with the Professional Role Delineation Project of the National Center for Health Education with funding from the U.S. Centers for Disease Control and the Health Resources Administration.[76] This project built on a foundation of previous work by national committees to specify the content and standards of professional training for health education specialists[77] and for other health workers applying health education.[78]

The scope, diversity, and boundaries of health education and health promotion are illustrated by the various labels used for their programs and activities, such as motivation programs, behavior modification, health counseling, and communications (see Fig. 1.2).

The term *motivation*, as in *motivational programs*, has been used in fields such as family planning and social marketing to refer to the activities generally included in health education programs.[79] Motivation programs are often combined with incentive schemes designed to appeal more directly to economic motives for changes such as consumption of products or services or family size

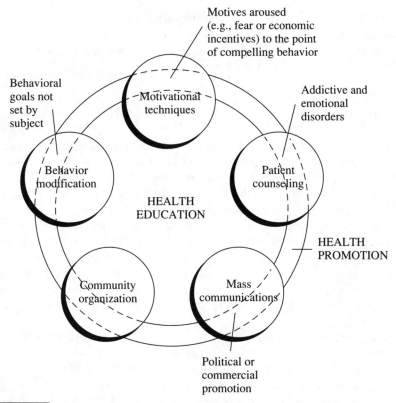

FIGURE 1.2

The overlapping spheres of health education and health promotion, and of specific strategies that fall sometimes inside and sometimes outside the boundaries of health education and health promotion.

limitation.[80] From a formal psychological standpoint, this usage of the term *motivation* is incorrect. Motivation is something that happens within the person, not something that is done *to* the person by others. It is a construct that has reference to the internal dynamics of behavior, not to the external stimuli. Thus motivation programs are more correctly identified as programs based on the use of motive-arousing appeals. Strictly speaking, we can appeal to people's motives, but we cannot motivate them. Motivational strategies qualify as means of health education under our definition as long as motives are not aroused to the point at which behavior is compelled. At that point, the condition of voluntariness, essential to our definition, has been violated. A clear example is the rural family planning program in India in which transistor radios, a considerable economic pressure in that setting, were offered to poor village men to induce them to submit to sterilization by vasectomy. This example falls within the scope of health promotion, but it falls outside the definition of health education because it goes beyond learning as the basis for voluntary change.

OF MEANS AND ENDS

The defining characteristic of health education is thus the voluntary participation of the learners in determining their own health practices. This is not merely a philosophical tenet. *The cumulative evidence from decades of research in education and other fields tell us that the durability of cognitive and behavioral changes depends on the degree of active rather than passive participation of the learner.* In addition, there are practical and strategic reasons to emphasize the voluntary nature of health education. It helps to avoid public resistance or reaction to programs that might be perceived as propagandistic, manipulative, coercive, politically or commercially directed, paternalistic, or threatening. But when the goals of the program are urgent enough or important enough to the community, some of the noneducational features of health promotion are justified and acceptable.

Other forms and methods of health education define its scope: community organization, in-service training, consultation, group work, computer-assisted instruction, noncomputerized teaching machines and audiovisual methods, patient teaching, health fairs, exhibits, libraries, conferences, and routine interactions between health providers and consumers. The scope of health promotion, however, is defined as much by its expected outcomes as by its methods and forms. The changes in health-related behaviors that can result from health education and other health promotion methods are numerous and varied.

A review of the population control policies and programs of the People's Republic of China provides an excellent opportunity to examine the distinctions and overlaps between health education and health promotion. Each married couple in China was offered the option of taking the one-child pledge. They were given extensive education through mass media, small groups, and counseling to develop their understanding of China's population problem, the country's economic and developmental goals that are affected by population growth, the advantages and disadvantages of small and large families, and the government's offer of bonuses and incentives to help offset the perceived disadvantages of having only one child. All of this is essentially educational. The couple had free choice to accept or reject the pledge. If they took it, they received economic advantages, including special provisions for the first-born child such as priority housing and preschool enrollment. If the couple subsequently had a second child, the bonuses were withdrawn. The economic aspect of this program is the promotional component that lies outside the scope of health education. The program was judged a partial success in making progress toward the national goals of population control, improved maternal and child health, productivity, and, at least for urban couples, quality of life. It received a poor press in the West, where China's prerogatives to set its own social goals for development and quality of life were judged in terms of Western values, and where some sensibilities were offended by the means employed.[81]

Where would you stand on the issues of means and ends in judging this program? Do the ends justify the means? What else could be done to strengthen the health education component to assure the informed consent and voluntary action of the Chinese couples? Has the promotional component of this policy gone too far?

One can judge the appropriateness of the *ends*, that is, the *purpose* of this policy, only by applying one's own values and societal norms. If those values arise from Western history and culture, they have evolved in the particular circumstances of Western countries, and to apply them to Asia, Africa, or the Middle East is a hazardous procedure. The only reliable criterion to use in judging a policy is the degree to which it meets the needs of the people it is supposed to serve. Clearly, that criterion can be applied only by knowing the needs of the people. Unless we ourselves are the target of the policy, we are again limited in our ability to judge the people's needs because the determination is made from our own perspective, filtered through our own perceptions. Our needs may be different from the needs of the Chinese population, and in the final analysis need is relative to perceived or felt need. Felt need is a subjective reality. In short, we can pass judgment on China's one-child policy only if we know how the Chinese themselves feel about the population problem and the developmental problems created by the population pressure in China.

So it is with any policy. Health professionals bring their own perception of the importance of health. They must consult the people who are the intended target of health programs to determine their perceptions of their needs, problems, and aspirations concerning quality of life. If professionals do not take this vital step, health policies remain sterile, technocratic solutions to problems that may not exist or that hold a low priority in the minds of the people. The danger is that such technocratic policies may waste resources on a "red herring" and so sabotage a real opportunity to address the people's true concerns. The Chinese family planning policy is an exotic example, easy to criticize on the basis of its means and ends. But the criticism of the means should be based on an understanding of the ends, and a criticism of the ends could appear sanctimonious coming from an outsider. Social assessment and ways to assure that the public's perception of its own problems, needs, and aspirations are taken into account as a first step in the planning process are discussed in Chapter 2.

THE PRECEDE–PROCEED MODEL

The ideas of intervention and support are important to the forgoing definitions of health education and health promotion. Organized health education activity intervenes in the process of development and change so as to maintain, enhance, or interrupt a behavior pattern or condition of living that is linked to improved health or to increased risks for illness, injury, disability, or death (Fig. 1.3). The behavior of interest is usually that of the people whose health is in question, either now or in the future. Equally important in the process of planning and developing the policies and programs are the behaviors of those who control resources or rewards, such as community leaders, parents, employers, peers, teachers, and health professionals.

Supports refer to the environmental conditions that health promotion seeks to leave in place following the intervention so that individuals, groups, or communities can continue to exercise their own control over the determinants of their health. New policies, regulatory provisions, and organizational arrangements represent environmental supports. Informed officials, committed legislators, concerned teachers, skilled parents, and understanding employers all can provide a supportive social environment, and each can be influenced by educational and political interventions. An increase in the proportion of the population who hold a favorable attitude toward the behavior that some individuals want to adopt provides a supportive environment in the form of normative enabling and reinforcing supports. For example, mass media can be used to raise the level of public awareness of the need to reduce fat in the diet, which in turn can produce a consumer demand for low-fat products in the marketplace, which in turn can cause restaurants and grocers to place more healthful products on their menus and shelves, which in turn can make the low-fat choice an easier choice for those who want to change their behavior.

Whether the health promotion program operates at the primary (hygiene and health enhancement), secondary (early detection), or tertiary (therapeutic) stage of prevention, it may accurately be seen as an intervention whose purpose is to short-circuit illness or enhance quality of life through change or development of health-related behavior and conditions of living (see Fig. 1.3). The PRECEDE framework takes into account the multiple factors that shape health status and helps the planner arrive at a highly focused subset of those factors as targets for intervention. PRECEDE also generates specific objectives and criteria for evaluation. The PROCEED framework provides additional steps for developing policy and initiating the implementation and evaluation process (Fig. 1.4).

PRECEDE and PROCEED work in tandem, providing a continuous series of steps or phases in the planning, implementation, and evaluation process. The identification of priorities and the setting of objectives in the PRECEDE phases

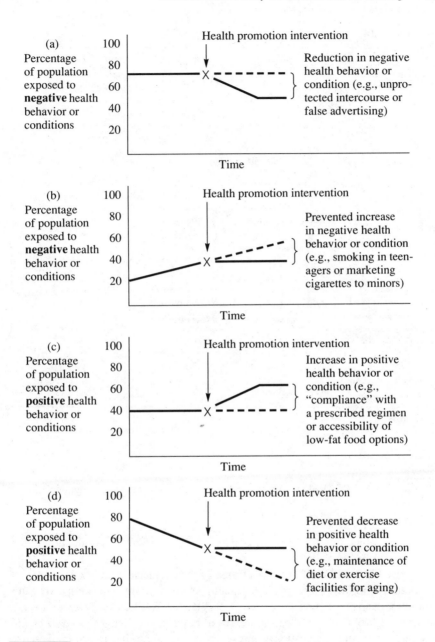

FIGURE 1.3

Examples of how health promotion interventions influence the prevalence or incidence of selected determinants of health.

PRECEDE

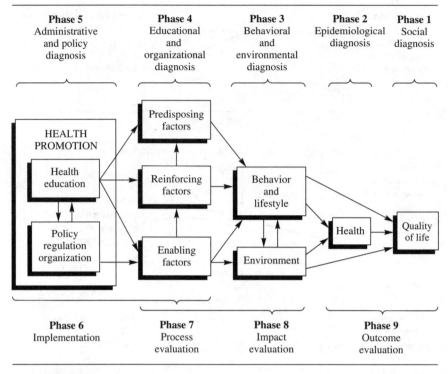

Phase 5	Phase 4	Phase 3	Phase 2	Phase 1
Administrative and policy diagnosis	Educational and organizational diagnosis	Behavioral and environmental diagnosis	Epidemiological diagnosis	Social diagnosis

Phase 6	Phase 7	Phase 8	Phase 9
Implementation	Process evaluation	Impact evaluation	Outcome evaluation

PROCEED

FIGURE 1.4

The PRECEDE–PROCEED model for health promotion planning and evaluation.

provide the objects and criteria for policy, implementation, and evaluation in the PROCEED phases.

PRECEDE–PROCEED is not offered as the exclusive road to quality health promotion. There *are* other models of health behavior, health education and health promotion, and procedures for planning.[82] PRECEDE–PROCEED is, however, a theoretically robust model that addresses a major acknowledged need in health promotion and health education: comprehensive planning. It is robust in the sense that it applies to health promotion in a variety of situations.[83] It has served as a successful model in a number of rigorously evaluated, randomized clinical and field trials[84]; as a guide to the development of local health department programs adopted by several state health departments[85]; as a federal guide to the planning, review, and evaluation of maternal and child health projects[86]; as an analytical tool for health education policy on a national and international scale[87]; as a model recommended by the National Committee for Injury Prevention and Control for planning and evaluating safety programs[88]; by the American Lung Association as a *Program Planning and Evaluation Guide for Lung Associations*[89]; by the American Cancer Society and the National Cancer Institute for a school nutrition and cancer education curriculum[90]; and as an organizational framework for curriculum development or training in health education for nurses,[91] pharmacists,[92] allied health professionals,[93] physicians,[94] and interdisciplinary training for behavioral scientists and health educators.[95] Other applications and validations of the model are mentioned or illustrated in subsequent chapters.

The PROCEED component of the model is of more recent inception and has had less exposure and testing. It is essentially an elaboration and extension of the administrative diagnosis step of PRECEDE, which was the final and least-developed link in the PRECEDE framework as presented in the previous edition of this book. The PROCEED framework has emerged with increasing detail in work on health promotion planning,[96] policy,[97] evaluation,[98] and implementation.[99]

BEGINNING AT THE END

One of the motivations to create the first edition of this book was the observation of two phenomena related to health education practice. First, many persons responsible for planning health education programs had more or less predetermined which intervention strategy they were going to employ. Second, in some instances, there was no apparent reason for choosing either the health issue to be addressed or the target population to be reached. Usually the practitioners seemed to select interventions based on which techniques they were most comfortable applying. Some were expert in mass media, some in community organization, some in group work. They tended to apply their preferred method even when it was not necessarily the most strategic or tactical choice.

That was then. Contemporary health education practice involves far less of that kind of grab-bag programming, primarily because demands for accountability require stronger justification for the expenditure of scarce resources. Health promotion falls prey to the grab-bag syndrome more frequently today because a much wider range of variously prepared professional, business, and commercial personnel find themselves planning programs in health promotion. The systematic and critical analysis of priorities and presumed cause–effect relationships can start the planner on the right foot in health promotion today, as it has health educators in the past decade.

The causal chain expected to be set in motion by a health promotion program is shown in schematic form in Figure 1.5. In this schema, the inputs are interventions (processes) and the outputs are the anticipated results of the interventions

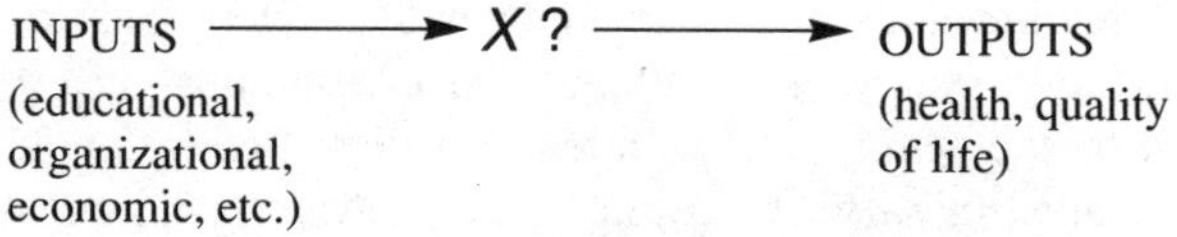

INPUTS ———————→ *X* ? ———————→ OUTPUTS
(educational,   (health, quality
organizational,   of life)
economic, etc.)

FIGURE 1.5

(changes in health or social conditions). Health practitioners, because of their activist orientation, have an understandable tendency to begin with inputs. Often they take a quick glance at the general problem at hand and then immediately begin to design and implement the intervention, health education, or other, assuming that the outcome will occur automatically.

The PRECEDE framework directs initial attention to outcomes rather than inputs. This forces the planner to begin the planning process from the *outcome* end. It encourages asking *why* before *how*. What at first seems to be the wrong end from which to start, from the standpoint of planning, is in fact the right one. You begin with the desired final outcome and determine what causes it—that is, what must *precede* that outcome (*X*? in Fig. 1.5). Stated another way, the factors important to an outcome must be diagnosed before the intervention is designed; if they are not, the intervention is based on guesswork and runs a great risk of being misdirected and ineffective.

THE EIGHT PHASES OF PRECEDE AND PROCEED

Working through PRECEDE and PROCEED is like solving a mystery. One is led to think deductively, to start with the final consequences and work back to the original causes. There are six basic phases to the procedure (see Fig. 1.4); evaluation of program impact and outcomes can extend it to seven or eight phases, depending on the evaluation requirements. To provide an overview, the phases are described in the following brief summary.

Phase 1. Ideally, one begins with a consideration of quality of life by assessing some of the general hopes or problems of concern to the target population (patients, students, employees, or consumers). This is best accomplished by involving the people in a self-study of their needs and aspirations. The kinds of social problems a community experiences are a practical and accurate barometer of its quality of life. Such problems can be ascertained by several methods, discussed in Chapter 2. Some of the indicators of these subjectively defined problems and priorities are listed in Figure 1.6.

Phase 2. The task of Phase 2 is to identify the specific health goals or problems that may contribute to the social goals or problems noted in Phase 1. Using available

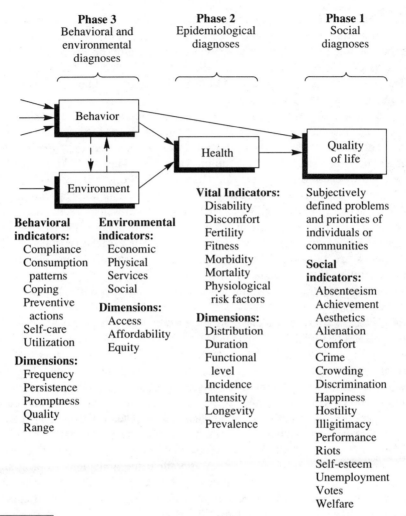

Phase 3
Behavioral and
environmental
diagnoses

Phase 2
Epidemiological
diagnoses

Phase 1
Social
diagnoses

Behavior

Environment

Health

Quality
of life

**Behavioral
indicators:**
Compliance
Consumption
patterns
Coping
Preventive
actions
Self-care
Utilization

Dimensions:
Frequency
Persistence
Promptness
Quality
Range

**Environmental
indicators:**
Economic
Physical
Services
Social

Dimensions:
Access
Affordability
Equity

Vital Indicators:
Disability
Discomfort
Fertility
Fitness
Morbidity
Mortality
Physiological
risk factors

Dimensions:
Distribution
Duration
Functional
level
Incidence
Intensity
Longevity
Prevalence

Subjectively
defined problems
and priorities of
individuals or
communities

**Social
indicators:**
Absenteeism
Achievement
Aesthetics
Alienation
Comfort
Crime
Crowding
Discrimination
Happiness
Hostility
Illigitimacy
Performance
Riots
Self-esteem
Unemployment
Votes
Welfare

FIGURE 1.6

Relationships, indicators, and dimensions of factors that might be identified in Phases 1, 2, and 3 of the PRECEDE diagnostic process or evaluated in the extension of PROCEED.

data, information generated by appropriate investigations, and epidemiological and medical findings, the planner ranks the several health problems. Based on methods outlined in Chapter 3, one selects the specific health problem most deserving of scarce educational and promotional resources. Examples of vital indicators or physiological measures of health factors and dimensions on which they might be measured are shown in Figure 1.6.

Many health professionals have the task of developing a program assigned to them after someone else, with or without having employed the systematic procedures of Phases 1 and 2, has concluded that a particular health promotion intervention is needed. A hospital administrator may order a smoking cessation program or a school principal may purchase an AIDS-oriented health education curriculum, sometimes without having assessed the need for and appropriateness of that particular intervention. When such a situation prevails, practitioners need to determine what assumptions have been made in relation to the cause–effect linkages implied in the first two phases. This precautionary action ensures that the assumptions are valid, or at least explicit and understood. It familiarizes the practitioner with crucial foundation information and the basis for the assumptions that have gone into the directive for a health promotion program.

Phase 3. Phase 3 consists of identifying the specific health-related behavioral and environmental factors that could be linked to the health problems chosen as most deserving of attention in Phase 2. Because these are the risk factors that the intervention is tailored to affect, they must be very specifically identified and carefully ranked. Notice in Figure 1.4 that we have linked behavioral and environmental factors to the *health* and to the *quality of life* boxes. **Environmental factors** are those external to an individual, often beyond his or her personal control, that can be modified to support the behavior, health, or quality of life of that person or others affected by that person's actions. Being cognizant of such forces enables planners to be more realistic about the limitations of programs consisting only of health education directed at the personal health behavior of the public. It also enables them to recognize that powerful social forces might be influenced when the principles of PROCEED are translated into organizational strategies applied by coalitions on the community, state, or national level. Even at the local level, health-related behaviors influenced by health education can include collective behavior directed at economic or environmental factors.

Phase 4. On the basis of cumulative research on health and social behavior, literally hundreds of factors could be identified that have the potential to influence a given health behavior. The PRECEDE model groups them according to the educational and organizational strategies likely to be employed in a health promotion program to bring about behavioral and environmental change. The three broad groupings are predisposing factors, reinforcing factors, and enabling factors (Fig. 1.7). **Predisposing factors** include a person's or population's knowledge, attitudes, beliefs, values, and perceptions that facilitate or hinder motivation for change. **Enabling factors** are those skills, resources, or barriers that can help or hinder the desired behavioral changes as well as environmental changes. They can be viewed as vehicles or barriers, created mainly by societal forces or systems. Facilities and personal or community resources may be ample or inadequate, as may income or health insurance, and laws and statutes may be supportive or restrictive. The skills required for a desired behavior to occur also qualify as enabling factors. Enabling factors thus include all the factors that *make possible* a desired change in behavior or in the environment. **Reinforcing factors**, the rewards received, and the feedback the learner receives from others following adoption of the behavior, may encourage or discourage continuation of the behavior.

The fourth phase thus consists of sorting and categorizing the factors that seem to have direct impact on the target behavior and environment according to the three classes of factors just cited. Study of the predisposing, enabling, and reinforcing factors automatically takes the planner on to decide exactly which of the factors making up the three classes deserve highest priority as the focus of intervention. The decision is based on their relative importance and the resources available to influence them.

Phase 5. Armed with the pertinent and systematically organized diagnostic information, the planner is ready for Phase 5, the assessment of organizational and administrative capabilities and resources for the development and implementation of a program. Limitations of resources, policies, and abilities and time constraints are assessed through methods suggested in Chapter 6. Some of these limitations and constraints can be offset by cooperative arrangements with other local agencies or larger organizations at state or national levels or through the development of coalitions and political alliances at the local level. All that remains then is the selection of the right combination of methods and strategies, the deployment of intervention staff, and the launching of the community organization or organizational development process.

The planning and launching considerations specific to each of the major settings for health promotion—communities, worksites, schools, and health care settings—are discussed and illustrated in Chapters 8–11, respectively.

Phases 6, 7, and 8. Listing evaluation as the last phase is misleading, for evaluation becomes an integral and continuous part of working with the entire model from the beginning. Although Chapter 7 presents a methodological discussion of the evaluation component of PROCEED, the criteria for evaluation fall naturally from the objectives defined in the corresponding steps in PRECEDE during the diagnostic process. These criteria are highlighted in Chapters 2–6. For example, the exposition of the social diagnosis in Chapter 2 emphasizes the importance of clearly stating program objectives so that the standards of acceptability are defined before, rather than after, the evaluation. Indeed, the PRECEDE model was first

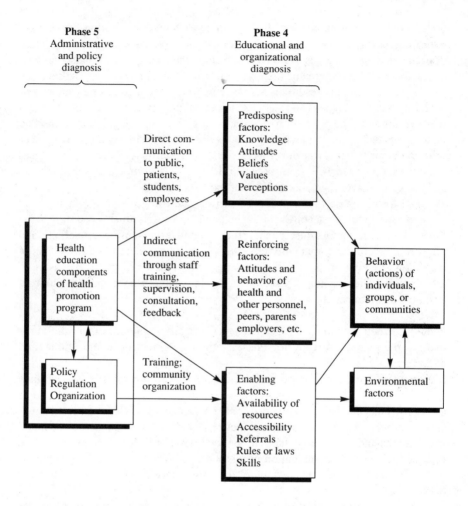

FIGURE 1.7

Phases 4 and 5 of PRECEDE address the strategies and resources required to influence the predisposing, reinforcing, and enabling factors influencing or supporting behavioral and environmental changes.

developed as an evaluation model,[100] evolving later into the planning framework presented in this book.

FOUNDATIONS: STAYING ON SOLID GROUND

The PRECEDE–PROCEED framework for planning is founded on the disciplines of epidemiology; the social, behavioral, and educational sciences; and health administration. Thus, successful completion of Phases 1 and 2, and portions of Phase 3, depends heavily on the use of epidemiological methods and information; working effectively through Phases 3 and 4 requires familiarity with social and behavioral theory and concepts; and handling the complex task of designing and implementing a health promotion program demands knowledge of political, educational, and administrative theory as well as experience. The PROCEED phase calls for some understanding of political and administrative science and community organization for entering the advocacy and implementation process, and of evaluation methods. In presenting this framework, we assume that the reader has had exposure to the several disciplines that constitute the scientific basis of health promotion.

Throughout the work with PRECEDE and PROCEED, two fundamental propositions are emphasized: (1) health and health risks are caused by multiple factors; and (2) because health and health risks are determined by multiple factors, efforts to effect behavioral, environmental, and social change must be multidimensional or multisectoral. The multidimensional nature of health promotion requires from program planners and administrators the kind of professional preparation or collaboration in which several scientific and professional disciplines are integrated. It is not surprising that planners occasionally become discouraged and even disenchanted as they wade through and try to synthesize the literature of biomedical science, behavioral science, economics, social and political science, education, and administration. The PRECEDE model can give direction and focus to such attempts at synthesis. The challenge is to pull together a variety of rapidly developing disciplines as a basis for understanding and in some way contributing to improvements in the quality of life. It is this challenge that sustains commitment and hope for health education and health promotion.

EXERCISES

1. What trends have you noticed in recent years, in your community or among your friends, in health behavior, conditions of living, and health concerns? Can you find any objective data to support your observations? If not, how would you go about verifying your subjective view of these trends?

2. Identify at least three national or international health campaigns or programs spanning a number of years. How do you account for the public concern with these different health problems at different times? What were the major features of the health promotion component of these programs? Why have different programs or problems at different times required different health promotion methods?

3. Identify and describe the demographic characteristics (geographic location, size, age and sex distribution, etc.) of a population (students, patients, workers, residents) whose quality of life you would like to improve. Follow the population you choose through most of the remaining exercises in this book. Look ahead at the upcoming exercises and make sure the population you choose is appropriate for the diagnostic and planning steps that will be required.

REFERENCES AND NOTES

1. Part of this chapter was adapted for "Health Promotion as a Public Health Strategy for the 1990s," *Annual Review of Public Health*, vol. 11, L. Breslow, ed. (Palo Alto, CA: Annual Reviews Inc., 1990), pp. 319–34. We are indebted to Sharon Dorfman, Johnathan Fielding, Bruce Simons-Morton, Denise Simons-Morton, and Jackie Wood for helpful reviews of earlier drafts.

2. Terms introduced in boldface type are defined in the glossary.

3. L. W. Green, M. W. Kreuter, S. G. Deeds, and K. B. Partridge, *Health Education Planning: A Diagnostic Approach* (Palo Alto, CA: Mayfield, 1980).

4. *Healthy People: The Surgeon General's Report on Health Promotion and Disease Prevention* (Washington, DC: U.S. Department of Health, Education, and Welfare, 1979).

5. J. P. Allegrante, "Potential Uses and Misuses of Education in Health Promotion and Disease Prevention," *The Eta Sigma Gamman* 18 (1986): 2–8; L. W. Green, "Health Promotion Policy and the Placement of Responsibility for Personal Health Care," *Family and Community Health* 2 (1979): 51–64.

6. M. Minkler, "Health Education, Health Promotion and the Open Society: An Historical Perspective," *Health Education Quarterly* 16 (1989): 17–30.

7. I. Kickbusch, "Approaches to an Ecological Base for Public Health," *Health Promotion* 4 (1989): 265–8; K. R. McLeroy, A. Steckler, and D. Bibeau, eds., "The Social Ecology of Health Promotion Interventions," *Health Education Quarterly* 15 (1988): 351–486.

8. L. Duhl, "The Healthy City: Its Function and Its Future," *Health Promotion* 1 (1986): 55–60; T. Hancock, "Beyond Health Care: From Public Health Policy to Healthy Public Policy," *Canadian Journal of Public Health* 76 (1985): 9–11; N. Milio, *Promoting Health Through Public Policy* (Philadelphia: F. A. Davis, 1981).

9. J. P. Allegrante and L. W. Green, "When Health Policy Becomes Victim Blaming," *New England Journal of Medicine* 305 (1981): 1528–9; N. Holtzman, "Prevention: Rhetoric or Reality," *International Journal of Health Services* 9 (1979): 25–39; J. B. McKinlay, "A Case for Refocusing Upstream – The Political Economy of Illness," in *Applying Behavioral Science to Cardiovascular Risk*, A. J. Enelow and J. B. Henderson, eds. (New York: American Heart Association, 1975), pp. 7–17.

10. L. W. Green, "National Policy in the Promotion of Health," *International Journal of Health Education* 22 (1979):161–8. See also L. W. Green, "Current Report: Office of Health Information, Health Promotion and Physical Fitness and Sports Medicine," *Health Education* 11 (1980): 28, "Health promotion is a combination of health education and related organizational, political and economic programs designed to support changes in behavior and in the environment that will improve health." This definition did not survive in the federal initiative because it encompassed "health protection," which was a separate strategy from health promotion in the government's policy directed at the physical environment including, for example, sanitation, fluoridation, toxic agent control, and occupational safety.

11. *Health Promotion: A Discussion Document on the Concept and Principles* (Copenhagen: World Health Organization Regional Office for Europe, ICP/HSR 602, Sept. 1984), reprinted in *Health Promotion* 1 (1986): 73–6; I. Kickbusch, "Lifestyle and Health," *Social Science and Medicine* 22 (1986): 117–24; D. Nutbeam, *Health Promotion Glossary* (Copenhagen: World Health Organization Regional Office for Europe, July 1985).

12. L. W. Green, "Determining the Impact and Effectiveness of Health Education as It Relates to Federal Policy," *Health Education Monographs* 6 (1978): 28–66.

13. M. W. Kreuter, "Activity, Health, and the Public," in *Academy Papers* (Reston, VA: Academy of Physical Education, Alliance for Health, Physical Education, Recreation and Dance, 1989), chap. 15; N. Wallerstein and E. Bernstein, "Empowerment Education: Freire's Ideas Adapted to Health Education," *Health Education Quarterly* 15 (1988): 379–94.

14. J. O. Mason, "Health Promotion and Disease Prevention: The Federal and State Roles," *Focal Points* 1 (1984): 1–2.

15. N. Freudenberg, "Shaping the Future of Health Education: From Behavior Change to Social Change," *Health Education Monographs* 6 (1978): 372–7; L. W. Green, "A Participant-Observer During a Period of Professional Change," in *Advancing Health Through Education: A Case Study Approach*, H. P. Cleary, et al., eds. (Palo Alto: Mayfield, 1984), pp. 374–81; idem, "Emerging Federal Perspectives on Health Promotion," in *Health Promotion Monographs*, no. 1, J. P. Allegrante, ed. (New York: Teachers College, Columbia University, 1981); M. W. Kreuter, "Health Promotion: The Public Health Role in the Community of Free Exchange," *Health Promotion Monographs*, no. 4, J. M. Dodds, ed. (New York: Teachers College, Columbia University, 1984); N. Parlette, E. Glogow, and C. N. D'Onofrio, "Public Health Administration and Health Education Training Need More Integration," *Health Education Quarterly* 8 (1981):123–46; A. Steckler, L. Dawson, R. M. Goodman, and N. Epstein, "Policy Advocacy: Three Emerging Roles for Health Education," in *Advances in Health Education and Promotion*, vol. 2, W. B. Ward, ed. (Greenwich, CT: JAI Press, 1987), pp. 5–27.

16. First International Conference on Health Promotion, "Ottawa Charter for Health Promotion," *Health Promotion* 1 (1986): iii–v.

17. D. Gerstein, ed. *Toward the Prevention of Alcohol Problems* (Washington, DC: National Academy Press, 1984); L. W. Green and J. Raeburn, "Health Promotion: What Is It? What Will It Become?" *Health Promotion* 3 (1988): 151–9; L. W. Green, *Community Health*, 6th ed. (St. Louis, MO: Times Mirror/Mosby, 1990); J. F. Mosher and D. H. Jernigan, "New Directions in Alcohol Policy," *Annual Review of Public Health* 10 (1989): 245–79; L. Wallack, "Health Educators and the New Generation of Strategies," *Hygie* 4(2) (1985): 23–30.

18. R. R. Faden, "Ethical Issues in Government Sponsored Public Health Campaigns," *Health Education Quarterly* 14 (1987): 27–38; L. E. Goodman and M. J. Goodman, "Prevention—How Misuse of a Concept Can Undercut Its Worth," *Hastings Center Report* 3 (1986): 26–38; L. W. Green, "The Theory of Participation: A Qualitative Analysis of Its Expression in National and International Health Policies," in *Advances in Health Education and Promotion*, vol. 1, pt. A, W. B. Ward, ed. (Greenwich, CT: JAI Press, 1986), pp. 211–36.

19. K. R. McLeroy, D. Bibeau, A. Steckler, and K. Glanz, "An Ecological Perspective on Health Promotion Programs," *Health Education Quarterly* 15 (1988): 351–77; M. Minkler, "Health

Education, Health Promotion, and the Open Society," op. cit. 16 (1989): 17–30.; M. C. Roberts, "Public Health and Health Psychology: Two Cats of Kilkenny?" *Professional Psychology: Research and Practice* 18 (1987): 145–9.

20. M. W. Kreuter, "Health Promotion: The Public Health Role . . . , op. cit.

21. L. W., Green, *Community Health*, 6th ed., op. cit., chap.18, pp. 477–9.

22. N. Bracht, ed., *Community Organization Strategies for Health Promotion* (New York: Sage, 1990); L. W. Green, "The Revival of Community and the Obligation of Academic Health Centers to the Public," in *Institutional Values and Human Environments for Teaching, Inquiry and Practice*, R. J. Bulger, S. J. Reiser, and R. E. Bulger, eds. (Des Moines: University of Iowa Press, 1990); L. W. Green and J. Raeburn, op. cit.; C. F. Nelson, M. W. Kreuter, N. B. Watkins, and R. R. Stoddard, "Planned Approach to Community Health: The PATCH Program," in *Community-Oriented Primary Care: From Principle to Practice*, P. A. Nutting, ed. (Washington, D.C.: Government Printing Office, U.S. Department of Health and Human Services, HRS-A-PE 86–1, 1987); R. D. Patton and W. B. Cissell, eds., *Community Organization: Traditional Principles and Modern Applications* (Johnson City, TN: Latchpins Press, 1990).

23. A. Fonaroff, *Community Involvement in Health Systems for Primary Health Care* (Geneva: World Health Organization, SHS/83.6, 1983); P. Freire, *Pedagogy of the Oppressed* (New York: The Seabury Press, 1970); L. W. Green, "Reconciling Policy in Health Education and Primary Health Care," *International Journal of Health Education* 24 (suppl.3, 1982): 1–11, 1982; L. W. Green, "The Theory of Participation . . . ," op. cit.; M. Minkler, "Citizen Participation in Health in the Republic of Cuba," *International Quarterly of Community Health Education* 1 (1980–81): 65–78; M. Minkler, S. Frantz, and R. Wechsler, "Social Support and Social Action Organizing in a 'Grey Ghetto': The Tenderloin Experience," *International Quarterly of Community Health Education* 3 (1982): 3–15; A. Steckler, L. Dawson, and A. Williams, "Consumer Participation and Influence in a Health Systems Agency," *Journal of Community Health* 6 (1981): 181–93; M. O. Tonon, "Concepts in Community Participation," *International Journal of Health Education* 23 (suppl., 1980): 1–13, 1980; J. G. Zapka and S. Dorfman, "Consumer Participation: Case Study of the College Health Setting," *Journal of American College Health* 30 (1982): 197–203.

24. R. Andersson, "Health Education at Local Level," in *Vigor* (Intl. Ed.), N. Ostby, ed. (Stockholm: Division for Health Education, National Board of Health and Welfare, 1985); B. Eklundh and B. Pettersson, "Health Promotion Policy in Sweden: Means and Methods in Intersectoral Action," *Health Promotion* 2 (1987): 177–94; J. Epp, "Achieving Health for All: A Framework for Health Promotion," *Health Promotion* 1 (1986): 419–28; A. Evers, "Promoting Health–Localizing Support Structures for Community Health Projects," *Health Promotion* 4 (1989): 183–8; D. Ingledew, "Target Setting for the Health of Populations: Some Observations," *Health Promotion* 4 (1989): 357–69; K. Leppo and T. Melkas, "Toward Healthy Public Policy: Experiences in Finland 1972–1987," *Health Promotion* 3 (1988): 195–203.

25. T. McKeown, *The Role of Medicine: Dream, Mirage or Nemesis*, 2nd ed. (Princeton, NJ: Princeton University Press, 1979); *Perspectives on Health Promotion and Disease Prevention in the United States* (Washington, DC: Institute of Medicine, National Academy of Sciences, 1978).

26. J. C. Burnham, "Change in the Popularization of Health in the United States," *Bulletin of the History of Medicine* 58 (Summer 1984): 183–97; C. Fellman and M. Fellman, *Making Sense of Self: Medical Advice Literature in Late Nineteenth-Century America* (Philadelphia: University of Pennsylvania Press, 1981); J. C. Riley, *The Eighteenth Century Campaign to Avoid Disease* (New York: St. Martin's Press, 1987); J. C. Whorton, *Crusaders for Fitness: The History of American Health Reformers* (Princeton, NJ: Princeton University Press, 1982).

27. G. Rosen, *A History of Public Health* (New York: MD Publications, 1958); D. C. Walsh and V. McDougall, "Current Policies Regarding Smoking in the Workplace," *American Journal of Industrial Medicine* 13 (1988): 181–90.

28. H. E. Sigerist, *The University at the Crossroads: Addresses and Essays* (New York: Henry Schuman, 1946); M. Terris, "What Is Health Promotion?" *Journal of Public Health Policy* 7

(1986): 147–51; L. W. Green, *Community Health*, 6th ed. (St. Louis: Times Mirror/Mosby, 1990), chap. 1.

29. C. E. A. Winslow, "The Untilled Fields of Public Health," *Science* 51 (1920): 23.

30. L. A. Aday, R. Andersen, and G. V. Fleming, *Health Care in the U.S.: Equitable for Whom?* (Beverly Hills: Sage, 1980); R. Andersen, M. Chen, L. A. Aday, and L. Cornelius, "Health Status and Medical Care Utilization," *Health Affairs* 6 (1987): 136–56; J. P. Bunker, D. S. Gomby, and B. H. Kehrer, *Pathways to Health: The Role of Social Factors* (Menlo Park, CA: Kaiser Family Foundation, 1989); J. Elinson, "Have We Narrowed the Gap Between the Poor and the Nonpoor?" *Medical Care* 15 (1977): 675–7; A. C. Marcus, L. G. Reeder, L. A. Jordan, and T. E. Seeman, "Monitoring Health Status, Access to Health Care, and Compliance Behavior in a Large Urban Community," *Medical Care* 18 (1980): 253–65, 1980; T. G. Rundall and J. R. C. Wheeler, "The Effect of Income on Use of Preventive Care: An Evaluation of Alternative Explanations," *Journal of Health and Social Behavior* 20 (1979): 397–406; B. Starfield, "Family Income, Ill Health and Medical Care of U.S. Children," *Journal of Public Health Policy* 3 (1982): 244–59.

31. J. H. Abramson, R. Gofin, J. Habib, et al., "Indicators of Social Class: A Comparative Appraisal of Measures for Use in Epidemiological Studies," *Social Science and Medicine* 16 (1982): 1739–46; H. P. Freeman, "Cancer in the Economically Disadvantaged," *Cancer* 64 (suppl., 1989): 324–34; L. W. Green and D. G. Simons-Morton, "Education and Life-Style Determinants of Health and Disease," in *Oxford Textbook of Public Health*, 2nd ed., W. W. Holland, R. Detels, and G. Knox, eds. (London: Oxford University Press, 1990); B. Starfield and P. P. Budetti, "Child Health Status and Risk Factors," *Health Services Research* 19 (1985): 817–86; U.S. Department of Health and Human Services, *Report of the Secretary's Task Force on Black and Minority Health* (Washington, DC: U.S. Government Printing Office, 1985).

32. *Report of the President's Committee on Health Education* (New York: Public Affairs Institute, 1973).

33. S. G. Deeds and P. D. Mullen, "Managing Health Education in HMOs: Part II," *Health Education Quarterly* 9 (1982): 3–95; P. D. Mullen and J. G. Zapka, *Guidelines for Health Promotion and Education Services in HMOs* (Washington, DC: U.S. Government Printing Office, 1982); P. D. Mullen and J. G. Zapka, "Health Education and Promotion in HMOs: The Recent Evidence," *Health Education Quarterly* 8 (1981): 292–315.

34. *Focal Points* (Atlanta: Bureau of Health Education, Centers for Disease Control, U.S. Department of Health, Education, and Welfare, July 1977).

35. L. W. Green, R. A. Goldstein, and S. R. Parker, eds., "Research on Self-Management of Childhood Asthma," *Journal of Allergy and Clinical Immunology* 72 (1983): 519–629; J. J. Kronenfeld, "Self-Help and Self-Care as Social Movements," in *Advances in Health Education and Promotion*, vol. 1, pt. A, W. B. Ward and Z. Salisbury, eds. (Greenwich, CT: JAI Press, 1986), pp. 105–27; L. S. Levin, "Forces and Issues in the Revival of Interest in Self-Care: Impetus for Redirection in Health," in *The SOPHE Heritage Collection of Health Education Monographs, Vol. 2: The Practice of Health Education*, B. P. Mathews, ed. (Oakland: Third Party Associates, 1982); pp. 268–73.

36. For composite, quantitative reviews of the cumulative evidence extant during this period, see E. C. Devine and T. D. Cook, "A Meta-Analytic Analysis of Effects of Psycho-Educational Interventions on Length of Postsurgical Hospital Stay," *Nursing Research* 32 (1983): 267–74; R. B. Haynes, D. W. Taylor, and D. L. Sackett, eds., *Compliance in Health Care* (Baltimore: Johns Hopkins University Press, 1979); S. A. Mazzuca, "Does Patient Education in Chronic Disease Have Therapeutic Value?" *Journal of Chronic Disease* 35 (1982): 521–9; P. D. Mullen, L. W. Green, and G. S. Persinger, "Clinical Trials of Patient Education for Chronic Conditions: A Comparative Meta-Analysis of Intervention Types," *Preventive Medicine* 14 (1985): 753–81; E. Mumford, H. J. Schlesinger, and G. V. Glass, "The Effects of Psychological Intervention on Recovery from Surgery and Heart Attacks: An Analysis of the Literature," *American Journal of Public Health* 72 (1982): 141–51; E. J. Posavac, "Evaluations of Patient Education Programs: A Meta-Analysis," *Evaluation and the Health Professions* 3 (1980): 47–62.

37. M. Terris, "What Is Health Promotion?" *Journal of Public Health Policy* 7 (1986): 147–51.

38. H. C. Boyte, *Community Is Possible: Repairing America's Roots* (New York: Harper and Row, 1984); L. W. Green, "The Theory of Participation...," op. cit. pp. 211–36.; D. P. Moynihan, *Maximum Feasible Misunderstanding: Community Action in the War on Poverty* (New York: Free Press, 1969).

39. P. L. Berger and R. J. Neuhaus, *To Empower People: The Role of Mediating Structures in Public Policy* (Washington, DC: American Enterprise Institute for Public Policy Research, 1977); L. W. Green, S. Werlin, H. Schauffler, and C. H. Avery, "Research and Demonstration Issues in Self-Care: Measuring the Decline of Medicocentrism," in *The SOPHE Heritage Collection of Health Education Monographs*, vol. 3, J. G. Zapka, ed. (Oakland: Third Party Publishing, 1981), pp. 40–69; L. S. Levin, "Lay Health Care: The Hidden Resource in Health Promotion," in *Health Promotion Monographs*, no. 3, K. A. Gordon, ed. (New York: Teachers College, Columbia University, 1983); L. S. Levin, A. Katz, and E. Holst, *Self-Care: Lay Initiatives in Health* (New York: Prodist, 1978); P. L. Schiller and L. S. Levin, "Is Self-Care a Social Movement?" *Social Science and Medicine* 17 (1983): 1343–52.

40. J. P. Allegrante and L. W. Green, "When Health Policy Becomes Victim Blaming," *New England Journal of Medicine* 305 (1981): 1528–9; R. Crawford, "You Are Dangerous to Your Health: The Ideology and Politics of Victim Blaming," *International Journal of Health Services* 7 (1977): 663–80.

41. R. Parkinson, L. W. Green, A. McGill, et al., *Managing Health Promotion in the Workplace: Guidelines for Implementation and Evaluation* (Palo Alto, CA: Mayfield, 1982). The background on development of the worksite health promotion movement is detailed further in Chapter 9.

42. A. J. Enelow and J. B. Henderson, eds., *Applying Behavioral Science to Cardiovascular Risk* (New York: American Heart Association, 1975).

43. L. W. Green and A. L. McAlister, "Macro-intervention to Support Health Behavior: Some Theoretical Perspectives and Practical Reflections," *Health Education Quarterly* 11 (1984): 323–39.

44. G. DeFriese, *Promoting Health in America: Breakthroughs and Harbingers* (Battle Creek, MI: W. K. Kellogg Foundation, 1989), p. 9.

45. Kaiser Family Foundation, *The Health Promotion Program of the Henry J. Kaiser Family Foundation* (Menlo Park: The Foundation, 1990); A. R. Tarlov, B. H. Kehrer, D. P. Hall, et al., "Foundation Work: The Health Promotion Program of The Henry J. Kaiser Family Foundation," *American Journal of Health Promotion* 2 (1987): 74–80.

46. See reviews and summaries, for example, in *Consumer Self-Care in Health* (Rockville, MD: National Center for Health Services Research Proceeding Series, DHEW Publication No. HRA 77–3181, 1977); F. Landry, ed., *Health Risk Estimation, Risk Reduction and Health Promotion* (Ottawa: Canadian Public Health Association, 1983); J. L. Schwartz, ed., *Progress in Smoking Cessation* (New York: American Cancer Society, 1978); American College of Preventive Medicine and Fogarty Center, *Preventive Medicine USA* (New York: Prodist, 1976); J. Steinfeld, W. Griffiths, K. Ball, and R. M. Taylor, eds., *Smoking and Health: Health Consequences, Education, Cessation Activities, and Government Action*, vol. 2 (Washington, DC: Department of Health, Education, and Welfare, NIH 77–1413, 1977).

47. A. J. Enelow and J. B. Henderson, eds., *Applying Behavioral Science to Cardiovascular Risk* (Dallas: American Heart Association, 1975); J. Cullen, B. Fox, and R. Isom, eds., *Cancer: The Behavioral Dimensions* (New York: Raven, 1976); J. D. Matarazzo, S. M. Weiss, J. A. Herd, et al., eds., *Behavioral Health: A Handbook of Health Enhancement and Disease Prevention* (New York: Wiley, 1984); E. J. Roccella and G. W. Ward, "The National High Blood Pressure Campaign: A Description of Its Utility as a Generic Program Model," *Health Education Quarterly* 11 (1984): 225–42; A. Somers, ed., *Health Promotion and Consumer Health Education* (Greenbelt, MD: Aspen Systems, 1976); W. Squyres, ed., *Patient Education: An Inquiry Into the State of*

the Art (New York: Springer, 1980); S. Weiss, A. Herd, and B. Fox, eds., *Perspectives on Behavioral Medicine* (New York: Academic Press, 1981).

48. J. M. Michaels, "The Second Revolution in Health: Health Promotion and Its Environmental Base," *American Psychologist* 37 (1982): 936–41; C. W. Taylor, "Promoting Health and Strengthening Wellness through Environmental Variables," in *Behavioral Health: A Handbook of Health Enhancement and Disease Prevention*, J. D. Matarazzo, S. M. Weiss, J. A. Herd, et al., eds. (New York: Wiley, 1984), pp. 130–49.

49. *Healthy People: The Surgeon General's Report on Health Promotion and Disease Prevention* (Washington, DC: U.S. Department of Health, Education, and Welfare, 1979); L. W. Green, "Toward National Policy for Health Education," in *Alcohol, Youth and Social Policy*, H. Blane and M. E. Chafetz, eds. (New York: Plenum, 1979), pp. 283–305; L. W. Green, "Healthy People: The Surgeon General's Report and the Prospects," in *Working for a Healthier America*, W. K. McNerney, ed. (Cambridge, MA: Ballinger, 1980), pp. 95–110.

50. M. A. LaLonde, *New Perspectives on the Health of Canadians* (Ottawa, Canada: Ministry of National Health and Welfare, 1974).

51. M. Terris, "The Epidemiologic Revolution, National Health Insurance and the Role of Health Departments," *American Journal of Public Health* 66 (1976): 1155–64; idem. "Public Health in the United States: The Next 100 Years," *Journal of Public Health Policy* 93 (1978): 602–8.

52. F. M. Andrews and S. B. Withey, *Social Indicators of Well-Being: Americans' Perceptions of Life Quality* (New York: Plenum, 1976); M. K. Chen, "The Gross National Health Product: A Proposed Population Health Index," *Public Health Reports* 94 (1979): 119–23; M. Terris, "Approaches to an Epidemiology of Health," *American Journal of Public Health* 65 (1975): 1037–45; C. T. Viet and J. E. Ware, Jr., "Measuring Health and Health-care Outcomes: Issues and Recommendations," in *Values and Long-Term Care*, R. L. Kane and R. A. Kane, eds. (Lexington, MA: Lexington Books, 1982). For an update on the progress toward new definitions and measures of health, see K. N. Lohr, ed., "Advances in Health Status Assessment: Conference Proceedings," *Medical Care* 27 (suppl., 1989): whole issue.

53. L. Davidson, S. Chapman, and C. Hull, *Health Promotion in Australia 1978–1979* (Canberra: Commonwealth of Australia, 1979); E. J. J. DeLeeuw, *Health Promotion: The Sane Revolution* (Maastricht, The Netherlands: Van Gorcum, 1989); Great Britain Expenditures Committee, *First Report from the Expenditures Committee. Session 1976–1977: Preventive Medicine* (London: Her Majesty's Stationery Office, 1977).

54. World Health Organization, *Alma-Ata 1978: Primary Health Care* (Geneva: World Health Organization, "Health for All" Series, no. 1, 1978).

55. L. W. Green, "Reconciling Policy in Health Education and Primary Health Care," *International Journal of Health Education* 24 (suppl. 3, 1982): 1–11; idem., *New Policies for Health Education in Primary Health Care* (Geneva: World Health Organization, 1986); idem., "The Theory of Participation . . . ," op. cit.

56. *New Approaches to Health Education in Primary Health Care: Report of a WHO Expert Committee* (Geneva: World Health Organization, Technical Report Series 690, 1983), pp. 40–1.

57. L. W. Green, "The Oversimplification of Policy Issues in Prevention," *American Journal of Public Health* 68 (1978): 953–4; idem, "To Educate or Not to Educate: Is That the Question?" *American Journal of Public Health* 70 (1980): 625–6; idem., "Individuals vs. Systems: An Artificial Classification That Divides and Distorts," *Health Link* (National Center for Health Education) 2 (1986): 29–30; J. M. Ottoson and L. W. Green, "Reconciling Concept and Context: A Theory of Implementation," in *Advances in Health Education and Promotion*, vol. 2, W. B. Ward, ed. (Greenwich, CT: JAI Press, 1987), pp. 339–68.

58. World Health Assembly, *New Policies for Health Education in Primary Health Care: Technical Discussions of the 36th World Health Assembly* (Geneva: World Health Organization, 1985).

59. M. F. Cataldo and T. J. Coates, eds., *Health and Industry: A Behavioral Medicine Perspective* (New York: Wiley, 1986); J. E. Fielding and P. V. Piserchia, "Frequency of Worksite Health Promotion Activities," *American Journal of Public Health* 79 (1989): 16–20; *National Survey of Worksite Health Promotion Activities: A Summary* (Washington, DC: U.S. Department of Health and Human Services, Public Health Service, Office of Disease Prevention and Health Promotion, 1987).

60. R. Y. Cohen, M. R. J. Felix, and K. D. Brownell, "The Role of Parents and Older Peers in School-Based Cardiovascular Prevention Programs: Implications for Program Development," *Health Education Quarterly* 16 (1989): 245–53; R. C. Ellison, A. L. Capper, R. J. Goldberg et al., "The Environmental Component: Changing School Food Service to Promote Cardiovascular Health," *Health Education Quarterly* 16 (1989): 285–97; B. R. Flay, "Psychosocial Approaches to Smoking Prevention: A Review of Findings," *Health Psychology* 4 (1985): 449–88; G. S. Parcel, B. G. Simons-Morton, and L. J. Kolbe, "Health Promotion: Integrating Organizational Change and Student Learning Strategies," *Health Education Quarterly* 15 (1988): 435–50; G. S. Parcel, B. G. Simons-Morton, N. M. O'Hara et al., "School Promotion of Healthful Diet and Physical Activity: Impact on Learning Outcomes and Self-reported Behavior," *Health Education Quarterly* 16 (1989): 181–99; B. G. Simons-Morton, G. S. Parcel, and N. M. O'Hara, "Implementing Organizational Changes to Promote Healthful Diet and Physical Activity at School," *Health Education Quarterly* 15 (1988): 115–30.

61. M. P. O'Donnell, "Definition of Health Promotion," *American Journal of Health Promotion* 1 (1986): 4–5.

62. M. P. O'Donnell, "Definition of Health Promotion: Part III: Expanding the Definition," *American Journal of Health Promotion* 3 (1989): 5.

63. L. Breslow and J. D. Egstrom, "Persistence of Health Habits and Their Relationship to Mortality," *Preventive Medicine* 9 (1980): 469–83; S. Epstein, "The Stability of Behavior: I. On Predicting Most of the People Much of the Time," *Journal of Personality and Social Psychology* 37 (1979): 1097–126; D. Mechanic, "The Stability of Health and Illness Behavior: Results from a 16-year Follow-up," *American Journal of Public Health* 69 (1979): 1142–5.

64. W. Bell, "Social Choice, Life Styles, and Suburban Residence," in *The Suburban Community*, W. Dobriner, ed. (New York: Putnam, 1958), pp. 225–42; G. Handel and L. Rainwater, "Persistence and Change in Working-Class Life Style," in *Blue-Collar World*, A. B. Shostack and W. Gomberg, eds. (Englewood Cliffs, NJ: Prentice-Hall, 1964), pp. 36–41.

65. J. D. Mattarazzo, "Behavioral Health: A 1990 Challenge for the Health Sciences Professions," in *Behavioral Health: A Handbook of Health Enhancement and Disease Prevention*, J. D. Mattarazzo, S. M. Weiss, J. A. Herd et al., eds. (New York: Wiley, 1984); A. F. Williams and H. Wechsler, "Interrelationship of Preventive Actions in Health and Other Areas," *Health Services Reports* 87 (1972): 969–76.

66. R. Andersen, *A Behavioral Model of Families' Use of Health Services* (Chicago: University of Chicago, Center for Health Administration Studies Research, Series No. 25, 1968); L. W. Green, *Status Identity and Preventive Health Behavior* (Berkeley: University of California School of Public Health, Pacific Health Education Reports, no. 1, 1970); J. Langlie, "Social Networks, Health Beliefs, and Preventive Behavior," *Journal of Health and Social Behavior* 18 (1977): 244–60.

67. J. R. Eiser, S. R. Sutton, and M. Wober, "Smoking, Seat-Belts, and Beliefs About Health," *Addictive Behavior* 4 (1979): 331–8; N. H. Gottlieb and L. W. Green, "Life Events, Social Network, Lifestyle and Health: An Analysis of the National Survey of Personal Health Practices and Consequences," *Health Education Quarterly* 11 (1984): 91–105; L. Kannas, "The Dimensions of Health Behavior Among Young Men in Finland," *International Journal of Health Education* 24 (1982): 146–55; B. L. Pesznecher and J. McNeil, "Relationship Among Health Habits, Social Psychologic Well-Being, Life Change and Alterations in Health Status," *Nursing Research* 24 (1975): 442–7; A. F. Williams and H. Wechsler, "Interrelationships . . .," op. cit.

68. J. Coreil and J. S. Levin, "A Critique of the Life Style Concept in Public Health Education," *International Quarterly of Community Health Education* 5 (1985): 103-14.

69. J. Allen and R. F. Allen, "Achieving Health Promotion Objectives through Cultural Change Systems," *American Journal of Health Promotion* 1 (1986): 42-9; R. Dwore and M. W. Kreuter, "Update: Reinforcing the Case for Health Promotion," *Family and Community Health* 2 (1980): 103-19; L. W. Green, *Toward a Healthy Community: Organizing Events for Community Health Promotion* (Washington, DC: U.S. Department of Health and Human Services, Public Health Service, Office of Disease Prevention and Health Promotion, 80-50113, 1980).

70. R. B. Dwore and M. W. Kreuter, "Update: Reinforcing the Case for Health Promotion," *Family and Community Health* 2 (1980): 103-19.

71. I. Kickbusch, "Health Promotion: A Global Perspective," *Canadian Journal of Public Health* 77 (1986): 321-6.

72. M. Terris, "Approaches to an Epidemiology of Health," *American Journal of Public Health* 65 (1975): 1037-45; M. L. Jasnoski and G. E. Schwartz, "A Synchronous Systems Model for Health," *American Behavioral Scientist* 28 (1985): 468-85.

73. L. W. Green, A. L. Wilson, and C. Y. Lovato, "What Changes Can Health Promotion Achieve and How Long Do These Changes Last?" *Preventive Medicine* 15 (1986): 508-21.

74. A. Viseltear, "A Short History of P.L. 94-317," in *Preventive Medicine USA*, American College of Preventive Medicine and Fogerty Center, eds. (New York: Prodist, 1976), pp. 825-37.

75. L. W. Green, "National Policy in the Promotion of Health," *International Journal of Health Education* 22 (1979): 161-8.

76. H. P. Cleary, "Issues in the Credentialing of Health Education Specialists: A Review of the State of the Art," in *Advances in Health Education and Promotion*, vol. 1, pt. A, W. Ward and Z. Salisbury (Greenwich, CT: JAI Press, 1986), pp. 129-54; A. C. Henderson, "Developing a Credentialing System for Health Educators," in *Advances in Health Education and Health Promotion*, vol. 2, W. B. Ward and S. K. Simonds, eds. (Greenwich, CT: JAI Press, 1987), pp. 59-91; A. C. Henderson, J. M. Wolle, P. A. Cortese, and D. I. McIntosh, "The Future of the Health Education Profession: Implications for Preparation and Practice," *Public Health Reports* 96 (1981): 555-60; *Preparation and Practice of Community, Patient and School Health Educators: Proceedings on Commonalities and Differences* (Bethesda: Bureau of Health Manpower, U.S. Department of Health, Education, and Welfare, HRA 78-71, 1978); *National Conference for Institutions Preparing Health Educators: Proceedings* (Washington, DC: U.S. Office of Health Information and Health Promotion, PHS 81-50171, 1981).

77. Society for Public Health Education, "Guidelines for the Preparation and Practice of Professional Health Educators," *Health Education Monographs* 5 (1977): 75-89.

78. World Health Organization, *Report of the Task Force on Health Education in Family Health* (Geneva: WHO Technical Report Series 45, 1979).

79. L. W. Frederiksen, L. J. Solomon, and K. A. Brehony, eds., *Marketing Health Behavior: Principles, Techniques, and Applications* (New York: Plenum, 1984); R. Manoff, *Social Marketing* (New York: Praeger, 1987).

80. L. W. Green, "Promoting the One-Child Policy of China," *Journal of Public Health Policy* 9 (1988): 273-83.

81. L. W. Green, "Promoting the One-Child Policy . . . ," op. cit.

82. For summaries of planning models in health promotion, see I. J. Bates and A. E. Winder, *Introduction to Health Education* (Palo Alto, CA: Mayfield, 1984); D. J. Breckon, *Hospital Health Education: A Guide to Program Development* (Rockville, MD: Aspen, 1982); D. J. Breckon, J. R. Harvey, and R. B. Lancaster, *Community Health Education: Settings, Roles, and Skills*, 2nd ed. (Rockville, MD: Aspen, 1989), chap. 11; M. B. Dignan and P. A. Carr,

Introduction to Program Planning: A Basic Text for Community Health Education (Philadelphia: Lea & Febiger, 1981); L. Ewles and I. Simnett, *Promoting Health: A Practical Guide to Health Education* (New York: Wiley, 1985), chaps. 6 & 7; G. D. Gilmore, M. D. Campbell, and B. L. Becker, *Needs Assessment Strategies for Health Education and Health Promotion* (Indianapolis, IN: Benchmark Press, 1989), esp. p. 13; J. S. Greenberg, *Health Education: Learner Centered Instructional Strategies* (Dubuque: Wm. C. Brown, 1987); M. Longe, *Innovative Hospital-Based Health Promotion* (Chicago: American Hospital Association, 1985); R. K. Manoff, *Social Marketing: New Imperatives for Public Health* (New York: Praeger, 1985); V. J. Marsick, "Designing Health Education Programs," in *Handbook of Health Education*, 2nd ed., P. M. Lazes, L. H. Kaplan, and K. A. Gordon, eds. (Rockville, MD: Aspen, 1987), chap. 1; R. S. Parkinson, L. W. Green, A. McGill et al., *Managing Health Promotion in the Workplace* (Palo Alto, CA: Mayfield, 1982); M. Pollock, *Planning and Implementing Health Education in Schools* (Palo Alto, CA: Mayfield, 1987); H. S. Ross and P. R. Mico, *Theory and Practice in Health Education*, (Palo Alto, CA: Mayfield, 1980); M. S. Strehlow, *Education for Health* (London: Harper & Row, 1983), chap. 6; B. K. Tones, "Past Achievement and Future Success," in *Health Education — Perspectives and Choices*, I. Sutherland, ed. (London, Allen & Unwin, 1979), chap. 12.

83. In the past, PRECEDE was called a framework. This was a caution against claiming too much for it as a model or a theory. A theory is "a set of interrelated constructs (variables), definitions, and propositions that presents a systematic view of phenomena by specifying relations among variables, with the purpose of explaining natural phenomena," from F. N. Kerlinger, *Behavioral Research: A Conceptual Approach* (New York: Holt, Rinehart & Winston, 1979). The primary purpose of PRECEDE was not to explain "natural phenomena" but to organize existing theories and constructs (variables) into a cohesive, comprehensive, and systematic view of relations among those variables important to the planning and evaluation of health education. Given the extensive application and validation of the framework in practice and in research, we now feel confident that it warrants being called a model. For further discussion of models and theories see K. Glanz, F. M. Lewis, and B. K. Rimer, eds., *Health Behavior and Health Education: Theory, Research, and Practice* (San Francisco: Jossey-Bass, 1990); L. W. Green, "Models of Health Education," in *Behavioral Health: A Handbook of Health Enhancement and Disease Prevention*, J. Matarazzo, S. M. Weiss, J. A. Herd et al., eds. (New York: Wiley, 1986); L. W. Green and F. M. Lewis, *Measurement and Evaluation in Health Education and Health Promotion* (Palo Alto, CA: Mayfield, 1986); S. B. Kar, "Communication for Health Promotion: A Model for Research and Action," in *Advances in Health Education and Promotion*, vol. 1, pt. A, W. B. Ward and S. B. Kar, eds. (Greenwich, CT: JAI Press, 1986), pp. 267–302; K. Lorig and J. Laurin, "Some Notions About Assumptions Underlying Health Education," *Health Education Quarterly* 12 (1985): 231–43; P. D. Mullen, D. Iverson, and J. Hershey, "Health Behavior Models Compared," *Social Science and Medicine* 24 (1987): 973–81; J. Rothman and J. E. Tropman, "Models of Community Organization and Macro Practice: Their Mixing and Phasing," in *Strategies of Community Organization*, 4th ed., F. M. Cox, J. Erlich, J. L. Rothman, and J. E. Tropman, eds. (Itasca, IL: F. E. Peacock, 1987), pp. 3–26.

84. J. L. Braily, "Effects of Health Teaching in the Workplace on Women's Knowledge, Beliefs, and Practices Regarding Breast Self-Examination," *Research in Nursing and Health* 9 (1986): 223–31; J. C. Cantor, D. E. Morisky, L. W. Green et al., "Cost-Effectiveness of Educational Interventions to Improve Patient Outcomes in Blood Pressure Control," *Preventive Medicine* 14 (1985): 782–800; L. W. Green, "Towards Cost-Benefit Evaluation of Health Education: Some Concepts, Methods and Examples," *Health Education Quarterly* 2 (suppl. 2, 1974): 34–64; L. W. Green, V. L. Wang, and P. Ephross, "A Three-Year Longitudinal Study of the Effectiveness of Nutrition Aides on Rural Poor Homemakers," *American Journal of Public Health* 64 (1974): 722–4; L. W. Green, A. Fisher, R. Amin, and A. B. M. Shafiullah, "Paths to the Adoption of Family Planning: A Time-Lagged Correlation Analysis of the Dacca Experiment in Bangladesh," *International Journal of Health Education* 18 (1975): 85–96; L. W. Green, D. M. Levine, J. Wolle, and S. G. Deeds, "Development of Randomized Patient Education Experiments with Urban Poor Hypertensives," *Patient Counseling and Health Education* 1 (1979): 106–11; M. J. Hatcher, L. W. Green, D. M. Levine, and C. E. Flagle, "Validation of a Decision Model for Triaging Hypertensive Patients to Alternate Health Education Interventions," *Social Science and Medicine* 22 (1986): 813–19; D. M. Levine, L. W. Green, S. G. Deeds et al., "Health Education for Hypertensive

Patients," *Journal of the American Medical Association* 241 (1979): 1700–3; L. Maiman, L. W. Green, G. Gibson, and E. J. Mackenzie, "Education for Self-Treatment by Adult Asthmatics," *Journal of the American Medical Association* 241 (1979): 1919–22; D. E. Morisky, D. M. Levine, L. W. Green, and C. Smith, "Health Education Program Effects on the Management of Hypertension in the Elderly," *Archives of Internal Medicine* 142 (1982): 1935–8; D. E. Morisky, D. M. Levine, L. W. Green et al., "The Relative Impact of Health Education for Low- and High-Risk Patients with Hypertension," *Preventive Medicine* 9 (1980): 550–8; D. E. Morisky, D. M. Levine, L. W. Green et al., "Five-Year Blood-Pressure Control and Mortality Following Health Education for Hypertensive Patients," *American Journal of Public Health* 73 (1983): 153–62; D. E. Morisky, N. M. DeMuth, M. Field-Fass et al., "Evaluation of Family Health Education to Build Social Support for Long-Term Control of High Blood Pressure," *Health Education Quarterly* 12 (1985): 35–50; B. Rimer, M. K. Keintz, and L. Fleisher, "Process and Impact of a Health Communications Program," *Health Education Research* 1 (1986): 29–36; J. Sayegh and L. W. Green, "Family Planning Education: Program Design, Training Component and Cost-Effectiveness of a Post-Partum Program in Beirut," *International Journal of Health Education* 19 (suppl., 1976): 1–20; V. L. Wang, P. Terry, B. S. Flynn et al. "Multiple Indicators of Continuing Medical Education Priorities for Chronic Lung Diseases in Appalachia," *Journal of Medical Education* 54 (1979): 803–11.

85. S. G. Brink, D. Simons-Morton, G. Parcel, and C. Tiernan, "Community Intervention Handbooks for Comprehensive Health Promotion Programming," *Family and Community Health* 11 (1988): 28–35; A. C. Gielen and S. Radius, "Project KISS (Kids in Safety Belts): Educational Approaches and Evaluation Measures," *Health Education* 15 (Aug.-Sept. 1984): 43–7; Health Education Center, *Strategies for Health Education in Local Health Departments* (Baltimore: Maryland State Department of Health and Mental Hygiene, 1977); *PATCH: Planned Approach to Community Health* (Atlanta: Centers for Disease Control, 1985); I. M. Newman, G. L. Martin, and R. Weppner, "A Conceptual Model for Developing Prevention Programs," *The International Journal of the Addictions* 17 (1982): 493–504.

86. L. W. Green, V. L. Wang, S. G. Deeds et al., "Guidelines for Health Education in Maternal and Child Health Programs," *International Journal of Health Education* 21 (suppl., 1978): 1–33.

87. N. Danforth and B. Swaboda, *Agency for International Development Health Education Study* (Washington, DC: Westinghouse Health Systems, March 17, 1978); L. W. Green, *New Policies for Health Education in Primary Health Care* (Geneva: World Health Organization, 1986); L. W. Green, R. W. Wilson, and K. Bauer, "Data Required to Measure Progress on the Objectives for the Nation in Disease Prevention and Health Promotion," *American Journal of Public Health* 73 (1983): 18–24.

88. National Committee for Injury Prevention and Control, *Injury Prevention: Meeting the Challenge* (New York: Oxford University Press), as a supplement to the *American Journal of Preventive Medicine*, vol. 5, no. 3, 1989. See also M. P. Eriksen and A. C. Gielen, "The Application of Health Education Principles to Automobile Child Restraint Programs," *Health Education Quarterly* 10 (1983): 30–55; D. A. Sleet, "Health Education Approaches to Motor Vehicle Injury Prevention," *Public Health Reports* 102 (1987): 606–8, for specific applications in injury prevention and control.

89. L. W. Green, *Program Planning and Evaluation Guide for Lung Associations* (New York: American Lung Association, 1987).

90. L. Light and I. R. Contento, "Changing the Course: A School Nutrition and Cancer Education Curriculum Developed by the American Cancer Society and the National Cancer Institute," *Journal of School Health* 59 (1989): 205–9. See also the broader ACS Plan for Youth Education: R. D. Corcoran and B. Portnoy, "Risk Reduction Through Comprehensive Cancer Education: The American Cancer Society Plan for Youth Education," *Journal of School Health* 59 (1989): 199–204.

91. A. Ackerman and H. Kalmer, "Health Education and a Baccalaureate Nursing Curriculum — Myth or Reality" (paper presented at the 105th annual meeting of the American Public Health

Association, Washington, DC, 1 Nov. 1977); M. S. Shine, M. C. Silva, and F. S. Weed, "Integrating Health Education into Baccalaureate Nursing Education," *Journal of Nursing Education* 22 (1983): 22–7.

92. D. Fedder and R. Beardsley, "Preparing Pharmacy Patient Educators," *American Journal of Pharmacy Education* 43 (1979): 127–9.

93. B. I. Bennett, "A Model for Teaching Health Education Skills to Primary Care Practitioners," *International Journal of Health Education* 20 (1977): 232–9; G. W. Simpson and B. E. Pruitt, "The Development of Health Promotion Teams as Related to Wellness Programs in Texas Schools," *Health Education* 20(1) (1989):26–8.

94. L. W. Green, "A Triage and Stepped Approach to Self-Care Education," *Medical Times* 111 (1984): 75–80; idem, "What Physicians Can Do to Increase Participation and Maintenance of Patients in Self-care," *Western Journal of Medicine* 147 (1987): 346–9; L. W. Green, M. E. Eriksen, and E. L. Schor, "Preventive Practices by Physicians: Behavioral Determinants and Potential Interventions," *American Journal of Preventive Medicine* 4 (suppl. 4, 1988): 101–7, reprinted in R. N. Battista and R. S. Lawrence, eds., *Implementing Preventive Services* (New York: Oxford University Press, 1988); R. S. Lawrence, "Summary of Workshop Sessions of the International Symposium on Preventive Services in Primary Care: Issues and Strategies," *American Journal of Preventive Medicine* 4 (suppl. 4, 1988): 188–9; D. M. Levine and L. W. Green, "Patient Education: State of the Art in Research and Evaluation," *Bulletin of the New York Academy of Medicine* 61 (1985): 135–43; idem, "Behavioral Change through Health Education," in *Prevention of Coronary Heart Disease: Practical Management of the Risk Factors*, N. M. Kaplan and J. Stamler, eds. (Philadelphia: Saunders, 1983), pp. 161–9; V. L. Wang, P. Terry, B. S. Flynn et al., "Multiple Indicators . . .," op. cit.

95. D. G. Altman and L. W. Green, "Area Review: Education and Training in Behavioral Medicine," *Annals of Behavioral Medicine* 10 (1988): 4–7; A. Fisher, L. W. Green, A. McCrae, and C. Cochran, "Training Teachers in Population Education Institutes in Baltimore," *Journal of School Health* 46 (1976): 357–60; D. M. Levine and L. W. Green, "Cardiovascular Risk Reduction: An Interdisciplinary Approach to Research Training," *International Journal of Health Education* 24 (1981): 20–5.

96. L. W. Green, *Program Planning and Evaluation Guide for Lung Associations* (New York: American Lung Association, 1987); idem., "Healthy People: The Surgeon General's Report and the Prospects," in *Working for a Healthier America*, W. K. McNerney, ed. (Cambridge, MA: Ballinger, 1980), pp. 95–110; D. C. Iverson and L. W. Green, "Drug Abuse Prevention from a Public Health Perspective—A Proposal for the 1980s," in *NIDA Drug Abuse Prevention Monograph*, W. Bukowski, ed. (Washington, DC: National Institute of Drug Abuse, Department of Health and Human Services, 1981); M. W. Kreuter, "Health Promotion: The Public Health Role . . .," op. cit.; M. W. Kreuter, G. M. Christenson, and A. DiVincenzo, "The Multiplier Effect of the Health Education–Risk Reduction Grants Program in 28 States and 1 Territory," *Public Health Reports* 97 (1982): 510–15; L. Kolbe, D. C. Iverson, M. W. Kreuter et al., "Propositions for an Alternate and Complementary Health Education Paradigm," *Health Education* 12 (May-June, 1981): 24–30; *Strategies for Promoting Health in Special Populations* (Washington, DC: Office of Disease Prevention and Health Promotion, 1981), reprinted in *Journal of Public Health Policy* 8 (1987): 369–423.

97. L. W. Green, *New Policies for Health Education in Primary Health Care* (Geneva: World Health Organization, 1986); idem., "National Policy in the Promotion of Health," 1979, op. cit.; idem, "Policies for Decentralization and Development of Health Education," *Revue Saude Publica* (Sao Paulo, Brazil) 22 (1988): 217–20.

98. R. Bertera and L. W. Green, "Cost-Effectiveness of a Home Visiting Triage Program for Family Planning in Turkey," *American Journal of Public Health* 69 (1979): 950–3; D. L. Bibeau, K. D. Mullen, K. R. McLeroy et al., "Evaluations of Workplace Smoking Cessation Programs: A Critique," *American Journal of Preventive Medicine* 4 (1988): 87–95; J. Cantor et al., "Cost-effectiveness . . .," op. cit.; H. Cohen, C. Harris, and L. W. Green, "Cost-Benefit Analysis of

Asthma Self-Management Educational Programs in Children," *Journal of Allergy and Clinical Immunology* 64 (1979): 155–6; L. W. Green, "Evaluation Model: A Framework for the Design of Rigorous Evaluation of Efforts in Health Promotion," *American Journal of Health Promotion* 1 (1986): 77–9; idem., "Research Agenda: Building a Consensus on Research Questions," *American Journal of Health Promotion* 1 (1986): 70–2; L. W. Green and F. M. Lewis, *Measurement and Evaluation . . .* , op. cit.; M. W. Kreuter, ed., "Results of Education Evaluation," *Journal of School Health* 55 (Oct. 1985): issue no. 8; M. W. Kreuter, G. M. Christenson, and R. Davis, "School Health Education Research: Future Uses and Challenges," *Journal of School Health* 54 (1984): 27–32; M. W. Kreuter, G. M. Cristianson, M. Freston, G. Nelson et al., "In Search of a Baseline: The Need for Risk Prevalence Surveys," *Proceedings of the Annual National Risk Reduction Conference* (Atlanta: Centers for Disease Control, 1981).

99. E. J. J. deLeeuw, *Health Promotion: The Sane Revolution* (Maastricht, The Netherlands: Van Gorcum, 1989); M. F. Cataldo, A. Herd, L. W. Green et al., "Preventive Medicine and the Corporate Environment: Challenge to Behavioral Medicine," in *Health and Industry: A Behavioral Medicine Perspective*, M. F. Cataldo and T. J. Coates, eds. (New York: Wiley, 1986), pp. 399–419; L. W. Green and D. Simons-Morton, "Education, Health Behavior and Health Promotion," in *Oxford Textbook of Public Health*, 2nd ed., W. W. Holland, R. Detels, and G. Knox, eds. (London: Oxford University Press, in press); M. W. Kreuter, G. M. Christenson, and A. DiVincenzo, "The Multiplier Effect . . . ," op. cit.; C. F. Nelson, M. W. Kreuter et al., "A Partnership Between the Community, State and Federal Government: Rhetoric or Reality?" *Hygie* (Paris) 5 (1986): 27–31; J. M. Ottoson and L. W. Green, "Reconciling Concept and Context . . . ," 1987, op. cit.; K. E. Powell, G. M. Christenson, and M. W. Kreuter, "Objectives for the Nation: Assessing the Role Physical Education Must Play," *Journal of Physical Education, Recreation and Dance* 55 (1984): 18–20.

100. L. W. Green, "Toward Cost-Benefit Evaluations of Health Education . . . ," 1974, op. cit.

Chapter 2

Social Diagnosis: Assessing Quality-of-Life Concerns

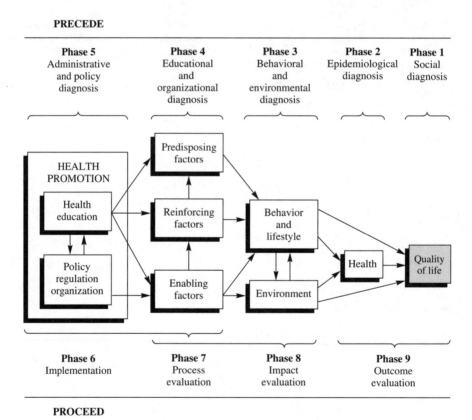

Health promotion typically occurs in community settings or in organizational settings that require policy decisions to support the programs.[1] Research and experience tell us that people's health and behavior and their perceptions of what is important are shaped, modified, and maintained by their interaction with the community or organizational environments in which they live and work. Your understanding of that social nexus before you intervene to change individuals or environments is both a moral and a strategic imperative. You can gain that understanding best by engaging the community actively in a self-study and social diagnostic process.

Nothing assures the success of a program more than to engage the people of a community in assessing their perceived problems, needs, and aspirations and their shared priorities for dealing with them. If you cannot find a way to link the health mission of your agency or program to the social goals and concerns of a target population or setting, you have little hope that the services you could offer that community will be valued or used. The social diagnostic phase of PRECEDE calls for attention and commitment to this critical aspect of planning. This chapter, which deals with social diagnosis (Phase 1 of health promotion planning), addresses two main issues: What is social diagnosis and why is it important? It then summarizes the methods and strategies that can be used to carry out this assessment of social and quality-of-life concerns.

THE PURPOSE AND IMPORTANCE OF SOCIAL DIAGNOSIS

Within the context of PRECEDE, we define **social diagnosis** (also called social needs assessment or social reconnaissance) as *the process of determining people's perceptions of their own needs or quality of life, and their aspirations for the common good, through broad participation and the application of multiple information-gathering activities designed to expand understanding of the community*. Several important assumptions implicit in this definition can be highlighted by elaborating on the specific terms in it.

The reference to *multiple* information-gathering activities highlights the fact that a useful social diagnosis is likely to require indicators and data from several sources. The published literature on quality of life and social indicators is extensive and growing.[2] Most scholars in those areas urge the use of multiple measures.

Community participation (or broad participation if the client system is other than a geographic community) is a foundation concept in social diagnosis and has long been a basic principle for health education and community development, though too often neglected in practice.[3] The notion of *expanded understanding* refers to a heightened awareness of the community's social, economic, cultural, and environmental concerns and goals. The new awareness benefits not only the health workers and volunteers, but also the other sectors whose cooperation is needed in health promotion and the people who will be affected by the program. All parties have something to learn. Maintaining this emphasis minimizes a *we/ they* mentality and helps nurture an *us* relationship.

One of the goals of health promotion programs is healthful living patterns and conditions that last. The behavioral and environmental changes induced by the program should have staying power. Programs conceived and developed apart from the spirit and day-to-day workings of a community are, by definition, outside that community. In such cases, when the initial resources dry up or the intervention period comes to an end, the program is not only over, it is gone! A program that never becomes a real part of the community generates no sense of community ownership and so has little or no chance of becoming a permanent part of the community fabric. To obtain a lasting effect, to achieve a positive shift in a community's health norms, genuine community participation and commitment are essential.

HEALTH AND SOCIAL PROBLEMS: A RECIPROCAL RELATIONSHIP

PRECEDE and PROCEED appear in most of the pictorial representations as a linear, cause-and-effect model. Inputs (health education, policy, regulation and organization) cause certain changes, which eventually lead to outcomes (improved quality of life). Of course, many of these linkages, especially the relationships between health and quality of life, are actually two-way streets. Another view is suggested in Figure 2.1, representing the relationships between health problems and quality of life at the individual and community levels. The arrows indicate that health can influence quality of life and social well-being at the same time that quality of life and social problems affect health. These cause–effect relationships can be mediated by social policy, social service interventions, health policy, and health programs.

The top arrow implies that social problems influencing the quality of life can lead to health problems or the motivation and ability to cope with health problems. This aspect of the reciprocal relationship is one that can be effectively addressed by health workers only in cooperation with social workers, recreation professionals, law enforcement, and other sectors who shape social policy and social service programs. This makes health promotion necessarily an intersectoral enterprise. The health sector cannot do it alone.

The bottom arrow indicates that social conditions and quality of life are themselves influenced by health problems that are amenable to modification by health policies and interventions for health improvement or maintenance. PRE-CEDE emphasizes the aspect of the reciprocal exchange represented by the bottom arrow, but the subsequent health promotion interventions affect the top arrow through behavioral and environmental changes. A recognition of this interrelatedness between social conditions and health status is critical to the

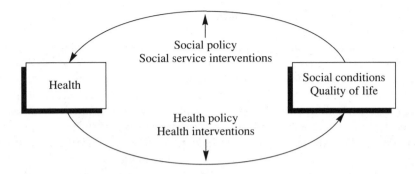

FIGURE 2.1

The relationships between health and social conditions are reciprocal.

improvement of each of them. Describing the limitations of Canada's health promotion programs, Dr. Carol Buck comments:

> It is instructive to observe what people worry about, because this gives one a sense of whether they understand the nature of their problem. What are people in this country worried about today? They are worried about nuclear war, pollution, unemployment, poverty and crime. Are they worried about health? Yes, and in particular about cancer, Alzheimer's disease, AIDS and the shortage of transplant organs. Since their worries about health are highly specific, they fail to see how closely health is connected with some of their other concerns. Until this connection is made, the actions necessary to create health will not be taken.[4]

The endorsement of these principles of participation, multisectoral orientation, and reciprocal causality by a World Health Organization Working Group on Concepts and Principles of Health Promotion reads as follows:

> *Health promotion involves the population as a whole in the context of their everyday life, rather than focusing on people at risk for specific diseases...*
>
> *Health promotion is directed towards action on the determinants or causes of health...*
>
> *Health promotion combines diverse, but complementary, methods or approaches*, including communication, education, legislation, fiscal measures, organizational change, community development and spontaneous local activities against health hazards.
>
> *Health promotion aims particularly at effective and concrete public participation*. This focus requires the further development of problem-defining and decision-making lifeskills both individually and collectively.
>
> While health promotion is basically an activity in the health and social fields, and not a medical service, *health professionals – particularly in primary health care – have an important role in nurturing and enabling health promotion.*[5]

CAN QUALITY OF LIFE BE MEASURED?

The social diagnosis starts by encouraging and assisting the community to assess its quality of life, not just its health concerns. This term, *quality of life*, like the concepts of *health* and *love*, is difficult to define and still more difficult to measure. Nevertheless, many approaches are available for assessing the quality of life in communities, both objectively and subjectively. Objective measures include social indicators, such as unemployment rates, and descriptions of such environmental features as housing density and air quality. More critical to the educational approach are subjective assessments, using information from the community members as a primary indicator of quality-of-life concerns. In this approach, the adjustment and life satisfaction of community members are surveyed. Typically, the components of adjustment are stressful life events and personal or social resources. Similarly, the components of life satisfaction are positive life experiences and personal or social resources.[6]

When the Kaiser Family Foundation conducted its social reconnaissance with the state of Mississippi, prior to making health promotion grants in that state, the major concerns of the population centered around quality of housing and economic development, which they related in part to the quality of schooling. These became central themes in the subsequent analysis of health problems and led to the coordination of planning with the Housing and Economic Development sectors of the state government and with the school boards of local communities.[7]

The subjective assessment of quality of life has the advantage of giving professionals a view of the situation through the eyes of the community residents themselves.[8] They tell us what is important to them and show us where health lies in the context of their lives. Health promotion seeks to promote healthful conditions that improve quality of life as seen through the eyes of those whose lives are affected. Health promotion might have instrumental value in reducing risks for morbidity and mortality, but its ultimate value lies in its contribution to the quality of life of those for whom it is intended. A true bottom line for health promotion depends on measuring advances in quality of life.

This bottom-line declaration will make some health officials uneasy, because they fear that health resources will be spent on nonhealth objectives. Your first task may be to help the head of your health agency understand that health promotion, more than health services and health protection, depends on the cooperation of other sectors. Unless the health sector can buy into the broader social goals of primary concern to the community and the other sectors, you may find your agency on the sidelines of the mainstream of community action and energy, isolated from the wellspring of community resources. You will be unable to attract the interest of the community to your agency's mission and unable to gain the cooperation of other nonhealth organizations in your programs. Relating health goals to the quality of life and social goals of the community is a measurement and marketing skill; those health organizations with the greatest viability in the years ahead will have perfected it.

In medical or nursing care, the counterpart of community social indicators or quality-of-life measures are health outcome measures other than biomedical. These may include ability to perform tasks of daily living, tolerance for side-effects of medications, energy level, and other indicators of well-being associated with but not identical to the medical condition.[9]

But is it possible, or even advisable, to quantify quality of life? Some claim that efforts to make explicit and generalize the factors that account for quality of life necessarily ignore the subtle differences in perceptions among the individual members or subgroups of a population. Others contend, and rightfully so, that it is inappropriate to impose one person's perception of wellness and satisfaction on another person who views those factors differently. It is precisely this concern that dictates the PRECEDE methods of conducting the social diagnosis. At the individual level, questionnaires and interviews can discern subjective quality-of-life concerns.[10] At the group or community level, group discussion and decision methods are required to arrive at consensus on priorities that reflect the concerns of all segments and allow people the opportunity to hear each other.

The fact that health education and health promotion programs are delivered either in community settings or in settings that require community or organizational support calls for analysis of the social conditions and perceptions held and shared at the community or organizational level. The social diagnostic phase in PRECEDE attempts to generate consensus on the shared priorities among the parties who are called upon to cooperate in the execution and maintenance of a health promotion program and those who will benefit from it.

HEALTH AS AN INSTRUMENTAL VALUE

Health is a good thing. Music, art, work, and play are good things, so is being a parent or a friend, and so too is eating. We value many good things in life, things that compete with each other for our time, interest, and energy. In fact, it is relatively rare for people to engage in what we label a *health-related behavior* primarily because they believe the behavior is going to make them live longer. More likely, their motivation can be explained in terms of how they expect the behavior to make them look, feel, or function. Health seems to be cherished because it serves other ends. The 1986 Ottawa Charter for Health Promotion puts it this way: "Health is seen as a resource for everyday life, not the objective of living."[11] The sociologist, Talcott Parsons, defined health as "the ability to perform certain valued social roles."[12] These functional views of health see it as a means to other ends and define health in terms of a person's ability to adapt to social and environmental circumstances.[13]

Because health is an instrumental rather than an ultimate value, it is essential for an analysis of a community's needs to consider not only health data but also what is valued besides health, and why. An added advantage of this broader approach is that the planner becomes sensitized to those values and those social and economic circumstances that seem to be the "prime movers" for action. For example, studies presented in Chapters 5 and 8 demonstrate that the decision to engage in physical activity is motivated by reasons other than health. Although the predispositions and enabling factors that influence the behavioral target are revealed during the educational diagnosis, early insight into those factors can help define the problem in broader social terms from the outset. "When problems are defined narrowly, subsequent analysis can only produce narrow and limited approaches to the problem."[14]

SETTING PRIORITIES

The need to set priorities and the need to engender community participation constitute two compelling and interrelated reasons for early attention to social diagnosis. When all the choices for health intervention look good, the health professional is like a kid in a candy store. When, in addition, resources are limited, one is in the familiar bind of trying to do too much with too little. If the health professional tries to set priorities without involving the community in the decision, the lower priorities will come back to haunt the program. The community will not ask "Why are you doing A?" but will ask "Why aren't you doing B?"

The problems a community faces all seem important, and all provide a meaningful challenge for creative programs. Health program priorities, and the subsequent allocation of resources to address them, are generally based on analysis of data indicating the pervasiveness of the problems and their human and economic costs. This is particularly evident in the development of health promotion policies at the international, national, state, and provincial levels.[15] Table 2.1 provides examples of priorities that have been set at the national level in developing the Year 2000 Objectives for the Nation in Disease Prevention and Health Promotion.[16] These 21 objectives look much like the 15 priorities in the 1990 Objectives for the Nation, which was developed using objective data on mortality rates and years of potential life lost as the criteria, without much consideration of the subjective priorities people might have for the less lethal problems.[17] The planning for the Year 2000 Objectives included regional hearings around the country. The strength of concerns expressed for reasons other than mortality brought several new issues into focus, notably improvement of mental health, preventing and controlling chronic disorders other than heart disease and cancer, and maintaining the quality of life of older people.

The priorities set forth in such national, state, and local policies and the data used to determine the priorities they address have been invaluable in helping

TABLE 2.1

Priorities for the year 2000 objectives for the nation in disease prevention and health promotion

Reduce tobacco use
Reduce alcohol and other drug abuse
Improve nutrition
Increase physical activity and fitness
Improve mental health and prevent mental illness
Reduce environmental health hazards
Improve occupational safety and health
Prevent and control unintentional injuries
Reduce violent and abusive behavior
Prevent and control HIV infection and AIDS
Prevent and control sexually transmitted diseases
Immunize against and control infectious diseases
Improve maternal and infant health
Improve oral health
Reduce adolescent pregnancy and improve reproductive health
Prevent, detect, and control high blood cholesterol and high blood pressure
Prevent, detect, and control cancer
Prevent, detect, and control other chronic diseases and disorders
Maintain the health and quality of life of older people
Improve health education and access to preventive health services
Improve surveillance and data systems

SOURCE: U.S. Department of Health and Human Services.

decision makers *recognize the potential health and social benefit that can accrue as a function of health promotion*. Table 2.2 shows how national data are used to demonstrate the years of productive life lost and the socioeconomic impact of selected health problems.[18]

Additional indicators of the social problems associated with specific diseases and causes of death include:

Complications: blindness, paralysis, amputations, side effects from drugs, activity limitation, disfiguration, disabilities, dizziness, imbalance,...
Direct costs: hospital care, physician and other professional fees, pharmaceutical costs, special equipment, long-term institutional care, days lost from work or major activity,...
Quality of life: for the afflicted individual—disability, missed opportunity

TABLE 2.2

Estimates of potentially postponable deaths, preventable years of life lost, and preventable economic costs by selected diagnostic categories.

(1)[a] Diagnostic category and deaths postponable	(2)[b] No. of deaths potentially postponable		(3)[c] Years of life lost potentially preventable		(4)[d] Economic costs $ billions potentially preventable	
All, 66%	1,260,000		23,000,000		$302 billion	
Injuries, 90%	144,000	(3)[e]	5,490,000	(2)[e]	75	(1)[e]
Circulatory diseases, 67%	665,000	(1)	8,385,000	(1)	57	(2)
Neoplasms, 67%	283,000	(2)	4,850,000	(3)	34	(3)
Respiratory diseases, 76%	98,000	(4)	1,359,000	(4)	25	(4)
Digestive diseases, 55%	41,000	(5)	779,000	(5)	23	(5)
Musculoskeletal, 30%	1,700		32,700		6	
Infectious diseases, 50%	38,000		708,000		5	

[a] Column (1) gives percentages of deaths estimated by Amler et al. to be postponable.
[b] Column (2) data are also from Amler et al.
[c] Column (3) data, which assume that deaths prior to age 73.5 are premature, were calculated by Foundation staff from estimates of Amler et al., which assume that deaths prior to age 65 are premature.
[d] Column (4) was obtained by multiplying the percentage in column (1) by the total cost for each diagnostic category, calculated by Rice et al.
[e] Rankings are shown in parentheses.
Source: Kaiser Family Foundation, *Health Promotion Program* (Menlo Park, CA: The Foundation, 1987); data based on Amler et al., *Closing the Gap: The Burden of Unnecessary Illness* (New York, Oxford University Press, 1987).[19]

for education, training, employment... For the family—transportation to health facility, financial and mental burden... For the community—greater dependency (welfare), reduced productivity, strain on facilities...

Such analyses have undeniable significance for policy decisions and have stimulated much of the government support for health promotion. The focus on mortality or morbidity as the basis for setting priorities, however, causes concern among those whose definition of health promotion includes quality-of-life factors not necessarily linked to mortality, or even to morbidity as traditionally measured in biomedical terms or to costs.

THE PRINCIPLE AND PROCESS OF PARTICIPATION

Priorities for health promotion often emphasize criteria other than morbidity and mortality, especially at the community and organizational levels. *Formal* planning at national and state levels, broader in scope and requiring more extensive logistical considerations for development, must rely almost entirely on quantitative, epidemiologic health information. One might therefore assume that the principle of participation, which is so necessary at the local level, is of lesser or even no importance at these more central levels. Not so. When policies and priorities set at level A depend for their execution on persons or institutions at level B, planners must make every effort to solicit active participation, input, and even endorsement from level B. Without such collaboration, the support and cooperation needed from level B are unlikely.

Failure to attend to this simple principle, even at the highest levels, is at once a foolish and a serious oversight. It is foolish in that participation requires only a simple act of courtesy and a modest expenditure of energy. The oversight is serious because it often produces a threat to the proposed program. Continued failure to call for a fully cooperative effort results in mistrust. It is this sentiment of mistrust that explains much of the tension frequently observed between agencies at the national and state or the state and local levels.[20]

Better even than plans formulated at central levels with input and consultation from "lower" or decentralized levels of the national or community structure are plans that have their origin and impetus from the grassroots. Figure 2.2 lays out an ideal sequence of steps, beginning with local initiative, in the planning, implementation, and evaluation process.[21] The steps fall into two broad categories of actions separated by the vertical dashed line: decentralized functions and centralized functions. By decentralized we mean the level of organization closest to where the people whose needs are in question live or work. This could be a work team in a factory, a department or a floor of workers in an office building, a plant within an industry, a classroom within a school, a school within a district, a neighborhood within a town or city, or a town within a county.

The Two Functional Levels. The steps to the left of the vertical line (see Fig. 2.2) are those initiated, implemented, and controlled by the "local" people. These decentralized functions are placed to the left rather than at the bottom of a vertical structure to break from the perception of hierarchical relationships characteristic of bureaucracies. True, many communities at the decentralized level must seek support from a smaller number of agencies or organizations at a more centralized level, as in the pyramid of a bureaucratic organization. But the relationship between the communities and the central organizations should not be viewed or approached as a bureaucratic relationship with the implicit top-down command and bottom-up reporting. In planning for health promotion, the ideal is for the initiative and the control to be vested at the most local level.

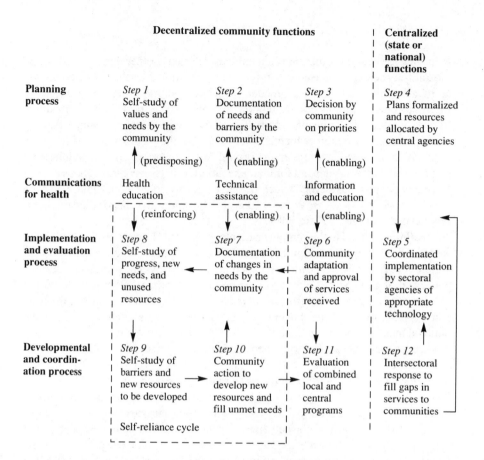

Decentralized community functions

Centralized (state or national) functions

Planning process

Step 1 Self-study of values and needs by the community

Step 2 Documentation of needs and barriers by the community

Step 3 Decision by community on priorities

Step 4 Plans formalized and resources allocated by central agencies

(predisposing)   (enabling)   (enabling)

Communications for health

Health education   Technical assistance   Information and education

(reinforcing)   (enabling)   (enabling)

Implementation and evaluation process

Step 8 Self-study of progress, new needs, and unused resources

Step 7 Documentation of changes in needs by the community

Step 6 Community adaptation and approval of services received

Step 5 Coordinated implementation by sectoral agencies of appropriate technology

Developmental and coordination process

Step 9 Self-study of barriers and new resources to be developed

Step 10 Community action to develop new resources and fill unmet needs

Step 11 Evaluation of combined local and central programs

Step 12 Intersectoral response to fill gaps in services to communities

Self-reliance cycle

FIGURE 2.2

The ideal sequence of steps in a systematic process of community social diagnosis, leading to centralized support, intersectoral cooperation, and ultimately self-reliance. [From L. W. Green, *Community Health*, 6th ed. (St. Louis, Times Mirror/Mosby College Publishing, 1990), with permission of the publisher.]

The Three Developmental Functions. Figure 2.2 also shows the steps progressing on three levels of development: planning on the first level, implementation and process evaluation at the second level, and developmental and coordination processes at the third level. Actually, the entire 12 steps could be considered developmental, and coordination ideally occurs at all stages. The third level might more properly be called the building of permanent capabilities and relationships, sometimes referred to as *institutionalization*. We avoid the latter term because of its implication that programs should become institutionalized. A more appropriate goal for health promotion programs is that the organizational and environmental supports (policies, regulations, funding mechanisms) should become institutionalized, but the people who provided the leadership should move on to other problems and needs, pursue other community goals and aspirations, rather than becoming locked into management responsibilities to maintain a program or an encrusted institution.

The Technical-Support Function. All this talk about local initiative, autonomy, participation, and control seems to imply that the necessary skills and technical knowledge to carry out a systematic social diagnosis and planning process are extant in the local group or community. This cannot be assumed for many of the disadvantaged and poor communities that need health promotion the most, at least not without some caveats. Much of the skill and knowledge needed may be found in the community with sufficient searching and encouragement, but it will remain dormant unless new circumstances or opportunity and information flush it out. Here health education has its most critical predisposing, enabling, and reinforcing functions: (1) *to arouse indigenous community awareness, concern, and initiative*, (2) *to provide technical assistance to those who wish to take initiative*, and (3) *to connect them with the sources of support needed from other levels of organization.* These functions are implied by the second row of Figure 2.2.

The Three Steps in Each Phase of PRECEDE. The social diagnosis consists of three steps that the community or the local group should be encouraged to go through independently or with the assistance of the external helping agency. These same three steps apply with some variation at each of the subsequent phases of PRECEDE — the epidemiological diagnosis, the behavioral and environmental diagnosis, and the educational diagnosis. The three steps are as follows:

1. Self-study by the community of its problems, needs, aspirations, resources, and barriers
2. Documentation of the presumed causes of the needs, or determinants of the desired goals
3. Decision on the priorities to be given to the list of problems, needs, or goals, based on perceived importance and presumed changeability and on formulation of quantified goals and objectives

The most important phase of planning in which the community needs to be actively involved in these three steps is the *social* diagnostic phase. The questions become more technical as the planning proceeds through the epidemiological, behavioral and environmental, and educational diagnoses. The necessity of professional staff work in reviewing the scientific literature to document the causes or determinants of the health, behavioral, and environmental problems or barriers becomes greater in the phases after the social diagnosis; the answers lie more in scientific fact than in values and local insight at the level of epidemiological and educational assessment. But failure to engage the community actively in these three steps in the social diagnostic phase can be most costly in the long-term effectiveness and viability of the health promotion program.

Step 3 in Figure 2.2 should involve a dialogue with professionals to assure some expertise in setting realistic priorities and goals based on scientific knowledge and prior experience. But the community's own aspirations and ambitions should rule. If professional health workers push people too far or discourage them too much from taking on larger problems or goals, the program becomes too much the property and responsibility of the professionals.

Centralized Functions. Step 4 shows the central agency or agencies—a state or national government agency, a foundation, or a headquarters of a private or voluntary health organization—that formalize the plans or proposals received from one or more local community groups into a strategic plan for allocation of its resources. The centralized resources include funding, material support, and technical assistance. Step 5 suggests the need for centralized agencies that share common interests in the same localities or social problems to coordinate their assistance to communities so that a harmonized flow of resources reaches the community. Too often the state and national organizations seeking to have their separate missions carried out at the local level compete unwittingly for the time and effort of precious talent and energy in needy communities. Intersectoral and interagency coordination at the central levels helps reduce the confusing and often redundant signals that communities receive.

Implementation and Evaluation. Steps 6–8 require central agencies to return selected implementation and evaluation functions to the community. Information and technical assistance are among the supports that communities need to be able to carry out these functions, as in some of the earlier diagnostic and planning functions. This goes beyond the social diagnosis phase, but it should serve the reader at this stage to have a picture of how the whole process of community organization and development for health promotion might play out.

The Self-Reliance Cycle. Steps 7–10 engage the community in a progressively greater degree of responsibility for managing and evaluating their own progress. By step 10, the competent community[22] has unearthed or developed its own indigenous resources to maintain the program[23] or to move on to the solution of other problems on its priority list.[24] Rather than turning back to central agencies for more support at that point, the community returns to step 7 and continues in the self-reliance cycle outlined by the dashed square in Figure 2.2.

Demonstration and Diffusion. Often the payoff of central support to local community projects from the point of view of the central agencies is not the solution of a local problem, but rather the demonstration of a problem-solving process by a typical community. The hope of most grant-making organizations is that their grants will inspire other communities or groups to emulate the example demonstrated by the grantees. To maximize this potential, evaluation of project impact and outcomes (step 11) becomes a central priority. The results of the evaluation can be inspirational to other communities but also can be instructive to the central agencies on how they can improve their coordination with other central organizations (step 12) and their technical assistance and support to other communities.

The series of steps just reviewed can be characterized and simplified as in Figure 2.3.[25]

SOCIAL DIAGNOSIS AS AN EDUCATIONAL PROCESS

Thus, in the planning of health promotion, the needs and resources are identified, causes assessed, priorities set, and goals pursued. To conduct an effective social diagnosis, one must apply the principle of participation and ensure the active involvement of the people who will be affected by the program being planned. The importance of this principle, echoed over the decades in the theories of psychology, education, and various other applied behavioral sciences, has been confirmed in community experience in three bodies of literature: the technical-assistance fields including notably public health (health education), family planning, and agricultural extension;[26] the community development and rural economic development literature from around the world, especially India;[27] and the concern with community involvement through *concientacion*, a phenomenon largely of Latin America in the 1960s and early 1970s.[28]

A convergence of these three traditions appears to be afoot. In some of the earlier policies supporting health education, the governments and the World Health Organization itself seemed more concerned with using health education to get people involved in *implementing* centrally planned programs. Later the concern was with health education to increase people's participation in the centralized *planning* of local programs.[29] That tendency was reversed with WHO's *New Policies for Health Education in Primary Health Care*.[30] During the same period, community development specialists who were addressing the plight of the rural poor were "shifting from the capital-investment growth models of the 1960s to the more people-centered basic-needs approaches . . . one of the most important and least understood of which is popular participation."[31]

The tradition of technical assistance in public health through health education can be broadened under the rubric of health promotion to combine the traditions of community development and *concientacion* whereby individual and community activation and development of human resources become ends in themselves. They can serve personal and community social needs primarily and thereby improve health indirectly. *Concientacion* is the Spanish word (which could perhaps be translated as *consciousness-raising*) for a process whereby poor people become

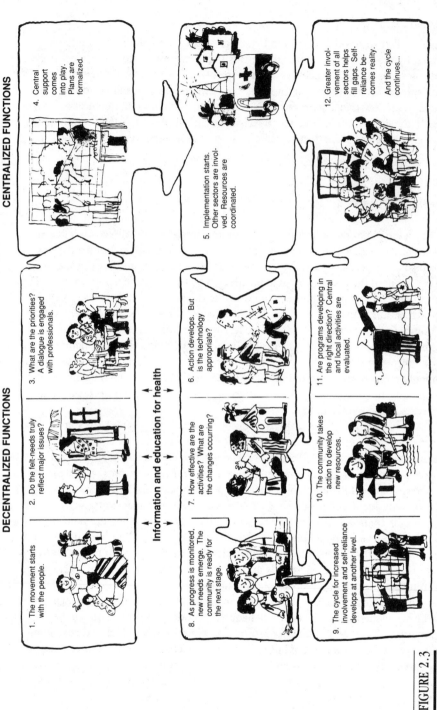

FIGURE 2.3

This simplified view of the flow chart in Figure 2.2 is not meant as a blueprint for planning, nor does it purport that communities should stop ongoing activities and start anew. Rather, it suggests that a practical approach for communities would be to support initiation in phases and to modify the process as experience develops. [From L. W. Green, *World Health*, Apr.–May: 13–17 (1983), with permission of the publisher.]

conscious of the political realities of their situation and take collective action to address issues of equity and social justice. They can be encouraged to take control of the determinants of their health through an educational and community organization process within the broader context of social, economic, and health policies,[32] as suggested by Figure 2.4. For this kind of empowerment and citizen control to occur, however, professionals must be willing to relinquish some of the power inherent in their positions and traditional roles. Above all they must be willing to listen and learn themselves. This could be the process occurring in Eastern Europe today.

Lichter and his colleagues applied the PRECEDE model but started with an epidemiological and educational diagnosis (assessing interests in health topics) rather than with a social diagnosis. Their experience demonstrated the practical utility of paying attention to community perceptions of needs and priorities in planning a health promotion program, and it demonstrated the need to start with an understanding of social or quality-of-life concerns before presuming the health topics to be ranked. They administered several brief surveys to assess needs and to help set priorities for a hospital-based community health promotion program in Dearborn, Michigan. Consumers and health professionals were independently surveyed to collect information about their perceptions of how important certain diseases were and what topics should be priorities for educational programs. There were only slight differences between consumers and health professionals in the ranking of the importance of disease topics, but the differences in their perceptions of which health topics should be addressed in educational programs were dramatic (Table 2.3). The health professionals, blinded by their scientific knowledge of the important relationship between health, disease, and cigarette smoking, identified smoking as the top priority; consumers ranked smoking 13th out of 15 choices. The consumers' first need was to gain a better understanding of health care insurance, a topic ranked 7th by the professionals.[33]

THE PARTNERSHIP APPROACH TO SOCIAL DIAGNOSIS

This and other discrepancies revealed in Table 2.3 serve to punctuate the question, "Whose priorities?" The question is not "Who was right?" Lichter's group was able to use their data as a point of departure for town meetings in which community members came together to reach a shared understanding of community health education needs. The problem of smoking would need to be addressed eventually, but a smoking intervention would meet a better reception eventually if the program had first addressed some of the community's more pressing concerns or combined the identified priorities in creative ways. The health promotion planners in this case might have found it easier to identify other community concerns with which to match the professional health priorities had they begun the joint planning process with a social diagnosis rather than a health topic priority assessment.

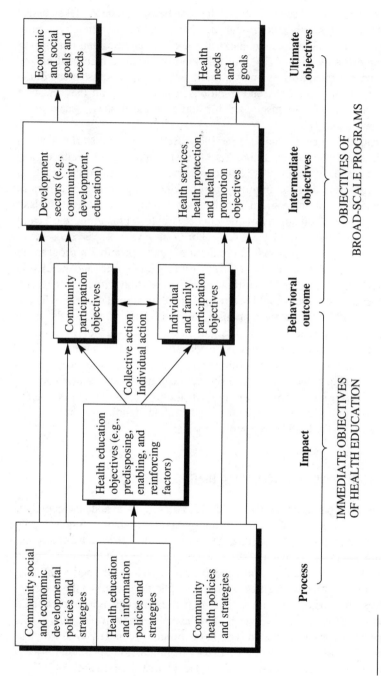

FIGURE 2.4

Health education, within the context of health promotion, can have as its first objective the predisposing, enabling, and reinforcing of individual and collective action to participate more actively in the community social development process. [From L. W. Green, *Community Health* (St. Louis: Times Mirror/Mosby College Publishing, 1990), with permission of the publisher.]

TABLE 2.3
Community versus professional ranking of concerns for various health topics.

Topic	Consumers		Professionals	
	Very concerned (%)	Rank	Very concerned (%)	Rank
Health care insurance	49	1	59	7
CPR	46	2	62	6
First aid	46	3	39	15
Use of medication	45	4	73	2
Accident prevention	43	5	52	10
Auto safety	43	6	63	5
Diet and nutrition	41	7	53	9
Immunization	40	8	64	4
Poison control	40	9	56	8
Stress management	37	10	45	11
Physical fitness	37	11	42	13
Weight control	33	12	41	14
Smoking	30	13	83	1
Birth control	29	14	44	12
Prenatal care	25	15	70	3

SOURCE: M. Lichter et al., *Health Care Management Review* 11 (1986): 75–87, with permission of the author.

The findings in the Michigan study would have been no surprise to Brazilian educational philosopher Paulo Freire, whose name is most widely associated with the *concientacion* movement. In 1970, he described two theoretical approaches to community change. One he characterized as *cultural invasion*, the other as *cultural synthesis*.

> In cultural invasion, the actors draw the thematic content of their action from their own values and ideology; their starting point is their own world, from which they enter the world they invade. In cultural synthesis, the actors who come from "another world" to the world of the people do not come as invaders. They do not come to teach or to transmit or to give anything, but rather to learn, with the people, about the people's world.[34]

He contended that those who are "invaded," irrespective of their level in society, rarely go beyond or expand on the models given them, implying that there is no internalizing, no growth. In the cultural synthesis approach, there are no imposed priorities: Leaders and people collaborate in the development of priorities and guidelines for action.

According to Freire, resolution of the inevitable contradictions between the views of leaders and the views of the people is only possible where the spirit of cultural synthesis predominates. "Cultural synthesis does not deny differences between the two views; indeed it is based on these differences. It does deny invasion of one by the other, but affirms the undeniable support each gives to the other."[35]

Although the metaphor of invasion may seem overly dramatic to some, Freire's view is widely shared. His theoretical framework provided the foundation of a unique program addressing the problems of poor health and isolation among low-income seniors. The program, based on social support and social action organizations, was developed and implemented for the elderly citizens living in single-occupancy hotel rooms in San Francisco's Tenderloin district. Minkler and her associates provide insightful analyses of how and why it was necessary to complement Freire's with other theoretical approaches.[36]

In international health education circles, community participation is a by-word. The 1983 WHO Expert Committee Report, *New Approaches to Health Education in Primary Care*, places great emphasis on what is termed *people-oriented health technology* but also counsels:

> While health care workers should not compel communities to accept the health technologies they propose, they should also not allow themselves to be forced into a situation where they have to abdicate their views on technical matters. The common ground between the two groups should serve as a basis for fruitful dialogue, which may lead to change, provided health workers keep in mind that sociocultural factors and beliefs are not necessarily for development.[37]

This point deserves careful attention: Health workers should take care not to abdicate their responsibilities while engaging the community in dialogue. In working hard to avoid being manipulative, one can go too far and be so fearful of falling into the trap of Freire's "cultural invasion," of imposing one's own agenda, that one is unable to offer constructive assistance. As a planner, you can do two things to avoid that situation. First, keep in mind the fact that you, the lay community, and your co-workers in other agencies and sectors are *partners*. Each can contribute technical or cultural experience and capacities to the task of making a difference. Second, make every effort to ensure that all the partners understand what you do and whom you represent. People are more willing to collaborate with you when they know what agency or group you represent and what its mission or agenda is. They need to know and understand what you can and cannot do — the technical capacities you have to offer as well as the limitations placed on you by your agency or employer. An understanding of these issues, which at first glance may seem irrelevant, helps clarify boundaries and roles and set realistic expectations for all parties.

Partnership implies complementarity of roles and contributions. Each partner can magnify the contribution of the others and through the partnership can leverage his or her own capabilities and resources. In the end, the partnership should evolve into full control by the community and its own professional and lay leadership. This will not happen easily if the partnership starts out with a "senior partner" from the outside and with the community in the role of "junior partner."

In summary, the process of social diagnosis should begin with more than token participation from the community and should lead toward full citizen control of the process, with helping agencies providing information and technical assistance as requested by the community.

METHODS AND STRATEGIES FOR SOCIAL DIAGNOSIS

When one is seeking ideas, methods, and strategies for planning, implementing, and evaluating health promotion programs, the literature of public health, the social and behavioral sciences, community development, and health education should be a first and continuing resource. By carefully examining the findings and methods of others, you can gain insights and sharpen your ideas for a social diagnosis.[38]

The literature illustrates the ways in which diverse methods of data collection have been used in social assessments: key informant interviews, community forums, focus groups, nominal group process, surveys, social indicators, archival research, and synthetic estimates from national data interpolated to the local level; all have been used as data sources. Because time and resources are precious, it is economic to retrieve existing information whenever possible, rather than generate new data. Federal, state, and local offices of housing and urban planning keep reasonably up-to-date summary records. Most of these data are in the public domain and easily accessible. A thorough social diagnosis, however, inevitably requires new and tailored information. It also calls for highly subjective and spontaneous information, which makes it difficult to gather by means of structured pencil-and-paper procedures.

METHODS TO ASSURE CITIZEN PARTICIPATION

Roesner compiled a list of 14 functions that community participation serves and cross-tabulated these with 39 techniques of gaining community participation.[39] Those techniques that serve the social diagnostic function include:

Charette: The assembly of interest groups for intensive meetings
Citizen's advisory committee: An ad hoc organization of citizens to present the ideas and attitudes of local groups
Citizen employment: The direct employment of client representatives

Coordinator: A single individual who provides a focal point for citizen participation

Fishbowl planning: An open planning process in which all parties can express their views before a proposal is adopted

Meetings convened by a community organization: Meetings organized to focus on a particular plan or project

Open-door policy (or **hotline**): A means of encouraging citizens to visit the local project office (or call) without prior appointment

Short conference: Intensive meetings organized around a detailed agenda

Workshops: Working sessions to discuss an issue and to reach an understanding regarding its role in the planning process

Total community participation cannot be expected nor should it be a goal of planning. As George Bernard Shaw put it:

> Every citizen cannot be a ruler any more than every boy can be an engine driver or a pirate king . . . If you doubt this—If you ask me 'Why should not the people make their own laws?' I need only ask you 'Why should not the people write their own plays?' They cannot. It is much easier to write a good play than to make a good law. And there are not a hundred men in the world who can write a good enough play to stand the daily wear and tear as long as a law must.[40]

Nevertheless, broad participation through a representation process should be sought in the assessment of needs because some of those least likely to be "skilled" at planning or "making laws" will be those most in need of health promotion.

THE RECONNAISSANCE METHOD FOR COMMUNITY SOCIAL DIAGNOSIS

A method first developed and recommended by Irwin T. Saunders,[41] and elaborated by Harold Nix,[42] called **social reconnaissance**, has been adapted more recently by the Henry J. Kaiser Family Foundation for use in engaging whole states in the Southern region of the United States in a process of assessing health promotion needs and priorities.

As defined by Nix,

> The community social analysis using the "reconnaissance sampling method" is a quick, efficient approach for determining relevant aspects of the social structure, processes, and needs of a community using leaders (general, locality and specialized) as informants or interviewees.[43]

This approach recognizes that changes in the determinants of health must be preceded by changes in the "social structure . . . the prevailing attitudes, values, aspirations, beliefs, behavior, and relationships in the community."[44] The host community is assisted, through its own agencies and organizations, to do the following:

1. Identify the felt needs or problems of the community (and other elements of social structure)
2. Rank in priority the need and problem areas to be dealt with
3. Organize or mobilize the community to deal with the chosen needs or problems
4. Study the identified needs or problems to determine specific goals or recommendations
5. Develop a plan of action to accomplish locally determined goals
6. Find resources needed to accomplish goals
7. Act or stimulate action to accomplish goals
8. Evaluate accomplishments

In this chapter we are focusing on the first four of these steps.

Application at the State Level. The Kaiser Family Foundation's application of the reconnaissance method in the South engages the Governor's Office, the State Health Department, the other state-level social service agencies, the state legislators, local and regional foundations, the United Way, the Chamber of Commerce, and other organizations in working through the first four steps. The Foundation then provides a planning grant to a selected state agency or coalition to complete the process down to the community level where projects would be developed (step 5) and funded by grants from the Foundation, other cooperating national and state organizations, and sometimes federal agencies (steps 6–8). The process assures greater support for the community projects from state-level organizations than they could expect if the Foundation funded community health promotion projects directly without state involvement.

Application at the Community Level. The same process and advantages apply at the community level, and even within large organizations (e.g., schools, worksites, or hospitals) where health promotion planning needs to be developed with broad participation in identifying needs and resources and setting priorities. The steps in applying the method can be delineated as follows:

Step 1. Identify an Entry Point. The point of entry to a host community can be a crucial decision, affecting all subsequent information and relationships. The official health agency is the logical starting point, but in some communities that agency may be part of the community's greatest concern and even a cause of some of the problems. The preferred entry point, when possible, is the chief executive official of the community: the governor, the mayor, the chairman of the town council, the county board of supervisors. The chief policy maker usually is an elected official. The city manager may be an appointed official but tends to have the confidence of the public. Entry at this level helps open doors at all levels and in all sectors. It avoids a premature focus on health problems when the first task is to understand the social structure and social concerns.

Step 2. Identify Local Cosponsors. An existing organization or an ad hoc group needs to support the study in one or more of the following ways identified by Nix:

1. Provide a representative group of local citizens to participate in an orientation or explanation session.
2. Provide a broadly representative sponsoring organization(s) or a community steering committee made up of representatives from different organizations and groups.
3. Support the research group as they make the study. This support should include or provide for:
   a. Assisting in the legitimization process
   b. Providing news releases on the proposed study giving purpose, sponsorship, and time
   c. Contacting each person to be interviewed
   d. In some cases, scheduling the interviews in some central place
4. Pay for or share the cost of publication of the study
5. Permit public release of the findings through various media such as newspapers, public meetings, and publication
6. Assure the use of the findings to stimulate study groups, program planning, and other community developmental efforts[45]

Step 3. Development of Research and Briefing Materials. Compilation of background data on the community, its leaders, its demography, its current affairs (based on content analysis of newspaper stories), and its social history and cultural traditions provides an archival account of the community's structure and trends. Summary of these analyses in a briefing book to be shared with participants puts everyone on an equal footing with regard to factual data. This briefing book ideally is produced by the host community group. On the basis of the findings of this archival analysis, questions to be asked of community leaders can be formulated for discussion and pretesting with the sponsoring group. These questions may form the basis of an interview schedule for private meetings with community leaders or an agenda for public meetings with community groups.

Step 4. Identification of Leaders and Representatives. The people to be interviewed must be able to speak either for the community power structure or for the population at large and the various segments of the population, especially the underrepresented segments. The **positional** approach to identifying leaders selects those who hold key positions in government, political, business, and voluntary organizations. The **reputational** approach tends to identify the more socially active among this same group of influential leaders but also picks up activists and opinion leaders who do not hold official positions. A combination of these two is recommended, with a careful eye to assuring the inclusion of minority and women's organizations and reputational polling among underrepresented groups.[46]

Step 5. The Field Interviews and Meetings. An intensive period of actual interviews and meetings with influentials, specialized leaders, subcommunity leaders, and leaders of underrepresented categories follows. Avoid spreading out this phase over too many weeks, during which local events could intervene to invalidate any comparisons between those interviewed early and those interviewed late. The number of individuals to be included in the sample of leaders ranges from 50 to 125, depending on the size and diversity of the community. Statewide initiatives require more participants to represent regional variations as well as the usual sources of diversity.

Step 6. Analysis, Reporting, and Follow-up. This step ideally is carried out by the local sponsoring group, with technical assistance as needed from the helping agency. The report should be made public through open meetings, the news media, and broad distribution of the written report. Community organizations are encouraged to select their own priorities among the top priorities to provide leadership in organizing a coalition or task force to pursue the issue further, mobilize resources, or prepare a grant proposal.

SPECIFIC QUANTITATIVE TECHNIQUES

Synthetic Estimates. Parcel and his co-workers used the PRECEDE framework to develop a series of problem- and cohort-specific community intervention guides.[47] In one such guide, *Smoking Control Among Women*, the social diagnosis focuses primarily on the financial burden and diminished worker productivity resulting from women who smoke. Based on extrapolation of national data, they devised worksheets that enable local planners to estimate the probable extent of this burden at their local level. The worksheets are displayed in Tables 2.4,[48] 2.5,[48] and 2.6.[49]

Increasing interest in community intervention as a viable strategy for preventing and controlling chronic diseases, injuries, and other health problems whose major contributing factors are behavior and the environment has created a need for

TABLE 2.4

Estimating the local prevalence of social problems related to smoking by women

- The social problems of smoking to our society include the financial burden of health care costs and lost worker productivity as well as its impact on human suffering.
- Scientists estimate that the annual total cost of smoking in the U.S. due to both direct costs of medical care and indirect costs of lost productivity is about $46 billion (1983 dollars).
- The yearly per capita cost of smoking is around $200.00. (Per capita means the average cost per person.)

The following calculations are for the geographic unit of:

A.1 IN OUR COMMUNITY THE TOTAL YEARLY COST OF SMOKING IS:

_____	×	$200.00	=	$ _____
total population of our community		estimated yearly per capita cost of smoking		estimated yearly total cost of smoking in our community

- Each nonsmoking adult pays about $100.00 in taxes and health insurance premiums for the medical needs of smokers.

A.2 IN OUR COMMUNITY THE COST OF SMOKING TO ADULT NONSMOKERS IS:

Step 1

_____	×	.70	=	_____
total population in our community 18 years or older		average proportion of adult population who DO NOT SMOKE		estimated number of adult nonsmokers in our community

Step 2

_____	×	$100.00	=	_____
estimated number of adult nonsmokers in our community		cost of medical needs of smokers		cost to nonsmokers (vis à vis taxes and insurance costs)

Source: G. S. Parcel et al., *Smoking Control Among Women: A CDC Community Intervention Handbook* (Atlanta: Centers for Disease Control, 1987), p. 13.

readily available, low-cost, small-area data (e.g., city and neighborhood). When actual data are not readily accessible, the use of synthetic estimates has utility (see Chapter 3).

Group Methods. Several group strategies have been used effectively to gather useful social diagnostic information. Three of these methods are highlighted here: (a) the nominal group process, (b) the Delphi technique, and (c) the focus group method.

To use **nominal group process**, one works with small groups to assess community perceptions of problems in a way that overcomes the usual unequal representation of opinions. The method consists of a series of small-group procedures designed to compensate for the dynamics of social power that emerge in most planning meetings. Those who use the method should keep in mind that its purpose is to identify and rank problems, not to solve them. The method, described as it applies to public health by Van de Ven and Delbecq,[50] is more effective than either the Delphi technique or the interactive or focus group process for generating ideas and getting equal participation from group members. Delbecq[51] summarizes the method as follows:

Step 1. Arrange the participants into groups of six or seven. The group size should not exceed seven to allow for appropriate interaction. Those selected as participants should be representative of, and knowledgeable about, the community in question.

Step 2. Pose a single question to the group, preferably in writing on a blackboard, overhead projector, flip-chart, or hand-out sheets. The question should be based on (a) the objectives of the meeting, (b) examples of the type of items sought, (c) the development of alternative questions, and (d) the pilot-testing of alternative questions with a sample group. One example of the type of question is the following: "What do you consider to be the major problems you are facing at this time?" Allow about 15 minutes for silent work on the question.

Step 3. Elicit individual responses in a round-robin fashion. First, one participant is asked to give a single response, the next gives a single response, and this continues until each participant has contributed a single response. As the responses are stated, they are written by the group leader on a blackboard or flip-chart, each item being given a number (1, 2, 3, etc.). The same process is repeated a second, then a third time, and so on, until all contributions have been recorded. This enables each group member to play a truly participating role. During this time, no discussion or critique is permitted regarding the form, format, or substance of a participant's response.

Step 4. Clarify the meaning of the responses. Take time for each response,

TABLE 2.5

Worksheet A for Table 2.4

- Smokers in the U.S. lose an estimated 146 million workdays due to smoking-related diseases (cancer, bronchitis, heart disease).
- Compared to nonsmokers, smokers:
  have an average 35% higher work absentee rate.
  cost approximately $300.00 more a year in insurance claims.
  have twice the rate of job-related accidents.
- It is estimated that the average smoker costs $1,000.00 in excess annual costs to an employer.

A.3 IN OUR COMMUNITY THE EXCESS COST OF SMOKING TO EMPLOYERS IS:

Step 1

_____   =   number of women ages 18–64 in our community

Step 2

_____   =   number from step 1 rounded to nearest 1,000
represents number of women of working age in our community

Step 3

_____ × .60   =   _____
number from step 2   average proportion of   estimated number of
                            women who work   women who work in our
                                                                 community

Step 4

_____ × .30   =   _____
number from step 3   average proportion of   estimated number of
                            women who smoke   working women who
                                                                 smoke in our community

Step 5

_____ × $1,000   =   _____
from step 4 estimated   estimated excess annual   estimated annual excess
number of working   employer cost per   cost to employers due to
women who smoke in   smoking employee   women employees
our community   smoking

TABLE 2.6

Summary sheet for reporting results of synthetic estimates of social problems related to smoking by women in a specific community

The summary sheets are provided as an aid in developing handouts or creating proposals. All of the rates and numbers for this community are estimates or averages based on national averages and assume the community is representative of the nation.

- The social problems of smoking to our society include the financial burden of health care costs and lost worker productivity as well as the impact on human suffering.
- Scientists estimate that the annual total cost of smoking in the U.S. due to both direct costs of medical care and indirect costs of lost productivity is about $46 billion (1983 dollars).
- The yearly per capita cost of smoking is around $200.00. (Per capita means the average cost per person.)

The following information is for the geographic unit of:

_____

In our community it is estimated that there is a $_____ yearly total cost of smoking (from Table 2.4).

- Each nonsmoking adult pays about $100.00 in taxes and health insurance premiums for the medical needs of smokers.

In our community there is an estimated cost of $_____ to nonsmokers of taxes and insurance for smokers (from Table 2.4).

- Smokers in the U.S. lose an estimated 146 million workdays due to smoking related diseases (cancer, bronchitis, heart disease.)
- Compared to nonsmokers, smokers:
  have an average 35% higher work absentee rate.
  cost approximately $300.00 more a year in insurance claims.
  have twice the rate of job-related injuries.
- It is estimated that the average smoker costs $1,000.00 in excess annual costs to an employer.

In our community there are an estimated number of _____ women who work, and of these an estimated _____ smoke. The estimated total excess cost per year to employers due to women employees smoking is $_____ (from Table 2.5).

SOURCE: G. S. Parcel et al., *Smoking Control Among Women: A CDC Community Intervention Handbook* (Atlanta: Centers for Disease Control, 1987), p. 15.

        to ask if it is clearly understood. Allow participants time to discuss the meaning of a particular response, the logic behind it, and even its relative importance. However, this is not the time for argumentation and lobbying. The group leader must direct the proceedings so that only clarification takes place.

Step 5. Conduct the preliminary vote. From the original listing of responses on the blackboard or flip-chart, participants are directed to select a stated number of items that they consider to be the most important (e.g., each participant is to select and rank 7 of the original 20 responses). This is accomplished by writing each of the statements selected on a separate card, and then rank-ordering them (in the example provided, seven points would be assigned to the most important item and one point to the least important). As a rule, group members can prioritize only five to nine items with some degree of reliability. Participants are asked to list the item number and the statement in the upper left-hand portion of the card. When all participants have accomplished this for the seven statements they have selected, they are then asked to rank the cards by placing the rank number in the lower right-hand portion of the card and underlining it. On the blackboard or flip-chart, the group leader then records the ranking assigned to the statement selected by each participant and sums up the votes after all participants have contributed their rankings. The item with the largest numerical total represents the top-priority issue.

In most instances, this is as far as one needs to go in the nominal group process. It can be extended to include additional discussion of the preliminary vote to assure accuracy.

The **Delphi technique**, which uses questionnaires, is also useful at the social diagnosis stage, especially if face-to-face meetings are impractical. In this method, a series of questionnaires is mailed to a small number of experts, opinion leaders, or informants. Differences of opinion among various key people can be resolved by the planner without forcing confrontation. Linstone and Turoff developed the method most fully[52] and Gilmore has provided a description of its application in health education:[53]

Step 1. Define the issue. A planning committee should develop a clear and concise statement as to the central issue to be addressed. For example: "The need to identify the top-priority barriers related to quality of life in this community."

Step 2. Establish who the participants will be. Individuals must be selected who are knowledgeable about the subject at hand. They must also be able to handle the written format that will be used. Because the process is accomplished by means of mailed materials, those involved can be widely dispersed. Using the mail system also prevents participants with high professional positions from influencing others, since they will not meet face-to-face as in the nominal group method. Usually from 15 to 30 participants nominated by the planning committee can provide the needed input.

Step 3. Develop the first questionnaire. This is the first mailing that goes out to the participants after they have agreed to become involved in the process. An introduction should clarify the central issue for the participant, who should also be given instructions for responding to an open-ended format. For example, the instruction might be "Please indicate on the enclosed form those items that you feel are the top-priority barriers to quality of life in this community." Also, it is important to give the participants a deadline (about two weeks later) for returning the first questionnaire. Upon the return of all questionnaires, the items are collated into appropriate categories representative of the items' meanings.

Step 4. Develop the second questionnaire. List the categories resulting from step 3 on the second questionnaire, with space for response next to them on the sheet. Commonly used categories of barriers from the first questionnaire can be presented to the participants so that they can rank or assign a value to the top seven as well as adding comments about any of the 20 categories. Again, a deadline for the return of the questionnaires should be set.

Step 5. Develop the third questionnaire. The values that participants assigned to each category on the second questionnaire are numerically added and entitled the *initial vote total*. Also, a summary of the participants' comments is prepared for each category receiving votes. The information is used to develop the third questionnaire, which also provides space for *final votes*. Upon the return of this third questionnaire, the totals for the *final vote* sections are calculated, leading to the arrangement of the categories in descending priority order.

Step 6. It is quite possible to construct a fourth questionnaire if the materials need to be more finely analyzed. Whether or not such a questionnaire is generated, a final report of the last questionnaire results should be sent to participants.

Some of the advantages of this process include being able to work with a variety of target group representatives, as long as they are considered to be knowledgeable about the issue of concern. It also means that large numbers can be handled, although having more than 30 respondents may not enhance results. During the process the participants remain anonymous to each other, thus protecting the generated ideas from the influences of group conformity, prestige, power, and politics.

Small-scale Delphi surveys to members of a target population can be economical and effective in estimating the prevalence and intensity of suspected concerns but are not efficient at the exploratory stage.

Surveys and Interviews. Surveys are perhaps the principal means used by health workers or any other group whose work depends on a better understanding of the beliefs, perceptions, knowledge, and attitudes of the people they serve. The quality of a survey is determined by several factors, including how valid and reliable the instrument is (does it consistently measure what it's supposed to?), how representative the sample is (can you generalize your results to the entire community or group?), and how the survey is administered (are the questions asked and coded (if necessary) in the same way for all the subjects interviewed?).[54]

The **focus group method** is the most popular interview strategy used in the application of social and behavioral sciences to practical enterprises. It has long been used by marketing groups as a means of obtaining perceptions of target groups and of testing ideas for the marketing of products.

Focus groups are informal sessions in which representatives of your target population are asked to discuss their thoughts on a specific topic or product. They can help you zero in on what should be the content, delivery, and appeal of your message or program to ensure that the program activities are timely, well constructed, and appropriate for the target population. Focus groups can be valuable during the various stages of your program: development of the work plan, review of materials, follow-up to determine why the activities were or were not attended, and so on.

Focus-group sessions last for one to one-and-a-half hours. The groups are usually small (8 to 12 persons per group), with particular emphasis placed on recruiting people who are representative of the community or target group of interest. The process requires a trained moderator. Following is a summary of the focus group method used in the Center for Disease Control's PATCH program:

USES OF FOCUS GROUPS

1. They can provide you with early impressions of your audience (baseline information).
2. They can help you determine which populations to target.
3. They can identify and clarify your audience's perceptions, misconceptions, and attitudes about specific topics, products, or messages.

4. The information can support other sources of qualitative data.

5. They can be used to critique materials such as pamphlets, public service announcements, and posters.

6. Feedback can be obtained on activities the planning team may want to undertake, as well as help with selection of a program theme (e.g., slogan), appeal (e.g., what would motivate people to participate), and potential role models.

ADVANTAGES OF FOCUS GROUPS

1. Since they are inexpensive, they may be used when quantitative data are not available, to interpret previously obtained quantitative results, or to generate hypotheses for future studies.

2. They can help to reduce distance between the target population and your planning team.

3. Probing is possible, thus allowing for follow-up responses.

4. The brainstorming and interaction may result in insights that would not be obtained if participants were interviewed individually.

5. Results can be assembled rather quickly.

6. The process allows the expression of honest and spontaneous responses rather than intellectual opinions.

LIMITATIONS OF FOCUS GROUPS

1. Data are not quantitative, and results should not be interpreted in a quantitative structure. For example, do not interpret as, "x percent said this and y percent said that."

2. Group members may not be representative of the target population—for example, when recruiting has identified qualified respondents in a mall or shopping center.

3. Responses may be influenced by the moderator and other participants.

4. Group members may be inhibited from discussing private topics in public.

5. The nature of the data precludes drawing firm conclusions.

6. Focus groups are subject to misuse through the absence of the required moderating skills and through misinterpretation of the data.

ARRANGING FOCUS GROUPS

1. For each topic, use a minimum of four groups. Ask the same questions in each group.

2. Group together participants with similar characteristics (e.g., do not mix *nonworking married women with children* and *working single women with no children*). Grouping by similar age is very important.

3. Keep recruitment instructions brief. Participants should not know exactly what they will be discussing. Follow up with a letter or phone call to remind each participant about the date, time, and place of the meeting.

4. Although you can recruit through churches or other organizations, it is best to recruit members of the target group as randomly as possible within the chosen setting.

5. It is better if group members do not know each other, so that they are more likely to be candid.

6. The group size should be 8–12. (Overrecruit to compensate for no-shows.)

7. Choose a convenient location, and try to create a relaxed, familiar atmosphere.

8. The group should last no more than 1½ to 2 hours.

9. Use rewards or incentives (e.g., $10–25, taxi fare, certificate of appreciation, refreshments).

10. Do not use the same people more frequently than every 6 months.

11. If appropriate, have a content expert available who can provide accurate information at the end of the meeting and correct any misinformation that might have come from participants. Of course, this should be done in a manner that will not embarrass a participant.

12. In addition to the moderator, you may want to have an observer present to note interactions, body language, and so on.

LEADING A FOCUS GROUP

1. As people arrive, provide name tags with first names only (to allow confidentiality). Give out index cards requesting information, including only very basic demographic information. The cards should also pose a number of leading questions so that participants can write their ideas about the topics to be discussed. Then, when you start asking questions, the group members will already have some ideas to discuss.

Seat the group in a circle or semicircle. Place "talkers" to your side to help avoid constant eye contact. Put shy people in front of you so they can be drawn into the discussion. Tape record or videotape the sessions, and announce that this is being done.

2. Opening remarks by the moderator should set the stage for the meeting. State the topic that will be addressed and the areas that need to be discussed. Make it clear that their input is important to the development of the new program. Introduce the rules for the session: Everyone should contribute; speak one at a time; people should say what they think, not what they think someone else wants to hear; and there are no right or wrong answers.

3. Avoid yes/no questions. Use questions that will give insight into what the participants think, what people in their neighborhood or social circle think, what media they attend to, what people they listen to, and what seems to influence their thoughts and behaviors. Address potentially sensitive questions to the group rather than to one person.

A MODERATOR SHOULD BE

- Properly trained and sufficiently experienced to guide focus groups.
- Informed about the project. This is more important than whether the moderator is viewed as being from the community; a moderator who understands the program can probe for the needed information.
- Able to express thoughts and feelings clearly.
- Able to draw reticent members into the discussion and keep more vocal ones from dominating the discussion.
- Encouraging and motivating. A good way to start is to have people tell a little about themselves, which also puts some demographics on tape.
- Receptive and flexible while maintaining control of the group; able to control side conversations and bring their topics to the forefront when they are pertinent.
- Attuned to the important information, not worrying if some topics are not covered.
- Intuitive, able to probe for further information to clarify a person's meaning.
- Culturally sensitive to the group and capable of fostering successful interpersonal communication. Participants must identify with the moderator.
- Empathetic; able to convey genuine interest in other people and have them feel they are talking with each other in a natural way.
- Kind but firm.

ANALYZING THE DATA

- First, listen to each session to get an overall impression of the discussion climate.
- Tabulate and organize discussion group findings and pertinent quotations.
- Evaluate differences between the thoughts, beliefs, and emotions of people of diverse characteristics.
- Analyze responses for inter- and intragroup homogeneity.[55]
- Add more focus groups if consistent patterns and trends are absent or if there are competing messages; in some cases, there may indeed be no common thread.
- Note what people said would motivate them.
- Note peoples' hesitations, silences, and emphases as well as their actual words used.
- Compare the tape and transcript to ensure that verbal and expressive content are included.
- Try categorizing some of the information into the three categories— predisposing, enabling, and reinforcing—to help the analysis.
- Remember that focus groups provide descriptive data, so be careful about generalizing the data.

PREPARING THE REPORT

- Best done by the person who conducts the focus group.
- Do not include statistical information in the report.
- Include in the format a statement of the purpose of the study, a list of key questions or topics, the number of participants, the methodological design, and a summary of the results.
- Describe each key question or topic using an introduction, summary, discussion, and conclusion, and include an analysis of both verbal and expressive content.

Focus groups can be thought of as operating in three domains, with focus on the *target audience*, the *media*, and the *opinion leaders*. For example, special interest groups (e.g., medical, community services) can be brought together and asked what they think a particular audience feels about a certain topic; use the group experience to recruit their help. A media group can help determine which methods are best for disseminating a message. Market researchers can help develop the script, cosponsor your program, and do the printing.

Focus groups can themselves help to organize the community. They can provide valuable insight into the target population that can guide the development of the program and intervention activities. This insight can help insure that planned activities are timely, well-conceived, and appropriate for the selected target population.

Another effective interview technique is the *central location intercept interview*. In this technique, interviews are conducted at locations in the community frequented by those who are likely to be the target of the program. This has two advantages: A high-traffic area can yield a number of interviews in a short time, and a central location for hard-to-reach target audiences is a low-cost means of gathering valuable information. A manual of methods for improving health communications describes intercept interviews as follows:

> A typical central location interview begins with the intercept. Potential respondents are stopped and asked whether they are willing to participate. Specific screening questions are then asked to see whether they fit the criteria of the target audience for the pretest. If so, they are taken to the interviewing station — a quiet spot at a shopping mall or other site — and are shown the pretest materials. Respondents are then asked a series of questions to assess recall, comprehension, and reaction to the items.[56]

Although the respondents intercepted through central location interviews may not be statistically representative of the entire target population, the sample is larger than that used in focus groups or individual in-depth interviews. Program planners often use the central location technique at the message development stage when assessments of comprehension, attention, believability, and other reactions are essential.

Unlike focus groups or in-depth interviews, the questionnaire used in central location intercept pretesting is highly structured and contains primarily multiple-choice or closed-ended questions. Open-ended questioning, which allows for free-flowing answers, should be kept to a minimum because it takes too long for the interviewer to record responses. As in any type of research, the questionnaire should be pilot tested before it is used in the field.

A number of marketing research companies throughout the country conduct central location intercept interviews in shopping malls. Clinic waiting rooms, churches, Social Security offices, schools, and other locations frequented by individuals representative of the target audience can also be used for this purpose. It is advisable to obtain clearances or permission to set up interviewing stations in these locations well in advance.

Using Public Service Data. Although sample surveys may be appropriate and feasible in the social diagnosis phase of health promotion planning, planners need not gather extensive statistical data that are not already available. The objectives of this phase can be achieved by interpreting and supplementing information from existing records, files, publications, and social indicators, and from informal interviews and discussions with leaders, key informants, and representative members of the target community.

Data on perceived needs and problems are more readily available than one might realize. For example, a rich source of this kind of data, and one that is often overlooked, is the broadcast media. Television and radio broadcasters are required by the Federal Communication Commission to ascertain community needs and concerns regularly and to offer public service programming to address those problems. For instance, in Baltimore, Maryland, a coalition of radio and television broadcasters employs an independent group to conduct public opinion surveys periodically to identify the needs and problems of the Baltimore area as seen through the eyes of those who live and work there. In addition, the coalition conducts monthly meetings with local government, religious, and neighborhood leaders to get their ideas about existing community problems. Most organizations will share their data when asked to do so, unless it has proprietary value.

INTERPRETING THE GATHERED INFORMATION

Once gathered, the quality-of-life indicators, both objective data and perceived needs, should be studied carefully to identify the factors that constitute the most formidable barriers to a desired quality of life. Some of the objective indicators can be calculated in terms of frequency counts, incidence rates, rates under treatment, utilization rates, and frequency distributions. Those that can be calculated can be compared with previous measures of the same indicators to ascertain trends or changes in problems. However, a quality-of-life assessment cannot be made solely on the basis of statistical analysis. Ultimately, the major resource for health planners during this important first phase in the diagnostic process is critical observation and good professional judgment. The final determination of quality-of-life concerns must be made by careful consideration of the available evidence, including the sentiments of the members of the community, the patients, students, workers, and citizens who are the intended benefactors.

"Taking the temperature and pulse" of the community is a consciousness-raising activity for the planner, for others in the planner's organization who will be involved in the overall health promotion program, and for the patients, students, workers, or citizens who have been engaged in the planning process. It reveals the reasons for the educational interventions.

In most situations it is probably not realistic for the health promotion planner to expect to be able to conduct a quality-of-life assessment before planning a program. Most programs are planned and delivered using procedures that are not fully systematic and well developed, often without continuity in staffing. Moreover, programs are usually instituted to meet a need that has caused sufficient concern to merit a call for educational attention. For example, alcohol and drug "units" or classes in school health education programs originated with the public's perception of the ill effects of alcohol and drug abuse on society. National and international population and family planning education programs are funded on the expectation that they will help reduce the social maladies that often accompany overpopulation and problem pregnancies. Self-care health education efforts are currently offered in the hope that program outcomes will include not only better health but also decreased medical costs and time lost from work due to illness, and increased self-esteem and personal control. Indeed, it is probably safe to say that most health education programs with any significant support from the general public are addressing health problems that have already been identified as potentially detrimental to quality of life.

Another problem is that staff changes often occur during the development of a program. Thus, many who conduct health education and health promotion activities, particularly those in clinical, school, and occupational settings, will be given the task of developing a program based on a quality-of-life assessment or social diagnosis (or something like it) already done by someone else. In fact, an epidemiological diagnosis (described in Chapter 3) may also have been completed, if only in the minds of an administrator or decision-making board. Because this situation is common in health promotion, especially in patient education and in some community health agencies, those who find themselves in it should make a special effort to become familiar with the information used by others in the assessment process. Such a review provides the crucial foundation information and orientation needed to keep perspective on the ultimate goal of the program. At the very least, participation of the target population in reaching some level of common concern, if not consensus, on the social purpose of the program should be sought.

SUMMARY

The identification and analysis of the social or economic problems or the aspirations of a target population or client system is a necessary first step in thorough health promotion planning. Health is not an ultimate value in itself except as it relates to social benefits, quality of life, or an organization's "bottom line." Health takes on greater importance to those who must support the program and those expected to participate in it when the connection between the health objective and some broader or more compelling social objective can be clearly seen. This chapter has presented a systematic series of steps and a variety of strategies and techniques that the planner can use to gather and analyze information about social problems, perceived quality of life, or bottom-line objectives in a population or client system.

The objectives of social diagnosis (Phase 1 of health promotion planning) can be summarized as follows:

1. To *engage* the community or client system as active partners in the social diagnostic process
2. To *determine* the subjective concerns with quality of life or conditions of living in the target population
3. To *verify* and clarify these concerns with analyses of existing social indicators and data available from newspaper files, census reports and vital records, and special surveys conducted by radio and television stations and marketing and social service agencies
4. To *document* the status of the target community in relation to those priority concerns for which there is a health component or cause
5. To *make explicit* the rationale for the selection of priority problems
6. To use the documentation and rationale to *justify* the further expenditure of health and other resources on the selected social problem or goal
7. Ultimately, to use the documentation and rationale as the bases on which to *evaluate* the program in cost–benefit terms.

These objectives apply, with minor adjustment, to each of the subsequent phases discussed in the next four chapters.

EXERCISES

1. List three ways you could (or did)[57] involve the members of the population you selected in Exercise 3 of Chapter 1 in identifying their quality-of-life concerns. Justify your methods in terms of their feasibility and appropriateness for the population you are helping.
2. How did (or would) you verify the subjective data gathered in Exercise 1 with objective data on social problems or quality-of-life concerns?
3. Display and discuss your real or hypothetical data as a quality-of-life diagnosis, justifying your selection of social, economic, or health problems to become the highest priority for a program.

REFERENCES AND NOTES

1. The term *community* henceforth refers either to the larger geographically defined community (neighborhood, town, city, county, district, or occasionally, a whole state, region, or country) or to the organizationally defined community (school, worksite, industry, church, clinic, hospital, or nursing home), through which communication and decisions must flow. See the Glossary. *Community* appears in some writings as a group of people who share a common interest. This use may apply

in patient education, self-help groups, and health promotion for dispersed groups. Electronic bulletin boards and satellite television open new possibilities for the interactive engagement of dispersed populations in health promotion planning to address their common concerns. Such electronic meetings have been held, for example, to involve chief executive officers of major companies in discussions of the potential for worksite health promotion programs in their industries.

2. R. A. Bauer, ed., *Social Indicators* (Cambridge, MA: MIT Press, 1966); J. C. Catford, "Positive Health Indicators – Toward a New Information Base for Health Promotion," *Community Medicine* 5 (1983): 125–32; W. J. Cohen, "Social Indicators: Statistics of Public Policy," *American Statistician* 22 (1968): 14–16; J. Dewey, *The Public and Its Problems: An Essay in Political Inquiry* (Chicago: Gateway Books, 1946); S. B. Kar, ed., *Health Promotion Indicators and Actions* (New York: Springer, 1989); S. Katz, ed., "The Portugal Conference: Measuring Quality of Life and Functional Status in Clinical Practice and Epidemiological Research," *Journal of Chronic Diseases* 40 (1987): issue 6; K. C. Land and S. Spilerman, eds., *Social Indicator Models* (New York: Russell Sage Foundation, 1975); M. Mootz, "Health (Promotion) Indicators: Realistic and Unrealistic Expectations," *Health Promotion* 3 (1988): 79–84; H. Noack and D. McQueen, "Towards Health Promotion Indicators," *Health Promotion* 3 (1988): 73–8: D. Patrick and P. Erickson, *Assessing Health-Related Quality of Life in General Population Surveys: Issues and Recommendations* (Washington, DC: National Center for Health Statistics, 1987); R. Wilson, "Do Health Indicators Indicate Health," *American Journal of Public Health* 71 (1981): 461. See also the journal *Social Indicators Research* and *American Journal of Community Psychology* for measurement issues and techniques.

3. B. Checkoway, "Community Participation for Health Promotion: Prescription for Public Policy?" *Wellness Perspectives: Research, Theory and Practice* 6 (1989): 18–26; A. Fonaroff, *Community Involvement in Health Systems for Primary Health Care* (Geneva: World Health Organization, SHS/83.6, 1983); F. Goldsmith and L. E. Kerr, "Worker Participation in Job Safety and Health," *Journal of Public Health Policy* 4 (1983): 447–66; L. W. Green, "The Theory of Participation: A Qualitative Analysis of Its Expression in National and International Health Policies," in *Advances in Health Education and Promotion*, vol. 1, pt. A, W. B. Ward, ed. (Greenwich, CT: JAI Press, 1986), pp. 211–36; R. B. Isely, "The Village Health Committee: Starting Point for Rural Development," *WHO Chronical* 31 (1977): 307–15; L. S. Levin, "Consumer Participation in Health Services," *Journal of the Institute of Health Education* (London) 9 (1971): 19–24; M. Minkler, "Citizen Participation in Health in the Republic of Cuba," *International Quarterly of Community Health Education* 1 (1980–1981): 65–78; D. Nyswander, *Solving School Health Problems* (New York: Oxford University Press, 1942); D. Nyswander, "Education for Health: Some Principles and Their Application," *California's Health* 14 (1956): 65–70; A. Steckler and L. Dawson, "Determinants of Consumer Influence in a Health Systems Agency," *Health Education Monographs* 6 (1978): 377–93; A. Steckler, L. Dawson, and A. Williams, "Consumer Participation and Influence in a Health Systems Agency," *Journal of Community Health* 6 (1981): 181–93; M. O. Tonin, "Concepts in Community Participation," *International Journal of Health Education* 23 (suppl., 1980): 1–13; J. G. Zapka and S. Dorfman, "Consumer Participation: Case Study of the College Health Setting," *Journal of American College Health* 30 (1982): 197–203.

4. C. Buck, "Beyond Lalonde; Creating Health," *Journal of Public Health Policy* 20 (1986): 444–57.

5. World Health Organization, *Health Promotion: A Discussion Document on the Concepts and Principles* (Copenhagen: WHO Regional Office for Europe, ICP/HSR 602, 1984).

6. These are sometimes associated with the term *wellness* to distinguish this focus of health promotion from conventional criteria of health. See D. F. Duncan and R. S. Gold, "Reflections: Health Promotion – What Is It?" *Health Values* 10 (May/June, 1986): 47–8; H. L. Dunn, *High Level Wellness* (Thorofare, NJ: Charles B. Slack, 1977); S. E. Goldston, R. H. Ojemann, and R. H. Nelson, "Primary Prevention and Health Promotion," in *Mental Health: The Public Health Challenge*, E. J. Lieberman, ed. (Washington, DC: American Public Health Association, 1975); M. S. Goodstadt, R. I. Simpson, and P. O. Loranger, "Health Promotion: A Conceptual Integration," *American Journal of Health Promotion* 1 (1987): 58–63.

7. Governor of Mississippi, *Social Reconnaissance: State of Mississippi* (Jackson, MS: Office of the Governor, 1989).

8. C. E. Basch, "Assessing Health Education Needs: A Multidimensional-Multimethod Approach," in *Handbook of Health Education*, 2nd ed., P. M. Lazes, L. H. Kaplan, and K. A. Gordon, eds. (Rockville, MD: Aspen, 1987), chap. 3.

9. M. Bergner, "Measurement of Health Status," *Medical Care* 23 (1985): 696–704; J. W. Bush, "Relative Preferences versus Relative Frequencies in Health-Related Quality of Life Evaluations," in *Assessment of Quality of Life in Clinical Trials of Cardiovascular Therapies*, N. K. Wenger, M. E. Mattson, C. D. Furber, and J. Elinson, eds. (New York: LaJacque, 1984), pp. 118–39; R. M. Kaplan, "Health-Related Quality of Life in Cardiovascular Disease," *Journal of Consulting and Clinical Psychology* 56 (1988): 382–92; K. N. Lohr, ed., "Advances in Health Status Assessment: Conference Proceedings," *Medical Care* 27 (suppl., 1989): issue no. 3; W. Squyres et al., *Patient Education and Health Promotion in Medical Care* (Palo Alto, CA: Mayfield, 1985).

10. N. M. Bradburn, *The Structure of Psychological Well-Being* (Chicago: Aldine, 1969); C. A. Donald and J. E. Ware, Jr., *The Quantification of Social Contacts and Resources* (Santa Monica, CA: Rand, 1982); H. J. Dupuy, "The Psychological General Well-Being Index," in *Assessment of Quality of Life in Clinical Trials of Cardiovascular Therapies*, N. K. Wenger et al., eds. (New York: LeJacque, 1984), pp. 170–83; L. K. George, Subjective Well-being: Conceptual and Methodological Issues," in *Annual Review of Gerontology and Geriatrics*, vol. 2, C. Eisdorfer, ed. (New York: Springer, 1981); pp. 345–82; S. M. Hunt, "Subjective Health Indicators and Health Promotion," *Health Promotion* 3 (1988): 23–34; W. J. Sauer and R. Warland, "Morale and Life Satisfaction," in *Research Instruments in Social Gerontology*, vol. 1, D. J. Mangen and W. A. Peterson, eds. (Minneapolis, MN: University of Minnesota Press, 1982); pp. 123–41; F. D. Wolinsky, R. M. Coe, D. K. Miller, and J. M. Prendergast, "Correlates of Change in the Subjective Well-being of the Elderly," *Journal of Community Health* 11 (1985): 93–107.

11. First International Conference on Health Promotion, "The Ottawa Charter for Health Promotion," *Health Promotion* 1(4) (1986): iii–v.

12. T. Parsons, "The Superego and the Theory of Social Systems," in *The Family: Its Structure and Functions*, R. L. Coser, ed. (New York: St. Martin's Press, 1964), pp. 433–49.

13. L. W. Green, *Community Health*, 6th ed. (St. Louis: Times Mirror/Mosby, 1990), chap. 2.

14. L. Wallack and N. Wallerstein, "Health Education and Prevention: Designing Community Initiatives," *International Quarterly of Community Health Education* 7 (1986–1987): 319–42.

15. B. S. Bloom and G. H. DeFriese, eds., *Cost-benefits, Cost-effectiveness, and Other Decision-making Techniques in Health Resource Allocation* (New York: Biomedical Information, 1983); A. J. Brennan, "Health Promotion: What's In It for Business and Industry?" *Health Education Quarterly* 9 (suppl., Fall 1982): 9–19; G. H. DeFriese, "Cost Effectiveness As a Basis for Assessing the Policy Significance of Health Promotion," *Advances in Health Education and Health Promotion*, vol. 1, pt. A, W. B. Ward, ed. (Greenwich, CT: JAI Press, 1986); pp. 7–21; J. M. McGinnis, "Trends in Disease Prevention: Assessing the Benefits of Prevention," *Bulletin of the New York Academy of Medicine* 56 (1980): 38–44; L. B. Russell, *Is Prevention Better Than Cure?* (Washington, DC: The Brookings Institution, 1986).

16. U.S. Department of Health and Human Services, *Promoting Health/Preventing Disease: Year 2000 Objectives for the Nation* (Washington, DC: Office of the Assistant Secretary for Health, Public Health Service, 1990). The list in this table was from the 1989 draft of the Objectives for the Nation document and so might differ slightly from the final list in the 1990 document.

17. Promoting Health/Preventing Disease: The 1990 Objectives for the Nation (Washington, DC: U.S. Department of Health and Human Services, Public Health Service, 1981).

18. R. W. Amler and H. B. Dull, *Closing the Gap: The Burden of Unnecessary Illness* (New York: Oxford University Press, 1987).

19. Kaiser Family Foundation, *Health Promotion Program* (Menlo Park, CA: The Foundation, 1987).

20. J. M. Ottoson and L. W. Green, "Reconciling Concept and Context: Theory of Implementation," in *Advances in Health Education and Promotion*, vol. 2, W. B. Ward and M. Becker, eds. (Greenwich, CT: JAI Press, 1987), pp. 353–82.

21. L. W. Green, *Community Health*, 6th ed. (St. Louis: Times Mirror/ Mosby, 1990), chap. 2.

22. L. S. Cottrell, "The Competent Community," in *Further Exploration in Social Psychiatry*, B. H. Kaplan, R. N. Wilson, and A. H. Leighton, eds. (New York: Basic Books, 1976), pp. 195–209; E. Eng, J. Hatch, and A. Callan, "Institutionalizing Social Support through the Church and into the Community," *Health Education Quarterly* 12 (1985): 81–92; J. Goeppinger and A. J. Baglioni, "Community Competence: A Positive Approach to Needs Assessment," *American Journal of Community Psychology* 13 (1985): 507–23.

23. R. M. Goodman and A. B. Steckler, "The Life and Death of a Health Promotion Program: An Institutionalization Case Study," *International Quarterly of Community Health Education* 8 (1987–1988): 5–21; A. Steckler and R. M. Goodman, "How to Institutionalize Health Promotion Programs," *American Journal of Health Promotion* 3 (1989): 34–44; idem., "A Model for the Institutionalization of Health Promotion Programs," *Family and Community Health* 11 (1989): 63–78; A. Steckler, K. Orville, E. Eng, and L. Dawson, *PATCHing It Together: A Formative Evaluation of CDC's Planned Approach to Community Health (PATCH) Program* (Chapel Hill, NC: Department of Health Behavior and Health Education, School of Public Health, University of North Carolina, 1989).

24. L. W. Green, "Comment: Is Institutionalization the Proper Goal of Grantmaking?" *American Journal of Health Promotion* 3 (1989): 44.

25. L. W. Green, "New Policies in Education for Health," *World Health* (April–May, 1983): 13–17.

26. E. C. Bivens, "Community Organization: An Old but Reliable Health Education Technique," in *The Handbook of Health Education*, P. M. Lazes, ed. (Germantown, MD: Aspen, 1979); G. P. Cernada, *Knowledge Into Action* (New York: Baywood Publishing Company, 1982); L. W. Green, "Theory of Participation . . ." op. cit.; D. M. Macrina and T. W. O'Rourke, "Citizen Participation in Health Planning in the U. S. and the U. K.: Implications for Health Education Strategies," *International Quarterly of Community Health Education* 7 (1986–1987): 225–39.

27. S. R. Arnstein, "A Ladder of Citizen Participation," *Journal of the American Institute of Planners* 35 (1969): 216–24; R. Dore and Z. Mars, *Community Development* (London: Croom Helm and UNESCO, 1981); D. Soen, "Citizen and Community Participation in Urban Renewal and Rehabilitation — Comments on Theory and Practice," *Community Development Journal* 16 (1981): 105–17. This body of literature is represented best in the *Community Development Journal*.

28. E. de Kadt, "Community Participation for Health: The Case of Latin America," *World Development* 10 (1982): 573–84; P. Freire, *Pedagogy of the Oppressed* (New York: The Seabury Press, 1970); M. Minkler and C. Cox, "Creating Critical Consciousness in Health: Applications of Freire's Philosophy and Methods to the Health Care Setting," *International Journal of Health Services* 20 (1980) 311–322; N. Wallerstein and E. Bernstein, "Empowerment Education: Freire's Ideas Adapted to Health Education," *Health Education Quarterly* 15 (1988): 379–94; D. Werner, "Health Care and Human Dignity," in *Health: The Human Factor: Readings in Health, Development and Community Participation*, S. B. Rifkin, ed. (Geneva: CMC, World Council of Churches, Special Series No. 3, 1980).

29. For a review of the U.S. "maximum feasible participation" experience during the 1960s, see D. P. Moynihan, *Maximum Feasible Misunderstanding: Community Action in the War on Poverty* (New York: The Free Press, 1969); for a review of the evolution of WHO policies on participation over four decades, see L. W. Green, The Theory of Participation . . . , op. cit.

30. World Health Assembly, *New Policies for Health Education in Primary Health Care: Background Document for the Technical Discussions of the Thirty-sixth World Health Assembly* (Geneva: World Health Organization, TD/HED/82.1, 1982).

31. J. M. Cohen and N. T. Uphoff, "Participation's Place in Rural Development: Seeking Clarity through Specificity," *World Development* 8 (1980): 213–35.

32. L. W. Green, *Community Health* (St. Louis: Times Mirror/Mosby, 1990), chap. 2.

33. M. Lichter et al., "Oakwood Hospital Community Health Promotion Program," *Health Care Management Review* 11 (1986): 75–87.

34. P. Friere, *Pedagogy . . .*, 1970, op. cit., p. 181.

35. Ibid., p. 183.

36. M. Minkler, "Building Supportive Ties and Sense of Community Among the Inner-city Elderly: The Tenderloin Senior Outreach Project," *Health Education Quarterly* 12 (1985): 303–14; M. Minkler, S. Frantz, and R. Wechsler, "Social Support and Social Action Organizing in a 'Grey Ghetto,' The Tenderloin Experience," *International Quarterly of Community Health Education* 3 (1982–1983): 3–15.

37. World Health Organization, *Expert Committee on New Approaches to Health Education in Primary Health Care* (Geneva: World Health Organization Tech. Rep. Series 690, 1983).

38. G. D. Gilmore, M. D. Campbell, and B. L. Becker, *Needs Assessment Strategies for Health Education and Health Promotion* (Indianapolis, IN: Benchmark Press, 1989).

39. J. B. Roesner, "Citizen Participation: Tying Strategy to Function," in *Citizen Participation Certification Community Development*, P. Marshall, ed. (Washington, DC: National Association of Housing and Redevelopment Officials, 1977), cited in D. Soen, "Citizen and Community Participation . . .," 1981, op. cit., p. 109.

40. G. B. Shaw, *The Apple Cart: A Political Extravaganza* (London: Constable and Co., 1930), pp. xiv–xv.

41. I. T. Sanders, *Preparing a Community Profile: The Methodology of a Social Reconnaissance* (Lexington, KY: Kentucky Community Series No. 7, Bureau of Community Services, University of Kentucky, 1950).

42. H. L. Nix and N. R. Seerley, "Community Reconnaissance Method: A Synthesis of Functions," *Journal of Community Development Society* 11 (Fall, 1971): 62–9.

43. H. L. Nix, *The Community and Its Involvement in the Study Planning Action Process* (Atlanta: Center for Disease Control, Public Health Service, CDC 78-8355, 1977), p.140.

44. Ibid., p. 141.

45. Ibid., pp. 143–4.

46. P. R. Mico, "Community Self-Study: Is There a Method to the Madness?" *Adult Leadership* 13 (1965): 288–92; H. L. Nix, *Identification of Leaders and Their Involvement in the Planning Process* (Washington, DC: U. S. Public Health Service Publication No. 1998, 1970); H. L. Nix, "Concepts of Community and Community Leadership," *Sociology and Social Research* 53 (1969): 500–10; H. L. Nix and N. R. Seerley, "Comparative Views and Actions of Community Leaders and Nonleaders," *Rural Sociology* 38 (1973): 427–8; D. J. Shoemaker and H. L. Nix "A Study of Reputational Leaders Using the Concepts of Exchange and Coordinative Positions," *The Sociological Quarterly* 13 (1972): 516–24.

47. S. G. Brink, et al., "Community Intervention Handbooks for Comprehensive Health Promotion Programming," *Family and Community Health* 11 (1988): 28–35; G. S. Parcel, et al., *Smoking Control Among Women: A CDC Community Intervention Handbook* (Atlanta: Centers for Disease Control, 1987); D. G. Simons-Morton, et al., *Promoting Physical Activity Among Adults: A CDC Community Intervention Handbook* (Atlanta: Centers for Disease Control, 1988).

48. Parcel, op. cit., p. 13.

49. Ibid., p. 15.

50. A. H. Van de Ven and A. L. Delbecq, "The Nominal Group as a Research Instrument for Exploratory Health Studies," *American Journal of Public Health* 62 (1972): 337–42.

51. A. L. Delbecq, "The nominal group as a technique for understanding the qualitative dimensions of client needs," CCinDD R.A. Bell, et al., editors, *Assessing Health and Human Service Needs* (New York: Human Sciences Press, 1983), pp 191–209.

52. H. A. Linstone and M. Turoff, *The Delphi Method: Techniques and Applications* (Reading, MA: Addison-Wesley, 1975).

53. G. D. Gilmore, "Needs Assessment Processes for Community Health Education," *International Journal of Health Education* 20 (1977): 164–73.

54. L. W. Green and F. M. Lewis, *Measurement and Evaluation in Health Education and Health Promotion* (Palo Alto, CA: Mayfield, 1986), chaps. 3–6 and 10; R. A. Windsor, T. Baronowski, N. Clark, and G. Cutter, *Evaluation of Health Promotion and Education Programs* (Palo Alto, CA: Mayfield, 1984), chap. 6.

55. E. Folch-Lyon and J. F. Trost, "Conducting Focus Group Sessions," *Studies in Family Planning* 12 (1981): 443–9.

56. E. B. Arkin, *Making Health Communication Programs Work: A Planner's Guide* (Bethesda, MD: Office of Cancer Communications, National Cancer Institute, NIH-89-1493, 1989).

57. It is recommended that these exercises be carried out with a real population accessible to the student or practitioner, but if this is impractical the exercises can best be followed with a well-described hypothetical population using actual census data and vital statistics from similar populations.

Chapter 3

Epidemiological
Diagnosis

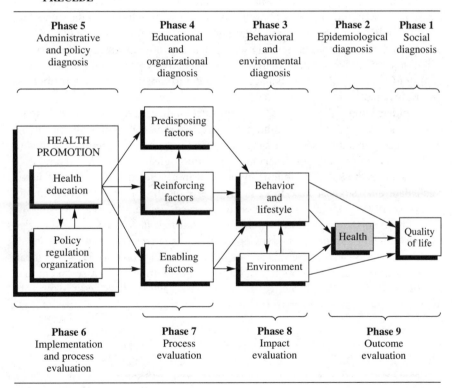

The preceding chapter urged that attention and sensitivity to the social and quality-of-life concerns of the target population are the best starting point for justifying and planning health promotion programs. This approach tends to be the best even when the priority concerns appear at first to have little to do with health.

Social problems, however, rarely command the sustained focus of a health promotion endeavor financed by the health sector unless a clear relationship to health can be demonstrated. (Unemployment, for example, might be ameliorated by health promotion, but a specific program in health promotion seldom tackles more than the health aspects of unemployment.) Health professionals invest their energies in improving the health status of certain groups or communities. Health outcomes constitute the most concrete long-range goals of most health promotion programs, even if those goals are explicitly justified in terms of the potential they have for contributing to the social or economic good. Thus, amid the multitude of problems that affect the common social good and quality of life, health professionals must direct their primary efforts toward the solution of health problems.

In this chapter we present Phase 2 of the PRECEDE framework, the **epidemiological diagnosis**.[1] This phase is concerned with pinpointing the important health problems of the target population. An epidemiological assessment is conducted to determine two things: (1) which health problems are important (measured objectively here, rather than by their subjectively perceived importance to quality of life) and (2) which behavioral and environmental factors contribute to the occurrence of those health problems.

Epidemiology, the study of the occurrence of disease in human populations, offers a methodology for determining the objective importance of health problems in a target population. By showing the magnitude and distribution of health problems in the population, descriptive epidemiological data suggest the relative importance of the health problems in terms of morbidity, disability, or mortality. Such data also suggest how the importance of health problems varies among subgroups of the population that differ in age, race, gender, lifestyle, housing, or exposure to specific behavioral or environmental risk factors. By assessing risk factors for health problems, analytic epidemiological investigation provides invaluable information about potential causes of those health problems, causes that can be the focus of health promotion programs. The epidemiological assessment thus identifies those health problems, and their risk factors, that deserve priority among the many problems a program might address.

RELATIONSHIP BETWEEN HEALTH AND SOCIAL PROBLEMS

What is the relationship between the epidemiological assessment and the social assessment? Two complementary approaches to analyzing the link between health and social problems can be offered here. The **reductionist** approach works from a broad social problem toward an assessment of the health components that contribute causally to that problem. The **expansionist** approach starts from a specified health problem and works to the larger social context within which that particular problem occurs.

THE REDUCTIONIST APPROACH

The reductionist approach consists of identifying priority health problems from a statement of social problems and an inventory of suspected determinants of the social problems. In the PRECEDE framework the social diagnosis, or quality-of-life assessment, is followed by an analysis of both health and nonhealth factors influencing the social problem. This can be considered the first step in the epidemiological assessment. Without this analysis you run the risk of targeting health problems that fail to make a difference in the social problem. If the social priority, for example, is drug-related crimes and you choose to focus on the health issue of cirrhosis of the liver, you are right on the mortality target with a leading cause of death associated with the most common drug (alcohol), but you missed the social target of drug-related crime by a mile.

Health professionals seldom use survey data on a community's perceived quality-of-life or social problems as a formal basis on which to decide which health problems deserve attention. Such surveys are routinely conducted by various public, private, and voluntary agencies with mandates other than health. Health agencies might gain greater public support and financing if they took greater pains to link their priorities more systematically with the community's quality-of-life or social concerns. In 1989, the three leading concerns of Americans according to various polls were crime, drugs, and AIDS. From a reductionist perspective, this list could be interpreted as drugs, drugs, and drugs. Much of the crime problem and much of the AIDS problem can be traced to drugs.

Existing surveys can be used to identify social problems affecting a particular population. For example, the health professional can use surveys on unemployment, substandard housing, illiteracy, welfare, isolation, or other social problems to determine which of those factors are the most prevalent, which have the highest perceived importance, and which persons or subpopulations fall into one or more of those categories. If the surveys contain information on health problems, the health professional can then determine the rates of health problems within each subgroup. These findings can be the basis for recommending priorities for health promotion programs directed at health problems, and (in cooperation with other sectors) directed at environmental factors, with the goal of ameliorating the social problems of greatest importance.

A review of the scientific and professional literature helps the health professional determine the relationship between health and social problems. For example, the relationship between health problems and the social problem of poverty is

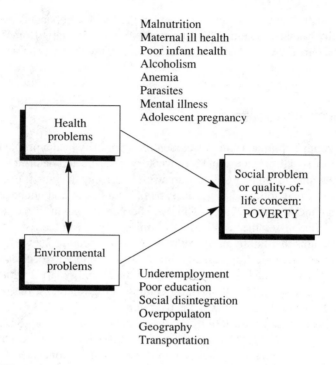

Malnutrition
Maternal ill health
Poor infant health
Alcoholism
Anemia
Parasites
Mental illness
Adolescent pregnancy

Health
problems

Social problem
or quality-of-
life concern:
POVERTY

Environmental
problems

Underemployment
Poor education
Social disintegration
Overpopulaton
Geography
Transportation

FIGURE 3.1

Examples of health and environmental factors contributing to poverty.

analyzed in a variety of works.[2] Figure 3.1 suggests how poverty can be separated into health-related and environmental factors. Such a categorization of factors can help in planning health promotion programs that are directed at health-related factors but designed within the broader environmental context.

The distribution and severity of health problems can be determined for each target population. For example, members of a rural community might suffer to a greater degree from parasitic infections, anemia, and malnutrition than people who live in an inner-city ghetto where alcoholism, mental illness, and adolescent pregnancy might predominate. In some southern states of the United States and in most developing countries, adolescent pregnancy is more common in rural areas and is a major factor in holding some families in an intergenerational cycle of poverty.[3]

The environmental factors that contribute to a social problem also vary with the makeup of the target population and its location: Migrant workers and their families might suffer from poor access to organized social support systems such as education and welfare. Poor roads or geographic isolation might contribute to poverty status, as might lack of jobs. In addition, social biases regarding racial or ethnic minority status frequently contribute to social and health problems.

Health professionals seldom have a mandate to address social-environmental factors that affect quality of life and may not be allowed to devote agency resources to do so. Nonetheless, it helps to be aware of the possible effect of the physical environment and of socioeconomic factors on potential solutions to a reciprocal poverty–health problem. Bureaucratic resistance to intervening in the environmental aspects of a problem must be overcome if the future of health promotion is to be relevant to the populations most in need of improved conditions of living. In the early years of the Mound Bayou Community Health Center, opened in Mississippi in the late 1960s, poor nutrition was a major problem in this population. The health center leadership thought it could be best attacked by encouraging community members to plant home gardens (with supplemental information on the nutritional preparation of food). Some initial bureaucratic resistance was eventually overcome, and the intervention resulted in improved nutritional status and improved living. Although health workers may not always be able to use the approaches that seem most direct, they can initiate cooperative efforts with other community agencies, they can advocate for policy changes, and they can refer people to community resources outside of the health sector.[4]

The reductionist approach can be used in epidemiological assessment when the social problem has been identified (as in Chapter 2) but the causes of the problem have not been clearly delineated. Usually, so many causes demand attention that health workers are in danger of frittering away their efforts. The reductionist approach serves health workers especially well in arriving at a few important but manageable problems by methods described later in this chapter.

THE EXPANSIONIST APPROACH

Health professionals often find themselves employed in situations for which a specific health problem—such as hypertension, tuberculosis, or obesity—with a particular target population has already been set as the priority, if not the sole mission, of the agency. Someone else has already reduced the ultimate social problem to a specified health problem on which this agency can make its contribution. Sometimes an agency has targeted a health problem according to previously established state or national priorities. Because of the scarcity of resources, it is essential even in these circumstances to weigh the importance of the assigned health problems against that of others. Surveying the scene from a larger perspective helps ensure that health promotion is focused on those problems whose reduction will yield the greatest social benefit. The assessment of how the assigned health problem fits into the larger health and social context is the expansionist approach.

One responsibility of the health professional is to interpret local data in the

light of medical and epidemiologic knowledge about cause-and-effect relationships and the natural history and distribution of the health problems in the
larger state or national population. Numerous documents describe in considerable
detail the nature, scope, and burden of health problems at the national level:
Canada's Health Promotion Survey and the *Canadian Health and Disability
Survey*[5]; *Advancing Australia's Health: Towards National Strategies and Objectives for Health Advancement*[6]; and annual publications of the U.S. Department of
Health and Human Services, including *Health, United States*[7] and the Department's monthly *Vital and Health Statistics* and weekly *Morbidity and Mortality
Weekly Reports* series. These provide national, regional, and state prevalence and
mortality data for the major health problems by age, gender, race, and location.
The *Source Book of Health Insurance Data*,[8] issued annually by the Health
Insurance Institute (New York), provides the latest statistics relating specific health
conditions to quality-of-life or economic factors, such as workdays lost due to each
disease category (see Table 3.1). Such data give health workers an idea of the
relative social impact of their assigned problem compared to a range of other
health problems.

For an example of the expansionist approach, consider the following. A health
educator has been asked to develop a safety education program for the control of
injuries to women over the age of 45 working in a large industry. A check of the
national figures (from Table 3.1) reveals that (1) noninjury problems account for a
larger number of workdays lost by women in this age group than injuries do and
(2) workdays lost for injuries are more prevalent for younger women and for
males. Even without support from local data, which are not often available, the
health educator is in a stronger position to argue for shifting attention to a different
health problem: to women in a different age group or to men in this or another age
group.

The expansionist approach is particularly useful when one is assigned an
oversimplified problem. Suppose a newspaper article announces an alarming
comparison between the local infant mortality rate and the state-wide rate. A
statement on the newspaper's editorial page denounces the quality of infant care in
local hospitals, and the city council calls for a corrective program directed at
neonatal care in the community hospital. Faced with this situation, a health
professional might analyze the following information:

- The two-county rural area within which the community is located is
  populated mainly by a low-income minority agricultural group that has a
  high rate of teenage pregnancy.
- The infant mortality rate in this community has remained at 24.9 per
  1,000 live births while there has been an overall decline in the state rate
  to 14.6 per 1000.
- The identified pregnancy outcome problems include premature birth, low
  birth weight, respiratory distress at delivery, and failure to thrive. The

TABLE 3.1

Workdays lost due to acute conditions in the United States

Acute conditions	Number of work-loss days (000,000)			Work-loss days per employed person		
	All ages 18 and over	Age 18–44	Age 45 and over	All ages 18 and over	Age 18–44	Age 45 and over
Both sexes						
All acute conditions	347	252	95	3.1	3.2	2.9
Infective and parasitic diseases	25	22	3	0.8	0.3	0.1
Respiratory conditions	111	81	30	1.1	1.1	1.0
Digestive system conditions	16	12	3	0.2	2.1	1.1
Injuries	119	85	34	1.1	1.1	1.0
All other acute conditions	18	11	17	0.2	0.1	0.2
Male						
All acute conditions	175	124	51	2.8	2.9	2.7
Infective and parasitic diseases	10	9	.9	0.2	0.2	0.1
Respiratory conditions	54	39	15	0.8	0.9	0.7
Digestive system conditions	8	6	3	0.2	0.1	0.2
Injuries	77	57	20	1.2	1.4	1.1
All other acute conditions	8	5	3	0.2	0.1	0.2
Female						
All acute conditions	172	128	44	3.4	4.0	3.1
Infective and parasitic diseases	15	13	2	0.3	0.4	0.2
Respiratory conditions	57	42	15	1.4	1.2	1.1
Digestive system conditions	7	7	.8	0.2	0.2	0.2
Injuries	42	28	14	0.8	0.5	1.0
All other acute conditions	9	6	4	0.2	0.2	0.3

NOTE: The data refer to the civilian, noninstitutional population. An acute condition is one that lasted less than 3 months and that involved either medical attention or restricted activity. A work-loss day is a day on which a currently employed person, 18 years of age and over, did not work at least half of his normal workday because of a specific illness or injury. In some cases the sum of the items does not equal the total shown, because of rounding.

SOURCE: *Source Book of Health Insurance Data, 1989* (New York: Health Insurance Association of America, 1989), p. 75; by permission of the publisher.

visiting nurse service also reports a high prevalence of maternal anemia and a high incidence of gastrointestinal infection and respiratory diseases in infants.

- Many mothers are at risk because of age (a disproportionate number between 14 and 17 years old), poor nutrition, lack of medical care, multiple pregnancies, and preeclampsia during pregnancy.
- Childhood health is poor: Injuries are common, and children look malnourished and report for school with handicapping conditions and no immunizations.

According to this information, the chief cause of the relatively high infant mortality rate in the area may not be deficiencies in the quality of neonatal care in community hospitals but may be poor prenatal care, poor maternal and infant nutrition, and lack of infant immunizations. Therefore, a decision to buy new, improved hospital equipment to care for neonates may actually be a more costly and less effective solution to the problem than a program of community outreach for prenatal health care, nutritional support, and childhood immunizations. By expanding his or her understanding of the problem and seeing the statistics in the broader context of relationships between health and social problems, the health professional can help the community address the problem more comprehensively and productively through prevention and health promotion rather than just through high-technology medical care.

This example illustrates two additional points. First, the relationship of health problems to quality of life can be readily discerned. High rates of adolescent pregnancy lead to high rates of school absenteeism, dropouts, and single-parent homes, often in lower-income brackets and in need of proportionately greater social services.

Second, the example suggests the vital importance of developing data for significant subgroups. In this population these are the low-income, minority, rural, teenage girls and their infants. In other populations the data might reveal a high prevalence of hypertension among black males or of lung cancer among white middle-aged males. Without such data, it is impossible for the health professional with a preassigned target problem to know which subpopulations should receive special attention and which health problems deserve higher priority than that assigned.

ASSESSING THE IMPORTANCE OF HEALTH PROBLEMS

To determine which health problems should receive priority, one has to describe and quantify health problems in sufficient detail. Going through this process serves three principal functions: (1) it helps to establish the relative importance of various health problems in the target population as a whole and in population subgroups; (2) it provides a basis for setting program priorities among the various health problems and subgroups; and (3) it aids in the allocation of responsibilities among collaborating professionals, agencies, and departments.

INDICATORS OF HEALTH STATUS IN POPULATIONS

The classic indicators of health problems are **mortality** (death), **morbidity** (disease), and **disability** (dysfunction). Sometimes discomfort and dissatisfaction are added, making a list of "five D's" including quality-of-life measures. In addition, there are positive indicators of health status such as life expectancy and fitness.[9] Mortality has been expressed increasingly in recent years as *years of potential life lost* (YPLL) to give greater weight to deaths at younger ages. This measure is more sensitive to the preventable mortality in childhood, youth, and the adult productive years.[10]

Comparative data on these indicators are available from a variety of sources, such as the National Center for Health Statistics, Centers for Disease Control, other agencies of the Department of Health and Human Services (or the ministries of health in other countries), local and state (or provincial) health departments, the Bureau of the Census (see the annual *Statistical Abstract of the United States*), professional journals and associations, and the World Health Organization.

MAKING COMPARISONS

To determine the relative importance of health problems, one makes comparisons. One can compare the data of interest for community X with other communities, the state, or the nation; one can compare data for different health problems within the same community; and one can compare data for various subgroups of the community, based on age, race, or gender. Such comparisons allow identification of health problems that are greater in this community than in other places or are most important within the community, or problems that plague specific groups within the community.

RATES

Data comparisons can be made only between like data: apples with apples, oranges with oranges. Expressing rates of death and disease uniformly as "number per thousand population per year" (for example) allows direct comparisons between populations of different sizes over different time periods.

Figure 3.2 compares the annual deaths per 1,000 population in New York City,

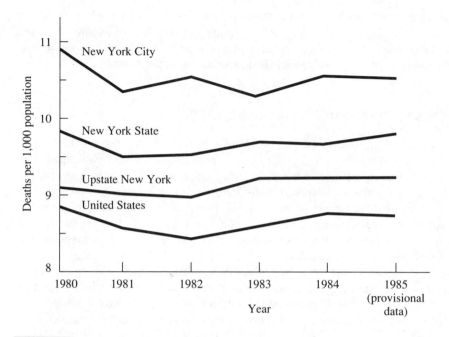

FIGURE 3.2

Death rates for New York City, New York State, Upstate New York, and the United
States, 1980–1985.

New York State, Upstate New York, and the United States. In addition to revealing
that New York City had the highest death rate, the data also show that after a drop
in the death rate for all four areas between 1980 and 1981, the rates leveled off and
remained stable; the relative differences in the death rates of the four areas
remained essentially the same during that period. With Figure 3.2 we can compare
information about areas that are very different in size and geography (city, state,
nation) because the deaths are presented using a common denominator – in this
case, deaths per 1,000 population.

The following explication of rates is adapted from training material for the
PATCH program, one of a variety of public health technical-assistance programs
to state and local health agencies provided by The Centers for Disease Control.
PATCH (*p*lanned *a*pproach to *c*ommunity *h*ealth) is a community-intervention
training program that follows the PRECEDE model. PATCH trainers report that
practitioners often find it helpful to review some of the basic terms one encounters
when using public health data, particularly rates.

It does not mean much to say, "In 1986 county X had 48 fatal injuries and its
state had 1,712." The state is much bigger than the county, the size of neither is

given, and so the numbers are not meaningful by themselves. You must first turn them into rates. A rate is the number of events (for example, fatal injuries) per 1,000 or 100,000 population. For example,

- divide the number of deaths in the county by the population of the county;
- divide the number of deaths in the state by the population of the state; then
- multiply the results by a multiple of ten to obtain a value for each that lies between 1 and 100.

These calculations yield the appropriate comparison: The injury death rate in county X is 55.8 deaths per 100,000, and that of the state is 36.4 deaths per 100,000. These figures indicate that the county has a higher rate of fatal injuries than the state as a whole, suggesting that further examination is warranted to see if county X really has more of a problem than the rest of the state or whether it only looks that way because of the county's age distribution. Adjusting rates to remove biases that result from different ages or other distributional characteristics of the populations will be taken up later.

The basic formula for a rate is $(X/Y) \times K$, where

X = numbers of events or cases

Y = population at risk for the event being studied

K = a constant value such as 100, 1,000, or 100,000 by which
      the rate is expressed (e.g., deaths per 1,000 population)

A further component of a rate is the time period during which, or the point in time at which, the numerator X and denominator Y were measured. One year is most commonly used to standardize the time period for comparison of rates.

Many events are expressed as rates: live births, infant deaths, mortality, etc. For all of them, the basic formula is rate $=(X/Y) \times K$; only the specific numbers change.[11]

Incidence and Prevalence. Two rates deserve particular discussion: incidence and prevalence. Both are measures of morbidity (disease) in the population, but there are important differences between the two measures. **Incidence** measures *new* cases of the disease within a certain time period, whereas **prevalence** measures the total number of existing disease cases at a particular *point* in time. Incidence rates for population groups are hard to come by, especially for chronic diseases, but the incidence rate is an important measure, allowing the determination of disease risk factors (discussed later). Most of the public health data systems that monitor health trends over time were designed many years ago for surveillance of communicable disease outbreaks. Consequently, most of the data available on incidence are based on information that is provided by physicians when they complete the forms required when they encounter a patient with a "reportable" disease.[12] Some states have begun to require physicians to report some specific noncommunicable diseases, such as occupational lung diseases or lead toxicity, so that health officials can intervene on environmental health threats.

Prevalence rates, available when and where surveys have been made, are not as good a measure of disease importance as incidence because they are complicated by the prognosis of the disease: Prevalence reflects both the incidence and the duration of disease. If diseases A and B have equal incidence rates, but disease A is mild whereas B is severe and causes early death, then disease A has a higher prevalence in the population. People live with the mild disease; they die with the severe one. Those who died are not around to be counted when the prevalence survey is done. Just looking at the prevalence rates could mislead you in determining which disease is more important.

This is illustrated by comparing common allergies with AIDS (acquired immunodeficiency syndrome). Allergies have a much higher prevalence than AIDS, due to both a higher incidence and a much milder disease course. It would certainly be incorrect to deduce from the higher prevalence that allergies are more important, because AIDS, the disease with the low prevalence, causes death. In another example, the prevalence of Type 1 (insulin dependent, juvenile onset) diabetes is much higher today than it was early in this century because improved treatment now allows those diabetics to live longer (and be counted). These examples illustrate that in comparing prevalence rates, one needs additional information about the severity and duration to determine which diseases are important. Although prevalence rates combine information about incidence and duration and so must be interpreted with care, they are important for planning health resources and programs.

From a health promotion perspective, prevalence rates on chronic diseases can be misleading in setting priorities for the future. They may identify the people whose behavior and living conditions 20 years ago caused the disease from which they died last year when the disease-specific rate was calculated. The data become available much too late to plan for primary prevention, and often too late for secondary prevention. Today we are tabulating the lung cancers, emphysema, and heart attacks of people who started smoking as many as 20 years ago, so we say that "smoking is the number one preventable cause of deaths in this country." Considering the dramatic declines in smoking in the past decade, we might be more accurate in saying that "smoking that began 10 to 20 years ago is the number one cause of deaths today." The proper criterion for setting a mortality-based priority in health promotion today would be today's number one cause of the deaths that will occur in the future. This cause may still be tobacco, or it may be alcohol, but more likely it is dietary fat.

The point is that prevalence data on chronic disease or on deaths this year are of limited use in targeting health promotion priorities to prevent the future diseases and deaths that are associated with today's lifestyles and conditions of living. The prevalence and trends of today's risk factors (behavioral, environmental) – rather

TABLE 3.2

Population attributable risk (PAR) summary for six risk factors, State of Michigan, 1983

Risk factor	Michigan adult prevalence, %	PAR deaths before age 65	PAR life years lost before 65
Smoking	32.4	3,444	38,106
Drinking	7.5 (heavy)		
	20.5 (moderate)	1,751	51,493
Seat belts[a]	86.5+ (use less than always)	546	17,736
Hypertension	20.6 (uncontrolled)	1,422	15,549
Exercise	65.1 (no regular exercise)	1,024	10,647
Nutrition/weight	17.7 (120% of ideal)		
	15.0 (111–119% of ideal)	4,088	45,485
Total		12,275	179,016

[a] Before seat belt law took effect

SOURCE: Michigan Department of Health, *Health Promotion Can Produce Economic Savings* (Lansing, MI: Center for Health Promotion, Michigan Department of Public Health, 1987), p. 7; by permission of publisher.

than today's mortality — would provide more reliable indicators of chronic-disease morbidity and mortality-prevention priorities. Unfortunately, most communities do not have good surveillance systems in place to monitor the risk factors on a continuous or periodic basis.[13]

Population Attributable Risk. A partial solution to the mortality-based priority-setting problem just described is provided by the knowledge and data accumulated over the past several decades on the quantitative risk of death associated with specific risk factors. When the prevalence of those risk factors is known, the projected number of deaths in the population can be estimated. Conversely, the number of deaths in each mortality category can be used to work back to an estimate of the number of those deaths attributable to each of the major risk factors.

Table 3.2 illustrates such a set of calculations by the Michigan Department of Public Health's Center for Health Promotion.[14] To take the smoking example in the first row of the table, a statewide survey in 1983 showed that 32.4% of Michigan adults were smokers. Smokers have a 10 times greater risk of getting lung cancer, and as we showed in Chapter 2, a relative risk of 2. of cardiovascular death. By combining the prevalence rate for smoking with the mortality from cancer, heart

TABLE 3.3

Return on dollar invested in health risk-factor interventions over working lifetime (ages 20–64) of those at risk, State of Michigan

Risk-factor intervention	$ Discount at 0%	$ Discount at 4%	$ Discount at 8%
Smoking	21.01	15.26	10.88
Hypertension	0.99	0.92	0.84
Nutrition/weight			
Moderate	0.34	0.26	0.18
Severe	0.62	0.48	0.36
Drinking			
Drinking/driving	1.40	1.30	1.19
Heavy drinking	3.17	2.68	2.24
Binge drinking	1.41	1.30	1.19
Sedentary (exercise)	0.42	0.35	0.27
Seat belt	105.07	105.07	105.07
Combined			
(nutrition/hypertension/exercise)	2.74	2.07	1.50

SOURCE: Michigan Department of Health, *Health Promotion Can Produce Economic Savings* (Lansing, MI: Center for Health Promotion, Michigan Department of Public Health, 1987), p. 9; by permission of publisher.

disease, lung diseases, stroke, and fires, each multiplied by a relative risk statistic, a product known as population attributable risk (PAR) is generated. This represents the mortality attributable to smoking. This can be expressed as the total number of deaths, the number of deaths before age 65 (responding to those policymakers who say, "Ya gotta go sometime"), or total years lost before age 65 (for those policymakers who worry most about productivity years lost).

Cost-Benefit Analysis from PAR. Once the mortality data have been interpreted in relation to risk factors of known prevalence, the population attributable risk data can be related back to the social diagnosis in a form that has additional meaning to policymakers: namely, **cost-benefit** analysis. The cost of starting and maintaining a smoking cessation program, for example, is known to the health department. The cost per person enrolled is easily calculated from the experience of the agency in maintaining such programs. On the benefit side, the medical costs associated with all diseases linked to a risk factor (e.g., smoking) and the lost income due to premature death before age 65 can be added to obtain a dollar estimate of the losses associated with each risk factor. Now, the potential benefits in dollars, divided by the costs of interventions to obtain those benefits, gives a cost-benefit ratio expressed as return on each dollar invested in the risk-factor intervention (Table 3.3)[15]

The bottom line on smoking, then, appears to be that with current rates projected into the future, smoking is important not just because of deaths today, but also because it will cause thousands of needless deaths and illnesses in the twenty-first century, and these deaths and illnesses would cost 10 to 21 times more than the cost of interventions to prevent them. We refer again to Table 3.3 when we discuss policy assessment in Chapter 6.

Sensitivity Analysis. The difference between the estimates of $10.88 and $21.01 in the return per dollar invested in smoking prevention programs is the difference between assuming a high discount rate such as inflation (which makes future dollars saved worth less today) and assuming a zero discount rate (which makes future dollars worth the same as current dollars). Many epidemiological analyses and policy analyses apply a range of assumptions similar to the two PAR columns in Table 3.2 and the three discount columns in Table 3.3 to determine how sensitive the results are to the various assumptions one might make in projecting current data to future circumstances or to another situation. This kind of range-finding is referred to broadly as **sensitivity analysis**.

Sensitivity and Specificity. Another type of sensitivity analysis in epidemiological assessments pertains to the use of mass screening results as the basis for generating estimates of the prevalence of a disease or condition in a population. If the test is able to detect virtually every case without fail, it is said to have high **sensitivity**. To take two extreme examples, death reporting by death certificates has high sensitivity, whereas physician reporting of communicable diseases has low sensitivity because it misses many of the cases of some diseases. The sensitivity concept is usually applied to laboratory and clinical tests such as mammograms and Pap smears for cancer, blood tests for serum cholesterol and sexually transmitted diseases, and blood pressure measures to detect and diagnose hypertension. Some of these tests can yield normal readings when in fact the person tested has the condition (i.e., a "false negative"). To that degree they lack sensitivity.

The related concept, **specificity**, measures the degree to which a screening test yields results that may be wrong in the other direction—positive when the case is negative (a "false positive"). A false positive might be better than a false negative, insofar as the person tested has not been missed when a treatable disease is present. Yet, tests with low specificity tend to be eschewed by health officials because of the high cost in following up on large numbers of false positives and because of the fear and shame that are aroused in people who have been told that their tests are positive. This emotional response is called the labeling problem of mass screening. It applies to the false positives and to the true positives because in both cases the people tested may overreact to being labeled as having a condition that they consider shameful or more dangerous than it may be.

Issues of sensitivity and specificity surround the use of mass screening to determine population prevalence rates and to detect cases early enough to be effectively treated. Cost-benefit considerations also enter the debate on mass screening when the cost of the tests run is high relative to the yield in number of treatable cases. These debates reach a crescendo when the disease in question is one that has social stigma and possible hiring, firing, or promotion consequences on the job. HIV testing and drug testing in the workplace have come to this juncture. Issues of sensitivity, specificity, cost-benefit, and labeling all pertain to the worksite debate on these tests, as well as to blood pressure screening and even fitness testing. Confidentiality of test results and assurances that results will not be used in personnel decisions can help overcome resistance but lack credibility in some corporate settings.

Finally, the concepts of sensitivity and specificity apply even within the evaluation of a health education effort to train lay people to recognize symptoms or signs of disease. The ability of women to identify lumps during breast self-examination has been expressed in terms of sensitivity and specificity.[16] These in turn can be related to demographic and socioeconomic characteristics to identify target populations in which the subsequent steps in the PRECEDE planning process can be focused.[17]

Age-Adjusted Rates. Rates may need other kinds of adjustment to make them equivalent for comparison. For example, data from different years or locations may need to be **age-adjusted** to account for different age distributions in the populations. Figure 3.3 shows the age-adjusted death rates for the United States for 1950–1980.[18] Because the rates are age-adjusted, the trends for decreasing death rates must be ascribed to some factor or factors other than the changing age structure of the nation. The differences among the races and between the sexes also can be ascribed to factors other than different age structures.

Specific Rates. To compare rates between subgroups or for various diseases, a **specific rate** is used. A specific rate is calculated for a specified population subgroup based on age, race, or sex. For example, a rate for 55–60 year olds is an **age-specific** rate. If the rate is further broken down by race it becomes an age-race–specific rate, such as a rate for black 18–24 year olds. Going a step further, we can break down the rate by sex to obtain an age-race-sex–specific rate: black 55–60-year-old men. Rates can also be calculated for particular causes of death. The rate of cancer deaths and the rate of lung cancer deaths are examples of cause-specific rates.

Comparison of rates in various groups can provide a clearer picture of the relative importance of health problems among those groups. If we examine the differences in cause-specific death rates between socioeconomic groups, we can

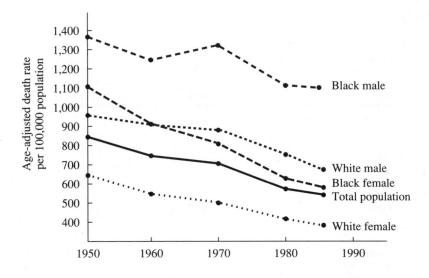

FIGURE 3.3

Age-adjusted death rates for all causes by sex and race, 1950–1986, United States.
SOURCE: National Center for Health Statistics, *Health, United States, 1988*
(Washington, DC: Government Printing Office), table 20.

identify causes of death that are more important for the poor or for the affluent. Comparison of rates within a group also can be instructive. For example, looking at death rates from unintentional injuries versus cardiovascular disease, we find that unintentional injuries have the greatest impact in children, whereas for the middle aged it is cardiovascular disease.

Data from Wisconsin show that males aged 12–17 (sex-age–specific) are at higher risk of dying than females and are much more likely to die of both intentional and unintentional injuries than their female counterparts. Tables 3.4 and 3.5 show, for both sexes, relatively high numbers of motor vehicle–related injuries, which constitute the principal cause of death for Wisconsin youth. National data for the same time period reflect a similar trend. This analysis illustrates another epidemiological technique for understanding trends and comparisons. In the Wisconsin statistics for this age group, the numbers are so small as to make a change of, say, one or two deaths by a particular type of injury a large percentage change. Such small numbers tend to make rates calculated from them unstable. A common technique to overcome this problem of small numbers is to combine the data for several years and average the resulting numbers to estimate the rate for a middle year.

Table 3.6 (from the *Report on the Secretary's Task Force on Black and Minority Health*)[19] shows infant mortality rates for blacks and nonminorities.

TABLE 3.4

Injury-related deaths among males ages 12–17, annual averages, Wisconsin, 1980–1984

Source of injury	Number[a]	Percent	Rate per 100,000 population
Motor vehicle	59	65.6	23.3
Drowning	9	10.0	3.5
Suffocation	3	3.5	1.3
Poisoning	2	2.7	0.9
Fire	2	1.8	0.6
Other sources	15	16.4	5.8
All injuries	90	100	35.4

[a] Deaths occurring in Wisconsin regardless of residency. Excludes homicides, suicides, and deaths for which intent was not determined. Rounded to whole numbers.
SOURCE: Adapted from unpublished data, Wisconsin Department of Health.

TABLE 3.5

Injury-related deaths among females ages 12–17, annual averages, Wisconsin, 1980–1984

Source of injury	Number[a]	Percent	Rate per 100,000 population
Motor vehicle	28	80.9	10.9
Poisoning	2	4.6	0.6
Drowning	1	2.3	0.3
Fire	1	1.7	0.2
Other sources	4	10.4	1.5
All injuries	35	100	13.5

[a] Deaths occurring in Wisconsin regardless of residency. Excludes homicides, suicides, and deaths for which intent was not determined. Rounded to whole numbers.
SOURCE: Adapted from unpublished data, Wisconsin Department of Health.

TABLE 3.6

Infant mortality rates for black and nonminority populations by state and selected counties within states

State	All	State Black	Non-minority	Key counties[a] Total	Black	Non-minority	Rest of state Total	Black	Non-minority
Alabama	15.1	21.6	11.6	15.9	21.6	10.7	14.0	21.3	12.6
Arkansas	12.7	20.0	10.3	13.9	20.0	9.5	11.3	19.9	16.9
California	11.1	18.0	10.6	11.8	19.7	16.7	10.6	16.1	16.6
D.C.	25.0	26.7	17.8	25.0	26.7	17.8	–	–	–
Florida	14.6	22.8	11.8	14.8	21.7	11.2	14.5	23.0	11.9
Georgia	14.5	21.0	10.8	16.2	20.8	11.8	10.8	22.6	9.5
Illinois	14.8	26.3	11.7	17.3	26.2	12.4	12.3	26.9	11.2
Indiana	11.9	23.4	10.5	14.8	23.5	11.5	10.8	23.1	10.3
Kansas	10.4	20.6	9.5	17.9	19.8	16.3	9.7	21.1	9.1
Kentucky	12.9	22.0	12.0	21.0	28.6	18.9	12.6	21.3	11.9
Louisiana	14.3	20.6	10.5	14.6	19.8	10.3	13.6	25.3	10.9
Maryland	14.0	20.4	11.6	18.1	21.5	14.5	10.7	16.5	10.2
Michigan	12.8	24.2	10.6	17.2	25.8	10.8	11.3	21.1	10.6
Mississippi	17.0	23.7	11.1	18.3	23.9	11.3	13.2	22.4	10.8
Missouri	12.4	20.7	11.1	18.1	22.9	12.1	11.7	19.2	11.0
New Jersey	12.5	21.9	10.3	16.4	23.1	9.7	12.0	21.3	10.4
New York	12.5	20.0	10.8	16.0	19.6	14.5	11.0	20.5	9.8
North Carolina	14.5	20.0	12.1	15.0	19.7	12.0	13.5	21.6	12.4
Ohio	12.8	23.0	11.2	17.7	28.5	12.5	12.0	20.6	11.0
Pennsylvania	13.2	23.1	11.9	19.3	22.9	15.8	12.1	23.4	11.5
South Carolina	15.6	22.9	10.8	16.8	23.8	11.1	11.1	15.1	10.1
Tennessee	13.5	19.3	11.9	15.0	19.9	10.9	12.7	17.5	12.2
Texas	12.2	18.8	11.2	14.3	20.0	11.8	12.0	18.6	11.1
Virginia	13.6	19.8	11.9	15.0	20.0	12.1	11.7	19.0	11.7

NOTE: Entries are deaths per 1,000 live births.
[a] Counties containing 20% or more of a single minority group.
SOURCE: *Report of the Secretary's Task Force on Black and Minority Health* (Washington, DC: U.S. Department of Health and Human Services, 1985).

TABLE 3.7

Mortality and social cost data assembled by North Carolina public health staff to make a case to the state legislature for permanent funding of health promotion

Cause of death	1985 total number of deaths (ages 18–64)	1985 years of life lost (below age 65)	Lifetime lost wages, $[a]	Lifetime lost state income tax, $[b]	Lifetime lost general sales tax, $[c]
Cardiovascular disease	5,436	52,941	725,291,700	36,254,585	9,317,616
Cancer	4,475	47,353	648,736,100	32,436,805	8,334,128
All accidents	2,013	58,943	807,519,100	40,375,955	10,373,968
Subtotal	11,924	159,237	2,181,546,900	109,077,345	28,025,712
All other causes [d]	4,679	79,351	1,087,138,700	54,355,435	13,965,776
Total	16,603	238,588	3,268,685,600	163,432,780	41,991,488

NOTE: Total population in North Carolina ages 18–64 is 3,928,097 based on extrapolation from 1970–1980 census data, N.C. Office of State Budget and Management.

[a] Based on 1982 average yearly income of $13,700. *Statistical Abstract for State Government, 1984.* Figures in this column represent what could have been contributed if these persons had lived to age 65.

[b] 5% derived from net income and net income tax paid, 1982. Ibid. Figures in this column represent what could have been contributed if these persons had lived until age 65.

[c] For a family of three (average in N.C., 1980), $176 is the estimated sales tax paid, 1982 (Federal Income Tax Form). Figures in this column represent what could have been contributed if these persons had lived until age 65.

[d] Includes diabetes mellitus, pneumonia/influenza, chronic obstructive pulmonary disease; chronic liver disease/cirrhosis; nephritis/nephrosis; suicide; homicide; all other causes.

SOURCE: Adapted from North Carolina Department of Health, unpublished data.

These data present a sober reminder of the disproportionate burden of death, disease, and disability carried by minorities. It can be seen that the differences between the black and nonminority rates are large, and they are consistently in the same direction.

At this point you may ask if all this attention to data is truly applicable in the real world of the practitioner. An affirmative response to this question can be seen in Table 3.7, prepared by staff of the North Carolina Department of Health in 1986. These data on mortality rates and their social costs were assembled to support legislation that would establish a permanent, state-funded health promotion and disease prevention program. The report was prepared and presented to the North Carolina General Assembly to inform them of important, preventable problems. In July 1987, the Assembly passed the legislation and provided a program budget. The Michigan data shown in Tables 3.2 and 3.3 also contributed powerfully to the passage of that state's Senate bill for a tobacco tax to support smoking prevention and other health promotion initiatives through the creation of the Center for Health Promotion.[20]

SETTING PRIORITIES FOR HEALTH PROGRAMS

Setting sound program **priorities** for health promotion depends on objectively constructed descriptions of prevailing health problems and how they manifest in the target population. To select one problem from several, the following questions should be answered:

1. Which problem has the greatest impact in terms of death, disease, days lost from work, rehabilitation costs, disability (temporary and permanent), family disorganization, and cost to communities and agencies for damage repair or loss and cost recovery?
2. Are certain subpopulations, such as children, mothers, blacks, or Hispanics, at special risk?
3. Which problems are most susceptible to intervention?
4. Which problem is not being addressed by other agencies in the community? Is there a need that is being neglected?
5. Which problem, when appropriately addressed, has the greatest potential for an attractive yield in improved health status, economic savings, or other benefits?
6. Are any of the health problems highly ranked as a regional or national priority? (State health agencies are developing priorities among health problems, often based on local epidemiologic data.)

Elaborating on the scope and impact of the health problems helps the planner get a clear focus on the problems of the target population and its subgroups. With sufficiently detailed information, the process can also help in selecting the strategies to be used and deciding whether a program is to be preventive, curative, rehabilitative, or some combination thereof. Consider the complex problem of motor vehicle injuries. Prevention efforts might consist of trying to reduce drunken driving, increasing the use of seat belts in combination with consistent enforcement of a 55-mile-per-hour speed limit, or employing strategies to improve road markings and conditions in areas where crashes are most common. The emphasis of a curative program might be on immediate emergency medical services (including transportation of injury victims to the appropriate facility). A rehabilitative effort might deal with disabilities resulting from injuries, thereby increasing the number of victims who regain productive lives and the speed with which they do so. Epidemiologic information provides insights on which facet or facets of the problem will (or will not) yield to intervention and on which focus — preventive, curative, or rehabilitative — should predominate.

ETIOLOGY: ASSESSING THE DETERMINANTS OF HEALTH

Once you have identified the most important health problems, you can turn to identification of the factors that contributed to those health problems. Factors that increase the probability of developing a disease or health problem are called **risk factors**. Health promotion programs can improve the health status of a population by working to decrease behavioral and environmental risk factors. The purpose of the second part of the epidemiological assessment is to identify the known risk factors for the priority health problems.

Health problems have behavioral, environmental, and genetic or biological causes (risk factors). The association of the most commonly targeted behavioral and environmental risk factors with the leading causes of death are shown in Table 3.8. Although the epidemiological diagnosis for health promotion is directed toward factors that are changeable, consideration must also be given to unchangeable factors such as genetic predisposition, age, gender, race or ethnicity, existing disease, physical or mental impairment, or climate. These factors do not lend themselves to intervention, but they must be taken into account to keep a perspective on the multiple determinants of the health problem being addressed and to identify high-risk population groups.[21]

Health promotion programs attempt to modify the behavioral and the environmental risk factors over which people can exert control through individual or collective action. Examples include smoking cessation, heart-healthy eating, seat belt use, and exercise, on the behavioral side; and include living conditions such as housing, transportation, food policies, and social norms or regulations on the environmental side. Such causes can be influenced by the behavior of health professionals, the public, and the individuals at risk. Communities, neighborhoods, or special-interest groups can organize, vote, boycott, lobby, or otherwise support or prevent certain environmental and technological changes.

Thus, behavior can influence health directly, through changes in personal behavioral risk factors or actions that will build fitness and host resistance, as suggested by arrow 2 in Figure 3.4. Behavior also can indirectly affect health by influencing environmental factors. People can exercise some control in exposing themselves to environmental risks (such as solar radiation), and in using health services, and they can work through community channels to change some of the environmental risk factors. Figure 3.4 diagrams these two additional paths by which behavior (individual and collective actions) can improve health. Health promotion interventions, presented in the PROCEED portion of this text, are concerned with using both avenues to change as well as with reducing the environmental risk factors themselves.

TABLE 3.8

The most common priorities for health promotion programs are the ten leading causes of death and the changeable risk factors associated with them

Risk Factors	Heart disease	Cancers	Stroke	Injuries (nonvehicular)	Influenza Pneumonia	Injuries (vehicular)	Diabetes	Cirrhosis	Suicide	Homicides	AIDS
Behavioral risk factors											
Smoking	•	•		•	•						
High blood pressure	•		•								
High cholesterol	•										
Diet	•	•					•				
Obesity	•	•					•				
Lack of exercise	•	•	•				•				
Stress	•		•	•		•			•		
Alcohol abuse		•		•		•		•	•	•	
Drug misuse	•		•	•		•			•	•	•
Seat belt nonuse						•					
Handgun possession				•					•	•	
Sexual practices											•
Biological factors	•	•	•				•	•			
Environmental risk factors											
Radiation exposure		•									
Workplace hazards		•		•		•					
Environmental contaminants		•									
Infectious agents		•			•						
Home hazards				•							
Auto/road design						•					
Speed limits						•					
Medical care access	•	•	•		•		•	•	•	•	
Product design				•							
Social factors[a]	•		•	•		•	•		•	•	

[a] This residual category of risk factors includes a variety of less well defined lifestyle factors and conditions of living related to social relationships, social support, social pressures, and socioeconomic status.[22]

SOURCE: Adapted from unpublished material, Centers for Disease Control, U.S. Department of Health and Human Services.

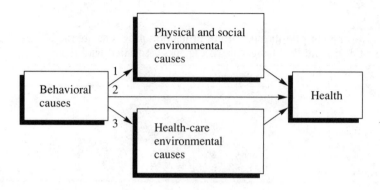

FIGURE 3.4

Three ways that behavior can influence health

WEIGHING THE RISK FACTORS FOR DISEASE

One of the purposes of epidemiology is to discover and calibrate the strength of risk factors for health problems. After much research, a consensus often develops about the strength of the association between a given risk factor and a specific health problem. The epidemiological assessment phase of PRECEDE includes identification of the known risk factors. The next phase in PRECEDE (Chapter 4), the behavioral and environmental assessment, determines which of those risk factors are present, and at what level, in the target population or community.

The health promotion planner should identify the known risk factors for those health problems that were prioritized in the first part of the epidemiological assessment. The epidemiological literature on the relative importance of specific risk factors listed in Table 3.8 is often summarized in consensus documents or federal publications, which planners can consult for information about a variety of health problems.[23]

If cardiovascular disease were found to be a priority health problem, the planner could consult consensus documents or review articles to generate a list of risk factors such as those shown in Table 3.9. The table presents the known risk factors for cardiovascular disease categorized by whether they are behavioral or not. Some are easy to classify in this way, and some more difficult. Smoking, heavy alcohol consumption, high fat diet, and sedentary lifestyle are clearly behavioral, whereas gender, age, and family history of heart attacks are clearly nonbehavioral. Other factors such as high serum cholesterol, obesity, high blood pressure, and stress, are not strictly behavioral but are associated with behavior. High blood pressure, serum cholesterol level, and obesity are all linked to eating habits; stress is associated with behaviors such as overworking, not taking time to relax, or not exercising enough.

TABLE 3.9
Risk factors for cardiovascular disease

Nonbehavioral	Behavioral	Related to behavior
Gender	Smoking	High blood pressure
Age	High-fat diet	Elevated serum cholesterol
Family history of disease	Heavy alcohol consumption	Stress
Diabetes	Sedentary lifestyle	Obesity

Lists of known risk factors, such as shown in Tables 3.8 and 3.9, help the program planner determine which risk factors will be most important for inclusion in a health promotion program. In the behavioral and environmental assessment, the next step in PRECEDE, the planner assesses those known risk factors in the target population for their prevalence and importance in order to set priorities among them for intervention.[24]

MEASURE OF DISEASE ASSOCIATION

To determine which factors increase the risk of developing disease, epidemiological studies employ measures of disease association. The health promotion planner should be familiar with these measures in order to understand epidemiological findings and the relative importance of the risk factors.

Measures of association relate the degree of exposure to a factor (a possible risk factor) to the development of the health problem of interest (e.g., disease or death). The most commonly used measure is **relative risk**. Relative risk compares the risk of people exposed to a factor developing the health problem to the risk of people not exposed. This is done by dividing the incidence of the health problem in the exposed population by that in the nonexposed:

$$\text{Relative risk} = \frac{\text{Incidence of the problem in those exposed to the risk factor}}{\text{Incidence of the problem in those not exposed to the risk factor}}$$

If the risk of developing the disease is greater in the exposed group, the relative risk is greater than 1. Thus, a relative risk tells you how many *times* greater the risk is in persons exposed to the risk factor. For example, the relative risk of developing coronary heart disease (CHD) in smokers compared with nonsmokers is about 2. Thus, smokers have two times the rate of CHD than nonsmokers; that

TABLE 3.10

Relative risk for coronary heart disease risk factors in middle-aged men

Risk factor	Relative risk
Smoking[a]	2.0
Hypertension	2.4
Elevated serum cholesterol	2–3 (depending on level of elevation)
Diabetes	2.5
Obesity	2.1
Physical inactivity[b]	1.9

[a] See ref. 25 in References and Notes at end of this chapter.
[b] See ref. 26 in References and Notes at end of this chapter.
SOURCE: Compiled by Denise Simons-Morton, M.D. Smoking and physical inactivity relative risk estimates are from the references cited. The other relative risk estimates are from W. B. Kannel et al., *Circulation* 70(1): 155A–205A, 1984.

is, they are twice as likely to develop the disease, or, stated still another way, they are 100% more likely to develop the disease.

The size of the relative risk indicates the comparative importance of the factor to the development of disease. If factor A has a relative risk of 10 for a particular disease and factor B has a relative risk of 2, then you conclude that factor A is the stronger risk factor. Table 3.10 shows the relative risks of developing CHD for several risk factors. Evidence that the risk factors have about the same impact on disease occurrence, and that the presence of more than one risk factor in the same people further increases the risk of disease, provides a rationale for interventions addressing multiple risk factors.

The relative risk also provides an indication of the importance of a factor in different population groups. For example, as seen in Table 3.11, the relative risk of CHD death due to cigarette smoking for 1-2 pack per day smokers depends on the age of the smoker: the older the smoker, the less the relative risk. Understanding this principle provides a rationale for allocating resources or directing program focus to younger age groups.

Strong epidemiological evidence that a factor does, in fact, increase risk for disease is provided when there is a **dose-response relationship**. Such a relationship is shown in Table 3.12 for smoking and CHD death: the higher the number of cigarettes smoked per day, the higher the relative risk.[27]

The relative risk is sometimes called the **risk ratio**, and you may see other terms in the epidemiological literature, such as odds ratio (OR), or relative odds, and the standardized mortality or standardized morbidity ratio (SMR). All are estimates of the relative risk that are also used as measures of association, and these various risk ratios can be interpreted in the same way.

TABLE 3.11

Relative risks for coronary heart disease death for smokers of 20–40 cigarettes per day, by age group for men and women

Age group (years)	Relative Risk	
	Men	Women
40–49	3.76	3.62
50–59	2.40	2.68
60–69	1.91	2.08
70–79	1.49	1.27

SOURCES: Adapted from S. M. Grundy et al., *Circulation* 97 (1987): 1340A–62A. Data are from E. C. Hammond and L. Garfinkel, *Archives of Environmental Health* 19 (1969): 167–82.

TABLE 3.12

Relative risks for coronary heart disease death by number of cigarettes smoked per day, men and women, 40–79 years old

Number of cigarettes smoked daily	Relative risk	
	Men	Women
Nonsmoker	1.00	1.00
1–9	1.45	1.07
10–19	1.99	1.81
20–39	2.39	2.41
40+	2.89	3.02

SOURCES: Adapted from S. M. Grundy et al., *Circulation* 97 (1987): 1340A–62A. Data are from E. C. Hammond and L. Garfinkel, *Archives of Environmental Health* 19 (1969): 167–82.

In addition to the relative risk, the prevalence of a risk factor in a population helps one determine the impact the factor has on a population. This is discussed in more detail in the next chapter.

AN EXAMPLE: COAL MINERS IN APPALACHIA

The following is an example of the use of health status indicators and measures of association in epidemiological assessment. The local chapter of the American Lung Association (ALA) wants to sponsor a health promotion program for a population of coal miners in two northern counties of West Virginia. Epidemiological data clearly suggest that the incidence of lung disease in coal miners in this area is greater than it is in other areas of the state, a situation the ALA would like to change. The important risk factor for lung disease in this area is, not surprisingly, frequent exposure to coal mining.

If the health problem is studied in terms of behavioral, environmental, and biological causes, certain additional epidemiological questions arise: Do all miners get lung disease? Who does and who does not get lung disease? Are all mine workers male? Do those who get lung disease have a family history of the disease? Answers to questions about these nonbehavioral factors (age, gender, and family history) identify the high-risk groups.

Once the high-risk groups have been identified, one asks questions about behavioral and environmental factors. Is there a higher incidence of disease in workers who are exposed to different levels of coal dust because, for example, they work in different mine locations? Are there mines in which better air circulation is associated with lower rates of lung disease? Is there a higher incidence of disease in smokers than in nonsmokers? Such questions can help the practitioner select the behaviors that will be the focus of the behavioral assessment and the environmental factors that will be examined in the environmental assessment.[28]

PROTECTIVE FACTORS FOR POSITIVE HEALTH

The relationships between risk factors and disease illustrated thus far (e.g., smoking causes lung cancer and heart disease) can be construed as "negative," driven by a preoccupation with disease. This raises the concern of some who believe that too much attention to these epidemiologic aspects result in a disease or health-problem approach (negative) rather than a health and wellness (positive) approach. We wonder how valid or productive this concern really is.

Attention to, and a working knowledge of, the complex factors that compromise our health and quality of life do not dictate that the subsequent effort to resolve the problem has to be accompanied by a negative tone. The positiveness of the health education or health promotion program continues to be, as it always has been, a manifestation of the method and sensitivity with which the program is planned and delivered, not of the data and information used to justify the public health importance of the problem that the program is trying to mitigate.[29]

The data drive the policy, and policy generates resources. The use of "negative" information (AIDS is a disease caused mainly by unprotected sex and sharing of needles; smoking causes lung cancer and heart disease; and high dietary fat and sedentary behaviors are associated with numerous preventable health problems) has been instrumental in helping pry loose resources needed for comprehensive school, community, and worksite programs. The availability of these resources has enabled wonderfully talented teachers, nurses, physicians, physical educators, and others to develop positive, upbeat wellness program in schools, communities, and worksites the world over.

Virtually all epidemiologic data derive from a problem focus. On the positive side, epidemiologic risk-factor studies, such as the classic research of Belloc and Breslow, can be turned around to emphasize the factors that can *improve* health. They analyzed data from large-scale surveys of American adults and concluded that at least seven personal health practices are highly correlated with physical health: sleeping seven to eight hours daily, eating breakfast most days, rarely or never eating between meals, being at or near the recommended height–adjusted weight level, being a nonsmoker, using alcohol moderately or not at all, and participating in regular physical activity.[30]

These findings lent support to the lifestyle construct discussed in Chapter 1, showing that a combination of factors was associated with good health, not just one behavior alone. The study also showed correlation between positive health practices and positive physical health, rather than the usual relationship between negative risk behavior and mortality and disease.

For the skeptics, Breslow and Engstrom followed up the people originally interviewed in 1965, examining mortality records 5½ and 9½ years later. They found that, for both men and women and in all age groups, those who had practiced more of the health behaviors were less likely to have died than those who practiced fewer. Indeed, at 9½ years, men who were engaging in all seven practices in 1965 had experienced 72 percent lower mortality than those who practiced zero to three of the behaviors; for women, the figure was 57 percent. Most of these relationships held when researchers controlled for 1965 income level and health status.[31]

These data on positive health practices or lifestyle lend credibility to estimates that at least 50 percent of all premature mortality is attributable to health behavior and provide scientific justification for an emphasis on lifestyle determinants of health, especially if lifestyle is interpreted to encompass conditions of living. The evidence of improved physical health status associated with combined health actions provides a rationale for the emphasis on behavior for those whose mission is not primarily mortality control and for those who seek a more comprehensive or holistic approach to health. Further analysis of the same cohort in subsequent years showed a powerful social factor operating in the protective effects. Friendship networks and social ties added to the protective effects of the behavioral factors in the lifestyle of the Alameda County (California) cohort.[32]

DEVELOPING HEALTH OBJECTIVES

When the health problem has been specifically defined and the risk factors identified, the next step is to develop the program objectives. This vital phase in program planning is often treated quite superficially, with unfortunate consequences for program implementation and evaluation.

Objectives are crucial; they form a fulcrum, converting diagnostic data into program direction. Objectives should be cast in the language of epidemiological or medical outcomes and should answer these questions:

- *Who* will receive the program? (Whose health is its focus?)
- *What* health benefit should they receive?
- *How much* of that benefit should be achieved?
- *By when* should it be achieved, or for *how long* should the program run?

Consider the maternal and child health data presented earlier in this chapter (in the section on the Expansionist Approach). The following program objective was developed, based on those diagnostic data and consonant with the mission or resources of the agency:

- The infant mortality rate in counties A and B will be reduced by 10 percent within the first two years and by an additional 15 percent the next three years, the rates will continue to decline until the state average is reached.

The target population (the *who*) is demographically implied (pregnant women) and geographically explicit (within counties A and B). The *what* is reduced maternal mortality. *How much* benefit is to be achieved and *how fast* are stated in stages: a 10 percent reduction in two years, a 25 percent reduction in a total of five years, and the program is to continue until the state average rate is achieved. (Note that the average rate for the state probably will go down concurrently, so the program has tackled a moving target.)

In developing program objectives, the planner should strive to set up the plan so that:

1. Progress in meeting objectives can be measured.
2. Individual objectives are based on relevant, reasonably accurate data.
3. Objectives are in harmony across topics as well as across levels.

The third of these conditions, that objectives be in harmony across topics, implies consistency. It means that objectives dealing with various aspects of a health problem (e.g., the objectives of a maternity program to improve nutrition, prenatal appointment compliance, weight and blood pressure control, and percentage of hospital deliveries) should be consistent with each other. Much work has gone into developing the *Model Standards for Local Health Departments*[33] as a source of exemplary objectives for community health programs consistent with the disease prevention and health promotion objectives for the year 2000. These model objectives can be adapted to the local circumstances, but they represent the consensus of national experts on what local health programs should be expected to achieve in the 1990s.

Objectives should also be coherent across levels, with objectives becoming successively more refined and more explicit, level by level. In the usual language of health planners, goals are considered to be more general than objectives. For example, the maternal and child health program objective just presented is in reality part of a three-tier hierarchy of concordant objectives consisting of an overall program goal, a set of more specific program objectives, and a number of even more specific objectives stated in behavioral terms. Health objectives arise from the epidemiological assessment, and behavioral objectives are developed in the next phase of PRECEDE, the behavioral and environmental assessment:

PROGRAM GOAL

- The survival rate of mothers, infants, and children will be raised through the optimal growth and development of children.

HEALTH OBJECTIVES

- The maternal mortality rate within counties A and B will be reduced by 10 percent within the first two years and an additional 15 percent the next three years, with reductions continuing until the state average rate is reached.
- The infant mortality rate will be reduced to the state average within ten years. Perinatal mortality rate will be reduced from 49 percent. Fetal death will be reduced from x percent to y percent in the same period.

BEHAVIOR OBJECTIVES

- In the two counties, 1,850 women under age 40 who have had two or more pregnancies will have two general health checkups in the first year of the program.
- Eighty percent of pregnancies in this group will be detected within the first trimester, and prenatal care with special diets will be instituted.
- Ninety-five percent of the pregnant women will be delivered by qualified medical personnel in obstetric facilities during the first year of the program.

Note that the objectives in this example, ranging from the broadest statement of program mission to the most immediate and precise target, are coherent. Achievement of each of the more specific and more immediate objectives will contribute causally to the achievement of the more general and more distant objectives and goals.

ENSURING KNOWLEDGEABLE COOPERATION

Detailing the health problem helps to harmonize the activities of the various individuals and groups involved in the program. Health education usually is part of a larger endeavor, engaging a variety of disciplines and perhaps several units within an agency. Hospital-based health programs, for example, might function across inpatient and outpatient units and might involve social service and nutrition departments. Programs based in a health department will often deploy staff from various personal-health-services units as well as from environmental protection and other sections.

The more heterogeneity there is among participants (and, therefore, perspectives), the greater the utility of sharply delineated statements of the problem. All participants in the activity need to share a full understanding of it. Understanding is further facilitated when program goals and subobjectives are thoroughly spelled out. A coalition of disparate agencies will remain together through difficult negotiations and disagreements on methods if they can be reminded of a common goal that all agree is worth the effort. We address this important issue in more detail in Chapter 6 and 8.

SUMMARY

This chapter highlights the relationship between health problems and social problems, the methods by which health problems are quantified and prioritized and the assessment of determinants of health.

Health professionals usually do not address social problems directly, but it is instructive to analyze the relationship between each health problem addressed by a program and the quality of life. Health problems should be described in detail using data from local, regional, state, and national sources interpreted against a background of current epidemiological knowledge as reflected in the literature. Particular attention must be directed toward identifying existing data on who is most affected (age, sex, race, residence), the ways in which they are affected (mortality, disability, signs, symptoms), and the most likely routes to improvement (impact of immunizations, treatment regimens, environmental alterations, behavioral changes). This information helps set program priorities for health problems that are both important and changeable.

The program's health priorities are expressed as objectives by specifying *who will benefit how much of what outcome by when*. A thorough epidemiological diagnosis is basic to the next phase of the PRECEDE framework: identifying the behavioral components of the health problem.

EXERCISES

1. List the health problems related to the quality-of-life concerns identified in your population in Exercise 3, Chapter 2.
2. Rate (low, medium, high) each health problem in the inventory according to
   (a) its relative importance in affecting the quality-of-life concerns and
   (b) its potential for change.
3. Discuss the reasons for your giving high-priority ratings to health problems in Exercise 2a in terms of their prevalence, incidence, cost, virulence, severity, or other relevant dimensions. Extrapolate from national, state, or regional data when local data are not available.
4. Cite the evidence supporting your ratings of health problems in Exercise 2b. Refer to the success of other programs and/or to the availability of medical or other technology to control or reduce the high-priority health problems you have selected.
5. Cite two uses for data generated by epidemiologic assessments other than for program planning, and give an example of each.
6. Write a program objective for the highest-priority health problem, indicating who will show how much of what improvement by when.

REFERENCES AND NOTES

1. We are indebted to Denise Simons-Morton, M.D., M.P.H., Department of Community Medicine, Baylor College of Medicine, for her special contributions to this chapter while she was a Postdoctoral Fellow at the Center for Health Promotion Research and Development, University of Texas Health Science Center at Houston.

2. National Center for Health Statistics, *Health, United States, 1988* (Washington, DC: U.S. Government Printing Office, DHHS-PHS-89-1232, 1989); F. P. Rivara, P. J. Sweeney, and B. F. Henderson, "A Study of Low Socioeconomic Status, Black Teenage Fathers and Their Nonfather Peers," *Pediatrics* 107 (1985): 648–56; D. Taylor, *Medicines, Health and the Poor World* (London: Office of Health Economics, 1982); World Bank, *World Development Report, 1983* (New York: Oxford University Press, 1983).

3. L. Schorr, *Within Our Reach: Breaking the Cycle of Disadvantage* (New York: Doubleday/Anchor, 1988).

4. S. Chapman, "Intersectoral Action to Improve Nutrition: The Roles of the State and the Private Sector. A Case Study from Australia," *Health Promotion International* 5 (1990): 35–44; B. Haughton, "Developing Local Food Policies: One City's Experiences," *Journal of Public Health Policy* 8 (1987): 180–91.

5. Health and Welfare Canada, *Canada's Health Promotion Survey: Technical Report* (Ottawa: Minister of Supply and Services Canada, 1988); Statistics Canada and Department of the Secretary of State of Canada, *Report of the Canadian Health and Disability Survey* (Ottawa: Minister of Supply and Services Canada, Catalog No. 82-555, 1986).

6. Australia, Department of Transport and Communication, *Road Crash Statistics Australia* (Canberra: Department of Transport and Communication, 1987); Australian Bureau of Statistics, *Deaths Australia* (Canberra: Australian Bureau of Statistics Cat. No. 3302.0, 1986); Better Health Commission, *Looking Forward to Better Health* (Canberra: Australian Government Printing Service, vols. 1–3, 1986).

7. National Center for Health Statistics, *Health, United States, 1988* (Washington, DC: U.S. Government Printing Office, DHHS-PHS-89-1232, 1989). This annual publication, in addition to its detailed tables comparing health status and health behavior statistics between regions, states, and demographic groups, also contains a detailed description of the sources and limitations of vital and health data systems of the federal government and various other national organizations (Appendix I), and a glossary of social and demographic terms used in health statistics. See also, for sources particularly relevant to health promotion, L. W. Green and F. M. Lewis, *Measurement and Evaluation in Health Education and Health Promotion* (Palo Alto, CA: Mayfield, 1986), pp. 128–45.

8. *Source Book of Health Insurance Data, 1989* (New York: Health Insurance Association of America, 1989), p. 75.

9. T. Abelin, Z. T. Brzenzinski, and V. D. Carstairs, eds., *Measurement in Health Promotion and Protection* (Copenhagen: WHO Regional Office for Europe, European Series, No. 22, 1987); M. Bergner and M. L. Rothman, "Health Status Measures: An Overview and Guide for Selection," *Annual Review of Public Health* 8 (1987): 191–210; J. Fries, L. W. Green, and S. Levine, "Health Promotion and the Compression of Morbidity," *Lancet* 1 (1989): 481–4; L. W. Green, "Some Challenges to Health Services Research on Children and the Elderly," *Health Services Research* 19 (1985): 793–815; R. R. Pate, "A New Definition of Fitness," *The Physician and Sports Medicine* 11 (1983): 77–82; B. Rimer, M. K. Keintz, B. Glassman, and J. L. Kinman, "Health Education for Older Persons: Lessons Learned from Research and Program Evaluations," in *Advances in Health Education and Promotion*, vol. 1, W. B. Ward, ed. (Greenwich, CT: JAI Press, 1986), pp. 369-96.

10. In use since 1982, Years of Potential Life Lost (YPLL) measure the impact of diseases and injuries that kill people before the customary age of retirement. It is computed as the sum of products over all age groups up to the age of 65, sometimes 75, each product being the annual number of deaths in an age group multiplied by the average number of years remaining before the age of 65 for that age group. See Centers for Disease Control, "Premature Mortality in the United States: Public Health Issues in the Use of Years of Potential Life Lost," *Morbidity and Mortality Weekly Report* 35 (suppl., 1986): 2S.

11. Division of Health Education, Center for Health Promotion and Education, Centers for Disease Control, *Reference Manuals: Planned Approach to Community Health* (Atlanta: Centers for Disease Control, 1988).

12. L. W. Green, R. W. Wilson, and K. Bauer, "Data Required to Measure Progress on the Objective for the Nation in Disease Prevention and Health Promotion," *American Journal of Public Health* 73 (1983): 18–24; M. W. Kreuter, G. M. Christianson, M. Freston, and G. Nelson, "In Search of a Baseline: The Need for Risk Prevalence Surveys," *Proceedings of the Annual National Risk Reduction Conference* (Atlanta: Centers for Disease Control, 1981).

13. L. W. Green, R. W. Wilson, and K. Bauer, 1983, op. cit.

14. Office of Health and Medical Affairs, Department of Management and Budget and Center for Health Promotion, Michigan Department of Health, *Health Promotion Can Produce Economic Savings* (Lansing, MI: Center for Health Promotion, Michigan Department of Public Health, 1987), p. 7.

15. Ibid., p. 9.

16. D. D. Celentano and D. Holtzman, "Breast Self-Examination Competency: An Analysis of Self-Reported Practice and Associated Characteristics," *American Journal of Public Health* 73 (1983): 1321-3; S. W. Fletcher, T. M. Morgan, M. S. O'Malley et al., "Is Breast Self-Examination

Predicted by Knowledge, Attitudes, Beliefs, or Sociodemographic Characteristics?" *American Journal of Preventive Medicine* 5 (1989): 207–16; J. G. Zapka and J. A. Mamon, "Breast Self-Examination in Young Women. II. Characteristics Associated with Proficiency," *American Journal of Preventive Medicine* 2 (1986): 70–8.

17. L. J. Brailey, "Effects of Health Teaching in the Workplace on Women's Knowledge, Beliefs, and Practices Regarding Breast Self-Examination," *Research in Nursing and Health* 9 (1986): 223–31; L. W. Green, "Site- and Symptom-Related Factors in Secondary Prevention of Cancer," in *Cancer: The Behavioral Dimensions*, J. Cullen, B. Fox, and R. Isom, eds. (New York: Raven Press, 1976), pp. 45–61; L. W. Green, B. Rimer, and T. W. Elwood, "Public Education," in *Cancer Epidemiology and Prevention*, D. Shottenfeld and J. Fraumeni, Jr., eds. (Philadelphia: W. B. Saunders, 1982), pp. 1100–10; J. A. Mamon and J. G. Zapka, "Breast Self-Examination by Young Women. I. Characteristics Associated with Frequency," *American Journal of Preventive Medicine* 2 (1986): 61–9; J. G. Zapka and J. A. Mamon, "Integration of Theory, Practitioner Standards, Literature Findings and Baseline Data: A Case Study in Planning Breast Self-Examination Education," *Health Education Quarterly* 9 (1982): 330–56.

18. National Center for Health Statistics, *Health, United States, 1988* (Washington, DC: Government Printing Office, DHHS-PHS-89-1232, 1989).

19. *Report of the Secretary's Task Force on Black and Minority Health* (Washington, DC: U.S. Department of Health and Human Services, 1985).

20. W. Sederburg, R. Ortwein, and W. Durr, *Michigan's Health Initiative* (Lansing, MI: Michigan State Legislature, no date); M. W. Kreuter, "Statement to the Michigan Senate Health Committee on Senate Bills 4 and 5," unpublished, Atlanta, Centers for Disease Control, Feb. 5, 1985; V. M. Hawthorne, G. Pohl, and G. V. Amburg, *Smoking is Killing Your Constituents: Deaths Due to Smoking by Michigan State Senate Districts* (Lansing, MI: Division of Health Education, Michigan Department of Public Health, November 1984).

21. For discussions and applications of the determinants of health and the Health Field Concept in health promotion, see L. W. Green, *Community Health*, 6th ed. (St. Louis: Times Mirror/Mosby, 1990), chap. 2; J. M. Raeburn and I. Rootman, "Towards an Expanded Health Field Concept: Conceptual and Research Issues in a New Era of Health Promotion," *Health Promotion: An International Journal* 3 (1988): 383–92.

22. For discussions and examples of these social factors as risk factors for disease and premature death, see G. K. Beauchamp and M. Moran, "Dietary Experience and Sweet Taste Preference in Human Infants," *Appetite: Journal for Intake Research* 3 (1982): 139–52; N. H. Gottlieb and L. W. Green, "Life Events, Social Network, Life-style, and Health: An Analysis of the 1979 National Survey of Personal Health Practices and Consequences," *Health Education Quarterly* 11 (1984): 91–105; idem., "Ethnicity and Lifestyle Health Risk: Some Possible Mechanisms," *American Journal of Health Promotion* 2 (1987): 37–45; J. E. Keil, "Incidence of Coronary Heart Disease in Blacks in Charleston, South Carolina," *American Heart Journal* 108 (1984): 779; L. Polissar, D. Sim, and A. Francis, "Survival of Colorectal Cancer Patients in Relation to Duration of Symptoms and Other Prognostic Factors," *Diseases of the Colon and Rectum* 24 (1981): 364–9.

23. Examples of consensus documents include *Healthy People: The Surgeon General's Report on Health Promotion and Disease Prevention* (Washington, DC: U.S. Department of Health, Education, and Welfare, 1979); Food and Nutrition Board, National Research Council, *Diet and Health* (Washington, DC: National Academy Press, 1989); R. W. Amler and H. B. Dull, *Closing the Gap: The Burden of Unnecessary Illness* (New York: Oxford University Press, 1987); U.S. Preventive Services Task Force, *Guide to Clinical Preventive Services* (Philadelphia, PA: Williams and Wilkens, 1989); Committee on Trauma Research, *Injury in America: A Continuing Public Health Problem* (Washington, DC: National Academy Press, 1985).

24. For further examples of and distinctions between the epidemiological and the sociobehavioral and environmental levels of assessment in health promotion planning, see L. W. Green, B. Rimer, and T. W. Elwood, "Biobehavioral Approaches to Cancer Prevention and Detection," in *Perspectives on Behavioral Medicine*, S. Weiss, A. Herd, and B. Fox, eds. (New York: Academic Press, 1981),

pp. 215–34; L. W. Green, F. M. Lewis, and D. M. Levine, "Balancing Statistical Data and Clinician Judgments in the Diagnosis of Patient Educational Needs," *Journal of Community Health* 6 (1980): 79–91; D. E. Morisky, D. M. Levine, J. C. Wood et al., "Systems Approach for the Planning, Diagnosis, Implementation and Evaluation of Community Health Education Approaches in the Control of High Blood Pressure," *Journal of Operations Research* 50 (1981): 625–34; V. L. Wang, P. Terry, B. S. Flynn et al., "Multiple Indicators of Continuing Medical Education Priorities for Chronic Lung Diseases in Appalachia," *Journal of Medical Education* 54 (1979): 803–11.

25. Office on Smoking and Health. *Health Consequence of Smoking: Cardiovascular Disease* (Washington, DC: U.S. Government Printing Office, 1987).

26. K. E. Powell, P. D. Thompson, and C. J. Caspersen et al., "Physical Activity and the Incidence of Coronary Heart Disease," *Annual Review of Public Health* 8 (1987): 253–87.

27. S. M. Grundy, P. Greenland, J. A. Herd, J. A. Huebesch et al., "Cardiovascular and Risk Factor Evaluation of Healthy American Adults: A Statement for Physicians by an Ad Hoc Committee Appointed by the Steering Committee, American Heart Association," *Circulation* 97 (1987):1340A–62A. Data from E. C. Hammond and L. Garfinkel, "Coronary Heart Disease, Stroke, and Aortic Aneurysm: Factors in the Etiology," *Archives of Environmental Health* 19 (1969):167–82.

28. For more detail and results on a similar epidemiological assessment applying PRECEDE, see V. Wang, P. Terry, B. S. Flynn et al., "Multiple Indicators of Continuing Medical Education Priorities for Chronic Lung Disease in Appalachia," *Journal of Medical Education* 54 (1979): 803–11; R. A. Windsor, L. W. Green, and J. M. Roseman, "Health Promotion and Maintenance for Patients with Chronic Obstructive Pulmonary Disease: A Review," *Journal of Chronic Disease* 33 (1980): 5–12.

29. L. W. Green, R. Wilson, and K. Bauer, "Data Required to Measure Progress on the Objective for the Nation in Disease Prevention and Health Promotion," *American Journal of Public Health* 73 (1983): 18–24; L. W. Green, "Some Challenges to Health Services Research on Children and the Elderly," *Health Services Research* 19 (1985): 793–815.

30. N. B. Belloc and L. Breslow, "Relationship of Physical Health Status and Health Practices," *Preventive Medicine* 1 (1972): 409–21; N. B. Belloc, "Relationship of Health Practices and Mortality," *Preventive Medicine* 3 (1973): 125–35.

31. L. Breslow and J. D. Egstrom, "Persistence of Health Habits and Their Relationship to Mortality," *Preventive Medicine* 9 (1980): 469–83.

32. L. F. Berkman and L. Breslow, *Health and Ways of Living: The Alameda County Study* (New York: Oxford University Press, 1983). For more on the social support factor, see J. M. G. Cwikel, T. E. Dielman, J. P. Kirscht, and B. A. Israel, "Mechanisms of Psychosocial Effects on Health: The Role of Social Integration, Coping Style and Health Behavior," *Health Education Quarterly* 15 (1988): 151–73; M. Minkler, "The Social Component of Health," *American Journal of Health Promotion* 1 (1986): 33–8; P. Thoits, "Conceptual, Methodological and Theoretical Problems in Studying Social Support as a Buffer Against Life Stress," *Journal of Health and Social Behavior* 23 (1982): 145–59; B. Wallston, S. Alagna, B. DeVellis, and R. DeVellis, "Social Support and Physical Health," *Health Psychology* 2 (1983): 367–91.

33. *Model Standards: A Guide for Community Preventive Health Services*, 2nd ed. (Atlanta: Centers for Disease Control, 1985).

Chapter 4

Behavioral and Environmental Diagnosis

PRECEDE

Phase 5 Administrative and policy diagnosis	**Phase 4** Educational and organizational diagnosis	**Phase 3** Behavioral and environmental diagnosis	**Phase 2** Epidemiological diagnosis	**Phase 1** Social diagnosis

Phase 6 Implementation	**Phase 7** Process evaluation	**Phase 8** Impact evaluation	**Phase 9** Outcome evaluation

PROCEED

125

W e have described health promotion as a process of enabling people to increase control over the determinants of their health and thereby to improve their health. We have defined the strategy of health promotion as any combination of educational and environmental supports for actions and conditions of living that are conducive to health. Those actions may be the personal health behavior and lifestyle adaptations of individuals and families, the advocacy of policy to assure healthful living conditions, or direct intervention by individuals or groups to improve environmental living conditions. Phase 3 of the PRECEDE planning process calls for an analysis of those personal and collective actions that are most pertinent to controlling the determinants of health or quality-of-life issues selected in the preceding phases. This chapter outlines the steps in conducting a behavioral assessment and then the steps in conducting an environmental assessment.

Simply stated, **behavioral diagnosis** or behavioral assessment is a systematic analysis of the behavioral links to the goals or problems that were identified in the epidemiological or social diagnoses. The **environmental diagnosis** is a parallel analysis of factors in the social and physical environment, other than specific actions, that could be causally linked to the **behavior** that was identified in the behavioral diagnosis, or directly to the outcomes of interest (health or quality of life).

In the matter of definitions, we depart from the distinction made between health promotion and health protection in the United States health policy initiative.[1] In the federal policy documents, health promotion is directed at the lifestyle and behavioral determinants of health (for both individuals and communities) whereas health protection is directed at the physical **environment** in order to control potential threats to health and safety through engineering. Because health promotion components exist in health protection, and vice versa, we do not attempt to maintain this rigid distinction but favor the European and World Health Organization use of the term *health promotion*, which encompasses both the behavioral and environmental determinants of health.

WHY AN EMPHASIS ON BEHAVIOR?

Health workers of all disciplines and professional roles share the long-term goal of improving the health and quality of life of the people they serve. To succeed, they must have the active and effective participation of the people whose health they seek to improve. Behavior is thus a critical variable in the relationship between professional or program interventions on one hand and health or quality-of-life outcomes on the other. Virtually all members of a target population, other than terminally comatose patients, can play an active role in improving their health. Even surgical patients can make a major difference in their post-operative recovery outcomes—for example, by following specific instructions for breathing, coughing, and moving while in bed.[2] Behavior is an inescapable influence in most of medicine and all of health promotion.

The extent to which behavior can decrease a person's years of potential life can only be inferred from the association of behavior with the leading causes of death (see Fig. 3.4); but as distinct from environmental, genetic or biological, and technological (medical) influences, the loss due to behavior has been roughly estimated at 50% or more.[3] At least half of the mortality in this country, by this estimate, is attributable to behavioral or lifestyle causes. This estimate is derived by working backward from the distribution of annual deaths in a population to the risk factors associated with each of those causes, a process parallel to PRECEDE. What this estimate does not address are the causes of behavior and the interaction of behavior and environment in their influence on health.

MEASUREMENT OF BEHAVIORS IN POPULATIONS

Recognition of the role of behavior in determining health has inevitably produced a rapid growth of survey activity to assess the distribution patterns of health behavior. For example, to provide a means of monitoring progress on the 1990 objectives for the nation, the National Center for Health Statistics created and administered a major health promotion/disease prevention supplement to the National Health Interview Survey in 1979 and 1985, with a follow-up scheduled for 1990. Among other things, the Supplement assesses all the principal behavioral risk factors associated with the leading causes of death, disease, and disability in the United States.[4] A similar survey was developed by the Canadian Health and Welfare Department, using PRECEDE as part of the conceptual framework.[5] Comparisons of the U.S. and Canadian adult populations were published in 1988.[6] These data now provide a set of baselines and norms for comparison of community survey results. Most communities, however, cannot afford to administer the full questionnaire.

Shorter or more specialized behavioral surveys are conducted at state, provincial, and local levels.[7] The Centers for Disease Control has developed a Behavioral Risk Factor Surveillance System (BRFSS), which continually assesses the prevalence of behavioral risks in the majority of U.S. states. In addition to state-level assessments, the BRFSS questionnaire has been applied extensively at the local level.[8] School-based surveys to obtain similar data on children and youth have been conducted nationally in Canada and the United States.[9]

The Department of Public Health in Toronto (Ontario) applied the BRFSS as a part of a community survey, the results of which have been used to guide health policy and programs to meet the needs of Toronto residents. Tables 4.1 and 4.2 display the percentages of persons sampled, by age and sex, who engage in selected behavioral risks and preventive health practices. The health leaders of Toronto described their use of this kind of behavioral data as follows:

TABLE 4.1

Percentage of persons sampled who engage in selected behavioral risks, Toronto, Canada, 1983

Risk factor (N, number sampled)	All ages			Age 15–34			Age 35–54			Age 55 and older		
	Both sexes %	Male %	Female %	Both sexes %	Male %	Female %	Both sexes %	Male %	Female %	Both sexes %	Male %	Female %
Alcohol consumption (N=976)												
Heavy drinker	9	14	5	7	13	3	12	17	8	7	12	5
Moderate drinker	35	42	31	37	43	32	39	43	35	29	36	25
Light drinker	41	32	47	43	34	51	38	29	45	39	33	42
Abstainer	15	12	17	13	10	14	11	11	12	25	19	27
Cigarette smoking (N=978)												
Current smoker	36	41	32	37	42	32	38	46	32	31	30	32
Former smoker	22	25	20	17	13	19	21	22	20	33	55	22
Never smoked regularly	2	3	2	2	3	1	4	2	5	2	2	2
Never smoked	40	32	45	45	42	47	37	30	43	33	12	44
Physical exercise (N=981)												
Sedentary	7	7	7	5	5	5	10	9	10	9	9	8
Somewhat active	11	9	13	8	7	9	11	10	12	18	14	21
Moderately active	33	28	36	19	15	22	35	34	35	55	52	56
Active	49	55	44	69	74	65	45	47	43	18	25	15
Hypertension												
Diagnosed	15	13	17	7	8	7	12	13	11	33	25	37
Medication prescribed (N=149)	69	56	77	20	6	35	68	76	56	90	81	93
Medication compliance (N=104)	93	100	90	100	100	100	91	100	80	93	100	91
Uncontrolled (N=104)	31	32	30	29	0	33	30	31	30	31	35	30
N, total	981	410	571	448	197	251	283	128	155	250	85	165
Percentage of total sample	100	42	58	46	20	26	29	13	16	25	9	17

SOURCE: Adapted from *The City of Toronto Community Health Survey: A Description of the Health Status of Toronto Residents* (Toronto: City of Toronto Department of Public Health, July 1984).

One outcome of the Community Health Survey will be its use for planning program interventions with identifiable groups of City residents. Until recently, the Health Department has had morbidity data only at the aggregated level, that is, for the City as a whole. Even when it was possible to examine the information at the census tract level (for areas of 2,500 to 8,000 people) we could not link a range of characteristics of individuals (such as socio-demographic features) with their health status. This survey therefore expands the Department's profile of the health of citizens of the City of Toronto. It becomes part of an integrated data base that will enable us to target groups of citizens who suffer ill health and identify in which areas of the City they reside.

For example, we may determine from the future analysis of our survey data that 15-24 year old men in 'XYZ' ethnic group in the City of Toronto drink or smoke excessively compared to other 15-24 year old men. From our census data we will know in which Health Areas, and even census tracts, these young men would most likely reside and, thus, where health promotion efforts would most likely be effective. We can then efficiently target a specific health promotion program/aimed at reducing the health risk factor found in these areas of the city in 'XYZ' language and in a form that is socially and culturally geared to this specific group.[10]

The data presented in Chapter 3 on health status and health practices lend support to the estimate that at least 50 percent of premature mortality (years of potential life lost) is attributable to health behavior. Although some skeptics question the precision of that estimate, they cannot escape the dominant count of behavioral risk factors associated with the 12 leading causes of death summarized in Table 4.3. Most of the risk factors shown for these 12 causes of death, which account for the vast majority of all deaths and medical care costs in Western countries, are directly controllable through the behaviors of individuals, families, organizations, and communities, and through social policies and environments supporting such behaviors.

Behavioral diagnosis is directed toward specific behaviors, but health problems have nonbehavioral causes, which also must receive careful consideration. These include the personal factors that are least controllable by individual or collective action but that do contribute to health problems. Among the least modifiable or controllable factors are genetic predisposition, age, gender, existing disease, physical and mental impairment, and places of work and residence, which encompass various social and environmental factors beyond the control of the individual.

Some of the nonbehavioral risk factors beyond the control of individuals do lend themselves to community intervention; and to a lesser degree, individuals can avoid or limit their exposure to environmental risks such as solar radiation, lead paint, and ambient smoke. We discuss some of these risks in the environmental diagnosis section in this chapter and some in the educational diagnosis section in the next chapter. The significance of the nonbehavioral risk factors here is that they contribute to the goals and problems of health and quality of life.

TABLE 4.2

Percentage of persons sampled who engage in preventive health practices, Toronto, Canada, 1983

Health practice (N, number sampled)	All ages			Age 15–34			Age 35–54			Age 55 and older		
	Both sexes %	Male %	Female %	Both sexes %	Male %	Female %	Both sexes %	Male %	Female %	Both sexes %	Male %	Female %
Seat belt use (N=977)	74	71	77	72	69	75	73	70	75	80	79	81
Annual blood pressure checkup (N=976)	79	72	84	76	68	82	76	69	82	88	86	88
Dentist visit within last year	61	53	67	67	60	72	63	47	75	49	47	50
Dental floss or water pick use daily	19	13	22	21	14	26	20	13	26	12	12	13
Pap test within the last year (N=569)	–	–	53	–	–	66	–	–	55	–	–	32
Annual breast exam by physician (N=568)	–	–	62	–	–	67	–	–	68	–	–	49
Regular breast self-examination	–	–	20	–	–	19	–	–	17	–	–	26
N, total	981	410	571	448	197	251	283	128	155	250	85	165
Percentage of total sample	100	42	58	46	20	26	29	13	16	25	9	17

SOURCE: Adapted from *The City of Toronto Community Health Survey: A Description of the Health Status of Toronto Residents* (Toronto: City of Toronto Department of Public Health, July 1984).

TABLE 4.3

Prominent controllable risk factors for leading causes of death in the United States

Cause of death	Risk factors
Heart disease and stroke	Smoking, high blood pressure, elevated serum cholesterol, diabetes, obesity, lack of exercise
Cancer	Smoking, alcohol misuse, diet, solar radiation, ionizing radiation, worksite hazards, environmental pollution
Unintentional injuries other than motor vehicle	Alcohol misuse, smoking (fires), product design, home hazards, handgun availability
Motor vehicle injuries	Alcohol misuse, lack of safety restraints, excessive speed, automobile design, roadway design
Pneumonia and influenza	Smoking, infectious agents
Diabetes mellitus	Obesity (for adult-onset diabetes)
Cirrhosis of the liver	Alcohol ingestion
Suicide	Handgun availability, alcohol or drug misuse, stress
Homicide	Handgun availability, alcohol or drug misuse, stress
AIDS	Sexual practices, drug misuse, exposure to blood products

NOTE: The listed causes of death account for the vast majority of all mortality and morbidity in the more developed societies.

The health practitioner who takes into account the contribution of non-behavioral factors to health problems will be better able to

- maintain perspective on the multiple determinants of the health problem or goal,
- select and rank the behavioral and environmental determinants to become the targets of the program, and
- identify factors for which strategies other than health education (e.g., political, regulatory organizational interventions directed at control of the social or physical environment) may be developed and concurrently used as part of the total health promotion strategy.

Health policies that ignore the influence of nonbehavioral factors, placing all the responsibility for health protection on the individuals whose health is threatened, are vulnerable to the charge of "blaming the victim." Recognizing the nonbehavioral causes of health problems acknowledges that there are other threats to health besides the behavior of the victim.

Most of the modifiable nonbehavioral causes of health problems are either environmental (air, water, roads, fluoridation, etc.) or technological (adequacy of medical care, health facilities). These factors can themselves be influenced by behavior, of the public, the victim, or, especially, by collective action. Communities, neighborhoods, or special-interest (e.g., self-help) groups can organize, vote, boycott, lobby, and otherwise support or prevent certain environmental and technological changes. Thus, behavior can influence health in three ways, one direct and two indirect, as shown in Figure 3.4.

THE FIVE STEPS IN BEHAVIORAL DIAGNOSIS

The steps in behavioral diagnosis are described using the following illustrative situation: A local health department has just completed a quality-of-life assessment and epidemiological diagnosis. On the basis of the findings, the director wants to allocate some of her resources to the health problem of cardiovascular disease. She gives a planning team, which includes community representatives, the task of developing a demonstration project to reduce the incidence of cardiovascular disease in the community. Epidemiological diagnosis has suggested that the intervention should include a component aimed at asymptomatic youth and young adults. The behavioral diagnosis comes next.

STEP 1 SEPARATING BEHAVIORAL AND NONBEHAVIORAL CAUSES OF THE HEALTH PROBLEM

The planner's first step is to delineate the behavioral and nonbehavioral causes of the health problem. One begins by reviewing the known risk factors for the disease in question, as identified in the epidemiological diagnosis (see Tables 3.8 and 3.9). Smoking, heavy alcohol consumption, high-fat diet, and sedentary lifestyle are clearly behavioral, whereas gender, age, and family history of heart attacks are clearly nonbehavioral. High serum cholesterol, obesity, high blood pressure, and stress are not strictly behavioral factors, yet they are obviously closely tied to behaviors. High blood pressure, serum cholesterol, and obesity are linked to eating habits; stress is associated with behaviors like working in a chaotic environment, having interpersonal conflicts, and not exercising enough.

STEP 2 DEVELOPING AN INVENTORY OF BEHAVIORS

The next step in the sequence is to refine the list of behavioral factors into two lists, one of preventive behaviors (primary, secondary, and tertiary) and one of the associated actions or treatment procedures:

a. Identify the behaviors associated with promoting health, preventing the health problem, or controlling the sequelae of the health problem. A useful typology is presented in Table 4.4, which shows a broad classification of various types of health behaviors.[11] Each of these types of behavior that is identified as associated with the health problem would then need to be analyzed further by specifying the particular actions to be undertaken for its accomplishment.

b. Identify and list sequentially the actions or treatment procedures for the health goal or problem. What are the steps that people have to take to reach their goal or to "comply" with the recommended method of prevention or treatment? Each step in a procedure can be identified as a particular behavior.

The major aim of step 2b is to generate an inventory of highly specific behaviors that can be used as the basis for specifying the behavioral objectives of the program. Table 4.5 shows such a list. Notice that many of the behaviors appear as both preventive and treatment behaviors. This is not at all unusual, and the information is valuable. If a single behavioral problem, such as smoking, appears in both parts of the inventory, a change in the behavior (stopping smoking) increases the probability of health improvement through both primary and secondary prevention. (*Primary prevention* consists of actions taken in the absence of signs or symptoms; *secondary prevention* is directed toward early detection and treatment.)

This list consists of several distinct behaviors, yet it is still crude and relatively nonspecific with respect to the actual behavioral steps one would have to take to achieve any one of these goals. Some of the behaviors comprise several specific behaviors and so can themselves be broken down into other lists of behaviors. For example, achieving or maintaining desirable weight results from such behaviors as buying low-calorie foods, cooking with less fat, serving smaller portions, eating fewer portions, and minimizing sugary desserts.

For the purpose of steps 2b, 3, and 4, the list in Table 4.5 is specific enough; but to translate the behaviors into behavioral objectives, they must be broken down into the actual steps that people must take to achieve each behavioral goal. One approach to analyzing behavior in more specific terms is to develop a flow chart of causation or transition from the beginning to the end of a behavioral process or event. For example, the behavior of taking a prescribed medication is preceded by other discrete behaviors such as seeking medical care, obtaining a prescription, and seeing that the medication is modified should that become necessary, as in the control of high blood pressure. This behavioral cycle could be sabotaged at many points—for example, if the hypertensive patient fails to keep the appointment at which prescriptions are to be renewed or changed. The broken-appointment cycle can be analyzed into a series of causes and effects (Fig. 4.1). This level of specificity makes it possible to separate concrete behavioral events from non-behavioral factors so that educational and administrative interventions can be accurately targeted to the people or the events and conditions that influence behavior. Training of staff, adjustment of appointment schedules, and child care or transportation provisions all could be identified as relevant interventions by the behavioral assessment reflected in the broken-appointment cycle.

TABLE 4.4

A typology of health-related behaviors

Behaviors	Definitions
Wellness behavior	Any activity undertaken by an individual, who believes himself to be healthy, for the purpose of attaining an even greater level of health.
Preventive health behavior	Any activity undertaken by an individual, who believes himself to be healthy, for the purpose of preventing illness or detecting it in an asymptomatic state.
At-risk behavior	Any activity undertaken by an individual, who believes himself to be healthy but at greater risk of developing a specific health condition, for the purpose of preventing that condition or detecting it in an asymptomatic state.
Illness behavior	Any activity undertaken by an individual, who perceives himself to be ill, to define the state of his health and discover a suitable remedy.
Self-care behavior	Any activity undertaken by an individual, who considers himself to be ill, for the purpose of getting well. It includes minimal reliance on appropriate therapists, involves few dependent behaviors, and leads to little neglect of one's usual duties.
Sick-role behavior	Any activity undertaken by an individual, who considers himself to be ill, for the purpose of getting well. It includes receiving treatment from appropriate therapists, generally involves a whole range of dependent behaviors, and leads to some degree of neglect of one's usual duties.
Family planning behavior	Any activity undertaken by an individual to influence the occurrence or normal continuation of pregnancy.
Parenting health behavior	Any wellness, preventive, at-risk, illness, self-care, or sick-role behavior performed by an individual for the purposes of ensuring, maintaining, or improving the health of a conceptus or child for whom the individual has responsibility.
Health-related social action	Any activity undertaken by an individual singularly or in concert with others (i.e., collectively) through organizational, legal, or economic means, to influence the provision of medical services, the effects of the environment, the effects of various products, or the effects of social regulations that influence the health of populations.

SOURCE: Adapted from L. J. Kolbe, in *Health Education and Youth: A Review of Research and Development*, in G. Campbell, ed. (Philadelphia: Falmer Press, 1984), as printed with permission in L. W. Green, *Annual Review of Public Health* 5 (1984): 215–36.

TABLE 4.5
Inventory of behaviors associated with reduction of mortality from cardiovascular disease

Preventive behaviors

1. Maintain or attain desirable weight.
2. Stop smoking (or don't start).
3. Stop heavy drinking (or don't start).
4. Continue or begin regular exercise.
5. Reduce consumption of foods high in saturated fats.
6. Avoid excessive, constant stress and/or do relaxation exercises.
7. Participate in high blood pressure and cholesterol screening programs.

Treatment behaviors

1. Make informed decisions regarding medication and surgery.
2. Keep scheduled appointments with health care providers.
3. Take medications as prescribed.
4. Maintain or reduce weight as prescribed.
5. Stop smoking.
6. Cut down alcohol consumption as prescribed.
7. Continue or begin regular exercise as prescribed.
8. Reduce consumption of foods high in saturated fat or sodium, as prescribed.

The broken-appointment cycle depicted in the figure illustrates a causal and sequential chain of behavior: The broken appointment means the patient will miss the medical assessment and advice needed to stay on a preventive or therapeutic course. The planner must ask, "Why are appointments made but not kept?" The motivation was there, but the behavior was somehow thwarted. Rather than leaping to the motivational question at this phase of the PRECEDE planning process, the planner should keep the focus on the behavior of other actors, including physicians, receptionists, and clinic administrators. The environmental circumstances surrounding the broken-appointment problem also should be assessed.

Chapter 11 presents a related example. The flow chart in Figure 11.1 shows several paths the individual can follow: recognition of symptoms, to seeking medical diagnosis, to obtaining a prescription, to either using, misusing, or not using the prescribed treatment. Each step involves one or more specific behaviors for which behavioral objectives and interventions can be designed, some for the public at large, some for patients, and some for the drug manufacturers, physicians, nurses, pharmacists, and other professionals and sectors relating to the issue.

STEP 3 RATING BEHAVIORS IN TERMS OF IMPORTANCE

With an extensive list of behaviors in hand, the next step is to reduce the list to a manageable length by establishing which behaviors are the most important and eliminating the least important. The following broad criteria provide guidelines for this task. The importance of a behavior is indicated if data are available showing that (1) the behavior occurs frequently and (2) is clearly linked to the health problem. Behaviors are also considered important if a strong theoretical case can be made for their being causally related to a health problem; in the absence of adequate data, such a relationship can be inferred from a thorough literature review. Based on these tests, a rationale is developed for selecting the behavior as a target of intervention.

Using the relative risk ratios in Chapter 3 (Table 3.10) and the prevalence data from surveys such as those mentioned at the beginning of this chapter, we can estimate the relative importance and prevalence of each behavior. In Table 4.6, eight key behaviors are ranked in terms of their importance as behavioral targets

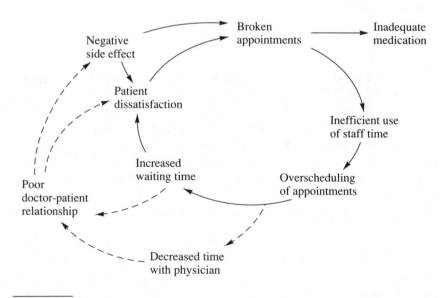

FIGURE 4.1

The broken appointment cycle

TABLE 4.6
Rating the relative importance of behaviors associated with cardiovascular disease prevention

Important	Basis for rating behavior
Smoking	Very strong risk ratio, high prevalence
Eating high-fat foods	Strong risk ratio, very high prevalence
Lack of exercise	
High stress	
	All unrelated to the desired outcome:
Less important	primary prevention
Not monitoring blood pressure	
Not adhering to medical prescription	
Not keeping medical appointments	
Making uninformed decisions about treatment	

for a primary prevention program to reduce the incidence of cardiovascular disease. The basis for these ratings is information on their incidence in the target population and the strength of their association with the disease.

STEP 4 RATING BEHAVIORS IN TERMS OF CHANGEABILITY

The fourth step in a behavioral diagnosis is rating behaviors in terms of changeability. How susceptible to change are the behaviors that have been selected? Even though a behavior is extremely important to a health problem, it is not a suitable program target unless there is reasonable expectation that it can be changed through health promotion. For example, it is claimed that excessive stress is associated with cardiovascular disease. A health promotion program directed to stress reduction would need to alter the major sources of stress, including the home and the workplace. How feasible is that for a health promotion program? The answer to such questions, about the environmental changes needed to support risk-factor changes, are deferred until we discuss environmental assessment later in this chapter.

Judgments about changeability must also include careful consideration of the time factor: How much time does the program have to show change? More deeply rooted and widespread behaviors are likely to take longer to change, making the time factor more important. Questions about time as a program resource, like other resource questions, can be answered more definitively at Phase 5 (Administrative and Policy Analysis, Chapter 6); at this phase, the judgments on changeability can be based primarily on evidence that the behavior has responded to interventions in previous studies and programs.

A few rules of thumb can help in determining the potential for behavior change. High changeability is probable when behaviors are still in the developmental stages or have only recently been established; low changeability is likely for behaviors that are deeply rooted in cultural patterns or lifestyles, and for behaviors that have been found not to change in previous attempts. Most resistant to change, or subject to the highest relapse rates, are those behaviors that have an addictive component (misuse of tobacco, alcohol, or drugs), those with deep-seated compulsive elements (compulsive eating or compulsive work), and those connected to strong family patterns or routines (eating, work, and leisure).

Behaviors that are not ruled out by applying these simple criteria can be further analyzed for changeability using another approach. This procedure, called the *attribute method*, examines the characteristics of the behavior that makes it easier or less easy to adopt, using criteria from the literature on the adoption of innovations.[12] The method is illustrated for the behaviors associated with cardiovascular disease in Table 4.7. Note that a total changeability score can be obtained by adding horizontally across the columns, scoring +1 for a plus sign and −1 for a minus sign. A more refined score can be obtained if the relative importance of the criteria can be estimated, allowing weighting factors to be applied. This procedure recognizes that not all criteria are equally important in determining the changeability of a behavior.[13]

By testing behaviors for changeability we come a step closer to an informal decision of which behaviors should be slated for intervention. Table 4.8 illustrates final changeability ratings for the case of cardiovascular disease, after taking into consideration the foregoing tables. Among the behaviors, only smoking prevention receives a high rating. Although arguments can be made against such a conclusion, findings in the literature on primary prevention of cardiovascular disease are, in fact, insufficiently consistent to place any of the other behaviors in the high changeability category with any confidence.

STEP 5 CHOOSING BEHAVIORAL TARGETS

With the behaviors ranked in terms of importance and changeability, the planner is ready to select the behavior or behaviors that will be the focus of the educational intervention. To facilitate that selection, we recommend that the ratings for importance and changeability be arranged in a simple fourfold table, as shown in Figure 4.2.

Depending on the program objectives, the behavioral objectives are more likely to derive from quadrants 1 and 2. Evaluation is crucial when you are uncertain about whether change will occur. Behaviors found in quadrant 3 are unlikely candidates except when there is political need to document change, as is the case when administrators or advisory committees need evidence of achievement. When such a need exists, the behaviors should be given priority on a

TABLE 4.7
Relative changeability based on perceived attributes of selected preventive health behaviors

Health behavior	Relevance	Social approval	Advantages	Complexity	Compatibility with values, experiences, and needs	Divisibility or trialability	Observability
1. Quitting smoking	+	+	+	−	−	+	+
2. Controlling weight	+	+	+	−	+	+	+
3. Controlling blood pressure	+	+	−	−	−	+	−
Taking medication	+	+	−	−	−	+	−
Maintaining low-sodium diet	+	+	−	−	−	+	−
4. Maintaining low-cholesterol diet	+	+	+	−	+	+	+
5. Exercising	+	+	+	0	+	+	+
6. Having preventive medical examinations	+	+	0	−	+	−	+

Note: + = positive, − = negative. Changes since the first edition in 1980 reflect changes in social norms and technologies. The only change in a negative direction has been in the complexity dimension of having preventive medical examinations. This is a manifestation of decreased support for indigent care and inaccessibility of health services to the rural and disadvantaged segments of the population in the United States.

Source: Adapted from L. W. Green, "Diffusion and Adoption of Innovations Related to Cardiovascular Risk Behavior in the Public," in *Applying Behavioral Sciences to Cardiovascular Risk*, A. Enelow and J. B. Henderson, eds. (New York: American Heart Association, 1975).

TABLE 4.8

Rating the changeability of behaviors associated with cardiovascular disease

Changeability	Basis for rating behavior
Most changeable	
Smoking	Recent trends and new research
Less changeable	
Eating foods with high fatty-acid content	These practices are deeply rooted in
Overeating	culture, social relationships, and lifestyle.
Exercise	Previous attempts to change them have had limited success.

temporary basis only. If no behaviors appear in quadrant 1, but the health problem is urgent, then extensive educational and behavioral research and evaluation is justified. This is often how agencies and foundations determine their own research priorities.

Figure 4.3 shows how the behaviors generated in the sample problem would be placed in the matrix. Only smoking appears in quadrant 1, and quadrant 2 carries three behaviors important in preventing cardiovascular disease. However, for none of these behaviors is there consistent, conclusive evidence of significant,

	More important	**Less important**
More changeable	High priority for program focus (quadrant 1)	Low priority except to demonstrate change for political purposes (quadrant 3)
Less changeable	Priority for innovative program; evaluation crucial (quadrant 2)	No program (quadrant 4)

FIGURE 4.2

Matrix of health behaviors

	More important	Less important
More changeable	Smoking	Medical treatment, related behaviors
Less changeable	Eating foods with high fatty-acid content Overeating Lack of exercise	Not relaxing

FIGURE 4.3

Matrix of health behaviors in the sample problem, cardiovascular disease prevention in youth

lasting change in response to educational interventions. We can imagine the following likely scenario for the planning meeting to select behaviors as the focus of the program.

- A team member cautions against spreading limited resources too thinly by choosing several behaviors.
- It is agreed that *one* behavior must be chosen.
- During the discussion that follows, smoking, fat consumption, and physical activity surface as possible targets.
- Research evidence is cited indicating that lack of physical activity, smoking, and high cholesterol are equally important as cardiovascular risks.
- It is pointed out that, in the general population, twice as many people are physically inactive as smoke or have high cholesterol.
- The notorious difficulty of inducing sedentary adults to undertake appropriate physical activity is mentioned.

There is an informed and reasoned back-and-forth discussion of the available evidence and the relative merits of each behavior. Then:

- One of the community representatives on the panel asks, "What about the community residents themselves? What do they see as the most important or interesting behavior?"
- This leads to a discussion of the need and feasibility of a community survey to determine the actual prevalence of the key behaviors and their perceived importance to the community.

A survey is conducted, leading the planners to select smoking as the target behavior for the program.

STATING BEHAVIORAL OBJECTIVES

Once the target health behavior has been identified, you are prepared to take the final step in this phase of planning: stating **behavioral objectives**. At this stage, precision is vital. The impact of health promotion efforts is jeopardized when behavioral objectives are vague or grossly conceived. Given the scarcity of health education resources, vagueness is a luxury that cannot be afforded. Instances of "intangible" and unmeasurable target behaviors generally reflect inadequacy in how the behavioral components of the health problem have been delineated. Phrases such as "improve health habits" and "increase the use of health services" are insufficiently specific to stand as useful behavioral objectives, and program efforts aimed at such diffuse targets are likely to be scattered. The result is that too little effort is directed at any one behavior to make a difference.

For this reason, when behavioral change is possible and appropriate, utmost care must be taken in stating the objectives precisely. Each behavioral objective should answer the questions:

- *Who?* The people expected to change
- *What?* The action or change in behavior or health practice to be achieved
- *How much?* The extent of the condition to be achieved
- *When?* The time in which the change is expected to occur

What might be the behavioral objectives for the sample problem of car-diovascular disease? Recall that the target behavior is smoking. In addition, the planning team has determined that the program should be implemented in county A because it is demographically representative of the state and similar to several other counties in adjoining states. The *who* will consist of all residents aged 20–35 in county A. The *what* will be a reduction in the prevalence of cigarette smoking. *How much* will be established as 20 percent.[14] *When* is defined as the proposed time of follow-up evaluation, such as 2 years for the sample program discussed here. Concisely stated, then, the behavioral objective will read: "County residents aged 20–35 will show a 20 percent reduction in the prevalence of cigarette smoking within 2 years of program implementation."

WHY AN EMPHASIS ON ENVIRONMENT?

In addition to the behavioral and biological factors that determine health, a complex array of environmental influences must also be assessed, using pro-cedures similar to those in steps 1–5 for behavior. The manageability of this diagnosis depends on having a good epidemiological diagnosis from phase 2 of

PRECEDE, as with behavioral diagnosis. A finite number of important environmental risk factors for a given health problem can be identified; but if the question is "What environmental influences on health exist?", then the analysis becomes at least a lifetime undertaking.

If the scope of environmental determinants of health becomes so encompassing and complex as to be impractical for health promotion planning, we recommend concentrating attention on those aspects of the environment that are: (1) more social than physical (e.g., organizational and economic), (2) interactive with behavior in their impact on health, and (3) can be changed by social action and health policy.

A useful classification for the environmental diagnosis comes from G. E. Dever, who divides the environment into three components: physical, social, and psychological. In the health context, the physical environment includes hazards such as air, noise, and water pollution, with potential consequences that include hearing loss, infectious diseases, gastroenteritis, cancer, emphysema, and bronchitis. To this list can be added the possibility of lung damage from acid rain and genetic mutation from some radiation. Dever combines the social and psychological dimensions of environmental health and outlines the major functions to include behavior modification, perceptual problems, and interpersonal relationships. He states that

> ...crowding, isolation, rapid...change, and social interchange may contribute to homicide, suicide, decisional stress, and environmental overstimulation...The health problems relative to the environment will only be rectified by imposing standards and controls on the responsible agencies and industries.[15] (p. 458)

The relation of the social environment to health is emerging as an important area for research and a priority for intervention. The Health Education Unit of the World Health Organization's Regional Office for Europe proposes two important objectives: (1) to try to control not only physical and environmental risks but also risks arising from the social environment, and (2) to encourage and support those factors in the environment that "cushion" individuals and help them cope with the social structure.[16]

One other distinction helps narrow the health promotion focus of this book. Much of health promotion, unlike health education, concerns the passage of laws to regulate or constrain behavior that threatens the health of others. We consider the initial stimulation of public interest and support for such legislation or regulation to be a function of health education; the political and organizational efforts to gain passage of such legislation to be the function of health promotion beyond health education; and the enforcement of such laws to be the function of health protection. In short, the promotion of health policy is health promotion; the enforcement of those health policies that require the restraint of individual behavior is health protection.

In general, the priority concern of most health education professionals is to plan a solid health education program for a classroom or a group of patients within a supportive institutional context. For them, the environmental diagnosis is an additional burden on the PRECEDE planning process that may well be the straw that breaks the camel's back. Thus, we recommend detailed consideration of this assessment phase only for those who have responsibility for implementing, organizing, and evaluating broad-scale health promotion programs. This puts the environmental diagnosis more squarely into the framework of PROCEED. If the environmental assessment is to be used later, it must precede the development and implementation of policy, regulation, and organization; so we keep it in PRE-CEDE as an optional step.

THE FIVE STEPS IN THE ENVIRONMENTAL DIAGNOSIS

The steps in environmental diagnosis parallel the steps in behavioral diagnosis; and, in fact, the first step is the same.

STEP 1 SEPARATING BEHAVIORAL AND NONBEHAVIORAL CAUSES OF THE HEALTH PROBLEM

This step produces a list of behavioral factors and a list of nonbehavioral factors.

STEP 2 ELIMINATING NONBEHAVIORAL CAUSES THAT CANNOT BE CHANGED

From the list of nonbehavioral factors identified in Step 1, we now eliminate the genetic, demographic, and historical factors in which little if any change can be expected, even with sweeping policy reforms. The result is an inventory of organizational, economic, and environmental factors that are known to contribute to the health or quality-of-life problem or goal, either directly or indirectly through behavior.

STEP 3 RATING ENVIRONMENTAL FACTORS IN TERMS OF IMPORTANCE

The inventory of environmental factors influencing the health goal or problem is likely to be too long to be manageable within the scope of a health promotion program or policy change. Select the factors that are more important than others according to one or both of the two criteria: (1) the strength of the relationship of the environmental factor to the health or quality-of-life goal or problem; (2)

the incidence, prevalence, or number of people affected by the environmental factor.

STEP 4 RATING ENVIRONMENTAL FACTORS IN TERMS OF CHANGEABILITY

Now you narrow the inventory further by eliminating those environmental factors that have the least chance of yielding to intervention through policy, regulation, or organizational change.

A critical analysis of changeability should include some consultation with community members and leaders to assess the political will to make changes. Environmental factors often prove to be important to the community for purposes other than health. For example, a common dilemma is the occupational hazard that can only be eliminated at the risk of losing the industry that supplies jobs for the community. Recall the West Virginia mining example discussed in Chapter 3. Because the lung disease may be largely attributable to the mining work, there may be no way to eliminate that hazard without eliminating the jobs. When the hazard cannot be eliminated, we usually resort to behavioral solutions, such as wearing protective equipment and going for periodic screening.

This step is most efficient if you apply it only to those environmental factors that survived the importance rating in the previous step; there is little to be gained from a critical analysis of the changeability of an environmental factor that has been deemed relatively unimportant in its causal link to the health or quality-of-life goal or problem. Alternatively, you could apply the changeability criterion first and save time by applying the importance test only to the factors that are most easily changed.

STEP 5 CHOOSING ENVIRONMENTAL TARGETS

The analytic method that was used in selecting behavioral targets can be applied here. Referring to Figure 4.2, we find that the same four quadrants would yield a distribution of environmental factors that would be more or less important and more or less changeable. The policy implication for action on factors in each quadrant would pertain equally to the environmental factors.

The only exception might be greater weight that could be given to quadrant 3, where the environmental factor is apparently changeable but relatively low in objective importance. As P. Slovic and others have pointed out in their research on risk perception, the subjective importance of an environmental factor for the community is often greater than the objective evidence for its relationship or causal link to the health goal or problem.[17] This might call for giving some priority to working with the community to bring about change in that environmental factor in order to help build their confidence and experience in making policy and organizational, economic, or environmental change.[18]

STATING ENVIRONMENTAL OBJECTIVES

With the priorities set for the environmental factors to be changed, the final step in this phase of the diagnostic planning process is to state the objectives for environmental change in quantitative terms. The main departure from the formula for behavioral objectives is that the *who* is eliminated for most environmental objectives. For example, the coalition of agencies working to reduce air pollution might set as its environmental objective "The amount of carbon monoxide released into the atmosphere in our community will be reduced by 50 percent by the year 2000."

If the environmental or social change objective requires for its accomplishment the action of specific groups of people, behavioral objectives might be set for their actions as well. This relationship between environmental and behavioral objectives is reflected in the vertical arrows in the PRECEDE–PROCEED model.

SUMMARY

As a result of working through the first phases of the PRECEDE model (Chapters 2 and 3), we have laid three foundations of program planning:

1. The first step in health promotion planning should be an assessment of the quality of life or social goals and needs of the target population or client system.
2. Epidemiological assessment based on the quality-of-life assessment or social diagnosis can identify specific health problems and risk factors that impede or compromise quality of life.
3. Program objectives should be based on findings from the quality-of-life and epidemiological assessments.

Building on these foundations, this chapter takes the next step in the PRECEDE framework, showing how to identify the most fruitful behavioral and environmental targets for intervention. Because each chosen behavior generates an educational diagnosis and each environmental factor an organizational diagnosis, the planner must be parsimonious in selecting problems.

Concentrating on only the most fruitful areas curbs the multiplication of subsequent planning steps and their associated costs. This is facilitated by the use of rigorous criteria and the application of critical judgment in the epidemiological assessment. Strict and realistic examination of the importance and changeability of each potential target behavior and environmental condition cuts down on the need for subsequent diagnostic efforts. And, finally, the concise statement of objectives leads to greater specificity in program development and simplifies the evaluation process.

EXERCISES

1. For the highest priority health problem identified in your program objective (Exercise 6, Chapter 3), list the specific behaviors that might be causally related to achieving that objective in your population or client system.
2. Rate each behavior in your inventory as low, medium, or high according to (a) prevalence (using population data where possible), (b) epidemiological or causal importance (using relative risk ratios where possible), and (c) changeability (using evidence from previous research where possible).
3. Write a behavioral objective for your population (*who*), indicating to what extent (*how much*) they will exhibit the behavior (*what*) at a given point in time (*when*). Note that you can state *what proportion* of the population will exhibit the behavior as a measure of *how much*.
4. Repeat Exercises 1–3 for the environmental assessment (substituting *environmental* for *behavioral*).

REFERENCES AND NOTES

1. U.S. Department of Health and Human Services, *Promoting Health/Preventing Disease: Year 2000 Objectives for the Nation* (Washington, DC: U. S. Government Printing Office, 1990), and the 1990 objectives that proceeded from *Healthy People: Surgeon General's Report on Health Promotion and Disease Prevention* (Washington, DC: U.S. Department of Health, Education and Welfare, 1979). The separate category for health protection, which contained the environmental-regulatory objectives, gave the impression that health promotion was concerned only with behavior, not with the environment. The health promotion objectives themselves provide ample evidence to the contrary, with numerous "service and protection" objectives in the health promotion areas that addressed policy, regulatory, and organizational interventions required to reduce smoking, alcohol and drug misuse, and violent behavior, improve diet, increase exercise and fitness, and improve the vitality and independence of older people.

2. E. C. Devine and T. D. Cook, "A Meta-analytic Analysis of Effects of Psycho-educational Interventions on Length of Postsurgical Hospital Stay," *Nursing Research* 32 (1983): 267–74; E. Mumford, H. J. Schlesinger, and G. V. Glass, "The Effects of Psychological Intervention on Recovery from Surgery and Heart Attacks: An Analysis of the Literature," *American Journal of Public Health* 72 (1982): 141–51.

3. R. W. Amler and H. B. Dull, *Closing the Gap: The Burden of Unnecessary Illness* (New York: Oxford University Press, 1987); Centers for Disease Control, *The Ten Leading Causes of Death* (Atlanta: Centers for Disease Control, 1978); Centers for Disease Control, "Premature Mortality in the United States: Public Health Issues in the Use of Years of Potential Life Lost," *Morbidity and*

Mortality Weekly Report 35 (suppl., 1986): 2S; M. A. LaLonde, *A New Perspective on the Health of Canadians* (Ottawa: Ministry of National Health and Welfare, 1974).

4. O. T. Thornberry, R. W. Wilson, and P. M. Golden, "Health Promotion Data for the 1990 Objectives. Estimates from the National Health Interview Survey of Health Promotion and Disease Prevention: United States, 1985," *Advance Data from Vital and Health Statistics* 126 (Sept. 19, 1986), DHHS No. (PHS) 86-1250; R. W. Wilson and J. Elinson, "National Survey of Personal Health Practices and Consequences: Background, Conceptual Issues, and Selected Findings," *Public Health Reports* 96 (1981): 218–25. For a copy of the questionnaire, adapted for local use, see L. W. Green and F. M. Lewis, *Measurement and Evaluation in Health Education and Health Promotion* (Palo Alto, CA: Mayfield, 1986), appendix A; or *Toward a Healthy Community: Organizing Events for Community Health Promotion* (Washington, DC: U.S. Department of Health and Human Services, Office of Disease Prevention and Health Promotion, PHS 80-50113, 1980).

5. I. Rootman, "Canada's Health Promotion Survey," in *Canada's Health Promotion Survey: Technical Report*, I. Rootman et al., eds. (Ottawa: Minister of Supply and Services, 1988).

6. T. Stephens and C. Schoenborn, "Adult Health Practices in the United States and Canada," *Vital and Health Statistics* (Hyattsville, MD: National Center for Health Statistics, 1988).

7. L. A. Aday, C. Sellers, and R. Andersen, "Potentials of Local Health Surveys: A State-of-the-Art Summary," *American Journal of Public Health* 71 (1981): 835–40; C. Aneshensel, R. R. Frerichs, V. A. Clark et al., "Telephone Versus In-Person Surveys of Community Health Status," *American Journal of Public Health* 72 (1982): 1017–21; M. S. Chen, Jr., and D. Bill, "Statewide Survey of Risk Factor Prevalence: The Ohio Experience," *Public Health Reports* 98 (1983): 443–8; L.W. Green, R. W. Wilson, and K. Bauer, "Data Required to Measure Progress on the Objectives for the Nation in Disease Prevention and Health Promotion," *American Journal of Public Health* 73 (1983): 18–24; M. F. Weeks, R. A. Kulka, J. T. Lessler et al., "Personal Versus Telephone Surveys for Collecting Household Health Data at the Local Level," *American Journal of Public Health* 73 (1983): 1389–94.

8. P. L. Remington, M. Y. Smith, D. F. Williamson, et al., "Design, Characteristics, and Usefulness of State-Based Behavioral Risk Factor Surveillance: 1981-87," *Public Health Reports* 103 (1988): 366–75. Results of surveys in the participating states are reported and compared periodically in *Morbidity and Mortality Weekly Report* of the Centers for Disease Control (see, e.g., vol. 38, July 14 and August 4, 1989 issues).

9. "Results from the National Adolescent Student Health Survey," *Morbidity and Mortality Weekly Report* 38 (March 10, 1989): 147–50. A. J. C. King et al., *Canada Health Attitudes and Behaviors Survey: 9-, 12-, and 15-year Olds, 1984-85*. (Ottawa: Health and Welfare Canada, Health Promotion Directorate, 1986).

10. City of Toronto Department of Public Health, *The City of Toronto Community Health Survey: A Description of the Health Status of Toronto Residents* (Toronto: City of Toronto Department of Public Health, July 1984).

11. L. J. Kolbe, "Improving the Health of Children and Youth: Frameworks for Behavioral Research and Development," in *Health Education and Youth: A Review of Research and Development*, G. Campbell, ed. (Philadelphia: Falmer Press, 1984), pp. 7–32, as printed with permission in L. W. Green, "Modifying and Developing Health Behavior," *Annual Review of Public Health* 5 (1984): 215–36.

12. C. E. Basch, J. D. Eveland, and B. Portnoy, "Diffusion Systems for Education and Learning About Health," *Family and Community Health* 9(2) (1986): 1–26, esp. p. 18; E. M. Rogers, *Diffusion of Innovations*, 3rd ed. (New York: Free Press, 1983).

13. L. W. Green, "Diffusion and Adoption of Innovations Related to Cardiovascular Risk Behavior in the Public," in *Applying Behavioral Sciences to Cardiovascular Risk*, A. Enelow and J. B. Henderson, eds. (New York: American Heart Association, 1975).

14. Note that "how much" could also be set in terms of number of cigarettes consumed, on an individual basis (reducing each smoker's consumption by 20%) or on a population basis (reducing the average or overall smoking consumption by 20%). In addition, such quantitative aspects of program goals should be adjusted for secular trends, such as the steady national decline in smoking prevalence of about 1% per year. See National Center for Health Statistics, *Health, United States, 1989 and Prevention Profile* (Hyattsville, MD: Public Health Service, DHHS-PHS-90-1232, 1990), esp. p. 22.

15. G. E. Dever, "An Epidemiological Model for Health Policy Analysis," *Social Indicators Research* 2 (1976): 453–66.

16. Health Education Unit, Regional Office of Education, WHO Regional Office for Europe, "Lifestyles and Health," *Social Science and Medicine* 22 (1986): 117–24.

17. Committee on Risk Perception and Communication, National Research Council, *Improving Risk Communication* (Washington, DC: National Academy Press, 1989); V. T. Covello, D. von Winterfeldt, and P. Slovic, "Risk Communication: A Review of the Literature," *Risk Abstracts* 3 (Oct. 1986): 171–82; P. Slovic, "Informing and Educating the Public About Risk," *Risk Analysis* 6 (1986): 403–15.

18. A commitment to change environmental factors is a commitment to engage the political forces in the community or target area. The issues in taking on that responsibility as a health professional are discussed in Chapters 6 and 8. The issues tend to be most explosive in matters of environmental control. See, for example, N. Freudenberg, *Not in Our Backyards! Community Action for Health and the Environment* (New York: Monthly Review Press, 1984); idem., "Citizen Action for Environmental Health: Report on a Survey of Community Organizations," *American Journal of Public Health* 74 (1984): 444–8; idem., "Training Health Educators for Social Change," *International Quarterly of Community Health Education* 5 (1984–1985): 37–52.

Chapter 5

Educational and Organizational Diagnosis: Factors Affecting Health-Related Behavior and Environments

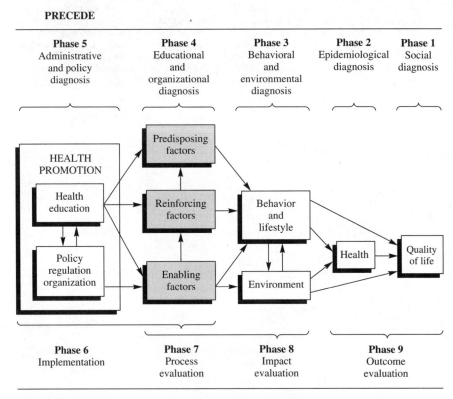

Phase 5	Phase 4	Phase 3	Phase 2	Phase 1
Administrative and policy diagnosis	Educational and organizational diagnosis	Behavioral and environmental diagnosis	Epidemiological diagnosis	Social diagnosis

Phase 6	Phase 7	Phase 8	Phase 9
Implementation	Process evaluation	Impact evaluation	Outcome evaluation

PROCEED

Thus far, the presentation of planning a health promotion program shows how an orderly sequence of social, epidemiological, behavioral, and environmental diagnosis can lead to a clear understanding of the actions and conditions of living affecting a population's aspiration, problem, or need. The next phase of the PRECEDE model – Phase 4, **educational and organizational diagnosis** – examines those behavioral and environmental conditions linked to health status or quality-of-life concerns to determine what causes them. The educational and organizational diagnosis identifies factors that must be changed to initiate and sustain the process of behavioral and environmental change; these factors will become the immediate targets or objectives of your program. They may be seen as the processes of change that must be activated or set in motion if the necessary behavioral and environmental changes are to occur.

Behaviors and environments to be influenced through health promotion programs include the full range of those classified in Chapter 4. The educational and organizational diagnosis in health promotion is concerned with factors influencing the behavior and conditions of living of the people at risk for the health problems identified in Chapter 3 and of those people who can influence environmental conditions; this phase of PRECEDE helps planners untangle the complex forces shaping health-related behavior and environmental conditions.

FACTORS THAT INFLUENCE BEHAVIOR

We can identify three categories of factors affecting individual or collective behavior, including organizational actions in relation to the environment, each of which has a different type of influence on behavior:

- **Predisposing factors** are those antecedents to behavior that provide the rationale or *motivation* for the behavior.
- **Enabling factors** are the antecedents to behavior that enable a motivation to be realized.
- **Reinforcing factors** are factors subsequent to a behavior that provide the continuing *reward* or incentive for the behavior and contribute to its persistence or repetition.

Any given behavior can be explained as a function of the collective influence of these three types of factors. The notion of *collective causation*, or *contributing causes*, is particularly important because behavior is a multifaceted phenomenon. This idea suggests that no single behavior, or action, is caused by just one factor. "'Tis a tangled web we weave" of causal factors, each increasing or decreasing the probability that the action will be performed, with every factor potentially affecting the influence of all other factors. Occasionally, exceptions to the combination rule do happen: A highly motivated behavior can sometimes overcome a deficit of resources and rewards; a highly rewarded behavior could occur in the absence of personal beliefs about its value or correctness. But for the average person, the three conditions—predisposing, enabling, and reinforcing—must be aligned for the behavior to occur and persist.

Any plan to influence behavior must consider all three sets of causal factors. For example, a program for disseminating health information to increase awareness, interest, and knowledge (predisposing factors) that does not recognize the influence of enabling and reinforcing factors, most likely will fail to influence behavior except in the segment of the population that has resources and rewards readily at hand (usually the more affluent people).

Figure 5.1 details some relationships among the three types of factors and shows how they can affect behavior through various pathways. For example, an adolescent may have a negative attitude toward smoking and believe that smoking is harmful (predisposing factors), which causes her not to smoke (the behavior); her nonsmoking may then be rewarded by her parents (reinforcing factors). Strong enforcement of local ordinances prohibiting sale of cigarettes to minors may lead to unavailability of cigarettes in her immediate environment (an enabling factor). Alternately, an adolescent may perceive peer pressure to smoke (a reinforcing factor) and notice the availability of cigarettes in stores (an enabling factor), both of which can result in a positive attitude toward smoking (a predisposing factor), which then causes her to smoke (the behavior), which is then reinforced by her peers (a reinforcing factor).

Normally, we expect the sequence to be as follows: A person has an initial reason, impulse, or motivation (predisposing factor) to pursue a given course of action. This first factor (arrow 1 in Figure 5.1) in the causal chain may be sufficient to start the behavior, but it will not be sufficient to complete it unless the person has the resources or skills needed to carry out the behavior. The motivation is followed by (arrow 2) deployment or use of resources to enable the action (enabling factor). This usually results in the behavior, followed by (3) a reaction to the behavior which is emotional, physical, or social (reinforcing factor). Reinforcement strengthens behavior (4), future resources (5), and motivation (6). The ready availability of enabling factors provides cues and heightens awareness and other factors predisposing the behavior (6). An exercycle in your home is more likely to prompt you to use it than one at the YMCA. Similarly, rewards and satisfactions from behavior make that behavior more attractive on the next occasion; today's reinforcing factor becomes tomorrow's predisposing factor (7).

Finally, perhaps most relevant to the environmental perspective of health promotion, the building up of social reinforcement for a behavior can lead to the enabling of behavior in the form of social support and assistance (arrow 5).

APPLICATION OF THE MODEL

The classification of factors affecting behavior into predisposing, reinforcing, and enabling categories makes it possible to group the specific features of the situation according to the types of interventions available in health education and health promotion:

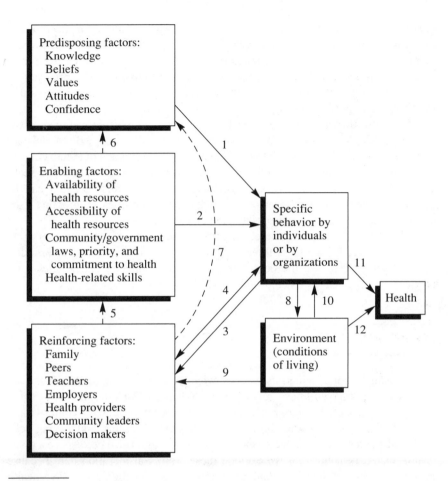

FIGURE 5.1

The causal relationships and order of causation for the three sets of factors influencing behavior. Solid lines imply contributing influence. Dashed lines imply secondary effects. Numerals indicate order in which actions or influences usually occur.

- Direct communications to the target population to strengthen the predisposing factors.
- Indirect communications through parents, teachers, clergy, community leaders, employers, peers, and others to strengthen the reinforcing factors.
- Community organization, political interventions, and training to strengthen the enabling factors.

Through educational and organizational diagnosis one identifies the prevalence or intensity of specific factors of each type while keeping in mind that there may be complex interactions among the factors. Those interactions need not be delineated in precise detail or for each person in a target population. The average or prevailing configuration, recognizing that personal factors differ from individual to individual, will suffice to plan an effective health promotion program for a population of community residents, students, patients, employees, or other relatively homogeneous group.

Countless theories have been developed that attempt to explain human behavior, yet no single theoretical model has been universally accepted. Models are constantly modified in response to new situations. The approach of identifying the predisposing, enabling, and reinforcing factors as determinants of behavior seeks a broad framework within which more formal theories and research can be organized. The rationale is based on several common theoretical themes that seem especially applicable and appropriate to health promotion.[1]

The PRECEDE model merely organizes the multitude of precursors into three categories. Within these three categories, the various concepts and models can be used in planning the details (e.g., messages, incentives, policies) of a particular component of a health promotion program.

PREDISPOSING FACTORS

Predisposing factors—which include knowledge, **attitudes**, **beliefs**, **values**, and perceived **needs** and abilities—relate to the motivation of an individual or group to act. They mostly fall in the psychological domain. They include the cognitive and affective dimensions of knowing, feeling, believing, valuing and having self-confidence or a sense of efficacy. Personality factors could also predispose a given health-related behavior, but we exclude these from consideration here because personality change does not lend itself readily to educational or other health promotion interventions short of psychotherapy.

Existing skills can, through the self-efficacy factor, predispose one to take action.[2] The extent to which people, organizations, or communities possess certain skills or capacities may predispose them to take certain actions, but for most purposes we classify skills as an enabling factor. Generally, we can think of predisposing factors as the "personal" preferences that an individual or group brings to a behavioral or environmental choice, or to an educational or organizational experience. These preferences may either support or inhibit behavior.

A variety of demographic factors—such as socioeconomic status, age, gender, and family size—predispose behavior. They are not in our list of predisposing factors only because they cannot be easily and directly influenced by a health promotion program. Such factors, however, are useful for *segmenting* populations into subgroups for which educational and organizational diagnoses of predisposing, reinforcing, and enabling factors would be conducted. Such an approach can help the planner determine whether different interventions should be planned for different groups.

For example, an educational and organizational diagnosis for moderate to vigorous physical activity would yield different results for children than for adults: For children an organizational enabling factor of importance is the type of activity required during physical education in school.[3] For adults an educational enabling factor would be new skills in setting flexible goals for participation in physical activity.[4] Another example is that predisposing factors for smoking cessation in women include attitudes and concerns about weight control and attractiveness, whereas those concerns are not so important in men.[5]

KNOWLEDGE OR AWARENESS

An increase in knowledge alone does not always cause behavioral or organizational change, but positive associations between changes in behavior and organizational variables were demonstrated in the early (Second World War) work of Cartwright,[6] in the most recent findings of the Stanford Five-Community Study,[7] and in countless studies conducted in the interim.[8] Health knowledge of some kind is probably necessary before a conscious personal health action can occur, but the desired health action will probably not occur unless a person receives a cue strong enough to trigger the motivation to act on that knowledge. A threshold level of knowledge may be necessary for some actions to occur, such as recognizing a symptom as abnormal, before one will go for a medical check; but after that level of knowledge is attained, additional information does not necessarily promote additional behavioral change.[9]

The same considerations influence organizational behavior. Knowledge influences organizational decisions by those in charge, but other strategic and political considerations must come into play in the implementation of those decisions. The applications of the PRECEDE model to policy decisions and to regulatory and organizational behavior are addressed in Chapter 6.

Motivation usually must come from sources other than, or in addition to, factual knowledge. School health curricula, for example, are frequently justified by reference to the simple, commonsense notion that knowledge is the best road to good health. Proponents of the opposing position argue that goals of knowledge are too "soft" and intangible to be used as criteria for program effectiveness in school health curricula. Furthermore, they state that contemporary students are disenchanted and bored by facts. Nonsense! Students are not turned off by facts; they are turned off by moralization, superficial coverage of subject matter, scare tactics, and tedious methods of presentation.

It is as ludicrous to say knowledge makes no difference as it is to say it makes all the difference. The appropriate perspective is a balanced one: Knowledge is a necessary but usually[10] not a sufficient factor in changing individual or collective behavior. And the same could be said for every other factor in the predisposing category. To repeat: A *combination* of factors defines motivation, and a *combination* of interventions defines health promotion.

A change in awareness or knowledge, like any other change in the complex system of predisposing factors, also brings about some change in other areas because of the human desire for consistency.[11] Behavior may not change immediately in response to new awareness or knowledge, but the cumulative effects of heightened awareness, increased understanding, and greater command (recognition and recall) of facts seep into the system of beliefs, values, attitudes, intentions, and self-efficacy, and eventually into behavior.

BELIEFS, VALUES, AND ATTITUDES

Beliefs, values, and attitudes are independent constructs, yet the differences between them are often fine and complex. Because we are concerned primarily with practice rather than research, we examine these factors in a practical way, trusting that those interested in more detailed analysis will look further in the theoretical and research literature.[12]

Beliefs. A *belief* is a conviction that a phenomenon or object is true or real. *Faith*, *trust*, and *truth* are words used to express or imply belief. Health-oriented belief statements include: "I don't believe that medication can work"; "Exercise won't make any difference"; "When your time is up, your time is up, and there's nothing you can do about it." If beliefs such as these are strongly held, to what extent will they interfere with good health? Can they be changed? Will changes facilitate health-promoting behavior?

The **Health Belief Model**, developed and assessed by various authors,[13] attempts to explain and predict health-related behavior in terms of certain belief patterns. The model is based on the following assumptions about behavior change:

1. The person must believe that his or her health is in jeopardy. For an asymptomatic disease like hypertension or early cancer, the person must believe that he or she can have it and not feel symptoms.
2. The person must perceive the *potential* seriousness of the condition in terms of pain or discomfort, time lost from work, economic difficulties, and so forth.
3. On assessing the circumstances, the person must believe that benefits stemming from the recommended behavior outweigh the costs and inconvenience and are indeed possible and within his or her grasp.
4. There must be a "cue to action" or a precipitating force that makes the person feel the need to take action.

This last point is fundamental to the entire model. Health education can provide the cue to action if the predisposing factors represented by the health beliefs are correctly diagnosed. Examples of specific applications and experimental tests of the Health Belief Model for educational diagnosis and evaluation can be found in studies of the determinants of each of the following health actions or health problems: AIDS and other sexually transmitted diseases,[14] contraceptive practices,[15] diabetes,[16] alcohol and driving,[17] child care and child health behavior,[18] participation in screening programs,[19] use of clinical health services,[20] dietary behavior,[21] asthma,[22] genetic counseling and screening,[23] breast self-examination,[24] immunization,[25] patient adherence to medical regimens,[26] smoking,[27] hypertension,[28] physician behavior in patient education and health promotion,[29] cardiac rehabilitation,[30] tuberculosis,[31] dental health behavior,[32] occupational therapy,[33] toxic shock syndrome,[34] exercise and physical activity,[35] miscellaneous preventive health practices,[36] general guidelines,[37] and other predisposing factors correlated with beliefs.[38]

Two of the dimensions of the Health Belief Model—belief in susceptibility and belief in severity of consequences—could be interpreted as **fear** of the disease or condition or behavior. Fear is a powerful motivational force, but it contains a dimension of anxiety beyond that in the belief. The source of such anxiety is the belief in susceptibility and severity *in combination with* a sense of hopelessness or powerlessness to do anything about a vague or diffuse threat. This combination produces a flight response that often manifests as denial or rationalization of the threat as unreal. Thus, arousal of fear in health education messages can backfire unless the fear-arousing message is accompanied by an immediate course of action the person can take to alleviate the fear.[39]

Values. The cultural, intergenerational perspectives on matters of consequence reflect the values people hold. Values tend to cluster within ethnic groups and across generations of people who share a common history and geographic identity. Ultimately, they are the basis for justifying one's actions in moral or ethical terms. Values underpin the right and wrong, the good and bad dimensions of people's outlook on specific behaviors. Consider this brief exchange between two people.

He: Did I hear you say that you are going to try skydiving?
She: Absolutely not!
He: Why not?
She: Because I value my life, that's why not!
He: Do you also value your health?
She: Of course I do.
He: Then why do you smoke cigarettes?
She: Because I enjoy smoking and it helps me relax.
He: If that's the case, can you honestly say that you really value your life?
She: Sure I can. It's not that I don't value my life and health but that I
      value other things too, among them the pleasure of smoking. What's
      wrong with that?

It goes without saying that personal values are inseparably linked to choices of behavior. In the preceding scenario, the person who values life, health, and cigarettes, too, reveals a conflict of values. Values often conflict with each other. According to the former Canadian Minister of National Health and Welfare, "Most Canadians by far prefer good health to illness, and a long life to a short one but, while individuals are prepared to sacrifice a certain amount of immediate pleasure in order to stay healthy, they are not prepared to forgo all self-indulgence nor to tolerate all inconvenience in the interest of preventing illness."[40]

In short-term health education or health promotion programs, one does not set out to *change* values. One seeks instead to help people recognize inconsistencies between their values (usually prohealth) and their behavior or environment (often antihealth). Recognizing deeply held values within ethnic groups, age groups, and other demographically defined subpopulations provides an immediate and efficient indicator of starting points for the analyis of predisposing factors in segments of the population.[41]

Attitudes. After *motivation*, one of the vaguest yet most frequently used and misused words in the behavioral sciences lexicon is *attitude*. To keep matters short and simple, we offer two definitions that, in combination, cover the principal elements of attitude. Mucchielli describes attitude as "a tendency of mind or of relatively constant feeling toward a certain category of objects, persons, or situations."[42] Kirscht viewed attitudes as a collection of beliefs that always includes an evaluative aspect;[43] that is, attitudes can always be assessed in terms of positive and negative. They differ from values in being attached to specific objects, persons, or situations and being based on one or more values. In the hierarchy posited by Rokeach, values are more deeply seated and therefore less changeable than attitudes and beliefs.[44]

Keep in mind the two key concepts: (1) Attitude is a rather *constant* feeling that is *directed toward an object* (be it a person, an action, a situation, or an idea); and (2) inherent in the structure of an attitude is *evaluation*, a good–bad dimension. We gain further understanding of the structure of an attitude by examining one technique frequently used to measure attitudes: the semantic differential.[45] This technique calls for people to respond to concepts by making a mark on a continuum between antonyms. Suppose we want to measure the attitudes expressed by the woman in the dialogue toward skydiving and cigarette smoking. Having heard her conversation with the man, we already have an idea about what her attitudes are; but let's measure them just the same.

Concept: Skydiving

good	___	___	___	___	X	___ bad
pretty	___	___	___	___	X	___ ugly
happy	___	___	___	X	___	___ sad

Concept: cigarette smoking

good	____	__X__	____	____	____	____	bad
pretty	____	____	__X__	____	____	____	ugly
happy	__X__	____	____	____	____	____	sad

From the conversation and from what we can see now in her response, it is clear that her attitudes toward skydiving and smoking are consistently in opposite directions. Because they are constant, they are probably strong. We can also see the woman's evaluation (in terms of good and bad) of the concepts: She avoided neutral responses on the continuum.

The relationships between behavior and constructs such as attitudes, beliefs, and values, though not completely understood, give ample evidence of their association. Analysis shows, for example, that attitudes are to some degree the determinants, components, and consequences of beliefs, values, and behavior. This alone gives sufficient reason to be concerned with attitudes, beliefs, and values as interrelated predisposing factors.

SELF-EFFICACY AND SOCIAL LEARNING THEORY

A relative newcomer to health behavior research is the concept of **self-efficacy** as a determinant of behavior. This concept from social learning theory has held special fascination for health educators[46] and others in health promotion[47] and in patient education.[48] The attractiveness of the self-efficacy concept in health promotion is probably because it expresses so succinctly the dominant purpose ascribed to health promotion. As declared by the Ottawa Charter,[49] health promotion is "the process of enabling people to increase control over, and to improve, their health." Self-efficacy implies a mental or cognitive state of taking control.[50]

"Inherent in the social learning conception is the idea that people self-regulate their environments and actions. Although people are acted upon by their environments, they also help create their surroundings."[51] This concept of reciprocal determinism is social learning theory's major departure from operant conditioning theory, which tends to view all behavior as a one-way product of the environment. Reciprocal determinism and its associated concepts of self-management and self-control make social learning theory ideally suited to the integration of the PRECEDE and PROCEED frameworks and the development of an educational approach to health promotion.

Learning takes place through three processes: (1) direct experience, (2) indirect or vicarious experience from observing others (modeling), and (3) the storing and processing of complex information in cognitive operations that enable one to anticipate the consequences of actions, represent goals in thought, and weigh evidence from various sources to assess one's own capabilities. Out of the third process comes a situation-specific self-appraisal that makes the individual more or less confident in taking on new behavior in situations that may contain novel, unpredictable, or stressful circumstances. Self-efficacy, then, is a perception of one's own capacity for success in organizing and implementing a pattern of behavior that is new, based largely on experience with similar actions or circumstances encountered or observed in the past.

In addition to its influence on behavior, self-efficacy affects thought patterns and emotional reactions that may alleviate anxiety and enhance coping ability. These interactions make enhanced self-efficacy particularly helpful to people attempting to quit smoking[52] and to modify other addictive and compulsive behavioral patterns where they have experienced failure and relapse,[53] including overeating.[54]

The self-efficacy variable has proved particularly useful in planning health promotion programs using mass media, with role models for the vicarious learning and modeling process and for instruction in self-control.[55]

Measurement instruments to assess self-efficacy have been developing gradually in recent years. Self-efficacy scales have been validated, for example, for health-related diet and exercise behaviors,[56] and for weight loss.[57] A review of the literature to identify the latest measurement advances is always advisable before embarking on a survey to assess any of the predisposing factors.

BEHAVIORAL INTENTION

Central to the theory of reasoned action[58] is the concept of **behavioral intention**. The theory of reasoned action holds that the final step in the predisposing process before actual action takes place is formulating a behavioral intention. This step is influenced by attitudes toward the behavior and by perception of social norms favorable to the behavior. These attitudes, in turn, are influenced by beliefs concerning the efficacy of action in achieving the expected outcomes and by the attitude toward those outcomes. Perception of social norms is influenced by beliefs about the strength of others' opinions on the behavior and by the person's own motivation to comply with those significant others.

Applications of the theory of reasoned action in health behavior studies can be found in the literature on dental health,[59] smoking,[60] recycling behavior,[61] alcohol,[62] drug abuse,[63] seat-belt use,[64] and contraceptive practices.[65] A school-based smoking prevention project in the Netherlands specifically integrated the theory of reasoned action with the PRECEDE model to design interventions that proved effective in reducing the uptake of smoking.[66] Longitudinal data from two cities in which surveys were conducted before and after the national HealthStyle campaign provided for a comparative analysis of the predictive power of several models including the theory of reasoned action (see Mullen et al., reference 13).

EXISTING SKILLS

A person may come to an educational situation already possessing the skills to take certain actions. Such skills may predispose the person to act in a particular way. For example, an experienced mother may already possess the skills for breastfeeding. When she gives birth to another child, those skills may predispose her to breastfeed that child. The mother has a high self-efficacy about breastfeeding because she has successfully breastfed in the past; she has formulated a behavioral intention to breastfeed because of her prior acquisition of skills. Thus, existing skills are closely tied to self-efficacy and behavioral intention.

Self-confidence and self-efficacy can be linked to skills that are already present and thus do not need to be learned for a specific health-behavior situation. For example, the ability to resist peer pressures is associated with nonsmoking in adolescents.[67] If a person does not possess the skills for a certain action, then the acquisition of those skills becomes an enabling factor for performing the action. Several smoking prevention programs have included skills training in resisting peer pressures to smoke to aid those students who do not already have those skills.[68]

ENABLING FACTORS

Enabling factors, often conditions of the environment, *facilitate* the performance of an action by individuals or organizations; included are the availability, accessibility, and affordability of health-care and community resources. Also included are conditions of living that act as barriers to action, such as availability of transportation or child care to release a mother from that responsibility long enough to participate in a health program. Enabling factors also include **new** skills that a person, organization, or community needs to carry out a behavioral or environmental change.

Enabling factors will become the immediate targets of community organization and training interventions in your program. They consist of the resources and new skills necessary to perform a health action and the organizational actions required to modify the environment. Resources include the organization and accessibility of health-care facilities, personnel, schools, outreach clinics, or any similar resource. Personal health skills, such as those discussed in the literature on self-care and school health education, can enable specific health actions.[69] Skills in influencing the community, such as through social action and organizational change, can enable actions directed toward influencing the physical or health-care environment.[70]

In a position paper on enabling factors, Milio contends that health behaviors of a population may be limited by the degree to which health resources are made available and accessible: "Organizational behavior . . . sets the range of options available to individuals for their personal choice-making."[71]

To plan interventions directed at changing enabling factors, the health promotion planner assesses the presence or absence of enabling factors in the community of interest. This calls for an organizational diagnosis of resources and an educational diagnosis of required skills.

THE HEALTH-CARE ENVIRONMENT

Enabling factors for health-care or medical-care behaviors include health-care resources such as outreach clinics, hospitals, emergency treatment rooms, health-care providers, classes in self-care, and other facilities, programs, or personnel. Cost, distance, available transportation, hours open, and so forth are enabling factors that affect the availability and accessibility of the health-care services.

Suppose a well-intended educational effort was successful in raising or appealing to the motivation of members of a target group to make greater use of medical services in their area, but the health-care providers in the area were not consulted. If they had been, they would have warned that existing facilities were overcrowded and that providers were overworked and unwilling to take on more work without an expansion of facilities and additional personnel.

What is the likely outcome? Participants in the program, deprived of services they need and were promised, may become discouraged and feel they have been "let down." Health-care providers may become angry and alienated from health education efforts because they were not considered and were made to look bad for not delivering promised services. A broken-appointment cycle like that shown in Figure 5.2 would likely develop.

As emphasized throughout this book, a health behavior has many causes, so one-dimensional efforts to affect behavior rarely produce the desired results. In this example, health education for better utilization of medical services, without attention to the enabling factors for that utilization, would fail to achieve its desired outcome.

OTHER ENVIRONMENTAL INFLUENCES

Environmental conditions can influence behavioral risk factors for disease, either healthfully or adversely. The availability, accessibility, and low cost of unhealthful consumer products are important enabling factors that adversely affect health behavior in the United States today. Examples include cigarette machines, which enable smoking by adolescents even where laws prohibit sale to minors; labor-saving devices, which foster sedentary lifestyles; fast food, which is convenient but often too high in salt and fat; and alcoholic beverages sold at sports events,

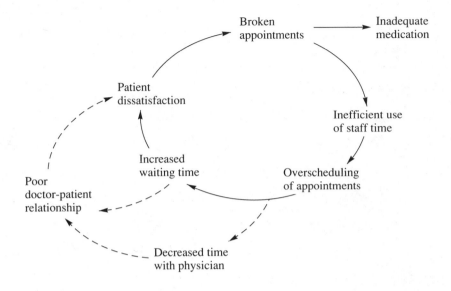

FIGURE 5.2

The broken-appointment cycle

which puts intoxicated fans in the driver's seat on the road home. Examples of environmental enabling factors that can counteract these adverse influences include the availability and low cost of smoking cessation programs, exercise facilities, and healthful food, and the enforcement of laws prohibiting alcohol sales to minors or during the second half of a sporting event.

For each priority behavioral-risk factor identified in the behavioral diagnosis, environmental enabling factors can be identified. For cigarette smoking, the environmental enabling factors that have been found to have an effect are cost of cigarettes, accessibility of cigarettes, smoking restrictions and bans, availability of smoking cessation and smoking prevention programs, and smoking cessation aids such as nicotine gum.[72]

Enabling factors that can discourage alcohol misuse among youth are leisure-time alternatives such as sports and recreation programs, after school activities, and alcohol-free social events; adult supervision; and regulation of alcohol sales through retail outlets.[73] Project Graduation demonstrated that chemical-free graduation celebrations can reduce the number of fatalities, alcohol- or drug-related injuries, and arrests for driving under the influence of alcohol.[74] Figure 5.3 shows the dramatic decline in teenage highway deaths associated with alcohol following the initiation of Project Graduation.

For encouraging physical activity in adults, the environmental enabling factors are programs that emphasize moderate, less strenuous exercise, and

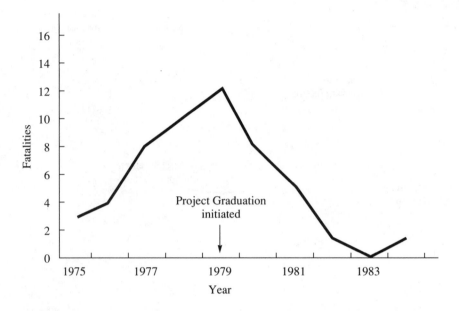

FIGURE 5.3

Motor vehicle–related fatalities among 15–19-year-old residents involving teenagers driving under influence of alcohol during graduation period, May 15–June 15, 1975–1984, in Maine. [From C. Mowatt, et al., *Morbidity and Mortality Weekly Report* 34 (1985): 233–5.]

increases in daily, lifestyle physical activity; accessibility of an exercise facility; low cost; and environmental opportunities for physical activity.[75]

NEW SKILLS

The term *skills* as used here refers to a person's ability to perform the tasks that constitute a health-related behavior. Skills for health promotion include abilities to control personal risk factors for disease, skills in appropriate use of medical care, and skills in changing the environment. Examples include the appropriate use of relaxation techniques and the ability to perform appropriate exercises, the use of the variety of medical instruments and diagnostic procedures frequently required in self-care programs, and the effective use of one's voting power and one's coalition-building and community-organizing potential to bring about change in one's neighborhood or community.

For each behavioral priority that is identified in the behavioral diagnosis, needed skills should be identified. For smoking prevention, the needed skills include resisting peer pressures to smoke, whereas for smoking cessation, the needed skills are coping and relaxation.[76] For physical activity, skills in flexible goal setting can increase adherence to an exercise program.[77]

Health promotion programs working to increase the ability of people to change their environment need to know whether the people possess skills for influencing organizations or their community. Included might be skills in community organizing, coalition building, fund raising, negotiating, working with the media, writing, and speaking.[78]

Assessing the extent to which members of the target population possess enabling skills can give the planner valuable insight into possible program components. Failure to consider the impact of enabling factors on the achievement of behavioral goals can lead to serious problems that threaten program success.

REINFORCING FACTORS

Reinforcing factors are those consequences of action that determine whether the actor receives positive (or negative) feedback and is supported socially after it occurs. Reinforcing factors thus include social support, peer influences, and advice and feedback by health-care providers. Reinforcing factors also include physical consequences of behavior, which may be separate from the social context. Examples include the feeling of well-being (or pain) caused by physical exercise and the alleviation of respiratory symptoms following the correct use of asthma medication.

Social benefits (such as recognition), physical benefits (such as convenience, comfort, relief of discomfort or pain), tangible rewards (such as economic benefits or avoidance of cost), and imagined or vicarious rewards (such as improved appearance, self-respect, or association with an admired person who demonstrates the behavior) all reinforce behavior. Reinforcing factors also include adverse consequences of behavior, or "punishments," that can lead to the extinction of a positive behavior. **Negative reinforcement** is the reward of alternative, wrong behaviors. For individuals, these might include the "high" that rewards the drug abuser, the relief of tension that rewards the smoker, or the masking of emotions that leads to compulsive eating. For organizations, these might include the profits that accrue from promoting a harmful product or the savings that accrue from using a pollutant in the manufacturing process. Changes in organizational behavior can be reinforced by tax incentives and penalties or fines that support non-polluting products or discourage polluting ones.

For each of the priority behaviors from the behavioral diagnosis, important reinforcing factors can be determined. For smoking cessation, for example, reinforcements may be sought in the form of social support from peers and spouse and advice from health-care providers.[79] Cigarette and alcohol advertising provides vicarious reinforcement for continuing to smoke or drink.[80] Family and spouse support, and advice and recommendations by health-care providers, are reinforcers for adherence to physical activity programs.[81]

Anticipation of reinforcement (or of punishment) can occur prior to a behavior. Such *anticipated* reinforcement influences the subsequent performance of the behavior. Social acceptance (or disapproval) thus can be a reinforcing factor. Some reinforcing factors that provide social reinforcement can become enabling factors if they generate ongoing social support, such as financial assistance or transportation, or even friendly advice. Reinforcement can also be *vicarious*, such as modeling a behavior after a television personality or an attractive person in an advertisement who seems to be enjoying the behavior.

The source of reinforcement, of course, varies depending on the objectives and type of program, as well as on the setting. In occupational health promotion programs, for example, reinforcement may be provided by co-workers, supervisors, union leaders, and family members. In patient education settings, reinforcement may come from nurses, physicians, fellow patients, and, again, family members.

Whether the reinforcement is positive or discouraging depends on the attitudes and behavior of significant people, some of whom will be more influential than others in affecting behavior. For example, in a high-school health education program, where reinforcement may come from peers, teachers, school administrators, and parents, which group is likely to have the most influence? Although there are no absolute answers to that question, research in adolescent behavior indicates that adolescent smoking, drinking, and drug-taking behavior is most influenced by approval from friends, especially a best friend.[82] Parental attitudes, beliefs, and practices, especially those of the mother, hold second place among social influences affecting the health status of adolescent children.[83]

Which people are significant may vary not only according to the setting but also according to a child's growth and development stage. The behavior of younger adolescents (grades 6–8) with respect to smoking appears to be influenced more by parents and that of older adolescents (grades 9–11) than by peers and siblings.[84]

Incremental and easily reversible changes in behavior are more likely to be reinforced by success. As people try to decrease salt consumption, they tolerate small steps toward a low-salt diet more easily than large steps; so small steps are more apt to be reinforced by their success. Large reductions in salt in each step tend to punish rather than reinforce. Consider, for example, the steps that can be taken toward the goal of a low-salt diet. These could be added one at a time, each after mastery of the previous step: salting only after tasting, decreasing salt in cooking, eliminating table salt, buying low-salt food products, and, finally, eliminating cooking salt.

Behaviors to influence environmental or health-care conditions also respond to reinforcing factors. Community or social support can reinforce individual actions to cooperate with or join advocacy groups seeking to influence these changes. Such support can also be provided by community residents, health-care providers, and health education or health promotion practitioners. A community change agent who does not have such support becomes discouraged, experiences "burnout," and as a consequence abandons his or her efforts.

Program planners must carefully assess reinforcing factors to make sure that program participants have maximum opportunities for supportive feedback for their new behaviors. Without such feedback, programs have less chance of sustained momentum and eventual success.

SELECTING FACTORS AND SETTING PRIORITIES

The core of PRECEDE's educational and organizational diagnosis phase is to select the predisposing, reinforcing, and enabling factors that, if modified, will help bring about the targeted health-related behavior and environmental change. This process has three basic steps: (1) identifying and sorting factors into the three categories, (2) setting priorities among categories, and (3) establishing priorities within the categories. Specific factors selected by this process form the basis for learning objectives and community organization objectives, which then lead to the selection of materials and methods for program implementation. If the program is well designed and carefully implemented, the probability is high that objectives will be met and target behaviors and environments modified.

STEP 1. IDENTIFYING AND SORTING

The list of causal factors initially identified for each behavior and environmental target should be as comprehensive as possible to help the planner avoid overlooking crucial determinants. Both informal and formal methods can be used to develop the list.

Informal Methods. The team assigned the responsibility for designing the intervention plan usually has educated guesses and hypotheses about the reasons why people behave in the desired manner. Members of the group at risk (the consumers or target population) can be helpfully involved in the planning at this point; their information and insight on their own behavior, attitudes, beliefs, values, and barriers to reaching the stated objectives are most relevant. Intensive interviews, informal group discussions, nominal groups, focus groups, panels, and questionnaires can provide useful data.[85]

The same methods of eliciting information can be used with staff who are involved in the delivery of the intervention and with people in agencies providing related services. Such people may suggest potential causes of behavior based on insights from their personal experience with the effects of agency or community resources, services, and operations. Systematic recording of the data will make this information useful and retrievable.

Brainstorming and the nominal group process are useful techniques for generating data on barriers to behavioral change.[86] A vital step in this phase of PRECEDE is sorting factors according to whether they have negative or positive effects. The negative effects must be overcome, and the positive effects can be built upon and strengthened.

Planners must be critical in accepting the assumptions of health-care providers on the predisposing factors of patients or clients. Some providers may interpret behavior that is different from their expectations as stemming from laziness, apathy, or ignorance. Generalizations of this sort do not help explain the behavior at issue. These characterizations only describe the behavior they are intended to explain. "Blaming the victim" can arise out of misunderstanding, poor communication, "burnout," or rationalization. The system may be at fault, rather than the patient.[87] On the other hand, "system-blaming" can arise out of frustration with the organizations and management of services, and this can be just as unproductive as putting all the responsibility for change on individuals.[88] The purpose of the assessment at this stage is not to fix blame or responsibility, but to take inventory of all the potential targets of change that might improve the situation.

Formal Methods. A search through relevant literature can yield information on cultural and social attitudes and descriptions of studies defining the impact of specific factors on health-related behavior.[89] For example, a market segment analysis to examine the beliefs and perceptions that adults have that may influence their exercise behavior found that (1) people are generally misinformed about the frequency, intensity, and duration of activity needed to obtain a cardiovascular benefit; (2) one's doctor is the most important referent regarding exercise; and (3) subjects did not perceive the health benefits of exercise to be as critical as the intrinsic, psychological, or emotional benefits.[90] Such a search may also yield items that can be used on surveys or to start a record-keeping system that will eventually become the basis for evaluation of the program.

Checklists and questionnaires are structured ways of collecting and organizing information from important individuals and groups. These can be used to measure knowledge, attitudes, and beliefs as well as perceptions of services. Zapka and Mamon conducted a formal study of the predisposing, enabling, and reinforcing factors associated with breast self-examination among college women on a university campus. Their analysis illustrates the formal application of survey methods to the sorting process.[91] Other formal surveys applying the PRECEDE model have been published and can be used in future assessments as a source of developed survey instruments and comparison data.[92]

Directories of available community resources are often compiled by planning agencies. These directories are particularly helpful when enabling factors are being examined. Utilization data from health care organizations and attendance records from agencies may also be available.[93] Surveys of community organizations can also be conducted, as recommended and detailed in a series of CDC community intervention handbooks.[94]

If planners have trouble deciding whether a factor is predisposing, enabling, or reinforcing, they should list it in all categories that might apply. The three categories are not mutually exclusive; a factor can appropriately be placed in more than one. A family may be predisposed to dieting, for example, and may reinforce (negatively or positively) that behavior once it has been undertaken. We do not want to define the categories so rigidly that PRECEDE becomes an academic debating point. The purpose of the categories is to sort the causal factors into three classes of targets for subsequent intervention according to the three broad classes of intervention strategy: direct communication to change the predisposing factors, indirect communication (through family, peers, teachers, employers, health-care providers) to change the reinforcing factors, and organizational or training strategies to change the enabling factors.

Later in the planning process, the specific educational and organizational activities and messages for each factor are devised based on your judgment of their importance as determinants of the desired outcomes. Then the category in which the factor falls makes a difference. For example, the design of messages, learning opportunities, and organizational strategies directed at families is different according to whether a family is seen as important in creating rewards to reinforce the behavior or providing financial support to enable the behavior.

A list at this point might look something like the one in Table 5.1, which shows both positive and negative factors related to reducing the sequelae of streptococcal throat infections in a preschool population. At the end of this chapter you will convert some of these factors into learning and resource objectives, which are statements of the immediate goals of health promotion programs. Those objectives must be achieved in order to obtain behavioral and environmental changes, which are the intermediate goals of the program. The behavioral and environmental objectives must be achieved if you hope to achieve health improvements or improvements in quality of life—the ultimate goals of the program.

STEP 2. SETTING PRIORITIES AMONG CATEGORIES

All the causes in a complete inventory for several behaviors cannot be tackled simultaneously. Decisions about which factors are to be the objects of intervention, and in what order, are therefore necessary.

One possible basis for establishing **priorities** among the three kinds of factors is developmental. For example, an HIV screening service must have its facility in operation and services available before it creates a demand for the services. The

TABLE 5.1

Classification of factors causing behavior

Behavioral objectives

Within three days of the initial manifestation of sore throat, 80 percent of the children in Hobbit's Preschool Program will have a throat culture done based on a swab taken by a parent.

The target group for the learning objectives will be the parents of the preschoolers, the parents' employers, relatives, and physicians, and the preschool personnel.

Predisposing factors

Positive	Negative
Attitudes, beliefs, and values: Mothers value child's health; mothers have been willing to use health services regularly. Knowledge: Mothers can read thermometers and determine temperatures; children are old enough to report sore throats.	Attitudes, beliefs, and values: Sore throats are not important; mothers feel that sore throats are temporary; mothers feel that sore throats do not have serious consequences and that there is no relationship between strep throat and sequelae.

Reinforcing factors

Positive	Negative
Teachers can identify ill children; teachers relate well to parents; physician has set up positive interaction with group; teachers and medical personnel encourage and support parents in taking throat swabs.	Mother's employers are not generous about time off for child's illness; grandmothers (or baby sitters) consider sore throats inconsequential and temporary.

Enabling factors

Positive	Negative
Mothers have thermometers in homes; clinic is close by; insurance reduces cost of follow-up visit. Throat swab kit for home use is available; clinic provides culture and analysis in three days; skill in swabbing is easily learned.	Cost of prescription penicillin regimen; teachers cannot take child to doctor; parent has to stay home with child or arrange for sitter because there is no preschool isolation room.

organizational enabling factors that provide the services and make them accessible have to precede the educational efforts to predispose people to use them. People do not adopt a set of behaviors to reduce a health risk if they are not aware that there is a risk. Belief in the immediacy of the risk and its implications have to be developed for the enabling resources to be utilized. Reinforcing factors cannot come into play until behaviors have been evidenced. Thus, for a community program, the enabling, predisposing, and reinforcing factors should be translated into interventions *in that order*. Different situations may require a different order of development, depending on the factors that already exist.

Some enabling factors have to be developed over a long period by means of community organization efforts, legislative pressure, and reallocation of resources. When that is the case, concerns of the basic target group may have to be postponed for months. In such cases the population so predisposed might be mobilized to support legislation or organizational development.

Some factors are difficult to work with because of agency policies or mandates. An agency may be restricted to activities related to one set of factors. A hospital may not have the personnel to contact families at home and may have to depend on another agency to undertake the task. A school system may be controlled by a ruling by a board of education that AIDS education can be taught only within classes on marriage and the family, and that discussion and provision of contraception is not a school responsibility.

Work on several factors can and should proceed simultaneously, however. Cooperation with the appropriate agency to establish a rehabilitation service for alcoholics, for example, can coincide with the mounting of a general information campaign throughout the community on the costs of alcoholism and the efficacy of treatment. By the time the service is operational, the climate is set for specific information about the type and availability of services.

STEP 3. ESTABLISHING PRIORITIES WITHIN CATEGORIES

Within the three categories of behavioral causes, factors can be selected for intervention using the same criteria as were used on the selection of the high-priority behaviors: importance and changeability.

Importance. Importance can be estimated by judging prevalence, immediacy, and necessity according to logic, experience, data, and theory. *Prevalence* asks, How widespread or frequent is the factor? If the factor identified is very widespread or occurs often, it should qualify for priority consideration. For example, if 80 percent of the students in a school system believe smoking is glamorous, then addressing that belief in an antismoking campaign should have much higher priority than if the belief is held by only 10 percent of students.

Immediacy asks, How compelling or urgent is the factor? Knowing the symptoms of a heart attack and what is needed to save a victim's life are an example of knowledge that has immediate consequences for people at high risk of heart attacks. Another type of immediacy concerns the relationship between the factor and the group at risk. If a group of adults believes no connection exists between strep throat and rheumatic heart disease, changing that belief is a high-priority goal if the adults are the parents of young children who are at high risk. It is not high priority if the adults are the parents of graduating seniors.

Necessity is based on the consideration that a factor may have a low prevalence but still has to be present for the change in behavior or environment to occur. If an outcome cannot be achieved without a certain factor, that factor deserves priority. Knowledge is often necessary though insufficient to bring about an action. It is difficult to envision an intravenous drug user giving up drugs to avoid AIDS without understanding how dirty needles can transmit HIV, or to envision a person committing himself or herself to a patient role without awareness of the illness, however minimal. Knowledge of exercise prescriptions is necessary for a person to participate in an aerobic conditioning program. Some beliefs also can be considered necessary. People who are supposed to present themselves for medical services must believe (however slightly) that the health professional can help alleviate the problem. A person who is attempting to stop smoking must believe smoking is harmful, at least to his or her social relations if not to health.

Changeability. Evidence of the changeability of a factor can be gained from looking at the results of previous programs. Assessments of changeability can also be made using techniques set forth in the literature. Rokeach, for example, posits a hierarchy in which beliefs are easier to change than attitudes and attitudes are easier to change than values.[95]

One also can analyze changeability and priority of factors according to a theory on stages in adoption and diffusion of innovations. This theory is based on work in communications and extensive experience in agriculture, education, family planning, and public health.[96] Behavior change is analyzed over time, and the stages through which behavior is adopted are observed at the individual and societal levels. Individuals pass through stages labeled *awareness, interest, persuasion, decision,* and *adoption.* When these stages are charted in a population or social system, they follow a pattern of prevalence or cumulative diffusion that looks like a series of increasingly flattened S-shaped curves.

In Figure 5.4 the five stages of adoption and the four groups of adopters identify points in time when different communication methods and channels are more or less effective. Identification of the stages allows the health promotion planner to match the most appropriate intervention strategy to the stage of the program recipients. For example, mass media are most efficient with innovators and early adopters, but outreach methods such as home visits are necessary with late adopters. Depending on the percentage of the population who have already adopted the health behavior at a given point in time, the relative changeability of the behavior in the remaining population is defined by this theory of diffusion.

Observability also influences changeability. If the factor is observable and can be demonstrated, a climate for others is set and their efforts are reinforced. As an example, consider the growing emphasis on nonsmoking in public meetings. Mass communications often can be utilized to promote reinforcing messages that support certain behaviors. The function of media, in such instances, is not to motivate but to reinforce.

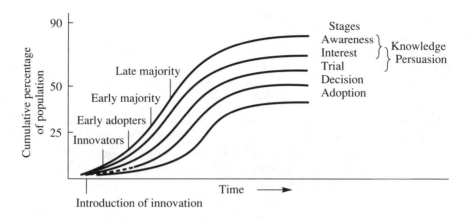

FIGURE 5.4

Five stages of adoption for four groups of adopters over time during diffusion of an innovation.

WRITING LEARNING AND RESOURCE OBJECTIVES

Writing learning and resource objectives is similar to writing behavior objectives, as presented in Chapter 4. Learning objectives define the predisposing factors and skills that will be the targets of intervention. They will also provide criteria for evaluation of the program. Resource objectives define the environmental enabling factors that should be in place at the end of a program.

Examples of learning objectives are shown in Table 5.2. Predisposing and enabling factors analyzed in Table 5.1 have been restated in terms of learning objectives for parents. Note the variations in the *how much* in these examples. It is usually possible to create a high level of knowledge. Often, over 90 percent of a given population can be made aware of a fact. A smaller percentage of those who are aware will believe the fact to be relevant, important, or useful. Not all of these will develop requisite skill to carry out recommended actions. Hence, if 60 percent of the population is expected to adopt a behavior, it is necessary to develop skills in 70 percent, establish health beliefs in 80 percent, and to create knowledge of the problem or recommendation in 90 percent or more.

This phenomenon accompanies the diffusion of any health practice. Figure 5.5 shows percentages of people during the early phases of the U.S. antismoking campaigns who were aware cigarette smoking is harmful, who were interested in doing something about it, and who had stopped smoking. By 1970 between 80 and 90 percent of the target group had become aware of the dangers of smoking;

TABLE 5.2

Examples of learning objectives based on predisposing and enabling factors analyzed in Table 5.1

Problem	Teaching parents to swab sore throats and submit swabs for throat cultures.
Target Group Parents	

Knowledge	By the end of the program period, 90 percent of the parents
	(a) will identify sore throat and fever as potential strep throat,
	(b) will identify throat swabs as necessary to determine whether strep accompanies sore throat,
	(c) can state the cure for strep throat,
	(d) can state that prescriptions are available at the clinic.
Beliefs	By the end of the program, 80 percent of the parents
	(a) will believe that the consequences of strep throat can be serious,
	(b) will believe that a cure is available,
	(c) will believe they can take action leading to identification and treatment of strep throat,
	(d) will believe that this series of steps will reduce the potential for further illness.
Skills	By the end of the program period, 70 percent of the parents
	(a) will be able to swab a child's throat,
	(b) will be able to return the swab to the clinic laboratory.

somewhat fewer than 50 percent had been able to stop smoking. It was clear at this point that further efforts were needed to increase the number of people willing to try quitting and to help those who wanted to be successful. It was also clear that little could be gained by continuing a program that only emphasized increasing awareness. This kind of historical trend analysis can be helpful in establishing an appropriate emphasis for a health promotion program.

One can also observe in Figure 5.5 that diffusion curves for awareness, interest, and adoption of smoking-cessation knowledge, persuasion, and behavior were similar to curves for corresponding early stages of the diffusion curves in Figure 5.4. If Figure 5.5 covered a longer period of time, it would show the increased rates of adoption of smoking-cessation behavior that developed between 1970 and 1980. By 1990, the rate of quitting had settled down to 33 percent trying to quit each year but only 20 percent being successful, which accounts for a 6 percent decrease of smokers. But new smokers recruited from the teenage group result in a net annual reduction of current smokers of only 1 percent.

Learning objectives can be developed not only for the target population but

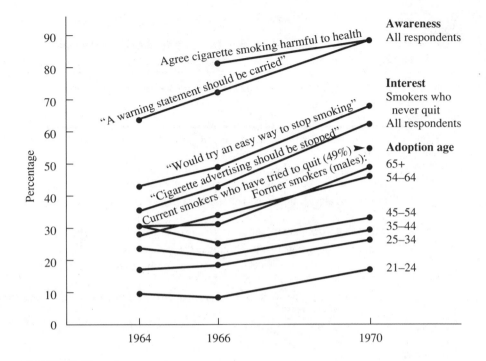

FIGURE 5.5

Adoption curve for smoking cessation. Percentages are given for those aware, those interested, and former smokers. [Adapted from L. W. Green, in *Applying Behavioral Science to Cardiovascular Risk*, A. J. Enelow and J. B. Henderson, eds. (New York: American Heart Association, 1975).]

also for those people who will reinforce the target population. For the example about throat cultures in preschool children, the preschool personnel might also be targets of intervention aimed at teaching them how to reinforce the parents. In addition, information about environmental enabling factors provides the basis for the development of resource objectives.

Examples of learning objectives for reinforcement and of resource objectives for environmental enabling factors are shown in Table 5.3. Note that the objectives address the reinforcing and environmental enabling factors that were defined in Table 5.1. Learning objectives for reinforcers and resource objectives are important components of a health promotion program that addresses all three categories of determining factors. Achievement of ongoing reinforcement and environmental resources can create a favorable situation in which the effect of the health promotion program continues even after the program is over.

Diffusion theory also provides a framework for diagnosis of reinforcing and

TABLE 5.3

Examples of learning and resource objectives based on reinforcing and enabling factors analyzed in Table 5.1

Problem	Teaching preschool personnel to reinforce and enable parents to swab sore throats of children

Target Group: Preschool Personnel

Learning objectives for reinforcement	By the end of the program period, 90 percent of the preschool personnel will

   (a) verbally reinforce mothers for swabbing their children's throats within 3 days of the initial manifestation of sore throat,

   (b) verbally reinforce mothers for returning swabs to the clinic laboratory,

   (c) inquire of parents about the results of throat swabs,

   (d) inform parents that prescriptions are available at the clinic,

   (e) administer prescribed medications according to instructions from the parent and physician,

   (f) inform other parents when a positive throat culture occurs in a preschool child.

Resource objectives for environmental enabling factors	By the end of the program period, 100 percent of the time the preschool personnel will make available for parents' use

   (a) throat swab kits,

   (b) thermometers,

   (c) laboratory slips for throat cultures.

---

enabling factors. For example, the presence of "No Smoking" sections in restaurants, an enabling factor for nonsmoking, has undoubtedly followed a diffusion curve. Warner presents an interesting analysis of smoking that supports the view that "nonsmokers' rights" have an extremely important influence on the current trend of decreased smoking in the population.[97] Reactions to smokers by nonsmokers, fueled by the nonsmokers' rights movement, can be considered reinforcing factors for nonsmoking. Attitudes and behaviors supportive of nonsmokers' rights have probably also followed a diffusion curve.

SUMMARY

This chapter examined the factors affecting behavior and the environment as these relate to health. We call this phase of PRECEDE the educational and organizational diagnosis because we identify those factors on which health education and community organization can have a direct and immediate influence, and thereby an indirect influence on behavior or environment. Three sets of factors were identified: predisposing, reinforcing, and enabling. Each plays a role in health-related behavior and organization. After identifying the factors, we suggested how to assess their relative importance and changeability. Use of these two criteria makes it possible to rank the various causes of health behavior in order of priority, and then to develop related learning and organizational objectives so that health promotion programs can focus where they will do the most good in facilitating development or changes of behavior and environment conducive to health.

Formulation of learning objectives follows from the identification of predisposing factors and skills; development of organizational and resource objectives follows from the identification of reinforcing and enabling factors.

EXERCISES

1. For one of the high-priority behaviors you selected in the previous chapter, make an inventory of all the predisposing, enabling, and reinforcing factors you can identify. For a priority environmental condition, list the enabling factors.
2. Rate each factor believed to cause the health behavior or environmental condition according to its importance and changeability. Give each factor a rating of low, medium, or high on each criterion.
3. Write learning or resource objectives for the highest-priority predisposing factor, enabling factor, and reinforcing factor.

REFERENCES AND NOTES

1. R. Andersen, *A Behavioral Model of Families' Use of Health Services* (Chicago: University of Chicago Center for Health Administration Studies Research Series, no. 25, University of Chicago Press, 1968); L. W. Green, "Toward Cost-Benefit Evaluations of Health Education: Some Concepts, Methods and Examples," *Health Education Monographs* 2 (suppl. 1, 1974): 34–64; idem., "Modifying and Developing Health Behavior," *Annual Review of Public Health* 5 (1984): 215–36; L. W. Green, B. Rimer, and T. W. Elwood, "Biobehavioral Approaches to Cancer Prevention and Detection," in *Perspectives on Behavioral Medicine*, S. Weiss, A. Herd, and B. Fox, eds. (New York: Academic Press, 1981), pp. 215–34; L. W. Green, "Health Education Models," in *Behavioral Health: A Handbook of Health Enhancement and Disease Prevention*, J. D. Matarazzo, S. M. Weiss, J. A. Herd, et al., eds. (New York: Wiley, 1984), pp. 181–98. See the first edition for other historical and theoretical roots of the PRECEDE model.

2. A. Bandura, *Social Learning Theory* (Englewood Cliffs, NJ: Prentice-Hall, 1977); idem., "Self-efficacy Mechanisms in Human Agency," *American Psychologist* 37 (1982): 122–47.

3. B. G. Simons-Morton, G. S. Parcel, N. M. O'Hara, et al., "Health-Related Physical Fitness in Childhood: Status and Recommendations," *Annual Review of Public Health* 9 (1988): 403–25.

4. D. G. Simons-Morton, S. G. Brink, G. S. Parcel, et al., *Promoting Physical Activity Among Adults: A CDC Community Intervention Handbook* (Atlanta, GA: Centers for Disease Control, 1988).

5. G. S. Parcel, D. G. Simons-Morton, S. G. Brink, et al., *Smoking Control Among Women: A CDC Community Intervention Handbook* (Atlanta, GA: Centers for Disease Control, 1987).

6. D. Cartwright, "Some Principles of Mass Persuasion: Selected Findings from Research on the Sale of United States War Bonds," *Human Relations* 2 (1949): 53–69.

7. J. W. Farquhar, S. Fortmann, N. Maccoby, et al., "The Stanford Five City Project: An Overview," in *Behavioral Health: A Handbook of Health Enhancement and Disease Prevention*, J. D. Matarazzo, S. M. Weiss, J. A. Herd, et al., eds. (New York: Wiley, 1984), pp. 1154–65; M. A. Winkleby, S. P. Fortmann, and D. C. Barrett, "Social Class Disparities in Risk Factors for Disease: Eight-Year Prevalence Patterns by Level of Education," *Preventive Medicine* 19 (1990): 1–12.

8. For example, A. J. Sogaard, "The Effect of a Mass-Media Dental Health Education Campaign," *Health Education Research* 3 (1988): 243–55.

9. M. H. Becker and J. Joseph, "AIDS and Behavioral Change To Reduce Risk: A Review," *American Journal of Public Health* 78 (1988): 394–410.

10. Awareness or new knowledge might appear to be the only thing required to obtain a change in behavior in situations where the other predisposing, enabling, and reinforcing factors are already in place. As Beverly Ware noted in her case study of the Ford Motor Company's medical screening and surveillance program, "Although there is little evidence that information alone achieves behavior change . . . considerable evidence exists to indicate that, in some kinds of situations, information is all that is needed to provide behavior change . . . This was such a case." B. G. Ware, "Occupational Health Education: A Nontraditional Role for a Health Educator," in *Advancing Health Through Education: A Case Study Approach*, H. P. Cleary, J. M. Kichen, and P. G. Ensor, eds. (Palo Alto: Mayfield, 1985), pp. 319–23. Quotation from p. 321.

11. R. P. Abelson, E. Aronson, W. J. McGuire, et al., *Theories of Cognitive Consistency: A Sourcebook* (Chicago, IL: Rand McNally College, 1968).

12. I. Ajzen and M. Fishbein, *Understanding Attitudes and Predicting Social Behavior* (Englewood Cliffs, NJ: Prentice-Hall, 1980); C.-A. Emmons, J. G. Joseph, and R. C. Kessler, et al., "Psychosocial Predictors of Reported Behavior Change in Homosexual Men at Risk for AIDS," *Health Education Quarterly* 13 (1986): 331–45; I. Janis, ed., *Counseling on Personal Decisions* (New Haven: Yale University Press, 1982); J. K. O'Connel, J. H. Price, S. M. Roberts, et al., "Utilizing the Health Belief Model to Predict Dieting and Exercising Behavior of Obese and Nonobese Adolescents," *Health Education Quarterly* 12 (1985): 343–51; G. S. Parcel and T. Baranowski, "Social Learning Theory and Health Education," *Health Education* 12(3) (1981): 14–18; V. J. Strecher, B. M. DeVellis, M. H. Becker, and I. M. Rosenstock, "The Role of Self-efficacy in Achieving Health Behavior Change," *Health Education Quarterly* 13 (1986): 73–92.

13. M. H. Becker, ed., "The Health Belief Model and Personal Health Behavior," *Health Education Monographs* 2 (1974): 324–473, whole issue; N. K. Janz and M. H. Becker, "The Health Belief Model: A Decade Later," *Health Education Quarterly* 11 (1984): 1–47; L. A. Maiman, M. H. Becker, J. P. Kirscht, et al., "Scales for Measuring Health Belief Model Dimensions: A Test of Predictive Value, Internal Consistency, and Relationship Among Beliefs," *Health Education Monographs* 5 (1977): 215–31. For a recent meta-analysis of studies testing the Health Belief Model, see J. A. Harrison, P. D. Mullen, and L. W. Green, "A Meta-analysis of Studies of the Health Belief Model," *Health Education Research* 5 (in press). For a validation of its predictive power in relation to other models including PRECEDE which encompasses the Health Belief Model, see P. D. Mullen, J. Hersey, and D. C. Iverson, "Health Behavior Models Compared," *Social Science and Medicine* 24 (1987): 973–81.

14. AIDS and other sexually transmitted diseases: C.-A. Emmons, J. G. Joseph, and R. C. Kessler, et al., "Psychosocial Predictors of Reported Behavior Change in Homosexual Men at Risk for AIDS," *Health Education Quarterly* 13 (1986): 331–45; J. Joseph, S. Montgomery, C.-A. Emmons, et al., "Magnitude and Determinants of Behavior Risk Reduction: Longitudinal Analysis of a Cohort at Risk for AIDS," *Psychology and Health* 1 (1987): 73–96; D. Nelkin, "AIDS and the Social Sciences: Review of Useful Knowledge and Research Needs," *Reviews of Infectious*

Diseases 9 (1987): 980–6; K. J. Simon and J. Das, "An Application of the Health Belief Model Toward Educational Diagnosis for VD Education," *Health Education Quarterly* 11 (1984): 403–18.

15. Contraceptive practices and family planning: M. E. Katatsky, "The Health Belief Model as a Conceptual Framework for Explaining Contraceptive Compliance," *Health Education Monographs* 5 (1977): 232–42; A. A. Fisher, "The Health Belief Model and Contraceptive Behavior: Limits to the Application of a Conceptual Framework," *Health Education Monographs* 5 (1978): 244–8.

16. Diabetes: T. E. Adamson and D. S. Gullion, "Assessment of Diabetes Continuing Medical Education," *Diabetes Care* 9 (1986): 11–16; M. Algona, "Perception of Severity of Disease and Health Locus of Control in Compliant and Noncompliant Diabetic Patients," *Diabetes Care* 3 (1980): 533–4; K. A. Cerkoney and L. K. Hart, "The Relationship Between the Health Belief Model and Compliance of Persons with Diabetes Mellitus," *Diabetes Care* 3 (1980): 594–8; R. Harris, M. W. Linn, and L. Pollack, "Relationship Between Health Beliefs and Psychological Variables in Diabetic Patients," *British Journal of Medical Psychology* 57 (1984): 253–9; W. J. Wishner and M. D. O'Brien, "Diabetes and the Family," *Medical Clinics of North America* 62 (1978): 849–56.

17. Injury control behavior: K. H. Beck, "Driving While Under the Influence of Alcohol: Relationship to Attitudes and Beliefs in a College Population," *American Journal of Drug and Alcohol Abuse* 8 (1981): 377–88; P. D. Mullen, D. C. Iverson, and J. Hersey, "Health Behavior Models Compared," *Social Science and Medicine* . . . op. cit.; M. P. Eriksen and A. C. Gielen, "The Application of Health Education Principles to Automobile Child Restraint Programs," *Health Education Quarterly* 10 (1983): 30–55; G. R. Webb, R. W. Sanson-Fisher, and J. A. Bowman, "Psychosocial Factors Related to Parental Restraint of Pre-school Children in Motor Vehicles," *Accident Analysis and Prevention* 20 (1988): 87–94. The seat-belt studies indicate that "cost versus benefits" beliefs (e.g., inconvenience) are more compelling than beliefs in susceptibility or severity of consequences in predicting seat-belt use.

18. Child health care and child health behavior: P. J. Bush and R. J. Iannotti, "A Children's Health Belief Model," *Medical Care* 28 (1990): 69–86; T. E. Dielman, S. L. Leech, M. H. Becker, et al., "Dimensions of Children's Health Beliefs," *Health Education Quarterly* 7 (1980): 219–38; D. S. Gochman and G. S. Parcel, eds., "Children's Health Beliefs and Health Behaviors," *Health Education Quarterly* 9 (1982): 104–270 (whole issue).

19. Participation in screening programs: M. H. Becker, M. M. Kaback, and I. M. Rosenstock, "Some Influences on Public Participation in a Genetic Screening Program," *Journal of Community Health* 1 (1975): 3–14; M. Calnan, "The Health Belief Model and Participation in Programmes for the Early Detection of Breast Cancer: A Comparative Analysis," *Social Science and Medicine* 19 (1984): 823–30; G. M. Hochbaum, "Why People Seek Diagnostic X-Rays," *Public Health Reports* 71 (1956): 377–80; S. S. Kegeles, "A Field Experiment Attempt to Change Beliefs and Behavior of Women in an Urban Ghetto," *Journal of Health and Social Behavior* 10 (1969): 115–24; J. B. King, "The Impact of Patients' Perceptions of High Blood Pressure on Attendance at Screening: An Extension of the Health Belief Model," *Social Science and Medicine* 16 (1982): 1079–82; J. R. C. Wheeler and T. G. Rundall, "Secondary Preventive Health Behavior," *Health Education Quarterly* 7 (1980): 243–62.

20. Use of clinical health services: M. H. Becker, C. A. Nathanson, M. D. Drachman, and J. P. Kirscht, "Mothers' Health Beliefs and Children's Clinic Visits: A Prospective Study," *Journal of Community Health* 3 (1977): 125–33; E. Berkanovic, C. Telesky, and S. Reeder, "Structural and Social Psychological Factors in the Decision to Seek Medical Care for Symptoms," *Medical Care* 19 (1981): 693–709; S. Kegeles, "Why People Seek Dental Care: A Test of Conceptual Formulation," *Journal of Health and Social Behavior* 10 (1969): 115–24; D. Lane, "Compliance with Referrals from a Cancer Screening Project," *Journal of Family Practice* 17 (1983): 811–17; E. Larson, E. Olsen, W. Cole, and S. Shortell, "The Relationship of Health Beliefs and Postcard Reminders to Influenza Vaccination," *Journal of Family Practice* 8 (1979): 1207–11; F. Leavitt, "The Health Belief Model and Utilization of Ambulatory Care Services," *Social Science and Medicine* 13A (1979): 105–12.

21. Dietary behavior: W. Aho, "Smoking, Dieting, and Exercise: Age Differences in Attitudes and Behavior Relevant to Selected Health Belief Model Variables. The Perceived Seriousness Is an Important Factor Influencing Behavior," *Rhode Island Medical Journal* 62 (1979): 85–92; M. H. Becker, L. Maiman, J. Kirscht, D. Haefner, and R. Drachman, "The Health Belief Model and Prediction of Dietary Compliance: A Field Experiment," *Journal of Health and Social Behavior* 18 (1977): 348–66; J. Hollis, G. Sexton, S. Connors, et al., "The Family Heart Dietary Intervention Program: Community Response and Characteristics of Joining and Nonjoining Families," *Preventive Medicine* 13 (1984): 276–85; J. O'Connell, J. Price, S. Roberts, et al., "Utilizing the Health Belief Model to Predict Dieting and Exercising Behavior of Obese and Nonobese Adolescents," *Health Education Quarterly* 12 (1985): 343–51.

22. Asthma: M. Becker, S. Radius, I. Rosenstock, et al., "Compliance with a Medical Regimen for Asthma: A Test of the Health Belief Model," *Public Health Reports* 93 (1978): 268–77; J. G. Bruhn, "The Application of Theory in Childhood Asthma Self-help Programs, *Journal of Allergy and Clinical Immunology* 72 (suppl., Nov. 1983): 561–77; S. Radius, M. Becker, I. Rosenstock, et al., "Factors Influencing Mothers' Compliance with a Medical Regimen for Asthmatic Children," *Journal of Asthma Research* 15 (1978): 133–49.

23. Genetic counseling or screening: R. Black, "Support for Genetic Services: A Survey. *Health and Social Work* 5 (1980): 27–34; M. Goldstein, S. Greenwald, T. Nathan, et al., "Health Behavior and Genetic Screening for Carriers of Tay-Sachs Disease: A Prospective Study," *Social Science and Medicine* 11 (1977): 515–20.

24. Breast self-examination: M. Calnan and S. Moss, "The Health Belief Model and Compliance with Education Given at a Class in Breast Self-examination," *Journal of Health and Social Behavior* 25 (1984): 198–210; J. Hallal, "The Relationship of Health Beliefs, Health Locus of Control, and Self Concept to the Practice of Breast Self-examination in Adult Women," *Nursing Research* 20 (1979): 17–29.

25. Immunization: K. Cummings, A. Jette, B. Brock, and D. Haefner, "Psychosocial Determinants of Immunization Behavior in a Swine Influenza Campaign," *Medical Care* 17 (1979): 639–49; E. Larson, E. Olsen, W. Cole, and S. Shortell, "The Relationship of Health Beliefs and a Postcard Reminder to Influenza Vaccination," *Journal of Family Practice* 8 (1979): 1207–11; I. M. Rosenstock, M. Derryberry, and B. Carriger, "Why People Fail to Seek Poliomyelitis Vaccination," *Public Health Reports* 74 (1959): 98–103; T. Rundall and J. Wheeler, "Factors Associated with Utilization of the Swine Flu Vaccination Program Among Senior Citizens in Tompkins County," *Medical Care* 17 (1979): 191–200.

26. Patient adherence to medical regimens: K. Cummings, M. Becker, J. Kirscht, and N. Levin, "Psychosocial Factors Affecting Adherence to Medical Regimens in a Group of Hemodialysis Patients," *Medical Care* 20 (1982): 567–80; W. Doherty, H. Schrott, L. Metcalf, and V. Iasiello, "Effect of Spouse Support and Health Beliefs on Medical Adherence," *Journal of Family Practice* 17 (1983): 837–41; J. Fincham and A. Wertheimer, "Using the Health Belief Model to Predict Initial Drug Therapy Defaulting," *Social Science and Medicine* 20 (1985): 101–5; L. W. Green, D. M. Levine, J. Wolle, and S. G. Deeds, "Development of Randomized Patient Education Experiments with Urban Poor Hypertensives," *Patient Counseling and Health Education* 1 (1979): 101–11; R. Harris, J. Skyler, M. Linn, et al., "Relationship Between the Health Belief Model and Compliance as a Basis for Intervention in Diabetes Mellitus," in *Pediatric and Adolescent Endocrinology: vol. 10, Psychological Aspects of Diabetes in Children and Adolescents*, Z. Loron and A. Galatzer, eds. (Basel: Karger, 1982), pp. 123–32; P. Hartman and M. H. Becker, "Non-compliance with Prescribed Regime Among Chronic Hemodialysis Patients: A Method of Prediction and Educational Diagnosis," *Dialysis and Transplantation* 7 (1978): 978–89; J. Hershey, B. Morton, J. Davis and M. Reichgott, "Patient Compliance with Antihypertensive Medication," *American Journal of Public Health* 70 (1980): 1081–9; J. Kirscht and I. Rosenstock, "Patient Adherence to Antihypertensive Medical Regimens," *Journal of Community Health* 3 (1977): 115–24; V. Nagy and G. Wolfe, "Cognitive Predictors of Compliance in Chronic Disease Patients," *Medical Care* 22 (1984): 912–21; E. Nelson, W. Stason, R. Neutra, et al., "Impact of Patient Perceptions of Compliance with Treatment for Hypertension," *Medical Care* 16 (1978): 893–906; J. Salloway, W. Pletcher, and J. Collins, "Sociological and Social-Psychological Models

of Compliance with Prescribed Regimens: In Search of Synthesis," *Sociological Symposium* 23 (1978): 100–21.

27. Smoking: W. Aho, "Smoking, Dieting, and Exercise: Age Differences in Attitudes and Behavior Relevant to Selected Health Belief Model Variables. The Perceived Seriousness Is an Important Factor Influencing Behavior," *Rhode Island Medical Journal* 62 (1979): 85–92; P. L. Ellickson and R. M. Bell, *Prospects for Preventing Drug Use Among Young Adolescents* (Santa Monica, CA: RAND, R-3896-CHF, 1990); S. Eraker, M. Becker, V. Strecher, and J. Kirscht, "Smoking Behavior, Cessation Techniques, and the Health Decision Model," *American Journal of Medicine* 78 (1985): 817–25; V. Giannetti, J. Reynolds, and T. Rihn, "Factors Which Differentiate Smokers from Ex-smokers Among Cardiovascular Patients: A Discriminant Analysis," *Social Science and Medicine* 20 (1985): 241–5; N. Gottlieb, "The Effect of Health Beliefs on the Smoking of College Women," *Journal of American College Health* 31 (1983): 214–21; L. Pederson, J. Wanklin, and J. Baskerville, "The Role of Health Beliefs in Compliance with Physician Advice to Quit Smoking," *Social Science and Medicine* 19 (1984): 573–80; R. Warnecke, S. Graham, S. Rosenthal, and C. Manfredi, "Social and Psychological Correlates of Smoking Behavior Among Black Women," *Journal of Health and Social Behavior* 19 (1978): 397–410; M. Weinberger, J. Greene, J. Mamlin, and M. Jerin, "Health Beliefs and Smoking Behavior," *American Journal of Public Health* 71 (1981): 1253–5.

28. Hypertension, high blood pressure control: L. W. Green, D. M. Levine, J. Wolle, and S. G. Deeds, "Development of Randomized Patient Education Experiments with Urban Poor Hypertensives," *Patient Counseling and Health Education* 1 (1979): 106–11; J. Hershey, B. Morton, J. Davis, and M. Reichgott, "Patient Compliance with Antihypertensive Medication," *American Journal of Public Health* 70 (1980): 1081–9; T. Inui, E. Yourtee, and J. Williamson, "Improved Outcomes in Hypertension After Physician Tutorials: A Controlled Trial," *Annals of Internal Medicine* 84 (1976): 646–51; J. King, "The Impact of Patients' Perceptions of High Blood Pressure on Attendance at Screening: An Extension of the Health Belief Model," *Social Science and Medicine* 16 (1982): 1079–91; J. Kirscht and I. M. Rosenstock, "Patient Adherence to Antihypertensive Medical Regimens," *Journal of Community Health* 3 (1977): 115–24; E. Nelson, W. Stason, R. Neutra, et al., "Impact of Patient Perceptions of Compliance with Treatment for Hypertension," *Medical Care* 16 (1978): 893–906; D. Taylor, "A Test of the Health Belief Model in Hypertension," in *Compliance in Health Care*, R. B. Haynes, D. W. Taylor and D. L. Sackett, eds. (Baltimore: Johns Hopkins University Press, 1979): 103–9; see also Table 5, pp. 458–9 in Haynes, Taylor and Sackett for a summary of those studies supporting and those not supporting relationships between the Health Belief Model and various compliance outcomes.

29. Physician behavior in patient education and health promotion: T. E. Adamson and D. S. Gullion, "Assessment of Diabetes Continuing Medical Education," *Diabetes Care* 9 (1986): 11–16; L. W. Green, M. P. Eriksen, and E. L. Schor, "Preventive Practices by Physicians: Behavioral Determinants and Potential Interventions," in *Implementing Preventive Services*, R. N. Battista and R. S. Lawrence, eds. (New York: Oxford University Press, 1988), pp. 101–7; T. Inui, E. Yourtee, and J. Williamson, "Improved Outcomes in Hypertension After Physician Tutorials: A Controlled Trial," *Annals of Internal Medicine* 84 (1976): 646–51; B. Maheux, R. Pineault, and F. Beland, "Factors Influencing Physicians' Orientation Toward Prevention," *American Journal of Preventive Medicine* 3 (1987): 12–18. See also Chapter 11 for related applications of the Health Belief Model.

30. Cardiac rehabilitation: B. Tirrell and L. Hart, "The Relationship of Health Beliefs and Knowledge to Exercise Compliance in Patients After Coronory Bypass," *Heart and Lung* 9 (1980): 487–93.

31. Tuberculosis: G. M. Hochbaum, "Why People Seek Diagnostic X-Rays," *Public Health Reports* 71 (1956): 377–80; G. M. Hochbaum, *Public Participation in Medical Screening Programs: A Social-Psychological Study* (Washington, DC: Public Health Service, PHS-572, 1959); C. D. Jenkins, "Group Differences in Perception: A Study of Community Beliefs and Feelings About Tuberculosis," *American Journal of Sociology* 71 (1966): 417–29; S. Wurtele, M. Roberts, and J. Leeper, "Health Beliefs and Intentions: Predictors of Return Compliance in a Tuberculosis Detection Drive," *Journal of Applied Social Psychology* 53 (1982): 19–21.

32. Dental behavior: S. S. Kegeles, "Why People Seek Dental Care: A Test of a Conceptual

Formulation," *Journal of Health and Human Behavior* 10 (1963): 166–73; G. Rayant and A. Sheiham, "An Analysis of Factors Affecting Compliance with Tooth-Cleaning Recommendations," *Journal of Clinical Periodontology* 7 (1980): 289–99; R. Tash, R. O'Shea, and L. Cohen, "Testing a Preventive-Symptomatic Theory of Dental Health Behavior," *American Journal of Public Health* 59 (1969): 514–21.

33. Occupational therapy: G. Kielhofner and C. Nelson, "A Study of Patient Motivation and Cooperation/Participation in Occupational Therapy," *Occupational Therapy Journal of Research* 3 (1983): 35–46.

34. Toxic shock syndrome: R. Riggs and M. Noland, "Awareness, Knowledge, and Perceived Risk for Toxic Shock Syndrome in Relation to Health Behavior," *Journal of School Health* 53 (1983): 303–7.

35. Exercise: W. Aho, "Smoking, Dieting, and Exercise: Age Differences in Attitudes and Behavior Relevant to Selected Health Belief Model Variables. The Perceived Seriousness Is an Important Factor Influencing Behavior," *Rhode Island Medical Journal* 62 (1979): 85–92; P. D. Mullen, J. Hersey, and D. C. Iverson, "Health Behavior Models Compared," *Social Science and Medicine*, op. cit.; J. O'Connell, J. Price, S. Roberts, et al., "Utilizing the Health Belief Model to Predict Dieting and Exercising Behavior of Obese and Nonobese Adolescents," *Health Education Quarterly* 12 (1985): 343–51; S. Slenker, J. Price, S. Roberts, and S. Jurs, "Joggers Versus Nonexercisers: An Analysis of Knowledge, Attitudes, Beliefs About Jogging," *Research Quarterly for Exercise and Sport* 55 (1984): 371–8; B. Tirrell and L. Hart, "The Relationship of Health Beliefs and Knowledge to Exercise Compliance in Patients After Coronary Bypass," *Heart and Lung* 9 (1980): 487–93.

36. Various preventive health practices: M. Becker, D. Haefner, S. Kasl, et al., "Selected Psychosocial Models and Correlates of Individual Health-Related Behaviors," *Medical Care* 15 (suppl.) (1977): 27–46; L. W. Green, "Should Health Education Abandon Attitude Change Strategies? Perspectives from Recent Research," *Health Education Monographs* 1(30) (1970): 25–48; J. Langlie, "Social Networks, Health Beliefs, and Preventive Health Behavior," *Journal of Health and Social Behavior* 18 (1977): 244–60.

37. General guidelines for the development of instruments to measure health beliefs: V. Champion, "Instrument Development for Health Belief Model Constructs," *Advances in Nursing Science* 6 (1984): 73–85; K. M. Cummings, A. M. Jette, and I. M. Rosenstock, "Construct Validation of the Health Belief Model," *Health Education Monographs* 6 (1978): 394–405; T. E. Dielman, S. L. Leech, M. H. Becker, et al., "Dimensions of Children's Health Beliefs," *Health Education Quarterly* 7 (1980): 219–38; L. W. Green and F. M. Lewis, *Measurement and Evaluation in Health Education and Health Promotion* (Palo Alto: Mayfield, 1986), pp. 101–46; A. Jette, K. Cummings, B. Brock, et al., "The Structure and Reliability of Health Belief Indices," *Health Services Research* 16 (1981): 81–98; L. A. Maiman, M. H. Becker, J. P. Kirscht, et al., "Scales for Measuring Health Belief Model Dimensions: A Test of Predictive Value, Internal Consistency and Relationships Among Beliefs," *Health Education Monographs* 5 (1977): 215–30.

38. Other predisposing factors correlated with health beliefs: J. Harrison and S. Carlsson, "Methodological Issues in Process and Outcome Studies: Psychophysiology, Systematic Desensitization, and Dental Fear," *Scandinavian Journal of Behaviour Therapy* 13 (1984): 97–116; J. King, "Psychology in Nursing, II. The Health Belief Model," *Nursing Times* 80 (1984): 53–5; J. Kirscht, M. Becker, and J. Eveland, "Psychological and Social Factors as Predictors of Medical Behavior," *Medical Care* 14 (1976): 422–31; R. Oliver and P. Berger, "A Path Analysis of Preventive Health Care Decision Models," *Journal of Consumer Research* 6 (1979): 113–22; E. Suchman, "Preventive Health Behavior: A Model for Research on Community Health Campaigns," *Journal of Health and Social Behavior* 8 (1967): 197–209; B. S. Wallston and K. A. Wallston, "Locus of Control and Health: A Review of the Literature," *Health Education Monographs* 6 (1978): 107–17.

39. S. H. Berman and A. Wandersman, "Fear of Cancer and Knowledge of Cancer—A Review and Proposed Relevance to Hazardous Waste Sites," *Social Science and Medicine* 31 (1990): 81–90; N. E. Miller, "Learning: Some Facts and Needed Research Relevant to Maintaining Health," in

Behavioral Health: A Handbook of Health Enhancement and Disease Prevention, J. D. Matarazzo, S. M. Weiss, J. A. Herd, et al., eds. (New York: Wiley, 1984), pp. 199–208.

40. M. Lalonde, *A New Perspective on the Health of Canadians* (Ottawa: Minister of National Health and Welfare, 1974), p. 8.

41. This approach to market segmentation and analysis is central to the marketing and social marketing fields. For examples of this application within the PRECEDE model, see J. A. Bonaguro and G. Miaoulis, "Marketing: A Tool for Health Education Planning," *Health Education* 14 (Jan-Feb, 1983): 6–11; and R. De Pietro, "A Marketing Research Approach to Health Education Planning," in *Advances in Health Education and Promotion*, vol. 2, W. B. Ward and S. K. Simonds, eds. (Greenwich, CT: JAI Press, 1987), pp. 93–118, esp. pp. 105-7.

42. R. Mucchielli, *Introduction to Structural Psychology* (New York: Funk & Wagnalls, 1970), p. 30.

43. J. P. Kirscht, "The Health Belief Model and Illness Behavior," *Health Education Monographs* 2 (1974): 387–408.

44. M. Rokeach, *Beliefs, Attitudes and Values* (San Francisco: Jossey-Bass, 1970).

45. G. E. Osgood, G. J. Cuci, and P. H. Tannenbaum, *The Measurement of Meaning* (Urbana: University of Illinois Press, 1961).

46. M. H. Bowler and D. E. Morisky, "Small Group Strategy for Improving Compliance Behavior and Blood Pressure Control," *Health Education Quarterly* 10 (1983): 57–69; N. M. Clark, "Social Learning Theory in Current Health Education Practice," in *Advances in Health Education and Promotion*, vol. 2, W. B. Ward and M. H. Becker, eds. (Greenwich, CT: JAI Press, 1987); pp. 251–75; L. W. Green, D. M. Levine, and S. G. Deeds, "Clinical Trials of Health Education for Hypertensive Outpatients: Design and Baseline Data," *Preventive Medicine* 4 (1975): 417–25; G. S. Parcel and T. Baranowski, "Social Learning Theory and Health Education," *Health Education* 12(3) (1981): 14–18; G. S. Parcel, J. G. Bruhn, and J. L. Murray, "Preschool Health Education Program (PHEP): Analysis of Education and Behavioral Outcomes," *Health Education Quarterly* 10 (1983): 149–72; V. J. Strecher, B. M. DeVillis, M. H. Becker, and I. M. Rosenstock, "The Role of Self-efficacy in Achieving Health Behavior Change," *Health Education Quarterly* 13 (1986): 73–92.

47. C. Peterson and A. J. Stunkard, "Personal Control and Health Promotion," *Social Science and Medicine* 28 (1989): 819–28.

48. F. M. Lewis, "The Concept of Control: A Typology and Health-Related Variables," in *Advances in Health Education and Promotion*, vol. 2, W. Ward and M. H. Becker, eds. (Greenwich, CT: JAI Press, 1987); pp. 277–309; K. Lorig and J. Laurin, "Some Notions About Assumptions Underlying Health Education," *Health Education Quarterly* 12 (1985): 231–43.

49. First International Conference on Health Promotion, "Ottawa Charter for Health Promotion," *Health Promotion International* 1(4) (1986): iii-v.

50. A. Bandura, "Self-efficacy Mechanisms in Human Agency," *American Psychologist* 37 (1982): 122–47.

51. D. H. Schunk and J. P. Carbonari, "Self-efficacy Models," in *Behavioral Health: A Handbook of Health Enhancement and Disease Prevention*, J. D. Matarazzo, S. M. Weiss, J. A. Herd, et al., eds. (New York: Wiley, 1984), pp. 230–47, quotation from p. 230.

52. M. M. Condiotte and E. Lichtenstein, "Self-efficacy and Relapse in Smoking Cessation Programs," *Journal of Consulting and Clinical Psychology* 49 (1981): 648–58; R. E. Glasgow, L. Schafer, and H. K. O'Neill, "Self-help Books and Amount of Therapist Contact in Smoking Cessation Programs," *Journal of Consulting and Clinical Psychology* 49 (1981): 659–67.

53. G. A. Marlatt and J. R. Gordon, eds., *Relapse Prevention: Maintenance Strategies in the Treatment of Addictive Behaviors* (New York: Guilford Press, 1985); V. J. Strecher, B. M.

DeVillis, M. H. Becker, and I. M. Rosenstock, "The Role of Self-efficacy in Achieving Health Behavior Change," *Health Education Quarterly* 13 (1986): 73–92.

54. R. G. Kingsley and J. Shapiro, "A Comparison of Three Behavioral Programs for the Control of Obesity in Children," *Behavioral Theory* 8 (1977): 30–3; G. S. Parcel, L. W. Green, and B. Bettes, "School-Based Programs to Prevent or Reduce Obesity," in *Childhood Obesity: A Biobehavioral Perspective*, N. A. Krasnagor, G. D. Grave, and N. Kretchmer, eds. (Caldwell, NJ: Telford Press, 1989), pp. 143–57.

55. H. de Vries, M. Dijkstra, and P. Kuhlman, "Self-efficacy: The Third Factor Besides Attitude and Subjective Norm as a Predictor of Behavioral Intentions," *Health Education Research* 3 (1988): 273–82; R. I. Evans, R. M. Rozelle, S. E. Maxwell, et al., "Social Modeling Films to Deter Smoking in Adolescents: Results of a Three-Year Field Investigation," *Journal of Applied Psychology* 66 (1981): 399–414. However, more skeptical conclusions about this application have been drawn from critical reviews of the literature and his own effectiveness study in Southern California by B. R. Flay, "Social Psychological Approaches to Smoking Prevention: Review and Recommendations," in *Advances in Health Education and Promotion*, vol. 2, W. B. Ward and P. D. Mullen, eds. (Greenwich, CT: JAI Press, 1987), pp. 121–80, esp. pp. 159–61.

56. J. F. Sallis, R. B. Pinski, R. M. Grossman, et al., "The Development of Self-efficacy Scales for Health-Related Diet and Exercise Behaviors," *Health Education Research* 3 (1988): 283–92.

57. M. Bernier and J. Avard, "Self-efficacy, Outcome, and Attrition in a Weight-Reduction Program," *Cognitive Therapy and Research* 10 (1986): 319–38; S. M. Glynn and A. J. Ruderman, "The Development and Validation of an Eating Self-efficacy Scale," *Cognitive Therapy and Research* 10 (1986): 403–20.

58. I. Ajzen and M. Fishbein, *Understanding Attitudes and Predicting Social Behavior* (Englewood Cliffs, NJ: Prentice-Hall, 1980); I. Ajzen and J. T. Madden, "Prediction of Goal-Directed Behavior: Attitudes, Intentions, and Perceived Behavioral Control," *Journal of Experimental Social Psychology* 22 (1986): 453–74.

59. A. J. Sogaard, "The Effect of a Mass-Media Dental Health Education Campaign," *Health Education Research* 3 (1988): 243–55.

60. K. E. Bauman and R. L. Chenoweth, "The Relationship Between the Consequences Adolescents Expect from Smoking and Their Behavior: A Factor Analysis with Panel Data," *Journal of Social Psychology* 14 (1984): 28–41; L. Chassin, C. C. Presson, M. Bensenberg, et al., "Predicting Adolescents' Intentions to Smoke Cigarettes," *Journal of Health and Social Behavior* 22 (1984): 445–55; J. Jaccard, "A Theoretical Analysis of Selected Factors Important to Health Education Strategies," *Health Education Monographs* 3 (1975): 152–67; I. M. Newman and G. L. Martin, "Attitudinal and Normative Factors Associated with Adolescent Cigarette Smoking in Australia and the United States of America: A Methodology to Assist Health Education Planning," *Community Health Studies* 6 (1982): 47–56; R. M. Page and R. S. Gold, "Assessing Gender Differences in College Cigarette Smoking: Intenders and Non-intenders," *Journal of School Health* 53 (1983): 531–5; H. de Vries, M. Dijkstra, and P. Kuhlman, "Self-efficacy: The Third Factor Besides Attitude and Subjective Norm as a Predictor of Behavioral Intentions," *Health Education Research* 3 (1988): 273–82.

61. G. J. Kok and S. Siero, "Tin-Recycling: Awareness, Comprehension, Attitude, Intention and Behavior," *Journal of Economic Psychology* 6 (1985): 157–73.

62. F. B. London, "Attitudinal and Social Normative Factors as Predictors of Intended Alcohol Abuse Among Fifth- and Seventh-Grade Students," *Journal of School Health* 52 (1982): 244–9; D. McCarty, S. Morrison, and K. C. Mills, "Attitudes, Beliefs and Alcohol Use: An Analysis of Relationships," *Journal of Studies on Alcohol* 2 (1983): 328–41.

63. R. Budd, S. Bleiner, and C. Spencer, "Exploring the Use and Non-use of Marijuana as Reasoned Actions: An Application of Fishbein and Ajzen's Methodology," *Drug and Alcohol Dependence* 11 (1983): 217–24; W. B. Lacy, "The Influence of Attitudes and Current Friends on Drug Use Intentions," *Journal of Social Psychology* 113 (1981): 65–76.

64. R. Budd, D. North, and C. Spencer, "Understanding Seat-Belt Use: A Test of Bentler and Speckart's Extension of the 'Theory of Reasoned Action'," *European Journal of Social Psychology* 14 (1984): 69–78.

65. A. R. Davidson and J. J. Jaccard, "Population Psychology: A New Look at an Old Problem," *Journal of Personality and Social Psychology*, cited by J. Jaccard, "A Theoretical Analysis of Selected Factors Important to Health Education Strategies," *Health Education Monographs* 3 (1975): 158.

66. H. de Vries and G. J. Kok, "From Determinants of Smoking Behaviour to the Implications for a Prevention Programme," *Health Education Research* 1 (1986): 85–94.

67. L. Chassin, E. Corty, C. Presson, et al., "Predicting Adolescents' Intentions to Smoke Cigarettes," *Journal of Health and Social Behavior* 22 (1981): 445–55; K. McCaul, R. Glasgow, H. O'Neill, et al., "Predicting Adolescent Smoking," *Journal of School Health* 52 (1982): 342–6.

68. G. Botvin and A. Eng, "A Comprehensive School-Based Smoking Prevention Program," *Journal of School Health* 50 (1980): 209–13; G. Botvin and A. Eng, "The Efficacy of a Multicomponent Approach to the Prevention of Cigarette Smoking," *Preventive Medicine* 11 (1982): 199–211.

69. D. Sobel and F. Hornbacher, *An Everyday Guide to Your Health* (New York: Grossman, 1973); G. S. Parcel, "Skills Approach to Health Education: A Framework for Integrating Cognitive and Affective Learning," *Journal of School Health* 66 (1976): 403–6. See, for example, the 22 skills contributing to self-management ability in children and adolescents outlined by C. E. Thoresen and K. Kirmil-Gray, "Self-management Psychology and the Treatment of Childhood Asthma," *Journal of Allergy and Clinical Immunology* 72 (suppl. Nov. 1983): 596–606.

70. See Chapters 6, 8, and 9 for more on these social action skills.

71. N. Milio, "A Framework for Prevention: Changing Health-Damaging to Health-Generating Life Patterns," *American Journal of Public Health* 66 (May 1976): 436. See also, N. Milio, *Promoting Health Through Public Policy* (Philadelphia: F. A. Davis, 1983), reprinted by the Canadian Public Health Association, 1987.

72. G. Parcel, D. G. Simons-Morton, S. Brink, et al., *Smoking Control Among Women: A CDC Community Intervention Handbook* (Atlanta: Centers for Disease Control, 1987). This and the other CDC Handbooks listed in the following citations apply the PRECEDE model to the assessment of needs and the planning of interventions for selected health problems and target populations. They provide detailed procedural guidelines on collecting and analyzing the data necessary to arrive at efficient judgments about the behavioral determinants and the predisposing, enabling, and reinforcing factors for behavioral change.

73. B. G. Simons-Morton, S. Brink, G. Parcel, et al., *Preventing Alcohol Misuse Among Adolescents and Young Adults: A CDC Community Intervention Handbook*, (Atlanta: Centers for Disease Control, 1989).

74. C. Mowatt, J. Isaly, and M. Thayer, "Project Graduation–Maine," *Morbidity and Mortality Weekly Report* 34 (1985): 233–5.

75. D. G. Simons-Morton, S. G. Brink, G. Parcel, et al., *Promoting Physical Activity Among Adults: A CDC Community Intervention Handbook* (Atlanta: Centers for Disease Control, 1988).

76. G. Botvin and A. Eng, "The Efficacy of a Multicomponent Peer-Leadership Approach to the Prevention of Cigarette Smoking," *Preventive Medicine* 11 (1982): 199–211; P. L. Ellickson and R. M. Bell, "Drug Prevention in Junior High: A Multi-Site Longitudinal Test," *Science* 247 (1990): 1299–1305; N. Gordon, "Never Smokers, Triers and Current Smokers: Three Distinct Target Groups for School-Based Antismoking Programs," *Health Education Quarterly* 13 (1986): 163–80.

77. D. G. Simons-Morton, S. G. Brink, G. S. Parcel, et al., *Promoting Physical Activity...*, 1988, op. cit.

78. M. I. Harrison, *Diagnosing Organizations: Methods, Models, and Processes* (Beverly Hills: Sage, 1987); A. M. Huberman and M. B. Miles, *Innovation Up Close: How School Improvement Works* (New York: Plenum Press, 1984); A. D. Kaluzny, A. Schenck, and T. Ricketts, "Cancer Prevention in the Workplace: An Organizational Innovation," *Health Promotion* 1 (1986): 293–9; R. Kantor, *The Change Masters* (New York: Simon and Schuster, 1983); G. L. Lippitt, P. Langseth, and J. Mossop, *Implementing Organizational Change* (San Francisco: Jossey-Bass, 1985); J. Porras and S. Hoffer, "Common Behavior Changes in Successful Organization Development Efforts," *Journal of Applied Behavioral Science* 22 (1986): 477–94.

79. M. E. Segall and C. A. Wynd, "Health Conception, Health Locus of Control, and Power as Predictors of Smoking Behavior Change," *American Journal of Health Promotion* 4 (1990): 338–44; R. Warnecke, S. Graham, S. Rosenthal, and C. Manfredi, "Social and Psychological Correlates of Smoking Behavior Among Black Women," *Journal of Health and Social Behavior* 19 (1978): 397–410.

80. S. Casswell, L. Stewart, and P. Duignan, "The Struggle Against the Broadcast of Anti-health Messages: Regulation of Alcohol Advertising in New Zealand 1980–87," *Health Promotion* 4 (1989): 287–96; C. Smith, J. L. Roberts, and L. L. Pendleton, "Booze on the Box – The Portrayal of Alcohol on British Television: A Content Analysis," *Health Education Research* 3 (1988): 267–72; L. M. Wallack, "Mass Media Campaigns in a Hostile Environment: Advertising as Anti-health Education," *Journal of Drug Addiction* 28 (1983): 51–63; K. Warner, *Selling Smoke: Cigarette Advertising and Public Health* (Washington, DC: American Public Health Association, 1986); A. Wyllie and S. Casswell, "The Response of New Zealand Boys to Corporate and Sponsorship Alcohol Advertising on Television," *British Journal of Addiction* 84 (1989): 639–46.

81. G. Godin and R. J. Shephard, "An Evaluation of the Potential Role of the Physician in Influencing Community Exercise Behavior," *American Journal of Health Promotion* 4 (1990): 255–9; N. Oldridge, "Compliance and Exercise in Primary and Secondary Prevention of Coronary Heart Disease: A Review," *Preventive Medicine* 11 (1982): 56–70.

82. S. L. Bailey and R. L. Hubbard, "Developmental Variation in the Context of Marijuana Initiation among Adolescents," *Journal of Health and Social Behavior* 31 (1990): 58–70; G. J. Botvin and A. McAlister, "Cigarette Smoking Among Children and Adolescents: Causes and Prevention," in *Annual Review of Disease Prevention*, C. B. Arnold, ed. (New York: Springer, 1982); L. Chassin, L. Mann, and K. Sher, "Self-awareness Theory, Family History of Alcoholism, and Adolescent Alcohol Involvement," *Journal of Abnormal Psychology* 97 (1988): 206–17; L. Friedman, E. Lichtenstein, and A. Biglan, "Smoking Onset Among Teens: An Empirical Analysis of Initial Situations," *Addictive Behaviors* 10 (1985): 1–13.

83. J. A. Best, S. J. Thomson, S. M. Santi, et al., "Preventing Cigarette Smoking Among School Children," *Annual Review of Public Health* 9 (1988): 161–201.

84. L. Chassin, E. Corty, C. Presson, et al., "Cognitive and Social Influence Factors in Adolescent Smoking Cessation," *Addictive Behaviors* 9 (1984): 383–90.

85. E. B. Arkin, *Making Health Communication Programs Work: A Planner's Guide* (Bethesda, MD: National Cancer Institute, 1989); G. D. Gilmore, M. D. Campbell, and B. L. Becker, *Needs Assessment Strategies for Health Education and Health Promotion* (Indianapolis, IN: Benchmark Press, 1989); R. Manoff, *Social Marketing* (New York: Praeger, 1986).

86. E. B. Arkin, *Making Health Communication...*, op. cit., pp. 95–6; C. E. Basch, "Focus Group Interview: An Underutilized Research Technique for Improving Theory and Practice in Health Education," *Health Education Quarterly* 14 (1987): 411–48; G. Gilmore, M. D. Campbell, and B. L. Becker, *Needs Assessment...*, op. cit., pp. 69–74. See Chapter 2 for more detail on focus group methods and applications.

87. R. R. Faden, "Ethical Issues in Government Sponsored Public Health Campaigns," *Health Education Quarterly* 14 (1987): 27–37; K. R. McLeroy, N. H. Gottlieb, and J. N. Burdine, "The Business of Health Promotion: Ethical Issues and Professional Responsibilities," *Health Education Quarterly* 14 (1987): 91–109.

88. L. W. Green, "Individuals Versus Systems: An Artificial Classification That Divides and Distorts," *Health Link* 2 (1986): 29–30.

89. Some authors refer to this level of needs assessment as behavioral diagnosis (the term we used for the previous phase of PRECEDE), but their intent is the same, to identify factors that influence behavior. For example, G. M. Arsham, "Behavioral Diagnosis for Patient Education," in *Patient Education in the Primary Care Setting: 1979 Proceedings*, P. LaVigne, ed. (Minneapolis: University of Minnesota, 1980); E. E. Bartlett, "Behavioral Diagnosis: A Practical Approach to Patient Education," *Patient Counseling and Health Education* 4 (1982): 29–35; C. D. Jenkins, "An Approach to the Diagnosis and Treatment of Problems of Health-Related Behavior," *International Journal of Health Education* 22 (suppl. 1979): 1–24; F. H. Kanfer and G. Saslow, "Behavioral Diagnosis," in *Behavior Therapy: Appraisal and Status*, C. M. Franks, ed. (New York: McGraw-Hill, 1969).

90. For examples of analyses of behavioral determinants specific to ethnic and other demographic groups, see N. H. Gottlieb and L. W. Green, "Ethnicity and Lifestyle Health Risk: Some Possible Mechanisms," *American Journal of Health Promotion* 2 (1987): 37–51; T. Stephens, D. R. Jacobs, Jr., and C. C. White, "A Descriptive Epidemiology of Leisure-time Physical Activity," *Public Health Reports* 100 (1985): 147–58; M. H. Weitzel and P. R. Waller, "Predictive Factors for Health-Promotive Behaviors in White, Hispanic, and Black Blue-Collar Workers," *Family and Community Health* 13 (1990): 23–34.

91. J. G. Zapka and J. A. Mamon, "Integration of Theory, Practitioner Standards, Literature Findings, and Baseline Data: A Case Study in Planning Breast Self-examination Education," *Health Education Quarterly* 9 (1982): 330–56.

92. L. W. Green and F. M. Lewis, *Measurement and Evaluation in Health Education and Health Promotion* (Palo Alto: Mayfield, 1986); see esp. chap. 6 for inventories and references on instrument selection and development, and Appendix C, pp. 331–41 for a questionnaire developed for the National Survey of Personal Health Practices and Consequences and adapted for community-level application. A Canadian national survey, also based on the PRECEDE factors, is described in I. Rootman, "Canada's Health Promotion Survey," in *Canada's Health Promotion Survey: Technical Report*, I. Rootman, et al., eds. (Ottawa: Minister of Supply and Services, 1988).

93. L. A. Aday and R. Eichhorn, *The Utilization of Health Services: Indices and Correlates* (Washington, DC: National Center for Health Services Research, DHEW Pub. No. HSM 73-3003, 1973). Such local sources of data can be most illuminating when contrasted with state or national data. A review of national data sources for the United States, organized according to the PRECEDE model factors influencing behavior, is provided by R. W. Wilson and D. C. Iverson, "Federal Data Bases for Health Education Research," *Health Education* 13(3) (1982): 30–34.

94. For example, G. S. Parcel, D. G. Simons-Morton, S. G. Brink, et al., *Smoking Control Among Women: A CDC Community Intervention Handbook* (Atlanta: Centers for Disease Control, 1987).

95. M. Rokeach, *Beliefs, Attitudes and Values* (San Francisco: Jossey-Bass, 1970).

96. E. M. Rogers, *Diffusion of Innovations*, 3rd ed. (New York: The Free Press, Macmillan, 1983). More refined analyses of the rates of change and diffusion for the successive stages of change and for different innovations are suggested in R. Crow, H. Blackburn, D. Jacobs, et al., "Population Strategies to Enhance Physical Activity: The Minnesota Heart Health Program," *Acta Medica Scandinavica* 711 (suppl., 1986): 93–112; L. W. Green, "Diffusion and Adoption of Innovations Related to Cardiovascular Risk Behavior in the Public," in *Applying Behavioral Sciences to Cardiovascular Risk*, eds. A. Enelow and J. B. Henderson (New York: American Heart Association, 1975).

97. K. E. Warner, "Cigarette Smoking in the 1970's: The Impact of the Anti-Smoking Campaign on Consumption," *Science* 211(13) (1981): 729–31; K. E. Warner, "Effects of the Antismoking Campaign: An Update," *American Journal of Public Health* 79 (1989): 144–51.

Chapter 6

Administrative and Policy Diagnosis: From PRECEDE to PROCEED

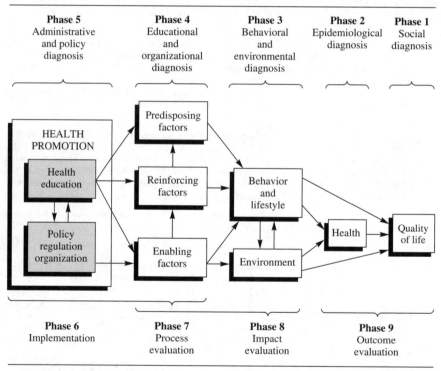

H aving identified in the preceding diagnostic steps the targets of development and change to be mobilized by your program, you stand ready now to convert your plan into health education interventions, policy, organization, and regulation. This requires several additional steps, some diagnostic and some political. The remaining diagnostic steps are those requiring an assessment of the budgetary and staff resources needed and available for the program, an assessment of barriers to be overcome in implementing the program, and an assessment of policies that can be used to support your program or that need to be changed to enable the program to proceed. These last diagnostic steps bring you to the final touches on your formal plan with a timetable, an assignment of resources and responsibilities, and a budget. The formulation of priorities, targets, objectives, timetables, and budgets, as described in this and previous chapters, completes the PRECEDE process. In this chapter,[1] you turn the corner from PRECEDE to PROCEED.

With a complete plan in hand, you PROCEED to implementation and evaluation. The implementation process draws immediately on the administrative diagnosis by reviewing the barriers identified and by initiating organizational, regulatory, and policy changes to overcome those barriers. Some of the barriers will be internal structures in the implementing organization. New policy or regulations can overcome these by reorganizing or reassigning responsibility within the organization. Other barriers will be in the behavior or operating procedures of this or other organizations whose cooperation is required. Here, the implementation of health promotion might gain cooperation through education of decision makers or through negotiation of exchange agreements—and sometimes through enforcement of existing agreements, rules, and laws—or the advocacy and promotion of new regulatory legislation. To determine the nature of agreements, rules, or laws, you assess current policy.

This chapter walks you through the administrative diagnosis and then to the implementation of the plan that evolves from that final set of diagnostic procedures. The evaluation plan to be developed in Chapter 7 also needs to be integrated into the formal program plan. The evaluation plan sometimes requires similar policy, regulatory, and organizational initiatives in order to be supported and implemented. All of these policy, regulatory, and organizational (the PRO in PROCEED) initiatives may be seen as enabling constructs for educational and environmental development (the CEED in PROCEED) that will support actions and living conditions conducive to health.

Some Definitions. Before plunging into the administrative diagnosis, some definitions should be considered. **Administrative diagnosis** refers here to an analysis of the policies, resources, and circumstances prevailing in the organizational situation that could facilitate or hinder the development of the health promotion program. **Policy** refers to the set of objectives and rules guiding the activities of an organization or an administration. **Regulation** refers to the act of implementing policies and enforcing rules or laws. **Organization** refers in this chapter to the act of marshalling and coordinating the resources necessary to implement a program. In Chapter 8, **community organization** is used to refer to the set of procedures and processes by which a population and its institutions mobilize to solve a common problem or pursue a common goal. **Implementation** refers here to the act of converting policies and program objectives into actions through administration, regulation, and organization.

ADMINISTRATIVE DIAGNOSIS

Your selection of educational methods in Chapter 5 was based, undoubtedly, on some conscious or unconscious consideration of resources at your disposal. Now you come more squarely and formally to the process of assessing those resources, matching resources to educational methods and strategies, and budgeting the time and material resources to implement the strategies.

STEP 1. ASSESSMENT OF RESOURCES NEEDED

The first step in the administrative diagnosis is to assess the resources required by the proposed educational methods and strategies. This entails an examination of the time frames for accomplishment of the objectives and of the types and numbers of people needed to carry out the program.

Time. The first and most critical resource is time. Time cannot be recovered once it is expended, it is inflexible in its supply, and it affects the availability and cost of all other resources. The time required has been estimated at several levels of the PRECEDE planning phases with the formulation of realistic objectives. Each objective states the time (date) by which that objective needs to be accomplished in order for the next higher level objective to be accomplished. Thus, certain educational and organizational objectives must be accomplished before certain behavioral and environmental objectives can be expected to materialize, and these in turn must occur before any palpable change in health or quality-of-life outcomes can be expected.

For example, suppose you have a set of predisposing educational objectives stating that a 60 percent increase in knowledge of an available vaccine, and a 50 percent increase in the prevalence of a belief in susceptibility should occur in the first 4 months of an immunization program. Your enabling objectives might include a 4-month target of dispatching 60 mobilized immunization stations, one in each school and shopping center in the community, and a 3-month target of obtaining commitments from 50 school principals and 10 shopping center managers. All these objectives must be accomplished within the time frames stated in

Activity	Feb	Mar	Apr	May	Jun	Jul	Aug	Sept
Preparation of material	X	X						
Pretest of material		X						
Production of material			X					
Dissemination				X				
First contact with schools		X						
Follow-up with schools			X					
First contact with managers		X						
Follow-up with managers			X					
Commitments from schools and managers				X				
Immunization stations organized					X			
Preschool immunizations						X	X	
Evaluation and follow-up							X	X

FIGURE 6.1

Representation of time requirements in the form of a Gantt chart for a school-entry immunization program.

order to achieve a behavioral objective of a 40 percent increase in the percentage of school children receiving measles immunization (from 90 percent previously immunized to 94 percent) at the end of 6 months. (Because this was a one-time behavior, you need not bother with an objective for reinforcing factors.)

These objectives clearly limit the time frame in which you must implement specific aspects of the program plan. A timetable or **Gantt chart** can be laid out, as in Figure 6.1, to show graphically the start and finish dates for each activity. It also shows the overlap of activities in time and the number of different activities that will be proceeding simultaneously during each period of time.[2]

From the Gantt chart the time requirements for each activity can be explicitly stated and placed in relation to every other activity, thereby enabling you to make an analysis not only of time requirements for each activity but also (reading down a column) of activity requirements for each period of time. This takes step 1 to the second resource, personnel.

Person	Week	1	2	3	4	5	6	7	8	9 ... 24	Total hours
Administrator		20	20	20	20	20	20	20	20	20 ...	480
Health educator		40	40	40	40	40	40	40	40	40 ...	960
Medical consultant		8	8	8	4	4				30	62
Graphic artist		8		8							16
Nurses										800	800
Secretary		20	20	20	20	20	20	20	20	20 ...	480

FIGURE 6.2

Personnel loading (hours) chart for 6-month immunization program.

Personnel. Staffing requirements take precedence over other budgetary considerations in the resource analysis because the personnel category generally constitutes the largest and most restricted line item in most budgets. People cost more than most resources and are more difficult to put in place than most equipment and material resources. Civil service and affirmative action hiring policies, union contracts, and due process in moving personnel all limit the flexibility and discretion with which you can mold this resource to your program needs. The personnel analysis is further complicated by the subtle considerations of talent, skills, personalities, and personal preferences and attitudes toward particular types of work to be done.

The Gantt chart from your time analysis (such as Fig. 6.1), can provide the basis for the first cut in analyzing personnel requirements. Each month's activities require certain types of people. These can be defined in your situation by the names of the existing personnel that you have in mind; but more properly they should be defined by the professional, technical, administrative, or clerical skills required. Here it is often useful to break the Gantt chart into smaller units of time—say, weeks, days, or even hours—depending on the overall duration and scope of the program. Your quantitative analysis of personnel requirements then might take the form shown in Figure 6.2.

The estimate of personnel hours required each week enables you to make a cost analysis of personnel, as well as a time allocation (loading) analysis that permits the administrator at the next higher level to consider where and when existing personnel might be reassigned to support the program without hiring new personnel. In the example shown in Figure 6.2, the personnel requirements include a half-time administrator and a full-time health education specialist throughout the program. The administrator might be a health education specialist with a masters degree and community experience. The other health educator, assigned to the communication and dissemination responsibilities, might hold a baccalaureate degree and have less experience. This kind of personnel analysis must be based on a matching of personnel with the administrative, educational, technical, and organizational requirements dictated by the process objectives outlined in Chapters 4 and 5.

Budget. The time and personnel requirements easily convert into cost estimates by multiplying each line in the personnel loading chart by an average hourly wage or salary estimate for each category of worker. Whether these personnel are hired, borrowed from another program within the same organization, or contracted as consultants (e.g., the medical consultant and graphic artist during the developmental phase, and the two full-time nurses during the final 10 weeks), the hourly costs should be recorded in the budget requirement at this stage because these are real requirements and therefore real costs to be anticipated. If they prove to be excessive for the organization, options for transfer of personnel, borrowing of personnel, recruitment of volunteers, donated services from other agencies, and other possibilities can be explored.

The other budgetary requirements include personnel benefits for salaried workers, materials or supplies, printing, postage, photocopying, telephone, equipment, data processing, and travel. Most organizations have a fixed overhead or indirect cost rate such as 20 percent or 50 percent. They add this average maintenance rate to any direct cost estimate to provide for administrative services of the front office, rental and upkeep of the building and offices, utilities, and sometimes local telephone or other fixed costs of the offices in which special projects are to be housed. For example, if the direct cost for a program is estimated at $10,000 in personnel and materials, the budget might be $12,000 to cover the usual 20 percent overhead the agency has established from experience to be its costs for office maintenance to support the personnel. An example of a preliminary budget is shown in Table 6.1.

STEP 2. ASSESSMENT OF AVAILABLE RESOURCES

Part of the educational diagnosis identified methods or materials appropriate to some of the educational objectives. Such materials and methods might need to be developed from scratch, as implied by the foregoing budget which provided for development and printing of a brochure to blanket the community with information about measles and the need to immunize children before school starts. Sometimes the material has been developed in a previous program or by a national or state agency that can make the material available at little or no cost to your agency. The costs that can be saved by using centrally developed educational materials or

TABLE 6.1

Initial budget estimates based on analysis of requirements, but before assessment of resources available

	Total hours	Hourly rate	Budget
Personnel			
Administrator	480	$25	$12,000
Health educator	960	20	19,200
Medical consultant	62	50	3,100
Graphic artist	16	12	192
Nurses	800	15	12,000
Secretary	480	10	4,800
		Total	51,292
Personnel benefits at 20% of salaries			10,258
Total personnel costs			61,550
Supplies			$7,900
Printing brochure		$2,000	
Postage (20,000 × .20 bulk rate)		4,000	
Office supplies		300	
Vaccination supplies (800 @ $2)		1,600	
Services			$3,900
Telephone		500	
Photocopying		400	
Data processing		3,000	
Travel			$880
Local (400 miles @ $.20)		80	
State conference		800	
Total direct costs			$74,230
Indirect costs (20% of direct costs)			14,846
Total budget estimate			$89,076

materials developed previously for another program can sometimes reduce a budget considerably, but the materials may not be tailored as specifically for the local situation or the current circumstances as would be desirable. Such trade-offs between costs and the ideal arrangements for your program will arise throughout the administrative and policy diagnoses.

Personnel. The likely circumstances for most health promotion programs developed within an organization to address that organization's mission are that existing personnel are expected to suffice in the implementation of the program. If the preceding diagnoses have produced a program design that requires more personnel than the sponsoring organization has available at your disposal, then you have the following choices:

1. Identify and seek part-time commitments from personnel from other departments or units within your organization. This will require commitments also from their supervisors if they are not authorized to allocate their own time. Temporary arrangements of this kind are common when the separate departments share common goals, which is often the case if the other department has the kind of personnel you need.

2. Retrain personnel within your department to take on tasks outside their usual scope of responsibility.

3. Explore the potential for recruitment of volunteers from the community. Short-term programs, in particular, can tap the underutilized pool of talent and energy available for volunteer effort for a worthy cause.[3]

4. Explore the potential for cooperative agreements with other agencies or organizations in the community to obtain help from their staff to fill in the gaps in your personnel.

5. Develop a grant proposal for funding, partial funding, or matched funding of your program by a government agency, a philanthropic foundation, or a corporate donor. The work you have done in following the PRECEDE planning process follows the logical format most granting agencies want to see in an application. With the addition of your evaluation plan and final budget request, you have a grant application in hand.

6. Appeal directly to the public for donations.

7. Price the service at a cost-recovery level of fees to be charged some or all users of the services. With options 6 and 7 you must be cautious that you stay within affordable limits, that you stay within range of market values for the services, and that you provide assurances that those in your priority target groups who might not be able to afford the services can still have access to them.

8. If none of the above seem appropriate, feasible, or sufficient, and if the program is to be a permanent or long-term commitment of the organization, then it is justifiable to pursue policy changes in the organization such that a more fundamental reorganization or redistribution of resources to your department or unit would be established before embarking on the program.

Other Budgetary Constraints. The foregoing options represent the main courses of action that can be pursued singly or in combination to close the gap between resources required and resources available within your organization to carry out the desired program. The same strategies for augmenting personnel might apply to

some other resources available from other departments or organizations as financial or in-kind contributions to the program.[4]

When resources cannot be found, the fall-back position, of course, is to trim
the sails on your program plan and propose more modest objectives and less
powerful methods of intervention. This course of action represents a compromise
on the plan and should be undertaken only with due consideration to the consequences for the integrity of the plan. Specific questions that should be asked before
giving up too many parts of the plan or levels of intervention with budget cuts are
the following:

1. *The Threshold Level.* Will the reduced level of resources still allow a
   sufficient level of intervention to achieve a threshold of minimally
   adequate impact to result in the achievement of subsequent objectives?
   The notion of a threshold level of resources suggests that there is a
   minimum level of investment below which the program will be too
   weak to achieve a useful result.[5] It is a theoretical notion with only a
   few documented examples of threshold levels in actual programs.[6]
2. *The Point of Diminishing Returns.* Is there a point of diminishing
   returns beyond which additional resources do not necessarily achieve
   commensurate gains in impact or outcome? If so, fewer resources
   might not hinder the achievement of at least some benefits. This, too, is
   largely a theoretical concept in health education and health promotion.[7]
   The same studies that were cited in the previous paragraph contain the
   limited data available on points of diminishing returns.
3. *Critical Elements.* Is there a critical element in the program plan,
   without which the objectives cannot be achieved? If so, will the budget
   cut or shortage of resources preclude achieving that one objective or
   element? In a worksite program to reduce lower-back injuries in nurses,
   for example, it might be determined that everything that can be done in
   the program depends on the nurses having release time from their
   duties to participate in the educational and exercise training program. If
   the hospital cannot provide the release time for these nurses, the
   director of occupational health is advised not to proceed with the
   program.
4. *Critical Expectations.* Can the target levels of the objectives be lowered
   without jeopardizing the integrity of the program or the expectations of
   the constituents or sponsors of the program? If the behavioral-change
   target can be reduced from 94 percent immunization of school-age
   children to 92 percent without risking a major outbreak of measles, the
   savings in outreach resources could be considerable because, as we
   have seen in the earlier discussions of diffusion theory, it gets harder
   and harder to reach those late adopters. An equivalent reduction in the
   target levels during the early phases of a program, say from 14 to 10

percent, would not yield a commensurate cost savings. The early adopters are easier to reach.

5. *Critical Timing and Cash Flow.* Can the target dates for the objectives be set back to spread the program effort over a longer period of time? This, by itself, will not save resources in the long run but will reduce costs in the initial year by shifting them to later periods. The initial costs could be the major budgetary barrier because of temporary fiscal circumstances. By slowing the pace of program implementation, some outlays could be delayed in anticipation of better budgetary times. This amounts to an adjustment of "cash flow."

6. *Critical Population Segments.* Can the types of people selected as priority target groups be reordered to give lower priority to the hard-to-reach? This is too often the most tempting adjustment in underfunded programs. Those who need the program the most are often the most expensive to reach and can least afford to subsidize the program with fees for service. This sometimes leads to a decision to make the underbudgeted program available on a first-come first-served basis. This should be a last resort in accepting a reduced budget because the integrity of the longer-term objectives is likely to be compromised. Although they cost more to reach per unit of education or service delivered, the poorer and more isolated segments of the target population will gain more in health improvement because they have more to gain if they are effectively reached.

STEP 3. ASSESSMENT OF BARRIERS TO IMPLEMENTATION

Besides resource constraints, there will be a host of other barriers to the smooth implementation of your program plan. The plan is not complete without some consideration of and provision for at least those barriers that can be acknowledged publicly. Some of the barriers will be essentially attitudinal, political, or power relationships that cannot politely be made a matter of public record in your formal plan, but you ignore them at the peril of your program.

Staff Commitment and Attitudes. Before a plan is complete, it needs to make the rounds to obtain comment and suggestions from those who will have a role in implementing it, especially if they have not been directly involved in formulating the plan up to this point. Staff members of the implementing agencies will be in the best position to anticipate barriers in their various roles and will welcome the opportunity to point out some of the pitfalls in your plan *before* they are asked to implement it. Their involvement at this stage, if they have not participated earlier in the planning, is essential to their commitment to the objectives and methods of the program. It does not guarantee their commitment; but without their participation in planning, their commitment and their attitude toward the program are almost certain to be undependable.

Goal Conflict. Plans that require a change in standard operating procedures place the goals and objectives of the new plans into question. If these are seen as conflicting with previously accepted goals and objectives, the conflict must be resolved through clarification of priorities.[8] As Ross and Mico put it, "The goals must accord with the client system's existing policy."[9]

Rate of Change. Incremental change is easier to implement than radical, ambitious, nonincremental changes.[10] Break your program plan's implementation steps down into bite-size, manageable pieces.[11]

Familiarity. Are the procedures and methods to be employed familiar to the staff members who must implement them? Do they depart radically from standard operating procedures? Even if skills are not at issue, unfamiliar methods and procedures require careful introduction and orientation to avoid being rejected, ignored, or poorly implemented.[12]

Complexity. A change requiring multiple transactions or complex relationships and coordination is more difficult to implement than single-action or single-person procedures.[13]

Space. One of the most precious commodities in many organizations is office space. If your program plan proposes to use existing office space for another purpose or to move staff members from one space to another, you are likely to be stepping on someone's toes. Space should be treated as a resource to be allocated according to rules or procedures similar to those suggested earlier for personnel and other budgetary items.

Community Barriers. Beyond your own organization, the community will respond to your proposed program at several levels. The principle of participation, emphasized throughout the previous chapters, should have cautioned you to take most of these potential reactive barriers into account in your planning. Even some of those who participated in your planning process will retain some misgivings about how your new program will affect them and their programs. Some of these misgivings will translate into passive resistance, some into subtle efforts to minimize, discredit, or even sabotage your program. The best protection against these defensive maneuvers in the community, besides earlier involvement in the planning, is to invite those organizations most threatened by your program to be co-sponsors or collaborators, sharing the credit and the public visibility of the program.

What remains after you have taken all these potential barriers and sources of opposition into account and after you have prevented or reduced those you can in the plan itself? The remaining barriers and sources of support to be assessed can be considered essentially political and structural barriers. These must be addressed in the final diagnostic phase, and some of them can be changed only through political processes because they lie beyond the direct control of your agency.

POLICY DIAGNOSIS

In the educational diagnosis of Chapter 5 you identified various enabling factors that influenced the high-priority health behaviors. In that chapter you assessed resources for the selected educational methods that would help develop the skills required to enable the behavior and for some community organization methods that would make resources more accessible to people whose motivation to act was frustrated by the inaccessibility of these enabling factors. Still, there were other enabling factors that direct educational efforts or appeals to the community could not be expected to change because they involved legal, political, or environmental conditions more or less "locked in" by current policy, regulations, and organization. These now become the focus of the policy diagnosis.

STEP 1. ASSESSMENT OF POLICIES, REGULATIONS, AND ORGANIZATION

Before your plan can be implemented, it must be examined from the standpoint of its fit with existing policy, regulation, and organization. Some of the barriers identified in the preceding administrative diagnosis revealed policy and organizational incompatibilities with your plan. Either your plan must adapt to the policy and organization, or you must seek change in the policy, the organization, or both. Your only other choice is to leave the organization and take your program plan to another. This option is available only if another organization stands ready with a similar mandate or mission, or if you are prepared to start a new organization.

The Issue of Loyalty. Before you bolt from your agency and resign your current position in favor of another organization that seems more sympathetic with your plan or compatible with your goals, consider carefully the ethics and practicalities. The ethics tend to be framed around issues of loyalty. Your organization has, after all, provided you a base from which to plan the program, has paid your salary or at least provided you with space and auspices for your effort during this period, and has put up with the hassles of participatory planning. You owe that organization at least the courtesy of advance notice before you leave, but you do not owe your conscience or your vision of a better future to the organization.[14] Too many potential change agents fail to bring about the improvements they are capable of offering in society or in their field because they misplaced their loyalty, vesting it in an organization rather than in the public's health.

The practicalities of choosing among organizational sponsors for a program plan, especially if the choice of a sponsor means moving yourself and possibly uprooting your family and severing other commitments, come down to realistic assessments of the stakes and the trade-offs. How important is the plan relative to the other things you can accomplish within your organization? Are you really the only one who can carry off the plan, or could you hand it off to the other organization? If you move to another organization, will your plan be compatible with the other contributions you can make to the field or to the community? Before bailing out, or jumping ship as it were, take another look at the remaining possibilities for change in the plan or in the policies of your organization that could make the plan workable. The remaining possibilities lie in the following policy analyses.

Consistency. Is your plan consistent with existing policy and organization? If so, you can strengthen your plan by documenting and communicating more effectively the specific policies it serves, ways in which it supports those policies and ways in which the policies can support the plan. Many new program plans are announced with an opening line invoking the organizational policy that authorizes or justifies the proposed program. The preamble to most new government plans or regulations, for example, cites the authorizing legislation or statute that makes the plan necessary or possible. This kind of preface or covering memo is often signed by the director or chief executive officer, giving the plan not only the force of legislation or policy but also the prestige or authority of the chief administrator.

If your plan is consistent with some policy of the organization but inconsistent with some other policy, then the policies themselves may be inconsistent or your plan may include one component that is inconsistent with policy. Your task in either case is to show how your overall plan serves the overall mission and policy of the organization, and then to seek an exception to the rule or a waiver of the specific policy from which your plan would deviate.

Flexibility. The first question you can ask about any policy that appears to be inconsistent with your program plan is how flexible is that policy. Most good policies have flexibility because it is impossible to know in advance all the problems and opportunities that an implementing organization or program will face.[15] The best test of flexibility is to find a previous program implemented under the policy and to examine its deviations, if any, from the policy. This will provide you with both an indicator of flexibility and a precedent to cite in defending your request for an exception or waiver of policy.

Administrative or Professional Discretion. The most common form of policy flexibility is that allowing an administrator or a professional who holds a particular position to use discretion in carrying out a policy.[16] Physicians are accorded considerable discretion by the policies of hospitals, nurses less but still a substantial amount. Other professionals have little discretion in patient care, but most have even greater discretion in implementing social policies. The policies themselves outside the patient care setting are more flexible than those governing patient care.

Schools tend to have more inflexible policies related to health than do institutions that deal more often with adults. Schools, in general, are second only to medical care settings in the rigidity of policies and regulations (protocols) intended to protect the wards of the institution and to protect the institution from liability.

STEP 2. ASSESSMENT OF POLITICAL FORCES

The political, regulatory, and organizational factors that might be altered through negotiation, persuasion, advocacy, and outright exercise of power are concerned with the making of policy rather than the implementation of plans, which has so far been the focus in this chapter.

Level of Analysis. The political milieu can be analyzed at both the intraorganizational level[17] and the interorganizational level.[18] Most of the suggestions for intraorganizational analysis and change that can be considered legitimate activities of the salaried insider have been presented in the foregoing sections of this chapter. If you are attempting to bring about change in another organization as an outsider, you have a greater need and justification for employing political methods because organizations resist change from without. In health promotion, the interorganizational level of analysis is particularly important because many of the programs and policies needed to alter lifestyles and environments are controlled by multiple organizations, some of them entirely outside the health sector.

Most of the community organization literature in health deals with the development of cooperation among organizations within the health sector.[19] The durable definition of community organization by Murray Ross emphasizes the cooperative element: "a process by which a community identifies its needs or objectives, ranks these needs or objectives, develops the confidence and will to work at these objectives, finds the resources (internal and external) and in so doing, extends and develops cooperative and collaborative attitudes and practices in the community."[20] The World Health Organization's global *Health for All* strategy also encourages cooperation but places the emphasis on "intersectoral" coordination in health policies.[21] Two of the rare case studies of how such intersectoral action has been developed in health promotion come from nutrition programs involving public and private sector cooperation in Australia[22] and the United States.[23]

The Zero-Sum Game. The political conflict perspective, contrary to the cooperation model of community organization, assumes that multiple, *independent* actors are in conflict over goals, resources, and actions. Their perceptions are determined by parochial priorities, goals, interests, stakes, and deadlines.[24] To the degree they are independent, the stakes are seen as a fixed pool of resources to be divided among the political sides. This means each transaction results in a gain for someone and a loss for someone else, a zero-sum game with a winner and a loser.

Systems Approach. Blending a systems approach with a political perspective, one can see the separate actors with their separate goals not as independent, but as *interdependent*.[25] This means that one's gain need not be another's loss because both depend on each other's success to make the community or system function effectively. Indeed, anyone's loss is everyone's loss in a system, with perhaps a few exceptions. One exception is where two or more individuals or organizations have identical goals and both depend on the same limited resources to pursue their goals. If both seek to maximize their goal without consideration for the other, and if one exhausts the finite resource on which both are dependent, then the other must suffer. Such is the purely competitive marketplace. Such is the circumstance of a fitness center in competition with another center in a neighborhood with a limited number of people who can afford to pay the membership or user fees. Their options are for one to move to another neighborhood, for both to recruit from a wider service area beyond the neighborhood, or to compete more aggressively through cost-cutting, price-cutting, and recruitment within the neighborhood.

True, the competitive market model helps produce innovation and efficiencies. It sometimes misses the mark, however, in social and health services because the "market" tends to be defined by those who can afford to pay for the services rather than those who need them the most. When the availability of resources for the service are limited and when the health of people may suffer for lack of the service, publicly supported (tax-based) services may be required to fill gaps in a private-sector dominated, market-driven service economy. A systems approach, not necessarily governmental but democratically planned and cooperatively negotiated, helps guard against the depletion of finite resources by a few.[26] It seeks to allocate resources in the most equitable and efficient fashion, to expand the market or service area, to provide for specialization within the market or service area, and to minimize duplication.

Those who enter the political arena do so because they have a stake in policy and must engage the conflict, sometimes even create it, to pursue their policy agenda.[27] Your purpose in diagnosing the politics of policy is to anticipate the political sides, the political actors, and the power relationships that will line up for and against the policies you or someone must promote to bring about the enabling support, regulation, and organizational or environmental changes required to achieve the health goals set for your program. After you have identified the sides, actors, and relationships, your remaining task is to propose a set of exchanges that will enable each of the sides or actors to gain something in a *win–win* rather than *win–lose* transaction.

Exchange Theory. One theory of organizational and political behavior is that people cooperate when the organization or policy allows each of them to pursue their individual goals and supports each of them in some way. They are willing, under those circumstances, to give up something in order to gain the stability and predictability of the organization or policy that serves them in some way. The key to a practical political analysis, following the systems and exchange approach, is to find the "something" that each can gain in exchange for organizational or policy change.[28]

Power Equalization Approach. The gains and sacrifices of exchange theory, unfortunately, are not equally distributed in a complex community or system. Some have less to gain and more to sacrifice than others. Some have more to gain, but relative to the sacrifice they would make, the gain seems trivial. At this point in political analyses, you must stand back from the attempt to make everyone happy and ask what is the common good. This raises the utilitarian ideal of John Stuart Mill who sought a political philosophy that would assure "the most good for the most people." Because power is unequally distributed in the community, the majority of people sometimes must make sacrifices or at least forgo their potential gains in favor of the gain of a few. This has been illustrated in relation to population and the environment by Garrett Hardin's "The Tragedy of the Commons."[29] When those sacrifices are basic human needs such as health, communities have the obligation to consider curtailment of the freedoms of the few who could exploit or harm others. This is done through legal and regulatory means when a protective law exists and by political means when the political will is strong enough to equalize the distribution of power long enough to get a new law or policy passed.

Power Educative Approach. The preferred means of bringing about policy and organizational changes, under the circumstances just described, is to educate community or organizational leaders, including those whose behavior is jeopardizing the health of others. This approach seeks to enlighten them to the harm that is being done and to appeal to their humanity and long-term interest in maintaining the community or system.[30] Implicit in this approach is the possibility of confrontation with legal action or political action if the situation is not corrected. Also implicit is the risk of bad publicity and sweeping legislative or regulatory reforms if the behavior does not change voluntarily.

Conflict Approach. If the educative approach fails, sometimes the only avenue left to equalize or tilt the balance of power on a political issue is organized confrontation and conflict in the form of strikes, petitions, boycotts, pickets, referenda, or legal action to bring about policy, regulatory, or organizational change. Similar effects on policy can be initiated through lobbying, organization of public interest groups to promote social action or to elect sympathetic candidates, and demonstrations or publicity to arouse public awareness and sentiment on the issue. This can become a program in itself, with a separate plan, or a part of a broader health promotion strategy.

Advocacy and Educating the Electorate. A growing health promotion literature on advocacy approaches to overcoming industry lobbying power, especially in the tobacco, alcohol, and environmental spheres, has developed in recent years.[31] Specific approaches, guidelines, resources, and strategies have been proposed for health educators and other professionals to use the media and to engage the political process more directly and more effectively on behalf of specific populations and health promotion issues, such as minorities,[32] the elderly,[33] increasing access to health services,[34] AIDS,[35] and the environment.[36] More general analyses and critiques of the role of health educators and other professionals in policy advocacy have been published in recent years.[37]

Empowerment Education and Community Development. A specific variation on the advocacy and education-of-the-electorate approaches represents a convergence of the self-care movement and the traditional community development approach in which the community takes much more of the initiative. In the **advocacy** approach, a politically skilled organization takes on the advocacy tasks on behalf of the community or interest group. In the **education of the electorate** approach, the outside organization or a small inside group take it upon themselves to educate the community to bring about political action. The **empowerment education** approach encourages people within the community to assume control over the entire process of educating themselves, defining their own problems, setting their own priorities, developing their own self-help programs, and, if necessary, challenging the power structure to remove hazards or to make resources available.[38]

Freudenberg's book *Not in Our Backyards!* presents case histories of chemical pollution of the environment and discusses actions taken by public groups and communities to protect themselves: the coalition building and various educational, legal, and legislative strategies that groups used on their own behalf.[39] A case study of a West Virginia experience describes a 6-year community self-help program that approximates the empowerment education approach.[40] The focus on a medical self-care model in this case study might have limited its clear reflection of the community organization and empowerment education approach, but the power of the participatory process in this community is thoroughly documented.[41]

More is presented on these policy, regulatory, and organizational components of health promotion planning in the application chapters.

IMPLEMENTATION

Much of the foregoing diagnostic process puts the planner in the midst of the implementation process. Where planning and policy formation leave off and implementation begins is virtually undefinable. As Mazmanian and Sabatier argue for their list of 16 variables influencing implementation, "the original policymakers can affect substantially the attainment of . . . objectives by utilizing the levers at their disposal to coherently structure the implementation process."[42] But trying to control implementation with more detailed and inflexible policy is like trying to control the growth and development of a child with more rules and restrictions. The program, like the child, needs room to breathe, to experiment, to adapt to new circumstances and people.[43]

Chase developed a 44-item checklist of factors to consider as obstacles to implementation.[44] Step 3 of the administrative diagnosis describes the most important of those barriers. The list of variables (each having a positive or facilitative and a negative or hindering possibility) shown in Table 6.2 should prove more useful to the implementor than the simple listing of barriers.

The importance of attention to implementation in health education and health promotion has been highlighted by the case study analysis of an evaluation performed on the School Health Curriculum Project.[45] Only 34 percent of the teaching/learning activities of the curriculum were implemented by the five teachers as they were intended to be implemented. This suggests the need for monitoring the implementation process as the first step in process evaluation, to be discussed in Chapter 7. It also suggests that policies and programs must provide for professional discretion and options so that they can be adapted to local situations and changing circumstances.

Training and supervision of personnel provide the best assurance of implementation. Each training program is an educational program in itself and deserves a similar planning process to that described by the behavioral, environmental, and educational diagnoses in the PRECEDE framework. Supervision can also be approached as an educational process: Behavior change goals can be set mutually by the supervisor and supervisee. Factors predisposing, enabling, and reinforcing the intended employee behavior can be analyzed periodically. And interventions can be planned to predispose, enable, and reinforce implementation through staff meetings, training, written materials, and rewards for high performance. Examples of PRECEDE applied to professional training in the medical care setting are presented in Chapter 11.

In the final analysis, textbooks can offer little on implementation that will improve upon a good plan, an adequate budget, good organizational and policy support, good training and supervision of staff, and good monitoring in the process evaluation stage, discussed in Chapter 7. The key to success in implementation beyond these six ingredients is experience, sensitivity to people's needs, flexibility in the face of changing circumstances, an eye fixed on long-term goals, and a sense of humor.

Most of these ingredients come with time and the opportunity to start small and build on success. The only shortcut to some of the required experience might be critical reading of case studies. Numerous case studies in health education and health promotion have been compiled in recent years.[46] A survey of practitioner and academic health education opinion of recommended readings[47] yielded case studies and program descriptions considered the best of the 1970s in Indian

TABLE 6.2

Effects on implementation of policy, implementing organization, political milieu, and the environment

Variables	Effects on implementation	
	Positive or facilitating	Negative or hindering
Policy		
Theory	Solid	Unproven
Assumptions	Defined	Unclear
Goals	Stated	Nonexistent
Change		
Amount	Small	Large
Rate	Incremental	Ambitious
Familiarity	Familiar	Unfamiliar
Centrality	Central	Peripheral
Complexity	Few transactions	Many transactions
Resources	Available	Nonexistent
Specification	Some	None
Flexibility	Alternative solutions	One right answer
Impact	Early stages	Later stages
Implementing organization		
Structure		
Goal	Relevant to policy	Irrelevant to policy
Task	Suitable	Unsuitable
Scale	Small	Large
Climate	Supportive	Unsupportive
Technical capacity		
Technology	Appropriate	Inappropriate
Resources	Available	Unavailable
Employee disposition		
Approach	Problem solving	Opportunistic
Motivation	Maintained	Declines
Values	Congruent	Incongruent
Attitudes	Favorable	Unfavorable
Beliefs	Faith in policy	No faith in policy
Employee behavior	Changeable	Resistant
Political milieu		
Power		
Strength	Strong	Strong
Support	Present	Absent
Environment		
Timing	"Right"	"Wrong"
Intended beneficiaries	Needs	No needs
Other organizations	Controllable	Uncontrollable

SOURCE: Adapted from J. M. Ottoson and L. W. Green, "Reconciling Concept and Context: Theory of Implementation," in *Advances in Health Education and Promotion*, vol. 2, W. B. Ward and M. H. Becker, eds. (Greenwich, CT: JAI Press, 1987).

health,[48] drug abuse prevention,[49] primary care settings,[50] dental health,[51] family planning,[52] worksite health education,[53] hospital health education,[54] mass media,[55] health fairs,[56] sex education,[57] health planning,[58] inner city and ethnic minorities,[59] a regional health education center,[60] and work with volunteers and the elderly.[61]

A flood of new case studies and program descriptions in the 1980s reflects the rapid growth and the changing emphasis in the field of health promotion. Some outstanding recent examples include the Tenderloin Senior Outreach Project,[62] a community organization project to stop herbicide spraying in Massachusetts,[63] issues encountered in developing health promotion coalitions and consortia,[64] a health education program about AIDS among seropositive blood donors in New York,[65] and another about AIDS in a minority high-risk community in Detroit.[66]

Hundreds of other program descriptions are buried in the text of articles reporting on program evaluations, some of which will come up in Chapter 7. These make useful reading for the theoretical rationale, the design of interventions, and the problems of implementation, but the descriptions are usually truncated in favor of space for reporting statistical results.

SUSTAINABILITY AND INSTITUTIONALIZATION

An increasing concern about the rapid growth and proliferation of health promotion programs in the past decade is the high probability that many programs will not survive long after the initial enthusiasm or external funding that launched them begins to wane.[67] Those programs directed at complex lifestyle changes and chronic disease risk factors cannot hope to have much impact on these outcomes, much less on morbidity and mortality, in a short period for large numbers of people. Short-burst programs can expect to have short-burst effects. It takes sustained interventions on a community- or institution-wide scale to make a significant change in the vital statistics of a community. Thus, sustainability of programs in health promotion becomes a greater issue than for some communicable disease control programs, for example, in which short campaigns can achieve a high level of immunization or other protection in the community.

On the other hand, one could argue that too much is made of the need to institutionalize health promotion programs. The continuation of a particular program might be less critical to the overall contribution to a community's health than the problem-solving ability and community competence that comes from successfully mounting and launching a series of short-term health promotion programs. It might be the cumulative and synergistic effect of many programs that brings about changes in the community norms, behavior, and conditions of living that are conducive to health. Those who successfully start programs often move on to start new programs, leaving the functions of the old programs to be divided and distributed among various departments, agencies, or institutions. If every program were institutionalized, most organizations would become stagnant and overwhelmed with obsolete programs.[68]

Nevertheless, some attention should be devoted at this stage of planning and early intervention leveraging. **Leveraging** refers to the use of initial investments and commitments to draw larger investments and commitments. A program that has come this far through the planning, approval, and implementation process has a chance of building on its initial successes to gain visibility and credibility for its sponsors, planners, or administrators. Other funding agencies will be drawn to innovative programs that have a good start. Other departments within an organization will want to associate themselves with an exciting and promising program. Other volunteers and professionals in the community will offer services to a high-profile program.

The leveraging approach to sustainability puts even more weight on the quality and thoroughness of the planning process that precedes implementation and on the effective involvement of key organizational and community leaders in that process. Now the principle of participation begins to pay off in sustained commitment to the program from multiple sources. According to Goodman and Steckler, "the more cells a particular health promotion program occupies, the more institutionalized it is."[69]

Cells refer here to the matrix of organizational subsystems in which the program can insinuate itself. If the program has interested parties, representation, or a presence in many different parts or departments of the organization or agencies of the community, it has already established many roots in the organization or community.

The other implication of the leveraging strategy for institutionalization is that evaluation data are even more eagerly awaited. Early evidence of how the program is taking hold, how it is being received, and what impact it is having on short-term objectives now becomes more than managerial data. It becomes political and marketing data in a world of competing interests. This makes fudging or inflating the data tempting for some program managers eager to make a good impression, but credibility depends on integrity. You gain more support as the program proceeds by presenting the strengths *and* the weaknesses of the program so that supporters can find some things to take pride in *and* some places where they can offer help.

All this brings the subject of evaluation to the table. The prospects for sustaining programs depend in part on evaluation results. The quality of program delivery depends on improvements signaled by short-loop feedback on materials, implementation, and reactions to components of the programs. Improved implementation, in turn, enhances the impact of the program on behavioral and environmental changes. And if the program has been well conceived, well planned, and well executed, the changes in behavior and environment should guarantee improvements in health and quality of life.

SUMMARY

The administrative diagnosis entails the assessment of resources required by your program, the resources available in your organization or community, and the barriers to implementation of your program. The policy diagnosis then asks what political, regulatory, and organizational supports and barriers can you change to facilitate your program and to enable the development of educational and environmental supports for community action. These steps took us from PRECEDE planning to PROCEED implementation. Evaluation, then, becomes part of both the plan and the implementation process.

Planning and policy in health education and health promotion can provide clarity of purpose, resources, and protection for the programs they produce, but they cannot mark every step on the path of implementation without retarding the very growth and development of the people they are intended to help. Plans and policies must leave enough flexibility and discretion for those who must implement the plans to adapt them to changing local circumstances, personalities, opportunities, and feedback from evaluation.

PRECEDE assures that a program will be *appropriate* to a person's or population's needs and circumstances. PROCEED assures that the program will be *available*, *accessible*, *acceptable*, and *accountable*. Only an appropriate program is worth implementing, but even the most appropriate program will fail to reach those who need it if it is unavailable, inaccessible, or unacceptable to them. PROCEED assesses resources required to assure the program's *availability*, organizational changes required to assure its *accessibility*, and political and regulatory changes required to assure its *acceptability*. Finally, evaluation assures that the program will be *accountable* to the policy makers, administrators, consumers or clients, and any other stakeholders who need to know whether the program met their standards of acceptability.

REFERENCES AND NOTES

1. We are indebted to Susan Brink, Dr.P.H., at the University of Texas Center for Health Promotion Research and Development, for her contributions to this chapter, and to Judith Ottoson, M.P.H., Ed.D., for her research on implementation and training, which provided a basis for parts of this chapter.

2. Software programs for microcomputer construction of Gantt charts and other tools for planning the flow of program activities are readily available. See, e.g., *Harvard Total Project Manager II* (Mountain View, CA: Software Publishing, 1986). See also, A. O. Awani, *Project Management Techniques* (New York: Petrocelli Books, 1983); M. Zeldman and S. Myrom, *How To Plan Projects and Keep Them on Schedule* (San Diego, CA: Integrated Software Systems, 1983).

3. R. Campbell and B. Chenoweth, "Health Education as a Basis for Social Support," *The Geron-*

tologist 21 (1981): 619–27; S. B. Hoffman, "Peer Counselor Training with the Elderly," *The Gerontologist* 23 (1983): 358–60; B. Rimer, M. Keintz, B. Glassman, and J. Kinman, "Health Education for Older Persons: Lessons from Research and Program Evaluations," in *Advances in Health Education and Promotion*, vol. 1, pt. B, Z. Salisbury, J. G. Zapka, and S. B. Kar, eds. (Greenwich, CT: JAI Press, 1986), pp. 369–96; B. M. Shannon, H. Smickiklas-Wright, B. W. Davis, and C. A. Lewis, "Peer Educator Approach to Nutrition for the Elderly," *The Gerontologist* 23 (1983): 123–6.

4. J. R. Miller, "Liaisons: Using Health Education Resources Effectively," in *Advancing Health Through Education: A Case Study Approach*, H. P. Cleary, J. M. Kichen, and P. G. Ensor, eds. (Palo Alto, CA: Mayfield, 1984), pp. 112–4; P. Mullen, K. Kukowski, and S. Mazelis, "Health Education in Health Maintenance Organizations," in *Handbook of Health Education*, P. Lazes, ed. (Germantown, MD: Aspen Systems, 1979).

5. L. W. Green, "Evaluation and Measurement: Some Dilemmas for Health Education," *American Journal of Public Health* 67 (1977): 155–61.

6. R. Bertera and L. W. Green, "Cost-Effectiveness of a Home Visiting Triage Program for Family Planning in Turkey," *American Journal of Public Health* 69 (1979): 950–3; D. B. Connell, R. R. Turner, and E. F. Mason, "Summary of Findings of the School Health Education Evaluation: Health Promotion Effectiveness, Implementation, and Costs," *Journal of School Health* 55 (1985): 316–21; A. J. Chwalow, L. W. Green, D. M. Levine, and S. G. Deeds, "Effects of the Multiplicity of Interventions on the Compliance of Hypertensive Patients with Medical Regimens in an Inner-city Population," *Preventive Medicine* 7 (1978): 51; L. W. Green, V. L. Wang, and P. Ephross, "A Three-Year Longitudinal Study of the Effectiveness of Nutrition Aides on Rural Poor Home-makers," *American Journal of Public Health* 64 (1974): 722–4; M. E. Hatcher, L. W. Green, D. M. Levine, and C. E. Flagle, "Validation of a Decision Model for Triaging Hypertensive Patients to Alternate Health Education Interventions," *Social Science and Medicine* 22 (1986): 813–9; L. W. Risser, H. M. Hoffman, B. G. Gordon, and L. W. Green, "A Cost-Benefit Analysis of Preparticipation Sports Examinations of Adolescent Athletes," *Journal of School Health* 55 (1985): 270–3.

7. J. E. Fielding, "Effectiveness of Employee Health Improvement Programs," *Journal of Occupational Medicine* 24 (1982): 907–16; L. W. Green, 1974, op. cit.; L. W. Green, 1977, op. cit.; V. L. Wang, P. Ephross, and L. W. Green, "The Point of Diminishing Returns in Home Visits to Rural Homemakers," in *The SOPHE Heritage Collection of Health Education Monographs*, vol. 3, J. Zapka, ed. (Oakland, CA: Third Party Publishing, 1981), pp. 155–73.

8. D. Van Meter and C. Van Horn, "The Policy Implementation Process: A Conceptual Framework," *Administration and Society* 6 (1975): 445–88.

9. H. S. Ross and P. R. Mico, *Theory and Practice in Health Education* (Palo Alto, CA: Mayfield, 1980), p. 222.

10. T. Smith, "Policy Roles: An Analysis of Policy Formulators and Policy Implementors," *Policy Sciences* 4 (1973): 297–307.

11. M. Schaeffer, *Designing and Implementing Procedures for Health and Human Services* (Beverly Hills: Sage, 1985).

12. N. H. Gottlieb, C. Y. Lovato, M. P. Eriksen, and L. W. Green, "The Implementation of a Restrictive Worksite Smoking Policy in a Large Decentralized Agency," (unpublished, 1990); D. Gustafson, *An Approach to Predicting the Implementation Potential of Recommended Actions in Health Planning* (Madison, WI: The Institute for Health Planning, 1979).

13. P. Berman and M. McLaughlin, "Implementation of Educational Innovation," *The Educational Forum* 40 (1976): 347–70; G. Chase, "Implementing a Human Services Program: How Hard Can It Be?" *Public Policy* 27 (1979): 385–435.

14. L. W. Green, "A Participant Observer in a Period of Professional Change," in *Advancing Health*

Through Education: A Case Study Approach, H. P. Cleary, J. M. Kichen, and P. G. Ensor, eds. (Palo Alto, CA: Mayfield, 1985), pp. 374–80.

15. M. Rein and F. Rabinovitz, "Implementation: A Theoretical Perspective" (Cambridge, MA: Joint Center for Urban Studies of MIT and Harvard University, Working Paper no. 43, 1977).

16. F. M. Lewis and M. V. Batey, "Clarifying Autonomy and Accountability in Nursing Service: Part 2," *Journal of Nursing Administration* 12 (Oct. 1982): 10–15.

17. G. Allison, *Essence of Decision* (Boston: Little, Brown, 1971); L. Bolman, and T. Deal, *The Political Frame* (Cambridge: Harvard Graduate School of Education, 1979); W. Williams and R. Elmore, eds., *Social Program Implementation* (New York: Academic Press, 1976).

18. E. Bardach, *The Implementation Game: What Happens After a Bill Becomes a Law* (Cambridge: MIT Press, 1977); E. Hargrove, *The Missing Link: The Study of the Implementation of Social Policy* (Washington, DC: The Urban Institute Paper 797–1, 1975).

19. N. Bracht, ed., *Community Organization Strategies for Health Promotion* (New York: Sage, 1990); D. J. Breckon, J. R. Harvey, and R. B. Lancaster, *Community Health Education: Settings, Roles, and Skills* (Germantown, MD: Aspen Systems, 1989), chap. 14; R. D. Patton and W. B. Cissell, eds., *Community Organization: Traditional Principles and Modern Applications* (Johnson City, TN: Latchpins Press, 1989).

20. M. Ross, *Community Organization: Theory, Principles, and Practice* (New York: Harper & Row, 1967), p. 14.

21. *Targets for Health for All* (Copenhagen: World Health Organization Regional Office for Europe, 1986).

22. S. Chapman, "Intersectoral Action to Improve Nutrition: The Roles of the State and the Private Sector. A Case Study from Australia," *Health Promotion International* 5 (1990): 35–44.

23. S. E. Samuels, "Project LEAN: Lowfat Eating for America Now," *American Journal of Health Promotion* 4 (1990): 435–40.

24. S. D. Alinsky, *Rules for Radicals: A Pragmatic Primer for Realistic Radicals* (New York: Vintage Books, 1972); G. Allison, op. cit., 1971.

25. R. Chin, "The Utility of System Models and Developmental Models for Practitioners," in *The Planning of Change*, 3rd ed., W. B. Bennis, K. D. Benne, R. Chin, and K. E. Corey, eds. (New York: Holt, Rinehart and Winston, 1976), pp. 90–102.

26. S. Levine, P. White, and N. Scotch, "Community Interorganizational Problems in Providing Medical Care and Social Services," *American Journal of Public Health* 53 (1963): 1183–95.

27. For example, S. D. Alinsky, op. cit., 1972; N. Freudenberg, *Not in Our Backyards! Community Action for Health and the Environment* (New York: Monthly Review Press, 1984); D. A. Stockman, *The Triumph of Politics: How the Reagan Revolution Failed* (New York: Harper & Row, 1986); R. Titmus, *The Gift Relationship from Human Blood to Social Policy* (New York: Vintage Books, 1972).

28. C. Argyris, *Integrating the Individual and the Organization* (New York: Wiley, 1964); T. J. Peters and R. H. Waterman, Jr., *In Search of Excellence: Lessons from America's Best Run Companies* (New York: Warner Books, 1984).

29. G. Hardin, "The Tragedy of the Commons," *Science* 143 (1968): 1243–6. See also, L. W. Green, *Community Health*, 6th ed., (St. Louis: Mosby, 1990), pp. 59–60.

30. M. F. Cataldo and T. J. Coates, eds., *Health and Industry: A Behavioral Medicine Perspective* (New York: Wiley, 1986), esp. pp. 399–419.

31. For example, T. Abelin, "Getting Health Promotion Off the Ground in Switzerland," *Journal of Public Health Policy* 9 (1988): 284–5; R. Blum and S. E. Samuels, eds., "Television and Teens:

Health Implications," *Journal of Adolescent Health Care* 11 (1990): issue no. 1; S. Casswell, L. Stewart, and P. Duignan, "The Struggle Against the Broadcast of Anti-health Messages: Regulation of Alcohol Advertising in New Zealand," *Health Promotion International* 4 (1989): 287–96; W. Farrant and A. Taft, "Building Healthy Public Policy in an Unhealthy Political Climate: A Case Study from Paddington and North Kensington," *Health Promotion International* 3 (1988): 287–92; A. McGuire, "There's Death on the Block, There's Hope in Congress," *Journal of Public Health Policy* 8 (1987): 451–4; P. A. Morgan, "Power, Politics and Public Health: The Political Power of the Alcohol Beverage Industry," *Journal of Public Health Policy* 9 (1988): 177–97; J. F. Mosher and D. H. Jernigan, "Public Action and Awareness To Reduce Alcohol-Related Problems: A Plan of Action," *Journal of Public Health Policy* 9 (1988): 17–41; L. M. Wallack, "Mass Media Campaigns in a Hostile Environment: Advertising as Anti-health Education," *Journal of Drug Addiction*, 28 (1983): 51–63.

32. For example, R. L. Braithwaite and N. Lythcott, "Community Empowerment as a Strategy for Health Promotion for Black and Other Minorities," *Journal of the American Medical Association* 261 (1989): 282–3; L. C. Liburd and J. V. Bowie, "Intentional Teenage Pregnancy: A Community Diagnosis and Action Plan," *Health Education* 20(5) (1989): 33–8; S. B. Thomas, "Community Health Advocacy for Racial and Ethnic Minorities in the United States: Issues and Challenges for Health Education," *Health Education Quarterly* 17 (1990): 13–19.

33. M. Minkler, "Building Supportive Ties and Sense of Community Among the Inner-city Elderly: The Tenderloin Senior Outreach Project," *Health Education Quarterly* 12 (1985): 303–14; M. Minkler and B. Checkoway, "Ten Principles for Geriatric Health Promotion," *Health Promotion International* 3 (1988): 277–86.

34. H. J. Geiger, "Community Health Centers: Health Care as an Instrument of Social Change," in *Reforming Medicine: Lessons of the Last Quarter Century*, V. Sidel and R. Sidel, eds. (New York: Pantheon, 1984).

35. N. Krieger and J. C. Lashof, "AIDS, Policy Analysis, and the Electorate: The Role of Schools of Public Health," *American Journal of Public Health*, 78 (1988): 411–5; T. G. Rundall and K. A. Phillips, "Informing and Educating the Electorate About AIDS," *Medical Care Review* 47 (1990): 3–13.

36. T. Dietz, P. C. Stern, and R. W. Rycroft, "Definitions of Conflict and the Legitimation of Resources: The Case of Environmental Risk," *Sociological Forum* 4(1) (1989): 47–70; N. Freudenberg, op. cit., 1984.

37. D. F. Collin, "Health Educators: Change Agents or Techno/Peasants?" *International Quarterly of Community Health Education*, 3 (1982–1983): 131–44; N. Freudenberg, "Shaping the Future of Health Education: From Behavior Change to Social Change," *Health Education Monographs* 6 (1978): 372–7; L. M. Hoffman, *The Politics of Knowledge: Activist Movements in Medicine and Planning* (Albany: State University of New York Press, 1989); M. Mahaffey and J. W. Hanks, eds., *Practical Politics: Social Work and Political Responsibility* (Silver Springs, MD: National Association of Social Workers, 1982); A. Steckler and L. Dawson, "The Role of Health Education in Public Policy Development," *Health Education Quarterly* 9 (1982): 275–92; A. Steckler, L. Dawson, R. M. Goodman, and N. Epstein, "Policy Advocacy: Three Emerging Roles for Health Education," in W. B. Ward and S. K. Simonds, *Advances in Health Education and Promotion*, vol. 2 (Greenwich, CT: JAI Press, 1987), pp. 5–28.

38. L. W. Green, "New Policies in Education for Health," *World Health* (April-May, 1983): 13–17; M. Minkler, op. cit., 1985; M. Pilisuk, S. Parks, J. Kelly, and E. Turner, "The Helping Network Approach: Community Promotion of Mental Health," *Journal of Primary Prevention* 3 (1982): 116–32; I. Shor and P. Freire, *A Pedagogy for Liberation* (Boston: Bergin and Garvey Publishers, 1987); C. Tjerandsen, *Education for Citizenship: A Foundation's Experience* (Santa Cruz, CA: Emil Schwarzhaupt Foundation, 1980); N. Wallerstein and E. Bernstein, "Empowerment Education: Freire's Ideas Adapted to Health Education," *Health Education Quarterly* 15 (1988): 379–94.

39. T. Dietz, P. C. Stern, and R. W. Rycroft, "Definition of Conflict and the Legitimation of Resources:

The Case of Environmental Risk," *Sociological Forum* 4(1) (1989): 47–70; N. Freudenberg, op. cit., 1984.

40. P. Schiller, A. Steckler, L. Dawson, and F. Patton, *Participatory Planning in Community Health Education: A Guide Based on the McDowell County, West Virginia Experience* (Oakland, CA: Third Party Publishing, 1987).

41. N. Wallerstein, [Book review of] "P. Schiller, A. Steckler, L. Dawson, and F. Patton, *Participatory Planning in Community Health Education: A Guide Based on the McDowell County, West Virginia Experience* (Oakland, CA: Third Party Publishing, 1987)," *Health Education Quarterly* 17 (1990): 119–21.

42. D. Mazmanian and P. Sabatier, *Implementation and Public Policy* (Glenview, IL: Scott, Foresman, 1983), preface.

43. J. M. Ottoson, and L. W. Green, "Reconciling Concept and Context: Theory of Implementation," in *Advances in Health Education and Promotion*, vol. 2, W. B. Ward and M. H. Becker, eds. (Greenwich, CT: JAI Press, 1987), pp. 353–82.

44. G. Chase, "Implementing a Human Services Program: How Hard Can It Be?" *Public Policy* 27 (1979): 385–435.

45. C. E. Basch, E. M. Sliepcevich, R. S. Gold, et al., "Avoiding Type III Errors in Health Education Program Evaluations: A Case Study," *Health Education Quarterly* 12 (1985): 315–35; see also, G. G. Wojtowicz, "A Secondary Analysis of the School Health Education Evaluation Data Base," *Journal of School Health* 60 (1990): 56–9.

46. R. W. Carlaw, *Perspectives on Community Health Education: A Series of Case Studies, Vol. 1, United States* (Oakland, CA: Third Party Publishing, 1982); H. P. Cleary, J. M. Kichen, and P. G. Ensor, *Advancing Health Through Education: A Case Study Approach* (Palo Alto: Mayfield, 1985); see also compilations by various resource centers and clearinghouses such as the American Hospital Association, the American Public Health Association, the CDC Center for Chronic Disease Control and Health Promotion, the U.S. Office of Substance Abuse Prevention, the Stanford Health Promotion Resource Center, the National Health Information Clearinghouse, and the Combined Health Education Data Base accessible through Medline.

47. T. L. Chen and G. P. Cernada, *Recommended Health Education Readings: An Annotated Bibliography* (Taipei: Maplewood Press, 1985). Abstracts of these selected case studies were published originally in sequential issues of the *International Quarterly of Community Health Education* (Baywood Publishing Company) between 1980 and 1984. The selections were made from a polling of faculty of graduate programs in community health education accredited by the Council on Education for Public Health and of practitioners who were members of the Society for Public Health Education in 1979–1980.

48. W. A. Bettes, "A Method of Allocating Resources for Health Education Services by the Indian Health Service," *Public Health Reports* 91 (1976): 256–60; P. Werden, "Health Education for Indian Students," *Journal of School Health* 44 (1974): 319–23.

49. P. G. Bourne, "Approaches to Drug Abuse Prevention and Treatment in Rural Areas," *Journal of Psychadelic Drugs* 6 (1974): 285–9.

50. B. Carlton and M. Carlton, "Defining a Role for the Health Educator in the Primary Care Setting," *Health Education* 9 (Mar./Apr., 1978): 22–3; J. Gittenberg, "Adapting Health Care to a Cultural Setting," *American Journal of Nursing* 74 (1974): 2218–21.

51. M. A. Thornton, "Preventive Dentistry in the Veterans Administration," *Dental Hygiene* 53 (1979): 121–4.

52. E. C. Cernada, Y. J. Lee, and M. Y. Lin, "Family Planning Telephone Services in Two Asian Cities," *Studies in Family Planning* 5 (1974): 111–4; G. Cernada, "The Case of the Unplanned Child," *Human Organization* 33 (1974): 106–9.

53. J. E. Fielding and S. Nelson, "Health Education for Job Corps Enrollees," *Public Health Reports* 91 (1976): 243–8.

54. F. B. Fiori, M. de la Vega, and M. J. Vacarro, "Health Education in a Hospital Setting: Report of a Public Health Service Project in Newark, New Jersey," *Health Education Monographs* 2(1) (1974): 11–29; R. A. Hinthorne and R. Jones, "Coordinating Patient Education in the Hospital," *Hospitals* 52 (1978): 85–8; L. V. Miller and J. Goldstein, "More Efficient Care of Diabetic Patients in a County-Hospital Setting," *New England Journal of Medicine* 286 (1972): 1383–91; A. W. Skiff, "Experiences with Methods for Patient Teaching from a Public Health Service Hospital," *Health Education Monographs* 2(1) (1974): 48–53.

55. I. M. Newman, G. L. Martin, and K. A. Farrell, "Changing Health Values Through Public Television," *Health Values* 2(2) (1978): 92–5.

56. N. D. Richie, "Some Guidelines for Conducting a Health Fair," *Public Health Reports* 91 (1976): 261–4.

57. J. M. Zapka and R. M. Mazur, "Peer Sex Training and Evaluation," *American Journal of Public Health* 67 (1977): 450–4.

58. M. D. Lightner, "The Health Education Coordinating Council," *Health Education* 7 (Nov./Dec. 1976): 25–6.

59. F. P. Li, N. Y. Schlief, C. J. Chang, and A. C. Gaw, "Health Care for the Chinese Community in Boston," *American Journal of Public Health* 62 (1972): 536–9.

60. A. A. Sorensen and J. S. Sinacore, "Developing a Regional Health Education Program," *Regional Health Education* 3(2) (1979): 79–84.

61. C. Cox, "A Pilot Study: Using the Elderly as Community Health Educators," *International Journal of Health Education* 22 (1979): 49–52.

62. M. Minkler, op. cit., 1985.

63. A. E. Winder, "The Mouse That Roared: A Case History of Community Organization for Health Practice," *Health Education Quarterly* 12 (1985): 353–63.

64. M. F. Davis and D. C. Iverson, "An Overview and Analysis of the HealthStyle Campaign," *Health Education Quarterly* 11 (1984): 253–72; R. S. DeFrank and P. M. Levenson, "Ethical and Philosophical Issues in Developing a Health Promotion Consortium," *Health Education Quarterly* 14 (1987): 71–7; D. Kemper, "The Healthwise Program: Growing Younger," in *Wellness and Health Promotion for the Elderly*, K. Dychtwald, ed. (Rockville, MD: Aspen, 1986), pp. 263–73; K. R. Pelletier, N. L. Klehr, and S. J. McPhee, "Town and Gown: A Lesson in Collaboration," *Business and Health* (Feb. 1988): 34–9; F. W. Schott, "WELCOM: The Wellness Council of the Midlands," in *A Decade of Survival: Past, Present, Future. Proceedings of the 20th Annual Meeting* (Washington, DC: Society of Prospective Medicine, 1985).

65. P. D. Cleary, T. F. Rogers, E. Singer, et al., "Health Education About AIDS Among Seropositive Blood Donors," *Health Education Quarterly* 13 (1986): 317–30.

66. L. S. Williams, "AIDS Risk Reduction: A Community Health Education Intervention for Minority High Risk Group Members," *Health Education Quarterly* 13 (1986): 407–21.

67. R. M. Goodman and A. Steckler, "A Model for the Institutionalization of Health Promotion Programs," *Family and Community Health* 11(4) (1989): 63–78.

68. L. W. Green, "Is Institutionalization the Proper Role of Grantmaking?" *American Journal of Health Promotion* 4 (1989): 44.

69. R. M. Goodman and A. Steckler, "A Framework for Assessing Program Institutionalization," *Knowledge in Society* 2 (1989): 57–71, quotation from page 69.

Chapter 7

Evaluation and the Accountable Practitioner

Entire textbooks and specific review articles have been published to address the scientific and technical issues of evaluation for each of the health problems and settings in the field of health promotion.[1] Obviously, one chapter can scarcely scratch the surface of program evaluation in this field, so we limit our scope to the tasks of **evaluation** as they are developed and carried out within the realities of program planning and management in the field.

Our discussion centers around nine questions: the embarrassing questions a professor, supervisor, agency head, board member, or legislator might ask; the tough questions posed by grant review panels; the innocent but penetrating questions a lay member of your planning committee or a program recipient could ask; and the questions raised by colleagues when you formally present findings from your health promotion program. Responses to the questions will illuminate some pathways that practitioners can follow when faced with the challenges and complexities—sometimes large, sometimes small—that inevitably accompany the evaluation of a program.

The good news for the accountable practitioner is that, having attended to the diagnostic steps of PRECEDE and PROCEED, you already have in hand most of the essential information you need for an evaluation.

1 WHY EVALUATE? THE VIEWS OF DIFFERENT STAKEHOLDERS

It should come as no surprise that the reasons given for evaluating differ depending on the perspective of the user or consumer of evaluative information. Where you stand on evaluation depends on where you sit on policy and program:

- The elected official needs evaluation results to demonstrate that a given program reached and served his or her constituents.
- The program manager uses information from evaluations to guide program decisions.
- The evaluation research specialist, behavioral scientist, or epidemiologist uses evaluation data to determine whether improvements in health outcomes were causally linked to a given intervention or a given behavioral change.[2]

As different as these viewpoints may appear, they are bound together by a common thread: the need to know what works. Each of these parties and other "stakeholders" can be helpfully informed by the products of evaluation. Their enlightenment, in turn, can provide support for continuing and improving useful programs and for discontinuing and reallocating resources from unproductive programs.[3]

---

2 IS EVALUATION REALLY NECESSARY?

Some of the stakeholders may be less interested in the evaluation of some programs than of others. The politician and the public are most interested in evaluations of the more costly and the more controversial programs. The program manager shares these interests but also needs some minimal level of evaluation for every program. The wider professional and scientific community is most interested in evaluation of the most innovative programs. Responsible professionals need to have something to show for their time and effort and so will seek some form of feedback on performance or impact.

The accountable practitioner or program manager approaches each new population and program combination as an experiment.[4] The PRECEDE diagnostic results supply the hypotheses, and the PROCEED implementation and evaluation steps supply a test of the hypotheses. Whether the evaluation is elaborate, extensive, and thorough or whether it is simple, limited, and superficial depends, then, on its cost, controversy, and innovativeness, but *some* evaluation is essential for accountable program managers and practitioners. If the PRECEDE planning process required few assumptions because there was much prior research, which linked with some certainty each cause and each effect in the causal chain, then the only evaluation necessary is the minimum required by the program manager to account for the expenditure of resources. If the PRECEDE linkages were tenuous, requiring some guesswork about cause–effect relationships, then a more elaborate evaluation may be in order to confirm or disconfirm the assumptions. The assumptions derived from educated guesswork represent hypotheses needing to be tested.

3 WHAT IS EVALUATION, REALLY?

Dictionaries generally define *evaluation* in two ways: to ascertain or judge the worth of something, and to examine carefully. Indeed, the primary tasks for the evaluator are "carefully examining" and "judging the worth" of methods, personnel, materials, or programs. In the context of health education and health promotion, we have defined **evaluation** simply as the *comparison* of an *object of interest* against a *standard of acceptability.*[5]

Objects of Interest. Objects of interest include any or all of the factors that one takes into account in applying the PRECEDE–PROCEED framework: measures of quality of life; health status indicators; behavioral and environmental factors; predisposing, enabling, and reinforcing factors; intervention activities; methods of delivery; changes in policies, regulations, or organizations; level of staff expertise; and quality of performance and educational materials. Any or all may be the objects of interest for evaluation. The interest in *program* evaluation per se is in some *change* in the object that can be associated with some change in program activity or input.

The Order of Interest. Each of the inputs, intermediate effects, and ultimate outcomes of health promotion programs can be objects of interest in an evaluation. Previous chapters have worked from right to left (against the arrows) along the causal chain implied by the PRECEDE model. It was a systematic search for root causes and preventive or promotive solutions. Evaluation, as described in this chapter, applies the same logic and model, but the order of attention is from left to right (with the arrows) from immediate policies, activities, resources, and implementation; to intermediate effects; and then to ultimate health outcomes and social benefits. The objects of interest are the same; the order of their examination and judgment is the opposite.

Objectives. The objects of interest in a well-developed PRECEDE plan are identified by the objectives. The term *objectives* derives from the term *object.* A hierarchy of objectives from ultimate social and health objectives, to intermediate behavioral and environmental objectives, and then to more immediate educational, organizational, regulatory, and policy objectives identifies the objects of interest in reverse order of immediacy. Recall that objectives had to state *who* is expected to experience *how much* of *what change* by *when.* The objects of interest center on the *who* and the *what change.*

4 WHAT ARE YOUR STANDARDS OF ACCEPTABILITY?

The standards of acceptability, following the same logic, are identified in the *how much* and *when* estimates in the objectives developed during the planning process. Standards state how an object of interest is expected to measure up. They also serve as targets, which, when attained or exceeded, signal success, improvement, or growth.[6] For health promotion programs, the standards are the expected *level* of improvement in social, economic, health, environmental, behavioral, educational, organizational, or policy conditions stated in the objectives.[7]

Now come the embarrassing questions — if the objectives were not explicit and specific enough about *how much* and *by when*. Legislators, directors, board members, and other policy makers and funding sources become impatient for results. They want to believe they made good investments in your program, but they need evidence to justify continuing the investment. Other priorities emerge over time, causing some of the policy makers to look for unproductive investments from which resources can be siphoned to fund new programs. Invariably, they expect more than their level of investment and the elapsed time should warrant, but you can fall back on the standards they accepted when they first funded the program if those standards are realistically and explicitly stated in the program objectives. Standards can be set in several ways.

ARBITRARY STANDARDS

Program managers or policy makers can simply declare that they want to see a given change: for example, a 50 percent rate of participation in program X by all employees. Seldom does such a seemingly arbitrary standard come from nowhere. The apparent fiat probably has some historical precedent or vague rationale in the mind of the perpetrator. The first task of the evaluator sometimes must be to decipher or trace the origin or rationale of an apparently arbitrary standard of acceptability.

SCIENTIFIC STANDARDS

At the other extreme lie the standards based on the state of the art as reflected by the latest published evaluations or randomized trials. Standards should be deemed acceptable based on justifications made from a review of the literature. For example, a practitioner charged with establishing a standard for a smoking cessation program would benefit greatly by consulting the data presented in Table 7.1 summarizing the quit rates for a variety of smoking cessation strategies at the

6-month and 1-year follow-ups.[8] The objectives for a program applying one or more of these methods might use these figures as the basis for estimating *how much* by *when*. Such scientifically based standards might more accurately be called "theoretical standards" because the formally tested methods in a review such as Table 7.1 can be only partially replicated in a real-world program. The scientific or theoretical standard says, in effect, "If everything in our program goes just as it did in the formal experiments with this method, here is the smoking cessation rate we should expect to achieve in 6 months and 1 year following the program."

HISTORICAL STANDARDS

The usual practice of administrators has been to set objectives for programs based on last year's performance in the same program, or on the temporal trend of outcomes in the program if it has gone on for a long period of time. This method applies most readily to outcome objectives that can be easily measured, such as birth rates, mortality rates, or attendance at clinics or other services where head counts are made routinely.

NORMATIVE STANDARDS

Setting objectives on the basis of what other such programs have achieved in similar communities, organizations, or populations applies a normative standard. Normative and historical standards can be readily constructed for program objectives and evaluation purposes when the object of interest is an outcome measured in routinely collected data such as vital events (births, marriages, deaths), hospital discharges, school attendance, communicable disease morbidity, ambient air quality, automobile crashes, and drug- or alcohol-related arrests. The most common standard for many community health promotion programs is the state average; and for many statewide health promotion programs, the national average.

COMPROMISE STANDARDS

Standards frequently emerge from a consensus process based on the informed opinions of experienced administrators, researchers, and practitioners and endorsement by recognized professional organizations or societies.[9]

CASE EXAMPLE: OBJECTIVES FOR THE NATION

Consider the U.S. *1990 Objectives for the Nation* in disease prevention and health promotion.[10] These objectives developed first as *scientific* standards based on extensive reviews of the literature carried out by federal government staff with the

TABLE 7.1

Summary of follow-up quit rates from 416 smoking cessation trials by method, 1959–1985

Intervention method	At least 6-month follow-up				At least 1-year follow-up			
	Number	Range	Median	Percentage ≤33%	Number	Range	Median	Percentage ≤33%
Self-help	11	0–33	17	18	7	12–33	18	14
Educational	7	13–50	36	71	12	15–55	25	25
Five-day plan	4	11–23	15	0	14	16–40	26	21
Group[a]	15	0–54	24	20	31	5–71	28	39
Medication	7	0–47	18	14	12	6–50	18.5	17
Nicotine chewing gum	3	17–33	23	33	9	8–38	11	11
Nicotine chewing gum and behavioral treatment or therapy	3	23–50	35	67	11	12–49	29	36
Hypnosis, individual	11	0–60	25	36	8	13–68	19.5	38
Hypnosis, group	10	8–68	34	50	2	14–88	–	50
Acupuncture	7	5–61	18	29	6	8–32	27	0
Physician advice or counseling	3	5–12	5	0	12	3–13	6	0
Physician intervention more than counseling	3	23–40	29	33	10	13–38	22.5	20

Physician intervention:							
Pulmonary patients	10	10–51	24	20	6	25–76	31.5	50
Cardiac patients	5	21–69	44	80	16	11–73	43	63
Risk factor	—	—	—	—	7	12–46	31	43
Rapid smoking	12	7–62	25.5	33	6	6–40	21	17
Rapid smoking and other procedures	21	8–67	38	57	10	7–52	30.5	50
Satiation smoking[b]	11	14–76	38	64	12	18–63	34.5	58
Regular-paced aversive smoking[b]	13	0–56	29	31	3	20–39	26	33
Nicotine fading[b]	7	26–46	27	29	16	7–46	25	44
Contingency contracting[b]	9	25–76	46	89	4	14–38	27	25
Multiple programs[b]	13	18–52	32	38	17	6–76	40	65

NOTE: Percentage ≤ 33% is percentage of trials with quit rates of at least 33%. Median not calculated for less than three trials. Caution: Quit rates provided suggest overall trends. Most quit rates were based on self-reports. Some quit rates were recalculated to include all subjects, but most quit rates were based on reports by investigators. Some quit rates omitted subjects who did not complete treatment or persons who did not reply to follow-ups. Definitions of follow-up may vary among trials.

[a] Three group trials had 5-month follow-ups.

[b] Other procedures may have been used, and some trials may be included in more than one method.

SOURCE: J. L. Schwartz, U.S. Dept. of Health and Human Services, National Institutes of Health, NIH Publication 87-2940 (Washington, DC: Government Printing Office, Apr. 1987), p. 130.

assistance of consultants. For many of the objectives, few formal evaluations could be generalized to the whole nation. *Historical* trends for some of these indicated a steady rise or a steady fall in the rates up through the late 1970s, which could be extrapolated or projected to estimate where we might be in 1990 if nothing were done to change the rate, and where the nation might be if we improved program performance. Some *normative* objectives could be set on the basis of what other western nations had accomplished, especially European countries whose infant mortality rates, for example, were generally better than those of the United States.[11]

These scientific, historical, and normative standards then were submitted to a group of experts at a national consensus conference that hammered out agreements on the most appropriate standards. The draft objectives for the nation were then distributed to several thousand organizations around the country for review and comment. The feedback from this process, finally, had to be reconciled back in the U.S. Office of Disease Prevention and Health Promotion. The final product was a set of 226 objectives reflecting some combination of scientific, historical, normative, and ultimately compromise standards of acceptability. A similar process has been followed in formulating the objectives for the nation in disease prevention and health promotion for the year 2000, with greater involvement of minority groups and state and local people at an earlier stage in the process. The structure and logical relationships of the 1990 objectives are shown in Figure 7.1.

Besides illustrating the various sources of standards of acceptability for objectives, the U.S. goal-setting experience brought home some other lessons concerning evaluation. One was that many goals had to be set in the absence of adequate data, because the most pressing problems for disease prevention and health promotion often were ones for which no data system was in place.[12] Program managers and practitioners must not be bullied by evaluators to limit the scope and objectives of their programs to those things that are measurable. This would trivialize most programs. Some of the more important and emergent problems, needs, and aspirations of a population will become measurable only when policy and programs give them enough attention to draw scientists and data collection agencies into the action arena. Within 5 years of the publication of the *1990 Objectives for the Nation*, most of the previously unmeasured objectives in health promotion had become covered by National Health Interview surveys.[13]

A second lesson learned in the 1990 objective-setting experience, later applied in the development of the *Year 2000 Objectives for the Nation*, was the need to tailor the objectives to special populations, particularly minorities, the elderly, and regional or local populations for whom the averages for the nation have the least relevance. Despite the best efforts to put the 1990 objectives through a consensus development process, the special populations still had to be consulted independently and their special needs addressed apart from the objectives and priorities for the majority.[14]

These lessons pertain equally to standards and objectives for local programs. Data will follow priorities. The statistics on minority populations, if they exist at

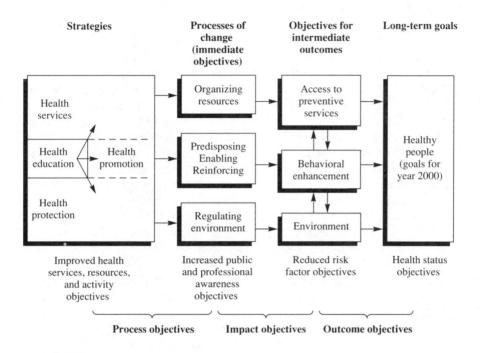

FIGURE 7.1

Approximate relationships among the objects of interest and the objectives for the nation in disease prevention and health promotion. [Adapted from L. W. Green, R. W. Wilson, and K. G. Bauer, *American Journal of Public Health* 73 (1983): 18–24, printed with permission of the publisher.]

all, simply get lost when the data are lumped with data on the majority; but it is often the needs of the minorities for health promotion that deserve the highest priority.

As emphasized throughout this book, participation is the linch-pin of effective programs. All participants and stakeholders in a program should have their views represented in the earliest planning activities, in establishing objectives, and in the implementation and evaluation of health promotion programs. Those views are essential to the collaborative dialogue needed if plausible, "acceptable" standards are to be set and respected.

CASE EXAMPLE: MODEL STANDARDS

The relationship of objectives to standards and the importance of collaborative input in establishing standards are vividly illustrated in *Model Standards: A Guide for Community Preventive Health Services*.[15] The Model Standards work was undertaken by collaborators from five organizations representing local, state, and national level public health interests: the American Public Health Association, the Association of State and Territorial Health Officials, the National Association of County Health Officials, the U.S. Conference of Local Health Officers, and the Centers for Disease Control of the U.S. Department of Health and Human Services. They hoped that the project would lead eventually to a norm wherein local-level health authorities use quantified measures of health and program processes to define program objectives and assess program impact. An evaluation of a state–local level negotiation process to implement the model standards in 18 local health agencies over a 2-year period in California concluded that "the use of Model Standards appeared to contribute to establishing program priorities, emphasizing the measurement of outcomes, improving the data management systems, and evaluating the current performance of programs."[16]

The standards, expressed either as program process or as risk-factor or health outcome objectives, were originally put forth as models for 34 prevention program areas. Tables 7.2 and 7.3 provide examples of the model standards for health education and chronic disease control, respectively. Note that the standards are expressed as either process or outcome objectives, an important distinction for program evaluation that will be discussed in detail later.

In establishing the model standards, the work group followed a flexible conceptual framework, a concept practitioners are well-advised to consider:

> ...standards must be significantly flexible to accommodate differences in the mix of preventable diseases and conditions facing communities...because of this variation in problems and service availability, it is neither useful or feasible to propose rigid, quantified national objectives for every community. Rather, a framework is presented that permits the quantification of objectives in every community irrespective of size, locale, nature of preventable problem, and present availability of preventive services.[17]

5 WHY IS EVALUATION SO THREATENING? OR WHY ME?

For some, the mere mention of the word *evaluation* brings discomfort. Perhaps it trumpets the possible detection of something gone awry or sounds a warning that scarce program resources may be diverted. Whatever triggers the anxiety, it can be considerably diminished by attending to a systematic planning process that precedes the implementation and evaluation of the program. Experienced evaluator Carol Weiss offers this insight:

> The sins of the program are often visited on the evaluation. When programs are well-conceptualized, and developed, with clearly defined and consistent methods of work, the lot of evaluation is relatively easy. But when programs are disorganized, beset with

TABLE 7.2

Examples of model standards for health education

Goal: Community residents will have the necessary knowledge, skills, capacity, and opportunity to improve and maintain individual, family, and community health; use preventive health services, practices, and facilities appropriately; understand and participate, where feasible, in decision making concerning their health care; understand and carry out prescribed medical instructions; and participate in community health decision making.

Focus	Process objectives	Indicators
Integration of health education services	**P-1**. By 19___ all community prevention programs will have an identifiable strategy for the use of health education, including at a minimum: a. Specification of population clusters with identifiable health problems or risks b. Assessment of behavior related to those problems c. Statement of educational objectives d. Educational methods to be employed with each target group e. Timelines for implementation f. Periodic evaluation of educational effectiveness Note: Health education programs to be effective must influence health practices in a positive direction, and the statement of educational objectives should be based on the cause-and-effect relationship between behaviors and health.	a. Existence and utilization of strategy b. Percentage of programs having identifiable strategy
Promotion of individual health maintenance	**P-2**. By 19___ the health education component of all community prevention programs will be conducted to provide the necessary knowledge, skills, and capacity to assure that individuals can do the following: a. Assume greater personal responsibility for improving and maintaining optimal health for themselves, their families, and their community: e.g., smoking cessation b. Use preventive services, practices, and facilities appropriately: e.g., well-baby care c. Participate in community health decision making d. Understand the nature of their work and the related health risks	a. Percentage of prevention programs in which (as relevant) there is an emphasis on increased individual responsibility for health b. Evidence of citizen participation in community health decision making c. Evidence of methods used for public education and information d. Documentation of individuals within the community participating in health promotion activities e. Existence of worker right-to-know legislation and programs

TABLE 7.3

Examples of model standards for chronic disease control

Goal: The community will experience a minimum of preventable illness, disability, and premature death; medical service utilization and attendant costs attributable to chronic diseases and conditions will be reduced.

Focus	Outcome objectives	Indicators
	O-1. By 19___ deaths due to _____ will be reduced to _____ among _____.	Cause-specific death rates
	O-2. By 19___ the prevalence of _____ will be reduced to _____ among _____. Note: Specific conditions or risk factors include the following: a. Smoking b. Uncontrolled hypertension c. Problem drinking d. Drinking and driving e. Nonuse of seat belts f. Poor nutrition: e.g., undernutrition and obesity g. Hypercholesterolemia h. Lack of physical fitness i. Occupational and environmental exposures	Prevalence of specific condition or risk factor
	O-3. By 19___ the incidence of _____ will be reduced to _____ among _____.	Incidence
	O-4. By 19___ preventable complications associated with _____ will be reduced to _____ among _____. Note: Specific chronic diseases or conditions include the following: a. Atherosclerotic, hypertensive, and other cardiovascular disease (e.g., coronary artery disease, rheumatic heart disease, stroke, myocardial infarction) b. Bone and joint disease (e.g., arthritis, osteoporosis) c. Cancer, specific sites (e.g., lung, breast, bladder, gastrointestinal tract, cervix, oral cavity) d. Chronic obstructive lung disease e. Cirrhosis f. Congenital anomalies g. Diabetes and other metabolic diseases h. Hearing impairment	a. Hospital admissions rate associated with specific preventable complication b. Hospital days of stay associated with specific preventable complication c. Disability days and restricted activity days associated with specific preventable complication d. Incidence or prevalence of specific preventable complication

disruptions, ineffectively designed, or poorly managed, the evaluation falls heir to the problems of the setting.[18]

The first antidote to evaluation anxiety, then, is good planning that precedes the evaluation. One of the benefits gained by working through the PRECEDE and PROCEED processes is that baseline data and objectives (or at least explicit assumptions about cause-and-effect relationships), so essential to carrying out a program evaluation, are built into the process. The care given to using valid and reliable measurement techniques in the diagnostic phases becomes valuable also for evaluation. A fully developed PRECEDE plan with social, health, behavioral, environmental, and educational objectives that are realistic, and with program activities and methods that are sound and targeted to those objectives, should lend itself easily to an evaluation that will detect the changes implicit in the objectives.

A second source of anxiety comes when evaluation places the program managers and practitioners in a posture of defensiveness, especially evaluations conducted by outsiders. This applies not only to social and health service workers but also to business evaluations.[19] Defensiveness can be overcome with greater integration of evaluation planning with program planning. Application of the diagnostic processes in PRECEDE helps practitioners cultivate an attitude and spirit of *inquiry*, a keystone principle for educational philosopher John Dewey.[20] Dewey's description of inquiry captures the essence of evaluation as an integral part of professional practice: an ongoing, self-corrective process through which we gradually gain a richer understanding of those things that shape our judgments. He felt that we must continually submit our judgments and claims to a "community of inquirers" because an effective democracy depends on a community of free and open-minded inquirers.

A third source of evaluation anxiety is the understanding that the program is too complex to be comprehended by evaluation and that the problems it seeks to change too complex to be affected by this program alone. Health promotion programs tend to grapple with problems that are at once biological and political, environmental and behavioral, individual and collective. Such complexity becomes even more difficult when geographic and population differences are taken into account. These circumstances demand that practitioners have the ability to make adjustments based on the differences inherent in the application of health promotion programs. The purpose of evaluation in health promotion must not be seen as finding the perfect program that can be packaged and parachuted into every community. The first purpose that evaluation should serve is to help improve and adapt the program to the circumstances at hand.

Health policy expert Mark Schlesinger emphasized the need for knowledge of local circumstances and for flexibility of programs to adapt to those circumstances when he cautioned decision makers to avoid the misperception that programs can be perfected prior to implementation and, once in place, left to run on automatic pilot.

Indeed, perhaps the most important legacy of the Great Society programs of the 1960s was not that they were ill-conceived, but that even relatively well-designed programs must be adapted to changing conditions and needs of their beneficiaries. For much of the two decades after their enactment, we allowed these programs to languish, and their effectiveness suffered as a result. In designing future programs, we must be sensitive to the need for flexibility and change based on program experience.[21]

Accountable practitioners actively share observations with others and understand that feedback from others generates information essential for program improvement. For them, part of the job is to ask questions: Is this program working toward achieving its objectives? Why is it working the way it is? How can we do it better, more efficiently, and perhaps at less cost? Or with less inconvenience to our clients? Evaluation that provides for this interactive, learning-oriented rather than judgment-oriented approach to new data not only will gain the support of practitioners but also will feed back more quickly and thoroughly into program improvements. This view approaches the "fourth-generation evaluation" described by Guba and Lincoln, where the first generation was measurement-oriented, the second description-oriented, and the third judgment-oriented.[22]

6 WHAT LEVEL OF OUTCOME IS APPROPRIATE AND SUFFICIENT TO INDICATE SUCCESS?

A health promotion program can be evaluated at one or more of three levels: process, impact, and outcome. The indicators and methodologies for detecting and comparing those indicators are different at each level (Figure 7.2). Note that we are using the term *impact* to refer to the immediate effect of a program or process and the term *outcome* to refer to the distant or ultimate effect. This usage conforms to established use in biomedical and health services research but is opposite to that in nonmedical fields of evaluation.

PROCESS EVALUATION

The first level is designated **process evaluation** because the information on the *process* of the program is the first to be available. The early detection of problems of implementation enables the program manager to make adjustments before the problems get out of hand. This is the time to experiment with methods, to "pilot" untried program components, and to debug new material for its readability, its cultural sensitivity, and its acceptability to the audience.[23]

Consider the following case. A rural cardiovascular prevention program had orchestrated multiple activities targeted at reducing selected risk factors for cardiovascular disease, including several related to hypertension. To take advan-

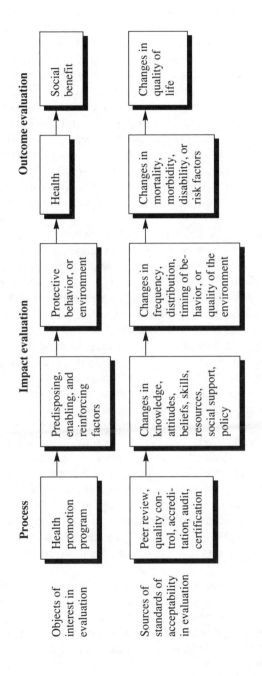

Process

Impact evaluation

Outcome evaluation

Objects of
interest in
evaluation

Health
promotion
program

Predisposing,
enabling, and
reinforcing
factors

Protective
behavior, or
environment

Health

Social
benefit

Sources of
standards of
acceptability
in evaluation

Peer review,
quality con-
trol, accredi-
tation, audit,
certification

Changes in
knowledge,
attitudes,
beliefs, skills,
resources,
social support,
policy

Changes in
frequency,
distribution,
timing of be-
havior, or
quality of the
environment

Changes in
mortality,
morbidity,
disability, or
risk factors

Changes in
quality of
life

FIGURE 7.2

Three levels of evaluation for accountability. [Adapted from L. W. Green and N. Gordon, *Health Education* 13 (1982): 4–10.]

tage of a national campaign effort, "May Is National Hypertension Month," special efforts were made to promote community participation in the various public information, screening, and counseling activities that accompanied the campaign. At a weekly program meeting early in May, intervention workers in the field reported that a sizable number of residents seemed to be interpreting the slogan to mean that May is the month you are at highest risk to get hypertension, just as January and February are the months you are mostly likely to come down with the flu![24] It is quite possible that persons with that perception might heed risk-reduction recommendations only in the month of May, mistakenly believing that such vigilance is unnecessary during the rest of the year.

In this example, staff were alerted to an unanticipated program effect by means of the weekly meetings designed to provide routine monitoring of the program processes. Had there been no commitment to review program process, the unanticipated reaction to the campaign could have led to behaviors directly opposite to those intended.

In process evaluation, the potential objects of interest include all program inputs, implementation activities, and stakeholder reactions. Inputs may include the policy or theoretical tenets of the program, the plausibility and specificity of program goals and objectives, and the resources (funds, personnel, space) allo-cated or expended. Implementation activities include staff performance, methods of data collection, regulatory and organizational activity, media that are distributed or broadcast, and events sponsored. Stakeholder reactions include the reviews of the program plans by boardmembers, focus group reactions of the intended recipients to the program materials, the level of participation among program recipients, and the response of collaborating organizations and the recipients to the program. The line between inputs and implementation is vague and, in the final analysis, probably unimportant for practical purposes.

The quality of the process can be determined by various methods: quan-titatively by periodic surveys, audits, and counts of services rendered; qualitatively by internal administrative surveillance of bookkeeping, contracts, and personnel, or by peer review, accreditation, certification, consumer reports; and other "external" or independent testing and observation.[25] The critical product from process evaluation is a clear, descriptive picture of the quality of the program elements being put in place and what is going on as the program proceeds. Numerous practical examples of innovative applications of process evaluation — also referred to as formative evaluation — can be found in the health promotion literature.[26]

Evaluation of implementation becomes all the more important when one is required to make a judgment about the program for possible exportation to other sites, or a judgment about the theory or policy upon which the program is based.[27] Such judgments usually must assume that the program has been implemented as prescribed by policy or theory and has reached the intended clients as designed. If that assumption is wrong — and it probably will be wrong, considering what was said earlier about the need for flexibility and adaptation of programs—then the evaluation will contain a Type III error.[28] The Type III error is a conclusion that the program is ineffective when in fact the program was never really implemented as designed. Process evaluation can help discern where the program's implementation has strayed from the policy, theory, or protocol, so that any generalization from the subsequent impact or outcome results can be interpreted in the light of known deviations from the intended program.

IMPACT EVALUATION

The second level, **impact evaluation**, assesses the immediate effect the program (or some aspect of it) has on target behaviors and their predisposing, enabling, and reinforcing antecedents, or on influential environmental factors.[29] The clarity, specificity, and plausibility of the behavioral and educational objectives generated in Phases 3 and 4 of the PRECEDE process provide the foundation for evaluating program impact.[30] A full-scale health promotion program should expect to find some impact on behavior, but components of the program, such as mass media, might not yield palpable behavioral impact if evaluated in isolation.[31]

OUTCOME EVALUATION

At the third level, **outcome evaluation**, the objects of interest are those health-status and quality-of-life indicators that were crafted in the earliest stages of the planning process. They are typically referenced in terms of mortality, disease, or disability rates for a given portion of the population. Social indicators—such as hunger, unemployment, homelessness, or elderly persons living independently— are often expressed as a percentage of the population. Examples of outcome evaluations where the PRECEDE model was applied can be found in recent published reports.[32]

The ability to detect changes in impact or outcome variables depends heavily on the specificity of the standards, the precision of their measurement, the size of the effect, and the size of the population or sample on which the measures are taken. These issues will be developed later in this chapter.

7 HOW MUCH PRECISION AND CONTROL DO YOU NEED?

In the PRECEDE process, you began by identifying a priority health or quality-of-life problem and then conduct a systematic search for the root causes holding the greatest promise of yielding social and health benefits, *assuming* that health promotion activities and resources can be mobilized and deployed to change those root causes. The justification for that assumption (that selected health promotion activities can have the desired effect) is usually based on a combination of the practitioner's vision and experience and the relevant findings from previously published studies. Impact and outcome evaluation studies should be considered when there is limited scientific evidence on the association between the desired outcome and the intervention selected.

The decision-making process in program planning and evaluation parallels the routine evaluations we make every day of our lives. When faced with a problem, we informally pose questions related to that problem, generate some options we might take to solve it, weigh the options, and act. The specific course of action we take frequently depends on the resources and time available and on the demands we feel for accountability to others for our actions.

Suppose you have an urgent need to haul some trash over a fair distance to a dump site. From among the following vehicles, you need to select one to haul the trash: a rental moving van, a small and sometimes unreliable pickup truck, a wheelbarrow, and a 1955 Corvette you are keeping for a friend. You can rule out the wheelbarrow because it's too small and the distance too far; and, assuming you want to keep your friend, you can rule out the use of the Corvette! That leaves the rental moving van and the small pickup truck. Although both will do the job, you note the van will be more efficient in that it can do the job in only one trip; you estimate three trips if you use the pickup. However, using the rental van will cost you more. Thus, the decision depends on factors like time and the availability of resources, as well as accountability to others.

The most pertinent question an evaluator can ask is, "What do I and other stakeholders need to know as a result of this evaluation?" The answer to that question enables the evaluator to determine, from the range of evaluation strategies available, which approaches are acceptable and which are not. Furthermore, among the approaches deemed acceptable, some are more appropriate than others, some more expensive, some more time-consuming, and some yield more data than necessary. One can err on the side of too little evaluation to satisfy the needs of stakeholders, and one can err on the side of wasting resources and time on unnecessary data and misplaced precision.

Consider two scenarios. In scenario A, a federal public health agency awards a sizable grant to a university with the intent of finding out whether a health promotion program consisting of a public education campaign and a physician education component leads to (1) an increase in the number of women who undergo mammographic screening, (2) an increase in the detection of early-stage breast cancer, and (3) a decrease over time in breast cancer mortality within the population exposed to the intervention.

In scenario B, a state or provincial health department makes some modest resources available to interested local health jurisdictions to determine if local health agencies could effectively implement some selected community-based primary prevention strategies that had been shown, through previous community trials, to be effective in delaying the onset of smoking in children ages 10–14.

The program planning process should be the same for both cases: the delineation of the health problem, the sound diagnoses of the salient behavioral and environmental factors and the probable precursors of those factors, the identification of specific program objectives at several levels, and the selection or development of intervention strategies targeted at those objectives. Even though the program planning activities will be quite similar, the evaluation questions posed in A and B are different, and tasks needed to carry out the respective evaluations will differ markedly in several ways.

WHEN OUTCOME IS THE FOCUS

In scenario A, among many possible process and impact evaluation questions that are likely to be posited, one outcome question is ultimate: Does exposure to this program result in reductions in breast cancer mortality? This is an evaluation *research* question. In Figure 7.3, it is question 3. The information needed to formulate an answer that can be given with confidence requires considerable effort.

Attributing changes in a population to a given program or program component requires evidence, or proof. The strength of that evidence depends on the evaluation methods used. The methods must be able to take into account the size of the sample studied, the validity and reliability of the measurements used, and the study design—that is, the method employed to control for the variety of factors that could be alternative explanations for those effects.

The selection of evaluation methods depends on a variety of complex factors and circumstances. Consider a few of the questions that the evaluation researcher must address:

What does the funding agency want?

Is the timeline realistic? How soon will impact or outcomes be measurable, relative to how soon they are expected?

How accessible is the population to be studied?

Will participants in the study be represented in the planning?

Is it possible or feasible to assign people randomly to the intervention to provide for an experimental study design? If not, what are the plausible alternatives?

What are the clearance and approval procedures for studies using human subjects?

Are standardized measurement instruments available to detect intermediate outcomes of interest or will new ones have to be developed and field tested?

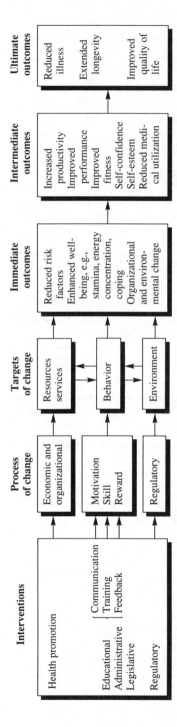

Primary question #2 (the usual program evaluation question): Do health promotion programs produce positive actions (behaviors, environmental changes, lifestyles)?

Do health promotion programs result in participants practicing presumably healthful lifestyles?

What are the elements of a successful program in each intervention area?

What environmental supports for behavior conducive to health are needed to supplement economic and educational effort to influence lifestyle?

Primary question #1 (the epidemiological question): Do actions (behavior, lifestyle) produce positive outcomes?

Do people with specific health practices and environmental conditions experience better health-related outcomes than other people?

Do people who practice presumably healthful lifestyles have lower health care costs than other people?

Do people who practice presumably healthful lifestyles have lower absenteeism or have higher productivity than other people?

Primary question #3 (the evaluation research question): Do people who change their behavior or lifestyle as a result of exposure to health promotion programs have positive outcomes compared with others?

Do people who modify their lifestyles through health promotion programs improve their health?

Do people who modify their lifestyles through health promotion programs reduce their health care costs?

Do people who modify their lifestyles through health promotion programs improve their productivity?

Do health promotion programs result in reduced health care costs and improved quality of life for individuals, social conditions for communities, or productivity for worksite programs? Will health promotion programs produce a positive return on investment for employers?

FIGURE 7.3

Approximate relationships among the objects of interest in evaluation of health promotion programs. [Adapted from L. W. Green, *American Journal of Health Promotion* 1(2) (1986): 70–2.]

What are the requirements for data collection (sample size, interviewing, record reviews, etc.), data analysis, and approvals (Institutional Review Boards and informed consent)?

Are the financial and staff resources adequate to carry out this study as intended?

It is impossible to contemplate these questions seriously without getting a feeling for the magnitude of effort demanded by such an undertaking. Without substantial technical and economic support, it is unrealistic and inappropriate to expect community programs, with modest resources and limited staff, to undertake such evaluation research tasks.

WHEN PROCESS IS THE FOCUS

In scenario B, a different question is raised. The state or provincial health department wants to determine if selected health promotion methods and protocols, previously demonstrated to be appropriate and effective in epidemiological, clinical, and evaluation research studies, could be implemented within the context of the routine services found in a local health department.

As in scenario A, one could generate a long list of interesting process and impact evaluation questions (see examples under primary question #2 in Figure 7.3) for the situation in case B. For example, *impact* evaluation might ask whether the intended school-aged population was being reached and, if they were, could the desired impact on their motivation or behavior be detected? A *process* evaluation might seek to identify characteristics that tend to differentiate teachers who faithfully employ the recommended methods from those who do not. A process variable that researchers increasingly include in program evaluations is the extent to which a practitioner applies a method as it has been previously applied and found effective in controlled studies.

The practitioners' "fidelity" to educational protocols and methods has been shown to be a variable accounting for differences in impact in several studies of health education.[33] Although fidelity *may* be important, program directors and practitioners need to be wary of demanding it too slavishly and interpreting it too literally. Striving to deliver the methods and protocols of the program *exactly* as prescribed in conclusions drawn from a model research project results in perfunctory practice.[34] The assumption that previous research on a given population, in a specific place and time, under the direction of research investigators, can justify the precise intervention that should be implemented in all populations and situations reduces the professional practitioner of health promotion to a technician, or worse, to a programmed automaton. Armed with diagnostic planning skills and the theoretical knowledge to interpret *why* a given method was effective, the inquiring practitioner will have the competence and confidence needed to make the procedural *adaptations* required with each new population or situation.

To answer process evaluation questions, as with other levels of evaluation, "objects of interest" must be compared against "standards of acceptability." Relevant objects of interest might include qualifications of staff, intensity and duration of instruction, access to and appropriateness of facilities, channels of communication, cultural sensitivity of instructional materials, the extent to which family and peer involvement is encouraged, the number of inspections made to enforce a nonsmoking regulation, and competence in applying appropriate community organization methods. The attainment of "standards of acceptability" could be assessed by the combined application of quantitative and qualitative methods.

Quantitative methods might include a record of the number and duration of the sessions conducted, the number of school-aged children reached, and a record of the times that mass-media messages were delivered and the type of message. Included among qualitative methods might be a description of the professional preparation, experience, and general qualifications of teachers and program staff who interact with program participants; reactions to the program by recipients, ascertained either by observation or by self-report; and observation of the program delivery.[35] Examples of qualitative and quantitative standards of acceptability for prevention programs for sexually transmitted disease (STD) are shown in Figure 7.4 at each of the three levels and for various target populations.

The complexities of sampling and research design demanded in scenario A do not apply in B, but the professional commitment to *rigor* does. Both approaches require attention to details, consistency and care in documentation, and objectivity in analysis and reporting. One reason for the poor reception of qualitative and process evaluation results is that they too often have been collected or reported with less rigor and objectivity than quantitative data, which are harder to mask with cosmetic prose.

8 WHAT DO EVALUATION DESIGNS ENABLE US TO DO?

Within the context of our earlier definition of evaluation, one can think of the design as the framework the evaluator uses to answer research questions and to provide a basis for comparing the object of interest against a standard of acceptability. Comparisons can be over time or between groups, or both.

An important purpose in selecting a study design is to reduce the possibility of errors in the interpretation of the results by maximizing the reliability and validity of the information collected in the evaluation. A measurement that is *reliable* is one that is consistent and stable; if you apply it once, and then repeat it a second time, or another interviewer or observer applies it the second time, the results will be the same (assuming that little happened between the two data points to alter the response). A measurement is *valid* when it yields an accurate or true measure of what it is supposed to measure; because of that, valid measures are also reliable.

Health Promotion's Target Population	Process Objectives and Measurements	Impact Objectives and Measures	Outcome Objectives and Measures
Adolescent students	Provision of accurate education about STDs to all junior and senior high school students by 1990 (nat.); Implementation of school based STD education programs for all junior and senior high school-aged students in the school district (local).	What percentage of students are able to recognize STDs, know how to protect against infection, and express intentions to use preventive measures.	Improve health status: By 2000, reported gonorrhea incidence should be reduced to a rate of 280 cases per 100,000.
High risk groups in the community	Identification of and establishment of contact with all high risk groups (e.g., gays, adolescents) in the community through hotlines and other outreach programs.	Increase in self-referrals and referral of sexual contacts for STD screening and treatment at an earlier stage; increase in general knowledge and practice of behaviors that decrease risk of STD contact.	By 2000, reported incidence of pelvic inflammatory disease should be reduced to a rate of 60 cases per 100,000 women.
General knowledge: subgroups within total populations	Provision of government funds and assistance for demonstration projects of community based STD prevention.	Data on what types of STD education approaches are most effective for particular organizational settings.	By 2000, reported incidence of primary and secondary syphilis should be reduced to a rate of 7 cases per 100,000 population per year, with a reduction in congenital syphilis to 1.5 cases per 100,000 children less than 1 year of age.
Health care professionals	Completion of the development and distribution, and assistance in the implementation, of the Quality Assurance Guidelines for STD Clinical Care; Provision of statewide continuing education workshops for health care professionals on how to identify high-risk individuals and how to educate patients for STD prevention (local).	By 1985, at least 95% of health care providers seeing suspected cases of STD should be capable of diagnosing and treating all recognized STDs. Increase in early referrals among private patients; increase in knowledge of STD prevention measures.	

FIGURE 7.4

Illustration of process, impact, and outcome evaluation levels to assess the effects of STD educational efforts. [Adapted from L. W. Green and N. Gordon, *Health Education* 13 (May/June 1982): 4–10.]

The following scene takes place in 1990: You ask a person her age and she responds, "30." Two weeks later you ask what her date of birth is and she replies, "June 1, 1960," which confirms her self-reported age. These two reports are consistent over time and may be correctly judged to be reliable. If later you discover that her birth certificate indicates that the actual date of birth was June 1, 1958, you know that the reliable verbal reports were not valid.

Practitioners will benefit by cultivating a working knowledge of this notion of validity because, among other things, it is of paramount importance in choosing among research designs. Consider this conversation between a program manager (PM), who coordinates a worksite health promotion program for a company called New Directions, and the chief executive officer (CEO) of the company.

CEO: My advisors have read the health promotion evaluation report. Good work.

PM: Thank you.

CEO: What do you consider the most important findings?

PM: We think there are two: (1) 24 percent of the those who signed up for the smoking cessation program are still not smoking after 2 months; and (2) of the 900 employees in the company, 250 turned out for at least one of the physical activity programs. Of those, 125 (50 percent) remain involved in regular aerobic activities.

CEO: Those are impressive findings. I'd like to consider implementing the program in the four regional offices of New Directions. However, the senior management staff has raised two questions that I can't answer; I hope you can. First, how do we know that the smoking cessation rates and the increases in physical activity are not the result of recent national campaigns and extensive local news reports? And second, if the evidence does show that our programs really do account for the differences noted, how do we know those programs will work in our various regional offices?

In the technical parlance of evaluation research, the CEO's staff was concerned about two, very basic "threats to validity." By wondering if other events (national campaigns and news reports) might explain the outcomes reported, they were questioning the **internal validity** of the claim that the positive changes in smoking and physical activity really were attributable to the program. The concern over whether similar results could be expected if the program is implemented in other New Directions sites raised the question of **external validity**. That is, how generalizable is the program? How confident can the CEO be about achieving similar results in the other regions?

The sections that follow give brief descriptions of six evaluation designs, ranging from the simple but often neglected collection of routine data on an ongoing basis to the collection of data in highly rigorous, highly controlled experimental settings. At the two extremes are the historical record-keeping approach, which is the least complex and is applicable to most programs, and the controlled experimental approach, which is usually impractical for most programs. Each has its own utility. Practitioners make their selections based on the evaluation questions and the data required to answer those questions. All designs can be implemented in two or three steps.

DESIGN A: THE HISTORICAL RECORD-KEEPING APPROACH

The record-keeping approach is the minimum that should be expected of any professional health promotion practitioner at any time. It yields tables, charts, or graphs that provide an ongoing account of what is occurring in a program. The procedure is manageable even under the most adverse operational circumstances. For example, it may be sufficient merely to count the number of people served each day and then add the daily figures to tabulate or chart the weekly, monthly, or yearly trends.

The first step is to construct a dummy graph showing the expected relationship between inputs and outcomes. The second step is to set up a record-keeping procedure to accumulate the data. The last step is to calculate and chart the data periodically, plotting the direction and magnitude of change taking place over time. How often should one tabulate and chart the data? That depends on the number of times the events being tabulated occur and how often you need to report trends to your stakeholders. An example of a design-A graph is given in Figure 7.5.

This figure demonstrates the sequential benefits of different educational and policy changes during three phases of a program conducted by a clinic for sexually transmitted diseases (STD) over a 2-year-plus period. The impact of each educational strategy can be noted in changes both in the absolute number of patients appearing at the clinic and in the composition of the patient population. The change in interviewing policy (C) was a change from asking patients to identify their sexual contacts to encouraging them to take the responsibility for seeing that their sexual partners received treatment. The behavioral impact in terms of the male/female ratio of patients at this point was most notable.[36] The ratios (looked at in combination with the graph) show increases in females and whites using the clinic until the numbers were closer to equal. Other examples of this simplest of designs for evaluation are listed in the bibliography.[37]

A similar evaluation of a venereal disease hotline in New Jersey permitted a cost-benefit analysis of the program. Records were kept of the number of calls handled by hotline operators during 1 year (process) and the number of clinic and emergency room visits for STD screening and treatment for 6 months following start of hotline operation (impact). Results showed that emergency room and clinic visits for STD care were 53 percent greater during the period when the hotline was operating than during the same time period of the year before the hotline's

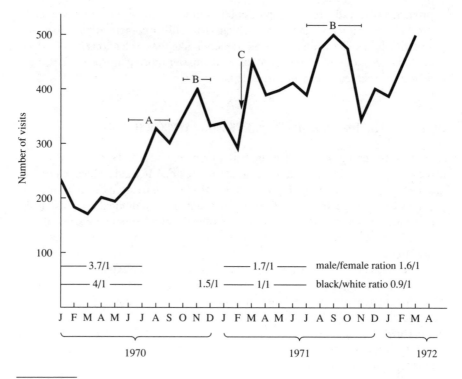

FIGURE 7.5

Example of design-A graph: Visits to a clinic. A, street groups contacted; B, radio announcements made; C, interviewing policy changed. [Adapted from John B. Atwater, *American Journal of Public Health* 64 (May, 1974): 433–7; printed with permission of American Public Health Association.]

existence. The cost per call in operating the hotline was calculated (process measure). Unfortunately, the cost-benefit evaluation was hampered by an absence of information about financial and person-power outlays for hotline publicity by the medical center, and by poor data on additional cost that resulted from the clinic and emergency room handling of STD patients.[38] This case illustrates the importance of building interagency cooperation for coordinated record-keeping into an evaluation plan to assure the availability of data needed.

DESIGN B: THE PERIODIC INVENTORY APPROACH

The inventory approach requires making a special effort periodically (rather than continuously) to collect data. Sometimes the prevailing record-keeping system does not incorporate the data required, and changing the system, perhaps expanding it, would be too disruptive to the service program. Rather than accumulating the data on an ongoing basis, as with design A, one can obtain the data by conducting special surveys.

The evaluator first sets target dates for the assessments and then identifies the expected target levels. Finally, the evaluator takes the surveys as a way of estimating the levels achieved at the selected points in time. Literature providing examples of the inventory approach is listed in the chapter notes.[39]

Comparisons in this design are "historical" in the sense that success is defined in relation to a prior period of performance in the same program or population. Often called the before-and-after design or the pre-posttest design, this *historical time-series* approach can be much more than just two measures, one taken before the start and one after the completion of the program. It is frequently used to take tests of knowledge gain or of attitude and behavior changes during a program in school and clinical settings.[40]

A variation on the continuous, uninterrupted program data marking approach is the *interrupted time-series* design. In this variation, the program is systematically stopped and started to see whether the impact or outcome measures (records or interviews) show corresponding changes. Figure 7.6 illustrates this method from a Dutch clinic, where the impact of advertising the existence of a VD hotline service was measured using a simple count of the number of calls per week relative to the starting and stopping of advertising.[41]

For some kinds of programs, such as smoking cessation programs, the critical points for measuring behavior are highly standardized.[42] Reviews of the literature reveal the times at which people are likeliest to drop out or relapse in programs dealing with such problems as smoking, hypertension treatment, antibiotic therapy, and oral contraceptive use.[43]

DESIGN C: THE COMPARATIVE HOW-WE-STACK-UP-AGAINST-OTHERS APPROACH

Evaluation by means of the comparative approach is an extension of the inventory or record-keeping design. The same procedures are followed, except that data from sources external to the program are obtained for comparison. One can usually identify similar data on programs in other places; borrow or copy the record forms used in these programs or buy into a common, standardized format for collecting such data; and do periodic comparisons between the programs on the same basis as design A or design B.

Various kinds of state or national data can be used for comparison. For example, the National Health Discharge Survey provides data derived from standardized questionnaires that can be compared with data collected in local programs. National norms suggest what health educators can expect in relation to breast examination, Pap smears, smoking cessation, and other health behaviors.[44] Comparability is an essential feature of cumulative evaluation. For this reason, it is better to use standardized formats for collecting data than to develop original questionnaires except where your data requirements are unique. Examples of the comparative or normative approach can be found in the literature.[45]

DESIGN D: THE CONTROLLED-COMPARISON QUASI-EXPERIMENTAL APPROACH

In the controlled-comparison approach, an evaluator first identifies a community or population similar demographically to the target population, but one *not* receiving the intervention program. The evaluator then applies design A or B in the intervention *and* comparison populations, and periodically collects relevant data to enable comparisons. One might want to compare the effects of various kinds of interventions in similar populations — in schools, for example, or in communities.

The community studies of Stanford, Minnesota, North Karelia, Texas, and Kentucky and Wales are the most notable contemporary examples of the latter application.[46] At Stanford, for example, the original three communities studied in the cardiovascular risk-reduction project included one in which an intensive educational effort had been made, another in which only a mass media effort was

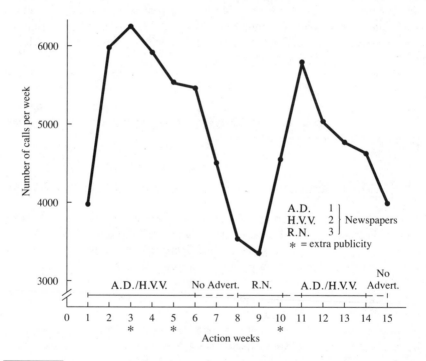

FIGURE 7.6

Illustration of the interrupted time-series design. [From J. Schuurmann and W. de Haes, *International Journal of Health Education* 23 (1980): 94–106.]

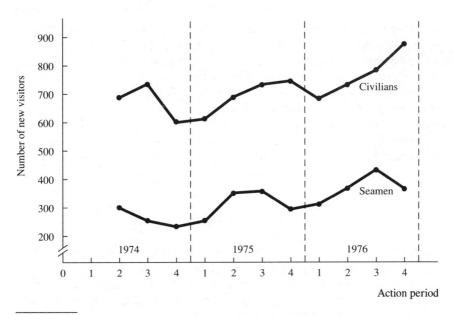

FIGURE 7.7

Illustrations of the controlled-comparison, quasi-experimental approach to evaluation in a Dutch seaport where civilians were exposed to media recruitment efforts of an STD clinic in 1975. [Adapted from J. Schuurman and W. de Haes, *International Journal of Health Education* 19 (1980): 94–106.]

made, and another in which neither effort was made, although there were comparable resources and facilities. The effectiveness of the strategies used in each of the three experimental communities and their various subpopulations was compared using impact and outcome data from surveys. Other examples of this approach can be found in the literature.[47]

The Rotterdam evaluation of the STD media/hotline campaign compared trends in new visits to the STD clinic during the intervention for civilians with those of seamen who were not likely to have been exposed to the campaigns and were thus a "control" group (see Fig. 7.7).[48] This example points out the importance of controlling for seasonal fluctuations or possible changes in the demographics of the population sampled when analyzing patterns of incidence and prevalence over long time periods.

DESIGN E: THE CONTROLLED-EXPERIMENTAL APPROACH

The controlled-experimental approach is comparable to the clinical trial in medical studies. It requires a formal procedure for random assignment of individuals within the target population to two (and sometimes more) groups. If there are two, one group receives the program (experimental group) and one does not (control group). Note that in this approach it must be possible and ethical to deny certain people the treatment. The control group typically receives "usual treatment" rather than nothing. Once the groups are set up but before the program is underway, the evaluator applies design A or B for both the experimental and the control groups. Often, baseline data are collected on all groups, but this is not essential. It depends on the kinds of change one hopes to detect. Records, observations, or survey data over time are then graphed to see how the groups compare at various points in the treatment.[49] Smoking cessation and weight control programs are often evaluated according to design E.

DESIGN F: THE EVALUATIVE RESEARCH PROJECT

The most complex of the evaluation designs, what might be described as a full-scale evaluative research project, is unlikely to be feasible in most community programs. Procedures are similar to those for design E, the controlled-experimental approach, except that multiple groups are randomized in factorial designs, and multiple measures are obtained on intermediate variables such as changes in knowledge, attitudes, and skills as well as on outcomes and impact variables such as behavior and health. Group tendencies are compared as are intragroup effects. The design can accommodate numerous refinements. For example, it can be used to detect the independent effects of the *components* of a program on selected impact and outcome variables. The program components in question have to be well-defined and the sample has to be large enough to enable the detection of changes in randomized subgroups that were systematically exposed to the program components independently and in combination.[50]

Such a design was used to demonstrate how the application of the PRECEDE model could produce changes not only in behavior but also in the mortality rates of low-income, urban black patients with high blood pressure.[51] This project provided much of the data on which the PRECEDE model was first tested formally. Experimental evaluation research studies of this nature are needed to continue to advance the knowledge base of health education and health promotion. However, because they require the application of complex, costly research designs, they are inappropriate undertakings for most community programs where the mission is service delivery.

Somewhere between the simplicity of design A, with its inconclusive but suggestive findings, and the expense and complexity of design F, is a level of evaluation with the appropriate degree of feasibility, practicability, and rigor. The trouble with the more complicated designs is that they usually have to be carried out under highly controlled conditions, which makes the behavioral circumstances unusual or unnatural.[52] Often it is necessary to remove people from their social milieu, the ordinary context for their behavior. It is seldom easy to find willing

participants for controlled, randomized experiments. Further, such designs require informed consent for those in the control group as well as those in the
experimental group. This usually requires health education for both groups, which
means the control group is not truly without a planned intervention.

In short, what one gains in internal validity through the more rigorous
randomized procedures one may sacrifice in feasibility and in generalizability of
findings. Can findings from highly controlled classroom, clinical, or community
trials be generalized to private practice and community-based programs?[53] Certainly one obvious factor is the extent to which the population or community
exposed to the program is like the one in the study; the closer the match, the
greater the likelihood of a generalizable effect. However, the most powerful
predictor of success in replicating the result is the ability of the practitioner(s) to
make the program adjustments and refinements required as a function of the
unique needs of their own target population. Thus, even when interventions have
been found effective in rigorously controlled studies, the practitioner considering
their use in a new population or situation still needs PRECEDE or some similar
assessment of needs and determinants to make the appropriate adjustment in the
interventions.

9 HOW MUCH IS ENOUGH?

Even with the best intentions, the processes of evaluation can be disruptive. And
no element of evaluation has more potential for disruption than the burden, real or
perceived, that accompanies the collection of data. Program participants, nonpar-
ticipants, and staff may resent being asked or required to complete questionnaires
(in person or by telephone); program and clerical staff are frequently asked to
carry an increased workload; some may interpret the costs of collecting *and*
coding as a drain on scarce resources that could have gone to the program; and staff
may perceive that the only beneficiary of the evaluation will be those academic
professors and doctoral students who secure their promotion, tenure, or degrees as
a result of the publications generated by the data collected by the program staff.

These problems cannot be completely eliminated; they emerge, more or less,
even under the best of circumstances. However, evaluators can minimize the
potential for disruption by developing, with input from program staff and key
stakeholders, a strategic plan for the evaluation. The following are key elements to
consider in developing that plan:

1. If possible, designate a staff member with responsibility for
   coordination of data collection.
2. Based on the measurable objectives delineated in the first four phases of
   the PRECEDE planning process, specify

TABLE 7.4

Example of a dummy table: Baseline smoking status compared with smoking status at year 1

Baseline smoking status	Year 1 smoking status		
	Never smoked	Former smoker	Current smoker
Never smoked			
Former smoker			
Current smoker			

(a) the hypotheses, derived from the objectives;

(b) a list of objects of interest representing independent variables or intervention strategies, methods, or materials;

(c) a list of objects of interest representing the dependent variables (anticipated impact or outcomes).

3. Construct several dummy tables or charts to help you visualize how the data may be organized and eventually summarized. Table 7.4 gives an example of a dummy table. Insert hypothetical numbers, percentages, or rates reflecting the standards of acceptability.

4. Make a list of the information you need.

5. Develop a timeline or work schedule for the remaining steps in the planning and execution of the evaluation, such as that shown in Figure 7.8.

6. Identify the data collection techniques that are appropriate and feasible for the information you need.

7. Identify: (a) the sources of existing data that may be used; (b) the existing data gathering instruments; and (c) the instruments that need to be developed.

8. Establish a data collection plan, including details on what data will be collected when and by whom.

9. Develop a plan for the reporting phase, including formal presentations of results, a final report, publication of papers and general dissemination plan.

Evaluators must be able to find the appropriate middle ground between undesirable extremes: falling prey to the temptation of data collection "over-kill" at one extreme and choosing methods and measures of minimal burden that provide useless information at the other. As usual, the best advice is to use common sense: Keep focused on the purposes and the audiences or stakeholders of the evaluation. Consider items 6 and 7 in the evaluation plan just described. Suppose you have completed the planning process and are ready to implement a community-based

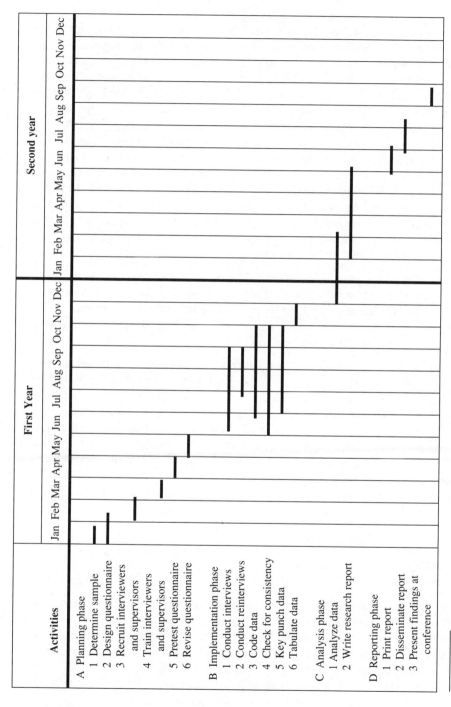

FIGURE 7.8

Example of a planning timeline.

health promotion program. Based on the epidemiological, behavioral, environmental, and educational diagnoses and the growing scientific evidence of its multiple health benefits, physical activity[54] is the intervention centerpiece of the program. Among other things, you want to determine whether, as a result of their exposure to the program, the participants increase their level of regular physical activity. You have selected a randomized control design that minimizes threats to internal validity, but you are uncertain how to measure potential changes in levels of physical activity. As you revisit the literature, you discover that physical activity has been measured by a wide range of questionnaires, which vary considerably in length and focus. Furthermore, you also learn that the scientists do not agree on which measures are the best.[55] Table 7.5 presents summary descriptions of 10 national probability surveys of physical activity. Under the column titled "Concept(s) of activity," note the diversity of focus and the implicit complexity of what is measured. For example, in the two National Health and Nutrition Examination Surveys (NHANES I and II), numbers 3 and 4, respectively, in Table 7.5, physical activity was measured by these two questions:

1. Do you get much exercise in things you do for recreation (sports, or biking, or anything like that), or hardly any exercise, or in between?
   (a) Much exercise (b) Moderate exercise (c) Little or no exercise
2. In your usual day, aside from recreation, are you physically very active, moderately active, or quite inactive?

Compare these with the questions presented in Table 7.6, which represent a *portion* of the questions taken from the Health Promotion/Disease Prevention Supplement to the National Health Interview Survey. If you choose to use these questions, you know that the data they generate will yield useful epidemiologic information about the frequency, intensity, and duration of activity. At the same time, you will recognize that such rich information requires resources that are often substantial and almost always underestimated. The evaluator's decision hinges on the response to two questions: (1) Precisely what is it we want to measure? (2) What measures are feasible given our capacities, time, and resources?

SUMMARY

This chapter highlights concepts and approaches to evaluation having particular utility for the health promotion practitioner. Program evaluation defines "the comparison of an object of interest against a standard of acceptability." The case has been made that professional commitment to accountability is best served by an inquiring practitioner who approaches the planning and implementation of each health promotion program as an experiment. The PRECEDE–PROCEED model produces a series of hypotheses about presumed relationships between interventions and outcomes. Evaluation provides the "test" of those hypotheses.

In the absence of a planned evaluation design that facilitates the collection and analysis of valid information, the processes and effects of a program are likely to go undetected. If accidentally detected, they tend to be over- or understated. Descriptions and examples of process, impact, and outcome levels of evaluation were presented, with emphasis on their practical application for the practitioner in the field. Several designs for evaluation were described in simple steps with examples listed in the reference notes for each design. By concluding the PRECEDE–PROCEED process with the results of an evaluation, the practitioners, program managers, and policy-makers are prepared to approach the next population or health problem armed with a better understanding of health promotion needs and effective ways to address them.

EXERCISES

1. Retrieve your program objective from Chapter 3, your behavioral and environmental objectives from Chapter 4, and three educational objectives from Chapter 5. For *each* objective, identify *two* different "standards of acceptability"; explain the strengths and weakness of each standard.
2. Using the circumstances described in the smoking and physical activity program offered at the company called New Directions (see section on evaluation designs), explain how you would answer the two questions posed by the CEO if you had employed (a) Design A, (b) Design C, (c) Design D.
3. Propose an evaluation plan for your program, indicating the data to be collected, the procedures for collection, and the comparisons you intend to make. Use charts or graphs with hypothetical data. As a part of the plan, include *two* design options, one that you would apply if research support is reasonable and the other if the resources are minimal.

TABLE 7.5

Selected national probability sample surveys assessing physical activity

Survey, date	Ages, sample size	Data collection methods	Agency doing fieldwork	Concept(s) of activity
1. Gallup, 1961 (May)	18+, 1,049 (1984)	Telephone interview	The Gallup Poll	Daily activity to keep fit
2. National Recreation Survey, 1965 (Sept–Oct)	12+, 7,194	80% face-to-face interview	Bureau of the Census	Participation in selected activities, last 12 months or last 3 months
1982–1983 (quarterly)	12+, 5,757	20% telephone interview (1982–1983)		
3. National Health and Nutrition Examination Survey I, 1972–1975	18–74, 13,628	Face-to-face interview	National Center for Health Statistics	"Much" activity, "little/no" activity
4. National Health Interview Supplement, 1975 (July–Dec)	20+, 11,741	Face-to-face interview	Bureau of the Census	Participation in 7 exercises and 15 sports
5. Perrier, 1978 (March)	18+, 1,510	Face-to-face interview	Louis Harris & Associates	Kilocalories calculated from frequency and intensity of 38 activities

6. General Mills, 1978 (month?)	18+, 1,254	Face-to-face interview	Yankelovich, Skelly & White, Inc.	Self-assessed change in activity, last 12 months
7. National Health and Nutrition Examination Survey II, 1976–1980	25–74, 8,615	Face-to-face interview (Behavior Questionnaire)	National Center for Health Statistics	"Much" activity, "little/no" activity
8. National Survey of Personal Health Practices and Consequences 1979 (spring) 1980 (spring)	20–64, 3,025 / 20–64, 2,453	Telephone interview	Chilton Research Services, Inc.	Never participate in any of 7 popular activities; self-assessed change in activity, last 24 months (1979) and last 12 months (1980)
9. Behavioral Risk Factor Surveys, 1981–1983	18+, 20,664	Telephone interview	State Health Departments	Kilocalories calculated from frequency, intensity, duration of most important activity
10. National Health Interview Survey Supplement, 1985 (Jan–Dec)	18+, 33,630	Face-to-face interview	Bureau of the Census	Kilocalories calculated from frequency, intensity, duration of 23 popular activities

SOURCE: T. Stephens, *Research Quarterly for Exercise and Sport* 58 (1987): p. 95.

TABLE 7.6

A segment of physical activity in the Health Promotion/Disease Prevention Supplement to the 1985 National Health Interview Survey

	b. How many times in the past 2 weeks did you [play/go/do] (activity in 2a)?	c. On the average, about how many minutes did you actually spend (activity in 2a) on each occasion?	d. (What usually happened to your heart rate or breathing when you (activity in 2a)? Did you have a small, moderate, or large increase, or no increase at all in your heart rate or breathing?
NOTE — ASK ALL OF 2a BEFORE GOING TO 2b–d.	NOTE: ASK 2b–d FOR EACH ACTIVITY MARKED "YES" IN 2a.		
Read to respondent: **These next questions are about physical exercise.** Hand calendar.			
2a. In the past 2 weeks (outlined on that calendar, beginning Monday, (date), and ending this past Sunday, (date), have you done any [of the following exercises, sports, or physically active hobbies) — [ ] 7			
YES NO			
(1) **Walking for exercise?** 1 [ ] 2 [ ]			
R2 Refer to age. 1 [ ] SP is 75 + (23) 14 / 8 [ ] Other (2)	(1) _____ Times 8–9	_____ Minutes 10–12	1 [ ] Small 3 [ ] Large / 2 [ ] Moderate 4 [ ] None 13
(2) **Jogging or running?** 1 [ ] 2 [ ] 15	(2) _____ Times 16–17	_____ Minutes 18–20	1 [ ] Small 3 [ ] Large / 2 [ ] Moderate 4 [ ] None 21
(3) **Hiking?** 1 [ ] 2 [ ] 22	(3) _____ Times 23–24	_____ Minutes 25–27	1 [ ] Small 3 [ ] Large / 2 [ ] Moderate 4 [ ] None 28
(4) **Gardening or yard work?** 1 [ ] 2 [ ] 29	(4) _____ Times 30–31	_____ Minutes 32–34	1 [ ] Small 3 [ ] Large / 2 [ ] Moderate 4 [ ] None 35
(5) **Aerobics or aerobic dancing?** 1 [ ] 2 [ ] 36	(5) _____ Times 37–38	_____ Minutes 39–41	1 [ ] Small 3 [ ] Large / 2 [ ] Moderate 4 [ ] None 42
(6) **Other dancing?** 1 [ ] 2 [ ] 43	(6) _____ Times 44–45	_____ Minutes 46–48	1 [ ] Small 3 [ ] Large / 2 [ ] Moderate 4 [ ] None 49
(7) **Calisthenics or general exercise?** 1 [ ] 2 [ ] 50	(7) _____ Times 51–52	_____ Minutes 53–55	1 [ ] Small 3 [ ] Large / 2 [ ] Moderate 4 [ ] None 56
(8) **Golf?** 1 [ ] 2 [ ] 57	(8) _____ Times 58–59	_____ Minutes 60–62	1 [ ] Small 3 [ ] Large / 2 [ ] Moderate 4 [ ] None 63
(9) **Tennis?** 1 [ ] 2 [ ] 64	(9) _____ Times 65–66	_____ Minutes 67–69	1 [ ] Small 3 [ ] Large / 2 [ ] Moderate 4 [ ] None 70
(10) **Bowling?** 1 [ ] 2 [ ] 71	(10) _____ Times 72–73	_____ Minutes 74–76	1 [ ] Small 3 [ ] Large / 2 [ ] Moderate 4 [ ] None 77
(11) **Biking?** 1 [ ] 2 [ ] 78	(11) _____ Times 79–80	_____ Minutes 81–83	1 [ ] Small 3 [ ] Large / 2 [ ] Moderate 4 [ ] None 84
(12) **Swimming or water exercises?** 1 [ ] 2 [ ] 85	(12) _____ Times 86–87	_____ Minutes 88–90	1 [ ] Small 3 [ ] Large / 2 [ ] Moderate 4 [ ] None 91
92	93–94	95–97	Small 98

REFERENCES AND NOTES

1. Detailed discussions on specific problems and examples of health promotion evaluations may be found in many of the publications cited in other chapters and elsewhere in this chapter. More general overviews of evaluation issues and techniques in health promotion can be found in the following publications: T. Abelin, Z. J. Brzezinski, and V. D. Carstairs, eds., *Measurement in Health Promotion and Protection* (Copenhagen: World Health Organization Regional Publications, European Series No. 22, 1987); M. T. Braverman, ed., *Health Promotion Programs* (San Francisco: Jossey-Bass, 1989); M. B. Dignan, *Measurement and Evaluation of Health Education* (Springfield, IL: Charles C. Thomas, 1986); A. Fisher, J. Laign, and J. Stoeckel, *Handbook for Family Planning Research Design* (New York: Population Council, 1983); B. R. Flay, "Efficacy and Effectiveness Trials in the Development of Health Promotion Programs," *Preventive Medicine* 15 (1986): 451–74; L. W. Green and F. M. Lewis, *Measurement and Evaluation in Health Education and Health Promotion* (Palo Alto, CA: Mayfield, 1986); S. B. Kar, ed., *Health Promotion Indicators and Actions* (New York: Springer Publishing Co., 1989); R. McCuan and L. W. Green, "Multivariate Statistical Methods for Evaluation of Health Education and Health Promotion Programs," in *Advances in Health Education and Promotion* vol. 3, W. Ward and F. M. Lewis, eds. (London: Jessica Kingsley, in press); D. Nutbeam, C. Smith, and J. Catford, "Evaluation in Health Education: A Review of Possibilities and Problems," *Journal of Epidemiology and Community Health* 44 (1990): 83–9; E. H. Wagner and P. A. Guild, "Primer on Evaluation Methods: Choosing an Evaluation Strategy," *American Journal of Health Promotion* 4 (1989): 134–9; R. A. Windsor, T. Baranowski, N. Clark, and G. Cutter, *Evaluation of Health Promotion and Education Programs* (Palo Alto, CA: Mayfield, 1984).

2. M. C. Alkin, R. Daillak, and P. White, *Using Evaluations: Does Evaluation Make a Difference?* (Beverly Hills: Sage Library of Social Research, vol. 76, 1979).

3. A. S. Bryk, ed., *Stakeholder-Based Evaluation* (San Francisco, Jossey-Bass, 1983); L. W. Green, "Three Ways Research Influences Policy and Practice: The Public's Right to Know and the Scientist's Responsibility to Educate," *Health Education* 18 (Aug/Sept 1987): 44–9; M. Q. Patton, *Utilization-Focused Evaluation* (Beverly Hills: Sage Publications, 1978).

4. D. T. Campbell, "Reforms as Experiments," *American Psychologist* 24 (1969): 409–29.

5. This definition is elaborated and applied variously in L. W. Green, "Toward Cost-Benefit Evaluations of Health Education: Some Concepts, Methods, and Examples," *Health Education Monographs* 2 (suppl. 1, 1974): 34–65; L. W. Green, "Evaluation and Measurement: Some Dilemmas for Health Education," *American Journal of Public Health* 67 (1977): 155–61; L. W. Green and I. Figa-Talamanca, "Suggested Designs for Evaluation of Patient Education Programs," *Health Education Monographs* 2 (1974): 54-71; L. W. Green and F. M. Lewis, *Measurement and Evaluation . . .*, op. cit., 1986; L. W. Green, "Evaluation Model: A Framework for the Design of Rigorous Evaluation of Efforts in Health Promotion," *American Journal of Health Promotion* 1(1) (1986): 77-9; M. W. Kreuter and L. W. Green, "Evaluation of School Health Education: Identifying Purpose, Keeping Perspective," *Journal of School Health* 48 (1978): 228–35.

6. Goal-oriented evaluation is the most common but not the only type of evaluation. See, for example, P. D. Mullen and D. C. Iverson, "Qualitative Methods for Evaluative Research in Health Education Programs," *Health Education* 13(3) (1982): 11–8 (also adapted as Chap. 7 in Green and Lewis, *Measurement and Evaluation . . .*, op. cit., 1986); M. Scriven, "Pros and Cons About Goal-free Evaluation," *Evaluation Comment* 3(4) (1972): 1–5.

7. The derivation of standards for evaluation from program objectives is described and illustrated most cogently by P. A. Guild, "Goal-oriented Evaluation as a Program Management Tool," *American Journal of Health Promotion* 4 (1990): 296–301.

8. J. L. Schwartz, *Review and Evaluation of Smoking Cessation Methods: The United States and Canada 1978-1985* (Washington, DC: Department of Health and Human Services, National Institutes of Health, NIH 87–2940, 1987).

9. "The history of public health might well be written as a persistent redefinition of the unacceptable," according to Sir Geoffrey Vickers, "What Sets the Goals of Public Health," *New England Journal of Medicine* 258 (1958): 12. Examples of "Standards of Acceptability" proffered by groups of professionals include: World Health Organization, *Health Program Evaluation: Guiding Principles* (Geneva, WHO, 1981); M. Franz, A. Kresnick, B. Maschak-Carey, et al., *Goals for Diabetes Education* (American Diabetes Association, Alexandria, VA, 1986); the series of six handbooks by IOX Assessment Associates, *Program Evaluation Handbooks: Diabetes Education, . . .Drug Abuse Education, . . .Nutrition Education, . . .Alcohol Abuse Education, . . . Physical Fitness Programs, . . .Stress Management* (Los Angeles, CA: IOX Assessment Associates, 1988); *Handbook for Evaluating Drug Abuse and Alcohol Prevention Programs* (Rockville, MD: Office of Substance Abuse Prevention, U.S. Department of Health and Human Services, DHHS (ADM) 87–1512, 1987). The most sweeping consensus development procedures resulting in national objectives made up of compromise standards of acceptability are the U.S objectives for the nation.

10. *Promoting Health/Preventing Disease: 1990 Objectives for the Nation* (Washington, DC: U.S. Department of Health and Human Services, 1981). Similar objectives for health promotion have since been developed in other national policies, e.g., in Sweden, Finland, the Netherlands, and the United Kingdom. See D. Ingledew, "Target Setting for the Health of Populations: Some Observations," *Health Promotion* 4 (1989): 357–69. The later U.S. objectives were released as this book went to press, *Healthy People 2000: National Health Promotion and Disease Prevention Objectives*, conference ed. (Washington, DC: Public Health Service, U.S. Department of Health and Human Services, 1990); J. M. McGinnis, "Setting Objectives for Public Health in the 1990s," *Annual Review of Public Health* 11 (1990): 231–49.

11. L. W. Green, "Healthy People: The Surgeon General's Report and the Prospects," in *Working for a Healthier America*, W. J. McNerney, ed. (Cambridge, MA: Ballinger, 1980), pp. 95–110; J. M. McGinnis, "Targeting Progress in Health," *Public Health Reports* 97 (1982): 295–307.

12. L. W. Green, R. W. Wilson, and K. G. Bauer, "Data Required to Measure Progress on the Objectives for the Nation in Health Promotion and Disease Prevention," *American Journal of Public Health* 73 (1983): 18–24.

13. R. Andersen, and R. Mullner, "Assessing the Health Objectives of the Nation," *Health Affairs* 9 (1990): 152–62; L. W. Green, R. Blakenbaker, F. Trevino, et al., "Report of the Subcommittee on Data Gaps in Disease Prevention and Health Promotion," *Annual Report of the U.S. National Committee on Vital and Health Statistics* (Washington, DC: National Center for Health Statistics, 1987); National Center for Health Statistics, *Health, United States, 1989* (Hyattsville, MD: Public Health Service, DHHS Pub. No. (PHS) 90–1232, 1990); U.S. Department of Health and Human Services, *The 1990 Health Objectives for the Nation: A Midcourse Review* (Washington, DC: Office of Disease Prevention and Health Promotion, 1986).

14. U.S. Department of Health and Human Services, *Promoting Health in Special Populations* (Washington, DC: Office of Disease Prevention and Health Promotion, 1981); reprinted in *Journal of Public Health Policy* 8 (1987): 369–423. See also Secretary's Task Force on Black and Minority Health, *Report of the Secretary's Task Force on Black and Minority Health* (Washington, DC: U.S. Department of Health and Human Services, 1985); and comment on the report by H. W. Nickens, "Health Promotion and Disease Prevention Among Minorities," *Health Affairs* 9 (1990): 133–43, esp. pp. 133–4. The year 2000 objectives process incorporated the focused attention to minority issues; see "The Nation's Health: Special Populations," *Healthy People 2000 . . .*, op. cit., 1990, pp. 29–43; J. O. Mason, "A Prevention Policy Framework for the Nation," *Health Affairs* 9 (1990): 22–9, esp. pp. 27–8.

15. *Model Standards: A Guide for Community Preventive Health Services*, 2nd ed. (Washington, DC: American Public Health Association, 1985). A later edition was in press at the time of this writing: *Healthy Communities 2000: Model Standards*, 3rd ed. (Washington, DC: American Public Health Association, in press).

16. C. Spain, E. Eastman, and K. Kizer, "Model Standards Impact on Local Health Department Performance in California," *American Journal of Public Health* 79 (1989): 969–74. Quotation from p. 969.

17. *Model Standards: A Guide for Community Preventive Health Services*, op. cit., 1985, p. 5.

18. C. H. Weiss, "Between the Cup and the Lip," *Evaluation* 1(2) (1973): 54.

19. O. W. Cummings, J. R. Nowakowski, T. A. Schwandt, et al., "Business Perspectives on Internal/External Evaluation," in *Evaluation Utilization*, J. A. McLaughlin, L. J. Weber, R. W. Covert, and R. B. Ingle, eds. (San Francisco: Jossey-Bass, 1988).

20. J. Dewey, *Logic: The Theory of Inquiry* (New York: Henry Holt, 1938). See also J. Dewey, *Moral Principles in Education* (Boston: Houghton Mifflin, 1909).

21. M. Schlesinger, "The Perfectability of Public Programs: Real Lessons from the Large-Scale Demonstration Projects (Editorial)," *American Journal of Public Health* 78 (1988): 899–902.

22. E. G. Guba and Y. S. Lincoln, *Fourth Generation Evaluation* (Newbury Park, CA: Sage Publications, 1989).

23. E. Doyle, C. A. Smith, and M. C. Hosokawa, "A Process Evaluation of a Community-Based Health Promotion Program for a Minority Target Population," *Health Education* 20(5) (1989): 61–4.

24. J. M. Kotchen, H.E. McKean, S. Jackson-Thayer, et al., "Impact of a Rural High Blood Pressure Control Program on Hypertension Control and Cardiovascular Mortality," *Journal of the American Medical Association* 255 (1986): 2177–82.

25. R. B. Bausell, ed., "Quality Assurance: Methods," *Evaluation and the Health Professions* 6(3) (1983): whole issue; L. W. Green and P. Brooks-Bertram, "Peer Review and Quality Control in Health Education," *Health Values* 2 (1978): 191–7; A. C. Henderson, "Developing a Credentialing System for Health Educators," *Advances in Health Education and Promotion*, vol. 2, W. Ward, ed. (Greenwich, CT: JAI Press Inc., 1987), pp. 59–91; S. G. Kernaghan and R. E. Giloth, *Tracking the Impact of Health Promotion on Organizations: A Key to Program Survival* (Chicago, IL: American Hospital Association, 1988); R. D. Luke and R. E. Modrow, "Professionalism, Accountability, and Peer Review," *Health Services Research* 17 (1982): 113–23; P. D. Mullen and J. G. Zapka, "Assessing the Quality of Health Promotion Programs," *HMO Practice* 3 (1989): 98–103; V. R. Neufeld and G. R. Norman, eds., *Assessing Clinical Competence* (New York: Springer, 1985); W. H. Nichols, C. J. Stewart, "Assessment of the Client-Centered Planning Approach in Continuing Education for Public Health Professionals," *Mobius* 3(3) (1983): 12–21; K. E. Young, C. M. Chambers, H. R. Kells, et al., *Understanding Accreditation* (San Francisco: Jossey-Bass, 1983); J. G. Zapka, "Management Functions of the Health Education Director: Examples of Data Management Activities," in *Advancing Health Through Education: A Case Study Approach*, H. P. Cleary, J. Kitchen, and P. Ensor, eds. (Palo Alto: Mayfield, 1985).

26. The following refererences provide a variety of methodological approaches to the evaluation of program process: S. E. Brunk and J. Goeppinger, "Process Evaluation: Assessing Re-Invention of Community-Based Interventions," *Evaluation and the Health Professions* 13 (1990): 186–203; J. R. Finnegan, Jr., D. M. Murray, C. Kurth, P. McCarthy, "Measuring and Tracking Education Program Implementation: The Minnesota Heart Health Program Experience," *Health Education Quarterly* 16 (1989): 77–90; S. M. Blake, R. W. Jeffrey, J. R. Finnegan, et al., "Process Evaluation of a Community-Based Physical Activity Campaign: The Minnesota Heart Health Experience," *Health Education Research* 2 (1987): 115–21; C. E. Basch, "Focus Group Interview: An Under-utilized Research Technique for Improving Theory and Practice in Health Education," *Health Education Quarterly* 14 (1987): 411–48. Recent examples in which the PRECEDE model was applied include: W. B. Brown, N. B. Williamson, and R. A. Carlaw, "A Diagnostic Approach to Educating Minnesota Dairy Farmers in the Prevention and Control of Bovine Mastitis," *Preventive Veterinary Medicine* 5 (1988): 197–211; S. R. Knox, B. Mandel, and R. Lazarowicz, "Profile of Callers to the VD National Hotline," *Sexually Transmitted Diseases* 8 (1981): 245–54; A. McAlister, P. Puska, J. T. Salonen, et al., "Theory and Action for Health Promotion—Illustrations from the North Karelia Project," *American Journal of Public Health* 72 (1982): 43–50; R. Michielutte and P. Beal, "Identification of Community Leadership in the Development of Public Health Education Programs," *Journal of Community Health* 15 (1990): 59–

68; S. A. Norman, R. Greenberg, K. Marconi, et al., "A Process Evaluation of a Two-Year Community Cardiovascular Risk Reduction Program: What Was Done and Who Knew About It?" *Health Education Research* 5 (1990): 87–97; J. K. Worden, B. S. Flynn, B. M. Geller, et al., "Development of a Smoking Prevention Mass-Media Program Using Diagnostic and Formative Research," *Preventive Medicine* 17 (1988): 531–58.

27. C. E. Basch, E. M. Sliepcevich, R. S. Gold, et al., "Avoiding Type III Errors in Health Education Program Evaluations: A Case Study," *Health Education Quarterly* 12 (1985): 315–31; J. M. Ottoson and L. W. Green, "Reconciling Concept and Context: Theory of Implementation," in *Advances in Health Education and Promotion*, vol. 2, W. Ward, S. K. Simonds, P. D. Mullen, and M. Becker, eds. (Greenwich, CT: JAI Press, 1987), pp. 353–82.

28. C. E. Basch, E. M. Sliepcevich, R. S. Gold, et al., "Avoiding Type III Errors in Health Education Program Evaluations: A Case Study," *Health Education Quarterly* 12 (1985): 315–31; D. Dobson and T. J. Cook, "Avoiding Type III Error in Program Evaluation: Results from a Field Experiment," *Evaluation and Program Planning* 3 (1980): 269–76; E. L. Rezmovic, "Program Implementation and Evaluation Results: A Reexamination of Type III Error in a Field Experiment," *Evaluation and Program Planning* 5 (1982): 111–18. In medical and health services research and evaluation, the Type III error would still be counted as an ineffective program because in these fields a distinction is made between efficacy and effectiveness. *Efficacy* refers to the achievement of intended results under ideal "laboratory" conditions. *Effectiveness* refers to the achievement of intended results in the field, where the program is in the hands of practitioners who will implement it with their own twist, adapting it to suit local circumstances. See B. R. Flay, "Efficacy and Effectiveness Trials in the Development of Health Promotion Programs," *Preventive Medicine* 15 (1986): 451–74.

29. Again, the line between the audience reactions in process evaluation and the antecedents to behavior in impact evaluation is fuzzy. Classification of an evaluation as process or impact within these overlapping spheres has little meaning or importance to anyone except a few evaluation experts. In the field, process evaluation and impact evaluations will tend to blend in their timing and methods. See L. C. Leviton and R. O. Valdiserri, "Evaluating AIDS Prevention: Outcome, Implementation, and Mediating Variables," *Evaluation and Program Planning* 13 (1990): 55–66; A. G. Ramirez and A. L. McAlister, "Mass Media Campaign—*A Su Salud*," *Preventive Medicine* 17 (1989): 608–21.

30. Examples of recent impact evaluations in which the PRECEDE model was used include: S. G. Brink, B. Simons-Morton, and D. Zane, "A Hospital-Based Infant Safety Seat Program for Low-Income Families: Assessment of Population Needs and Provider Practices," *Health Education Quarterly* 16 (1989): 45–56; P. J. Bush, A. E. Zuckerman, P. K. Theiss, et al., "Cardiovascular Risk Factor Prevention in Black School Children—2-Year Results of the Know Your Body Program," *American Journal of Epidemiology* 129 (1989): 466–82; M. A. Pentz, D. P. Mackinnon, J. H. Dwyer, et al., "Longitudinal Effects of the Midwestern Prevention Project on Regular and Experimental Smoking in Adolescents," *Preventive Medicine* 18 (1989): 304–21; D. M. Vickery, H. Kalmer, D. Lowry, et al., "Effect of a Self-care Education Program on Medical Visits," *Journal of the American Medical Association* 250 (1983): 2952–6; H. J. Walter, E. L. Wynder, "The Development, Implementation, Evaluation, and Future Directions of a Chronic Disease Prevention Program for Children—The Know Your Body Studies," *Preventive Medicine* 18 (1989): 59–71; B. L. Wells, J. D. DePue, T. M. Lasater, and R. A. Carleton, "A Report on Church Site Weight Control," *Health Education Research* 3 (1988): 305–16; R. A. Windsor, "Planning and Evaluation of Public Health Education Programs in Rural Settings: Theory into Practice," in *Advancing Health Through Education: A Case Study Approach*, H. P. Cleary, J. M. Kichen, and P. G. Ensor, eds. (Palo Alto: Mayfield, 1984), pp. 273–84.

31. S. Redman, E. A. Spencer, and R. W. Sanson-Fisher, "The Role of Mass Media in Changing Health Related Behaviour: A Critical Appraisal of Two Models," *Health Promotion International* 5 (1990): 85–102; L. M. Wallack, "Mass Media Campaigns: The Odds Against Finding Behavior Change," *Health Education Quarterly* 8 (1981): 209–60; B. R. Flay and T. D. Cook, "Evaluation of Mass Media Prevention Campaigns," in *Public Communication Campaigns*, R. E. Rice and W. J. Paisley, eds. (London: Sage, 1981), pp. 239–64. When the campaign's objective is to

influence policy through increased public awareness, then media success can be appropriately measured by tracking the number of news stories on the issue, legislative acts proposed and passed, or other political outcomes. See W. DeJong and J. A. Winsten, "The Use of Mass Media in Substance Abuse Prevention," *Health Affairs* 9 (1990): 30–46; L. Wallack, "Assessing Effects of Mass Media Campaigns: An Alternative Perspective," *Alcohol, Health and Research World* 5 (1980): 17–29.

32. For example, D. M. Levine, L. W. Green, S. G. Deeds, et al., "Health Education for Hypertension Patients," *Journal of the American Medical Association* 241 (1979): 1700–3; L. Maiman, L. W. Green, G. Gibson, and E. J. Mackenzi, "Education for Self-treatment by Adult Asthmatics," *Journal of the American Medical Association* 241 (1979): 1919–22; K. V. Mann, and P. L. Sullivan, "Effect of Task-Centered Instructional Programs on Hypertensives' Ability to Achieve and Maintain Reduced Dietary Sodium Intake," *Patient Education and Counseling* 10 (1987): 53–72; D. E. Morisky, D. M. Levine, L. W. Green, et al., "Five-Year Blood Pressure Control and Mortality Following Health Education for Hypertensive Patients," *American Journal of Public Health* 73 (1983): 153–62; P. B. Terry, V. L. Wang, B. S. Flynn, et al., "A Continuing Medical Education Program in Chronic Obstructive Pulmonary Diseases: Design and Outcome," *American Review of Respiratory Diseases* 123 (1981): 42–6; H. J. Walter, "Primary Prevention of Chronic Disease Among Children: The School-based 'Know Your Body' Intervention Trials," *Health Education Quarterly* 16 (1989): 201–14.

33. *Fidelity* has been identified as a factor influencing outcomes in several studies. It was a noteworthy variable in the findings presented in "The School Health Education Evaluation Study," *Journal of School Health* 55 (Oct. 1985): issue no. 6; see also K. D. McCaul and R. E. Glasgow, "Preventing Adolescent Smoking: What Have We Learned About Treatment Construct Validity?" *Health Psychology* 4 (1985): 361–87.

34. This is one of several paradoxes or dilemmas of evaluation in health education described in L. W. Green, "Evaluation and Measurement: Some Dilemmas for Health Education," *American Journal of Public Health* 67 (1977): 155–61. This problem of "fidelity" was discussed earlier in this chapter in relation to the "Type III error" in evaluation.

35. A pioneering text in qualitative evaluation is M. Q. Patton, *Qualitative Evaluation Methods* (Beverly Hills, CA: Sage, 1980); see also A. Steckler, "The Use of Qualitative Evaluation Methods to Test Internal Validity: An Example in a Work Site Health Promotion Program," *Evaluation and the Health Professions* 12 (1989): 115–33; R. M. Goodman and A. Steckler, "A Model for the Institutionalization of Health Promotion Programs," *Family and Community Health* 11 (1989): 63–78.

36. J. B. Atwater, "Adapting the Venereal Disease Clinic to Today's Problem," *American Journal of Public Health* 64 (1974): 433–7.

37. J. Bailey, "An Evaluative Look at a Family Planning Radio Campaign in Latin America," *Studies in Family Planning* 4 (1973): 275–8; L. W. Green, S. Werlin, H. Shauffler, and C. H. Avery, "Research and Demonstration Issues in Self-care: Measuring the Decline of Medicocentrism," *Health Education Monographs* 5 (1977): 161–89; E. H. Kwon, "Use of the Agent System in Seoul," *Studies in Family Planning* 2 (1971): 237–340; M. Drazen, J. S. Nevid, N. Pace, and R. M. O'Brien, "Worksite-based Behavioral Treatment of Mild Hypertension," *Journal of Occupational Medicine* 24 (1982): 511–4; N. P. Roos, "Evaluating Health Programs: Where Do We Find the Data," *Journal of Community Health* 1 (1975): 39–51; C. V. Spiegel and F. C. Lindaman, "Children Can't Fly: A Program to Prevent Childhood Morbidity and Mortality from Window Falls," *American Journal of Public Health* 67 (1977): 1143–6; K. E. Warner, "The Effects of the Anti-smoking Campaign on Cigarette Consumption," *American Journal of Public Health* 67 (1977): 645–50.

38. N. H. Bryant, W. Stender, V. Frist, and A. R. Somers, "VD Hotline: An Evaluation," *Public Health Reports* 91 (1976): 231–5.

39. R. L. Bertera, L. K. Oehl, and J. M. Telepchak, "Self-help Versus Group Approaches to Smoking Cessation in the Workplace: Eighteen-Month Follow-up and Cost Analysis," *American Journal of*

Health Promotion 4 (1990): 187–92; D. J. Bogue, R. Burs, and J. Mayo, *Communicating to Combat VD: The Los Angeles Experiment* (Chicago, IL: Community and Family Study Center Monographs, University of Chicago, 1979); R. H. Conn and D. Anderson, "D.C. Mounts Unfunded Program of Screening for Lead Poisoning," *HSMHA Health Report* (now *Public Health Reports*) 86 (1971): 409–13; J. C. Franz and R. J. Weisser, Jr., "Venereal Disease Education in West Virginia, USA," *British Journal of Venereal Diseases* 54 (1978): 269–73; D. Rosenblatt and L. Kabasakalian, "Evaluation of Venereal Disease Information Campaign for Adolescents," *American Journal of Public Health* 56 (1966): 1104–13; U.S. Department of Health and Human Services, *The 1990 Health Objectives for the Nation: A Midcourse Review* (Washington, DC: Office of Disease Prevention and Health Promotion, 1986). J. W. Williamson, S. Aronovitch, L. Simonson, et al., "Health Accounting: An Outcome-based System of Quality Assurance— Illustrative Application to Hypertension," *Bulletin of the New York Academy of Medicine* 51 (1975): 727–38.

40. This is usually referred to as formative evaluation when the purpose is to make adjustments in the program as it is developing. See, for example, C. E. Basch, "Preventing AIDS Through Education: Concepts, Strategies, and Research Priorities," *Journal of School Health* 59 (1989): 296–300; C. E. Basch, et al., 1985, op. cit.; H. Mendelsohn, "Some Reasons Why Information Campaigns Can Succeed," *Public Opinion Quarterly* 39 (1973): 50–61; D. Rosenblatt and L. Kabasakalian, 1966, op. cit.

41. J. Schuurman and W. de Haes, "Sexually Transmitted Diseases: Health Education by Telephone," *International Journal of Health Education* 23 (1980): 94–106.

42. U.S. Department of Health and Human Services, *The Health Consequences of Smoking Cessation: A Report of the Surgeon General*, (Washington, DC: PHS, Office on Smoking and Health, 1990); C. C. DiClemente, and J. O. Prochaska, "Self-change and Therapy Change of Smoking Behavior: A Comparison of Process of Change in Cessation and Maintenance," *Addictive Behaviors* 7 (1982): 133–42; S. M. Glynn, C. L. Gruder, and J. A. Jerski, "Effects on Treatment Success and on Mis-reporting Abstinence," *Health Psychology* 5(2) (1986): 125–36,; R. V. Leupker, V. E. Pallonen, D. M. Murray, and P. L. Pirie, "Validity of Telephone Surveys in Assessing Cigarette Smoking in Young Adults," *American Journal of Public Health* 79 (1989): 202–4; D. M. Murray and C. L. Perry, "The Measurement of Substance Use Among Adolescents: When Is the 'Bogus Pipeline' Method Needed?" *Addictive Behaviors* 12 (1987): 225–33; T. F. Pechacek, B. H. Fox, D. M. Murray, and R. V. Luepker, "Review of Techniques for Measurement of Smoking Behaviors," in *Behavioral Health: A Handbook of Health Enhancement and Disease Prevention*, J. Matarazzo, S. M. Weiss, A. Herd, et al., eds. (New York: Wiley, 1984); R. A. Windsor and C. T. Orleans, "Guidelines and Methodological Standards for Smoking Cessation Intervention Research Among Pregnant Women: Improving the Science and Art," *Health Education Quarterly* 13(2) (1986): 131–61.

43. L. W. Green and K. J. Krotki, "Class and Parity Biases in Family Planning Programs: The Case of Karachi," *Social Biology* 15 (1968): 235–51; A. Marlatt and J. A. Gordon, *Relapse Prevention* (New York: Guilford Press, 1985); J. S. Neill and J. O. Bond, *Hillsborough County Oral Polio Vaccine Program* (Jacksonville: Florida State Board of Health, monograph no. 6, 1964); V. L. Wang, P. Ephross, and L. W. Green, "The Point of Diminishing Returns in Nutrition Education Through Home Visits by Aides: An Evaluation of EFNEP," *Health Education Monographs* 3 (1975): 70–88; G. H. Ward, "Changing Trends in Control of Hypertension," *Public Health Reports* 93 (1978): 31–4.

44. R. W. Wilson and D. C. Iverson, "Federal Data Bases for Health Education Research," *Health Education* 13 (1982): 30–4.

45. For example, D. Douglas, B. Wertley, and S. Chaffee, "An Information Campaign That Changed Community Attitudes," *Journalism Quarterly* 47 (1970): 220–7; J. C. Franz, and R. J. Weisser, Jr., "Venereal Disease Education in West Virginia, USA," *British Journal of Venereal Diseases*, 54 (1978): 269–73; V. L. Wang, P. Terry, B. S. Flynn, et al., "Multiple Indicators of Continuing Medical Education Priorities for Chronic Lung Diseases in Appalachia," *Journal of Medical Education* 54 (1979): 803–11; R. A. Windsor, 1984, op. cit.

46. J. Farquhar, "The Community-based Model of Life Style Intervention Trials," *American Journal of Epidemiology* 108 (1978): 103–11; J. W. Farquhar, S. P. Fortman, J. A. Flora, et al., "Effects of Community-wide Education on Cardiovascular Disease Risk Factors—The Stanford 5-City Project," *Journal of the American Medical Association* 264 (1990): 359–65; S. Fortmann, P. Williams, S. Hulley, et al., "Effect of Health Education on Dietary Behavior: The Stanford Three-Community Study," *American Journal of Clinical Nutrition* 34 (1981): 2030–8; H. Blackburn, "Research and Demonstration Projects in Community Cardiovascular Disease Prevention," *Journal of Public Health Policy* 4 (1987): 398–421; Kotchen, et al., 1987; D. Nutbeam and J. Catford, "The Welsh Heart Programme Evaluation Strategy: Progress, Plans and Possibilities," *Health Promotion* 2 (1987): 5–18; A. G. Ramirez and A. L. McAlister, "Mass Media Campaign—*A Su Salud,*" *Preventive Medicine* 17 (1989): 608–21. For summary discussions and reviews of the evaluation designs of the cardiovascular disease prevention projects at Stanford, Minnesota, Pawtucket, and North Karelia, see Blackburn, 1987, op. cit.; a series of descriptions in J. D. Matarazzo, S. M. Weiss, J. A. Herd, et al., *Behavioral Health: A Handbook of Health Enhancement and Disease Prevention* (New York: Wiley, 1984); D. Nutbeam, C. Smith, and J. Catford, "Evaluation in Health Education: A Review of Possibilities and Problems," *Journal of Epidemiology and Community Health* 44 (1990): 83–9; S. Shea and C. E. Basch, "A Review of Five Major Community-based Cardiovascular Disease Prevention Programs. Part I: Rationale, Design, and Theoretical Framework," *American Journal of Health Promotion* 4 (1990): 203–13.

47. J. W. Farquhar, N. Maccoby, and P. D. Wood, "Community Education for Cardiovascular Health," *Lancet* 1(8023) (June, 1977): 1192–5; N. Maccoby, J. W. Farquhar, and P. D. Wood "Reducing the Risk of Cardiovascular Disease: Effects of a Community-based Campaign on Knowledge and Behavior," *Journal of Community Health* 23 (1977): 100–14.

48. J. Schuurman and W. de Haes, "Sexually Transmitted Diseases: Health Education by Telephone," *International Journal of Health Education* 23 (1980): 94–106.

49. R. A. Dershewitz and J. W. Williamson (1977), "Preventing Childhood Household Injuries: A Controlled Clinical Trial," *American Journal of Public Health* 67 (1977): 1148–53; D. L. Roter, "Patient Participation in the Patient-Provider Interaction: The Effects of Patient Question-asking on the Quality of Interaction, Satisfaction and Compliance," *Health Education Monographs* 5 (1977): 281–315; J. Sayegh and L. W. Green, "Family Planning Education: Program Design, Training Component and Cost-effectiveness of a Postpartum Program in Beirut," *International Journal of Health Education* 19 (suppl., 1976): 1–20.

50. J. Bailey and M. C. Zambrano, "Contraceptive Pamphlets in Colombian Drugstores," *Studies in Family Planning* 5 (1974): 178–82; T. W. Elwood, E. Ericson, and S. Lieberman, "Comparative Educational Approaches to Screening for Colorectal Cancer," *American Journal of Public Health* 68 (1978): 135–8.

51. L. W. Green, D. M. Levine, and S. G. Deeds, "Clinical Trials of Health Education for Hypertensive Outpatients: Design and Baseline Data," *Preventive Medicine* 4 (1975): 417–25; L. W. Green, D. M. Levine, J. Wolle, and S. G. Deeds, "Development of Randomized Patient Education Experiments with Urban Poor Hypertensives," *Patient Counseling and Health Education* 1 (1979): 106–11; M. E. Hatcher, L. W. Green, D. M. Levine, and C. E. Flagle, "Validation of a Decision Model for Triaging Hypertensive Patients to Alternate Health Education Interventions," *Social Science and Medicine* 22 (1986): 813–9; D. M. Levine, L. W. Green, S. G. Deeds, et al., "Health Education for Hypertensive Patients," *Journal of the American Medical Association* 241 (1979): 1700–3; D. E. Morisky, D. M. Levine, L. W. Green, et al., "Five-Year Blood-Pressure Control and Mortality Following Health Education for Hypertensive Patients," *American Journal of Public Health* 73 (1983): 153–62.

52. L. W. Green, "Evaluation and Measurement: Some Dilemmas for Health Education," *American Journal of Public Health* 67 (1977): 155–61; L. W. Green and F. M. Lewis, *Measurement and Evaluation in Health Education and Health Promotion* (Palo Alto, CA: Mayfield, 1986); R. A. Windsor, T. Baronowski, N. Clark, and G. Cutter, *Evaluation of Health Promotion and Education Programs* (Palo Alto, CA: Mayfield, 1984).

53. D. A. Bertram and P. A. Brooks-Bertram, "The Evaluation of Continuing Medical Education: A

Literature Review," *Health Education Monographs* 5 (Winter 1977): 330–62; I. Figa-Talamanca, "Problems in the Evaluation of Training of Health Personnel," *Health Education Monographs* 3 (Fall, 1975): 232–50; M. W. Kreuter and L. W. Green, "Evaluation of School Health Education: Identifying Purpose, Keeping Perspective," *Journal of School Health* 48 (Apr., 1978): 228–35; Guy W. Stuart, "Planning and Evaluation in Health Education," *International Journal of Health Education* 12 (1969): 65–76.

54. B. Simons-Morton, G. D. Parcel, N. M. O'Hara, et al., "Health-related Physical Fitness in Childhood: Status and Recommendations," *Annual Review of Public Health* 9 (1988): 403–25.

55. R. E. Laporte, H. J. Montoye, and C. J. Caspersen, "Assessment of Physical Activity in Epidemiologic Research: Problems and Prospects," *Public Health Reports* 100 (1985): 131–46; R. E. LaPorte, L. L. Adams, D. D. Savage, et al., "The Spectrum of Physical Activity, Cardiovascular Fitness and Health: An Epidemiologic Perspective," *American Journal of Epidemiology* 120 (1984): 507–17.

Chapter 8

Applications of PRECEDE–PROCEED in Community Settings

The PRECEDE model asks and helps answer *what*, *who*, and *why* questions. What are the quality-of-life, health, behavioral, and environmental problems or aspirations? Who has those problems or aspirations? Why do they have them (what are their causes or determinants)? PROCEED asks what resources, barriers, policies, regulations, and organizational factors need to be adjusted to make a program work and to set up an implementation and evaluation design. At this point, with plans in hand, the next task is to develop and deploy the combination of health education and environmental strategies likely to achieve the health promotion objectives. The way this happens varies according to the setting in which PRECEDE and PROCEED are applied.

This chapter examines the community as a setting for health promotion and some of the principles and techniques that practitioners have found most useful in successful community health promotion applications. Given reasonable resources, the chances are good that a community intervention will succeed if the practitioner (1) builds from a base of community ownership of the problems and the solutions, (2) plans carefully, (3) uses sound theory, meaningful data, and local experience as bases for program decisions, (4) knows what types of interventions work best for specific populations and circumstances, and (5) has an organizational and advocacy plan to orchestrate multiple intervention strategies into a complementary, cohesive program. The steps of PRECEDE and PROCEED – and the theoretical concepts, data, and local involvement required to work effectively through those steps – have given the practitioner a sound footing for items 1, 2, and 3. We now address items 3, 4, and 5.

THE COMMUNITY AS A MEDIUM FOR CHANGE

We begin by expanding the definition of the word *community* provided in Chapter 1, developing the distinctions between *community intervention* and *interventions in communities* and discussing practical guidelines for establishing and maintaining community coalitions. Examination of the process of community intervention in light of the principles of PRECEDE and PROCEED follows. We emphasize the use of multiple strategies for intervention and the rationale behind their coordinated application in the community.

DEFINING COMMUNITY

The term *community* is easily understood in common parlance. But when it is used in the context of health practice or research, its varied meanings force the use of an operational definition, even though operational definitions of community are sure to bring simultaneous cries of "too restricting" and "lacks precision"! As used in this chapter, *community* is defined in terms of two characteristics: structure and function. Structurally, a community is an area with geographic and often political boundaries that demarcate it as a district, county, metropolitan area, city, township, or neighborhood. Functionally, a community is a place where "members have a sense of identity and belonging, shared values, norms, communication, and helping patterns."[1] Effective community workers understand the dynamic social characteristics and the less dynamic cultural traditions of a community, and plan interventions with sensitivity to them. The structural aspect of the community delimits activity to a local focus, leaving the larger national, provincial, and state endeavors for consideration elsewhere.[2] Even so, this definition leaves room to roam.

For instance, it is fair to ask, how formal are the political boundaries and what do you mean by a neighborhood? Clearly, the *informal* political forces often exert more influence on policy formulation and program implementation than the formal political structures usually associated with official boundaries.[3] For example, it would be foolhardy to launch a health promotion program in the borough of Harlem, simply on the grounds that the mayor of New York City endorsed it, just as it would in London's Lewisham area, based on the support of that great British city's lord mayor.

Ultimately, the geopolitical scope of a program must be left to the prudent judgment and sensitive action of those working with the program, guided by the local people who know the culture and traditions of the community, and by PROCEED analyses of the resources available within the community and from other levels (state, provincial, or national) to support the program.[4]

COMMUNITY INTERVENTIONS AND INTERVENTIONS IN COMMUNITIES

They sound alike, but they are different. *Community interventions* seek small but pervasive changes that apply to the majority of the population; the approach is community wide. *Interventions in a community* seek more intensive or profound change in a subpopulation, usually within or from a specific community site such as the workplace, hospital or clinic, nursing home, or school; this approach is targeted. The objective of both approaches is to reduce the incidence of health problems or to improve the health status of the community.

The encouraging results from the large-scale family planning and immunization programs reported in the 1960s and early 1970s[5] and the cardiovascular and cancer community intervention trials initiated in the late 1970s and early 1980s[6] have been primarily responsible for the increasing number of community-based health promotion programs reported in the international literature. The environmental movement has sought a similar level of community-wide activation around issues such as recycling, toxic waste disposal, water conservation, and van pooling.[7] The AIDS epidemic and HIV infections have revived a parallel and converging interest in community approaches to health education.[8]

Most of the chronic disease demonstrations were designed to produce small changes in large populations, the idea being that the net effect of achieving a small percentage change in an entire population would yield more profound public health benefits than would strategies aimed exclusively at the 10 percent of the population deemed to be at highest risk. The target is the community and everyone in it. Public health analysts[9] provide the epidemiologic and sociologic justifications for supporting these population approaches. Others point out, however, that it should not be an either–or choice because both strategies have independent and additive effects.[10] The community-wide approach has the potential of complementing and supporting institution-based programs in five ways, as follows.

The Epidemiologic Case. In North Karelia (Finland), only 2 percent of the target population lost weight, but this amounted to 60,000 persons, far more than could have been reached through doctors' offices.[11] The Australian *Quit for Life* media campaign produced a measly 2.8 percent reduction in smoking prevalence,[12] which would be considered a failure by targeted smoking cessation program standards,[13] but it amounted to 83,000 fewer smokers in Sydney. A television and community organization effort to support smokers' quitting in Canada yielded a 2.9 percent reduction in smoking prevalence, which translated as 8,800 fewer smokers than expected from extrapolated trends in Canada.[14] The scattered and sporadic but relentless antismoking efforts in the United States between 1964 and 1978 produced a net annual smoking prevalence reduction of only 1 percent, but this produced in turn an estimated 200,000 fewer premature smoking-related deaths, with many more expected to be avoided as former smokers age through the 1980s and 1990s.[15]

These epidemiologic examples of the extensive, though proportionately small, benefits of community-wide or population interventions relative to the more effective but limited range of targeted, institutionally based interventions argue for a place at the health promotion table for community approaches.

The Social-Psychological Case. On the basis of their review of the research and experience of decades of work on sexually transmitted disease control, Solomon and DeJong conclude: "More than any other recommendation, we urge that AIDS risk-reduction strategies focus on establishing a social climate in which people feel that it is the norm and not the exception to adopt AIDS risk-reduction behavior."[16] This concept of building a social norm for behavior conducive to health lies at the heart of the social-psychological justification for community approaches to health promotion.[17] Clearly, the antismoking initiatives have succeeded in doing just that; designated drivers rather than drinking and driving appears to be making similar strides in becoming a norm; eating low-fat foods has begun to take on the mark of a social norm, at least in more affluent communities and their upscale restaurants.[18] The task now is to be sure these norms continue to diffuse to all segments of the community. This will require more targeted efforts in the high-risk sub-populations.

The social-psychological case does not argue for a choice between community-wide approaches and targeted approaches. It argues for a combination. As every social marketing and classroom-learning experience demonstrates, targeting or "market segmentation" assures that tailored, relevant, and effective teaching and persuasive messages reach individuals. But individual change can be powerfully *predisposed* by the individual's own perception that others have made the change successfully (role models) and with satisfaction (vicarious reinforcement). Furthermore, the individual process of making the change can be *enabled* by imitation and help from friends and *reinforced* by the approval of significant others, if enough social change is taking place around the individual (i.e., if other people and environmental circumstances are supporting the change in the same period of time). This is the fundamental thesis of "reciprocal determinism" in social learning theory.[19]

The combination of targeted and community approaches reconciles the debate between individualized approaches and system approaches, which some have characterized as a debate between health education and health promotion or between educational and environmental approaches.[20] Community approaches count on individual innovators to blaze the trail for social change, but communities must reinforce those changes and increasingly reach others by building greater environmental and normative supports for the changes. Ordinances to control smoking in public places, for example, support those who have quit smoking and protect them from exposure to the smoking behavior of others, while encouraging others to quit.

The task of community programs is to provide both the general environmental and the social supports for change through policies and mass media and the institutional interventions to strengthen psychological readiness through families, schools, worksites, and health-care settings where more individualized communications can be organized. Policies and mass media, in the long term, also help shape psychological readiness; institutional settings also provide ideal opportunities for social and environmental supports for change. The combination of interventions at multiple levels achieves the community diffusion effect necessary to reach those who cannot be reached personally by health professionals.

The Economic Case. A major barrier to reaching the less motivated and the more economically disadvantaged segments of the population *sometimes* is the accessibility and cost of the more healthful options. The market economy for food and fitness products, for example, tends to be driven by the consumer preferences of the more upscale and middle-income majority segments of the population than by the poorer and typically late-adopter segments. Until consumer demand in the more profitable middle-income majority segments of the population causes producers and distributors of food products to bring low-fat alternatives to the market, they are unlikely to produce or make these products accessible through fast-food restaurants and convenience grocery stores, where the poorer segments obtain much of their food.[21]

The Political Case. Just as the strength of numbers makes the epidemiological case, the strength of social norms makes the sociological case, and the strength of purchasing power makes the economic case for community-wide strategies in health promotion, the combination of these makes the political case. The policy changes needed to support behavior in some health promotion programs tend to favor numbers, norms, and money. The political power of the middle majority lies in the number of votes this segment of the population represents. The political power of social norms lies in the voter sentiments and public opinion reflected by broadly accepted norms. The political power of money lies in contributions to campaign funding and lobbying. The numbers and norms clearly give the middle majority of the population an advantage in democratic policy making.

Economic influence on politics might seem to favor the most affluent minority, but politicians increasingly feel pressures to diversify their sources of campaign funding and prefer many small donations from the mainstream over a few large donations from rich, special-interest groups. Gaining or holding elected office on the strength of a few large campaign donations leaves a politician with limited options and tainted integrity. Similarly, the lowest income minority of the population commands little political influence, having neither money nor numbers.

Health promotion strategies that increase broad public awareness, interest, and commitment, therefore, stand a much greater chance of gaining political support than those directed exclusively at either high- or low-income populations.

Programs and policy issues related exclusively to the needs of the poor and minority and other politically marginal groups gain less support in Congress, Parliament, and state or provincial legislatures than issues framed as affecting everyone. Wilson concludes from his analysis of policy in the United States:

> In the final analysis, the question of reform is a political one. Accordingly, if the issues are couched in terms of promoting economic security for all Americans, if the essential political message underscores the need for economic and social reform that benefits all groups in society, not just poor minorities, a basis for generating a broad-based political coalition to achieve such reform would be created. Minority leaders could play an important role in this coalition once they fully recognize the need to shift or expand their definition of racial problems in America and to broaden the scope of suggested policy programs to address them.[22]

SIZE, SCOPE, AND COMPLEXITY

From the point of view of intervention methods, the fundamental differences between *community interventions* and *interventions in communities* are two: (1) the comparative magnitude of the undertaking, which is determined by the size of the group or population for whom the program is intended and (2) the number of organizations and the *levels of organization* that need to be involved. Consequently, the quantitative aspects of the intervention process should vary mainly as a function of the size and scope of the program, but the added complexities of organizing and managing a community-wide program make the qualitative aspects quite different.

A commitment to a community intervention is a commitment to *big*. It implies that the planners have the staff (or committed volunteers), resources, and political influence to deliver on the task of involving all segments of the community, including the major channels of mass communication. From an evaluation standpoint, it means having the resources and capacity to collect and analyze the population-based data necessary to detect changes over time.

Health workers using interventions in a communty can take greater advantage of the strong reinforcement that group dynamics within institutions, support systems, and interpersonal channels of communication bring to a program. Such interpersonal and small-group interventions are more common, more manageable, and probably better understood than community-wide programs, as subsequent chapters show. Institution-based programs lend themselves better to systematic, controlled research and hence have a stronger research base. But community-wide programs have greater potential for making significant population changes, primarily as a result of reaching larger numbers of people through mass media and multiple channels of communication, of building widespread normative, economic, and political support for the changes, and possibly by stimulating change in a community's social fabric.

One reason to recognize the distinction between these two approaches is that goals and objectives set at the community level can lead to unrealistic expectations when the power to intervene is limited largely to isolated institutional settings. Consider this scenario.

Like most other communities of the United States, Eagerton's leading causes of death are heart disease and selected cancers. On the basis of the growing body of scientific evidence linking high dietary fat intake to these leading causes of preventable death, and given the availability of reasonably good baseline data indicating high rates of fat consumption in the community, a health promotion planning committee establishes the following as one of its health goals: By the year 2000 (10 years from the beginning of the program), residents of Eagerton will reduce their intake of dietary fat by 25 percent, from an average of 40 percent of calories to 30 percent of calories.

That is both a behavioral objective and a health objective. It is concise, it addresses a priority public health problem, and studies such as those conducted in five California communities[23] and in North Karelia, Finland[24] show that population approaches can result in substantial reductions in fat intake. Objectives like this one are consistent with mainstream disease prevention and health promotion policy efforts.[25] As discussed in Chapters 1 and 7, public health policy the world over is being driven by explicitly stated objectives aimed at reducing preventable health problems.

The question for the planners in Eagerton, however, is whether they can meet that objective within the context of Eagerton's circumstances. Do they have access to the economic and human resources required to launch and sustain the effort needed to reach the large numbers of people and to change people's complex food-consumption behavior. Let us say that Eagerton has a population of 100,000 and that the estimate of 40 percent of calories coming from dietary fat represents a normal distribution.[26] Planners in Eagerton are encouraged by the results from the intervention strategy in the North Karelia study, which reported 35 percent declines in milk and butterfat consumption for both men and women.[27] But the total reduction in the percentage of calories from fat was only 15 percent (from 40 to 34). Difficulties would arise if a community program goal of a 25 percent reduction were accepted when the best previous experience was a 15 percent reduction.

In the absence of adequate economic and personnel resources to carry out a community-wide program equaling that of North Karelia, Eagerton is setting itself up for disappointment. If the necessary resources are not committed, both the community members, whose expectations are high, and the leaders in the agency responsible for carrying out the program will be disillusioned. As they realize the impossibility of the task, staff morale will drop. To prevent such scenarios, planners must keep an eye out for the scope and realities of the intervention process. The goal of 25 percent reduction might be quite appropriate for specific clinical, school, and worksite subpopulations in Eagerton because the programs can exert considerable control over predisposing, enabling, and reinforcing factors within specific settings; but for the community as a whole, such a large reduction may be unrealistic because of the inability to control as many of these factors.

DEMONSTRATION AND DIFFUSION VALUE OF SMALLER PROGRAMS

In this discussion, the reader may be getting the idea that bigger is better, that using the *interventions in communities* strategy is less commendable than taking on the larger community interventions. Not necessarily. In fact, site- or area-specific interventions carried out within communities have great potential for long-term, positive social change. When these smaller intervention efforts are sensitively carried out within the envelope of the community, they tend to become focal points for attention. At first they may be viewed merely as curious experiments. But over time, curiosity gives way to genuine interest and imitation. As more people begin to get a sense that respectable individuals and organizations think the undertaking is a good thing, more people want in.[28] As more organizations adopt or extend components of the program, a multiplier effect is underway.[29]

The multiplier effect was documented in describing the three forces that accounted for health improvements in Mississippi from 1956 to 1981, especially among African-Americans. The first was the passage of federal laws providing for new human service entitlement for Food Stamps, Head Start programs, Medicare and Medicaid, and housing improvements. The second and third forces address the multiplier effect.

> A second force was the establishment of a variety of health services and health undertakings, originally by concerned external groups such as the Medical Commission on Human Rights and later by Mississippians themselves. These indigenous efforts were, in part, responses to innovations of outside origin, e.g., in maternal and child care. Overall, while some health projects like the Tufts University's Mound Bayou Health Center were well funded, long lasting, and capable of providing a variety of services to a defined Black population in the Delta, many projects were very small, ephemeral and maintained on shoestrings. Nevertheless, the health projects of the 1960's and the early 1970's introduced new concerns for health standards, often improved methods, and involvements of communities in the improvement of health. The third force arose out of the first two. It was the growth of valid health information among both races. This led to an awareness of health needs, enhanced capacities for self-help, and greater demands for quality from health services providers.[30]

The theoretical underpinnings of the health promotion methods and the application of those methods vary little between community interventions and interventions in communities. The differences are in the magnitude and complexity, and therefore the risk, of the application of intervention strategies. For community-wide (including statewide and nationwide interventions), the size and complexity of the undertaking call for a broad base of awareness and political support (produced by a social diagnosis in some instances). It requires the resources of more than one organization and the cooperation of more than one sector. Daunting as the challenge of community interventions may seem, strategic assessment and mobilization of broad public interest, concern, commitment, and resources can turn the "impossible dream" into a realistic community plan.

COMMUNITY PARTICIPATION

One thing that should not differ between community interventions and interventions in the community is the importance of the principle of participation, highlighted in Chapter 2. Early involvement of community members in identifying their own needs, setting their own priorities, and planning their own programs is, in itself, a form of intervention. It provides the opportunity for ownership, which can lead to a sense of empowerment and self-determination—those difficult-to-measure intangibles that so often make the difference between long-term success and failure.

Gaining broad-based community participation for the federally funded, large-scale research and demonstration efforts, however, has been problematic. Up-front community initiation and participation has been limited in the pioneering community-intervention trials mentioned earlier, for good reason. These were large scientific studies conceived and, for the most part, planned by public health officials at the federal level and by the professors who received the grants. Efforts to engage the community typically occurred *after* the planning had been started, if not completed. The protocol was approved by a national peer review panel, and the grant approved by a federal agency. Usually, the active participation of the community could come only after the grant was in hand. Asking communities and organizations to implement programs planned elsewhere and evaluated on someone else's terms might gain some followers, but often with commitments only "as long as the money lasts."

Academicians working on large community interventions are faced with a paradox. Public health workers cry out for the resources needed to bring prevention to the community. Decision makers are taken by the idea but want proof that it will make a difference. Guidelines for scientific trials and rigorously evaluated demonstrations are delineated by the federal government. Academics design proposals. "Participation" begins when key influentials in the target communities are informed of the university's intent to apply for the grant and their willingness to cooperate is secured.

This form of community participation is criticized as too little too late in the eyes of some. If community members are invited to participate in the implementation but not the policy and planning stages, they may feel as if they are being used as free labor for university-initiated projects. This dilemma reflects an inability to design unbiased scientific tests of community interventions without damaging the variable (active community participation) that is most likely to account for successful community structural and cultural change, as well as behavioral change in individuals.[31] Very early activation of the community in these instances may falsely raise community hopes and expectations should funding not be secured. Nevertheless, some communities go on from this aborted nudge to develop their own programs without external funding.

The scientific benefits of the early community studies may have justified their restraints on early and active participation of community members. The compelling evidence pointing to the benefits of community participation now demands a continuing search for funding mechanisms between levels of government and for procedures of grantmaking that require and facilitate greater community involvement.[32]

Changes in the organization of Local Community Services Centers in Quebec illustrates the intergovernmental problem of funding and community participation. The defenders of local autonomy opposed central government programming on the grounds that it would result in low-level adaptation to local needs, bureaucratization of services, and the discouragement of local participation. In response to these concerns, Bozzini commented:

> This danger is real, but the analysis should be freed from ideological preconceptions. First, nobody should, *a priori* be scandalized because the state offers, over the whole Quebec territory, a homogeneous set of services addressing the most prevalent needs of the citizens. Furthermore, centralized programming does not mean a lack of local autonomy in the ways of doing things; against this anti-institutional rhetoric, the present situation shows that this autonomy is quite large including locally determined styles of community organization.[33]

All of this suggests the need for practitioners to be clear in their understanding of what community participation means. Having several influential community authorities on a steering committee is politically wise and undoubtedly strengthens a program's chances for support, but it does not constitute community participation. At the same time, the small steering or planning committee is an essential first step, and pending the outcomes of that smaller group's deliberations, the formation of a broad-based coalition will follow.[34]

The commitment to community participation is felt, not talked about. The sincerity of the practitioner and the group he or she works with reflect to the community how genuine they are in their commitment to community participation. This suggests that health education, in the context of health promotion and development programs, has as a primary function the arousal of individuals and communities to demand partnership and a voice in assessing their own needs, setting their own priorities, and planning their own programs, not just implementing them.

COALITIONS: GROUPS TO BE RECKONED WITH

Whether meeting basic needs in Nigeria,[35] establishing preventive and curative services in northern Tanzania,[36] trying to establish healthy public policy in an impoverished inner-city area of London,[37] or sustaining a PATCH program in rural New York[38] or Ohio,[39] community coalitions emerge as an essential part of any community-based intervention program. Two types of relationships occur between groups and individuals within a community: *exchange* relationships between providers and consumers or professionals and clients and *coordinative* relationships in which the common interests of two or more groups are managed toward mutual ends. Coalitions operate on the basis of coordinative relationships. Coordinating organizations and coalitions provide the balance of power for multiple smaller organizations to counter the political and economic influence of major corporate or governmental bodies that hold exchange power.

> Research findings suggest that reputed community leaders gain influence over others by occupying economic and governmental positions of exchange, which allow them to control, in varying degrees, the lives of other people. In order to distribute effectively this influence over community-wide affairs, community leaders must participate actively in influential organizations of a coordinated nature which are composed of representatives of different interest groups and organizations.[40]

The coordinating organization may vary in size according to the region or situation, but the centrality of its function does not. Coalitions should be established in the earliest possible stages of planning. Early involvement sends a signal to the community at large that their interests are being represented, thus increasing the chance for ownership; it also automatically activates informal channels of communication, which leads to heightened community awareness and commitment.[41]

THE POLITICS OF COALITIONS AND COMMUNITY POWER

Communities are political places. For decades, academics[42] and political commentators[43] alike have used the metaphor of a "game" to describe politics. For the moment, set aside your social, epidemiologic, and behavioral diagnostic information, take off your public health hat, and let us talk politics.

In politics, as in games, there are rules. The game metaphor is not meant to cast politics as either frivolous or negative. Politics lay out the informal rules for the exchange of ideas and the negotiations for competing priorities in any social system. Those who want to initiate activities in a community, health promotion programs for instance, need to be mindful of those rules. The political game has many rules, and those rules vary from community to community. Here are some practical principles that will give you a feel for the game and its rules.

1. *There are never enough resources to cover all the demands for resources.* Your program is, figuratively speaking, in a competitive market. Thus, not only does a program have to meet the professional practice standards the planner sets for it, it also must have attributes that appeal to decision makers and to a large segment of their constituents.

2. *Often, the ultimate decision as to what resources will be allocated to what demand are made by those who are not expert in the issues.* Therefore, special efforts need to be made to insure that decision makers are informed by credible experts as to the value of your project.

3. *Although decisions are sometimes influenced by the sheer weight of popular clamor, they are often influenced by effective penetration of the inner circle of the decision makers.* Therefore, program advocates need to know how to gain access to that inner circle.

Even the entry-level practitioner quickly realizes that failure to pay attention to these and other political issues can prevent the best of programs from getting off the ground or, once initiated, from being sustained. Most health workers, however, especially those employed by official or governmental agencies, are discouraged, if not forbidden, from taking what might be construed as political action. Often they are informed that their program activities should remain "independent" of politics. Legally, this means campaigning for a political candidate or lobbying for legislation is prohibited on work time or in the name of your organization. Practically, it means avoiding any appearance of using public funds to influence legislative or electoral decisions.

Among other things, coalitions address the political issues that inevitably surface in community work. Coalitions thus relieve agencies of direct political action, but they carry the burden of having to represent the indirect political interests of their several members. As such, the process of selecting coalition members requires careful thought.

The extent to which decision makers support specific policies or programs depends in large part on signals received from groups to be reckoned with. What are the characteristics of "groups to be reckoned with"? They are well organized, are capable of mobilizing the support of large or influential constituencies, and have a clear and appealing agenda.

In culling the literature in search of the sine qua non rules that guide health promotion planners in the process of coalition building, one finds a few.[44] More plentiful are examples of effective innovations in coalition building, each crafted to address the unique needs and sensitivities of a unique community.[45] The following are practical reminders to consider in establishing and nurturing a community health promotion coalition for a specific community; they are not guaranteed guidelines.

1 Clarify the Agenda. Many of the people capable of making a difference at the community level are already making a difference. Therefore, they are busy people and are very selective about taking on new projects and activities. The aim of the coalition, its agenda, must be clear and appealing to gain the attention and interest of these busy people. It must elicit in the prospective coalition member sentiments such as "this is really important" or "this agenda ties in with our mission" or "I've heard Dr. Martha Francis (influential community figure) talk about this issue." Just recall how discomforted you have been on the occasions you have had to sit through a meeting with a loose and nondescript agenda. In general, the more concrete and specific the coalition's goal, the better. Of course, if the goal is too specific, it discourages the formation of a broad constituency. Nevertheless, given the choice between a vague, motherhood-and-apple-pie goal and a precise, well-understood goal, it is better to negotiate the expansion of a specific goal to encompass other activities than it is to start with a general agenda that runs the risk of having universal but lukewarm appeal.[46]

2 Seek Broad Representation. A coalition can serve the community program in several ways: to plan, advise, and counsel as to the selection of program priorities; to carry out political actions and strategies; and to communicate with a variety of groups and organizations.

Clarifying the key role(s) of the coalition provides insight to the planners on the matter of recruitment. Nix[47] has identified the following types of leaders as relevant to community health programs: (1) top-level community influentials who legitimize the program, (2) subarea (neighborhood) leaders if the program includes more than one area, (3) key health leaders, (4) leaders of the most influential organizations or companies, (5) leaders of factions and those who can act as go-betweens or links to several groups, (6) leaders of the target population (opinion leaders who represent the underserved, minority groups and those at high risk), (7) specialists with skills and knowledge relevant to the goals of the program, and (8) officials who control or support health programs (mayor, health director, commissioner, etc.).

Coalitions should seek to include representation from two other influential groups: the media and religious groups. A formative evaluation of CDC's PATCH program found that the most successful PATCH communities had media representation on the core group (coalition).[48] In addition to the obvious advantage of having direct contact with a principal communication channel within the community and the political support that can bring, the skills of the media representative can be invaluable in planning media elements for the program. Others have demonstrated the influential role religious groups and leaders can have on establishing community health promotion programs.[49]

After Yogi Berra and his New York Yankee teammates won their fourth World Series in a row, Yogi is quoted as saying "this is *déjà vu* all over again!" Practitioners need to be wary of giving community members the impression that the community effort they are undertaking is a brand new idea that will be the answer to their prayers. The fact is that most communities are already organized, and there is a very good chance that many of them have been down this road before; some probably serve on other community groups that also have a health agenda. By demonstrating interest and respect for prior experience, the practitioner can capitalize on current and past experiences of coalition members.

3 Pay Attention to Details. Establishing a strong, representative coalition with a common agenda is one thing, managing that coalition is another. What will you do when you enter a room full of the community's most influential people?

- Do your homework. Generally, work goes better and faster when you know and understand the people you work with. Prior to your first meeting, find out about coalition members' interests and hobbies as well as their professional background and health concerns.
- Attention to the details of coalition meetings should be a priority. If at all possible, schedule meetings at the same location and a time most convenient for the majority of the group. The meeting room should be as comfortable and pleasant as possible. Depending on the norms of the group, planners could think of creative ways to provide refreshments or food as appropriate.

4 The Crucial First Meeting. The first meeting is the most important one. It sets the tone for the coalition and establishes a model for the meetings to follow. Consider these steps for the first meeting:

- Establish the content of the agenda by asking the question, "What do we want the coalition members to leave the meeting with?" For the first meeting, the agenda should accomplish four things: (1) clarify the problem and convey an awareness that there is potential to resolve it, (2) facilitate knowing everyone who is on the coalition, understand what they can and cannot do, (3) clarify for members why this activity is a worthwhile endeavor for their organization or group, and (4) convey that the group staffing the coalition is well organized.
- Begin the meeting with a round robin of self-introductions limited to name, title, and organization or group representation, and perhaps why each person came. Keep it short, there will be opportunities for more detailed discussion at two points later in the meeting.
- Following the brief introductions, a presentation should be given about

the proposed program or activity by a respected person in the community, one who is articulate and has been well briefed on the details of the program to date. The presentation should include a clear statement of the problem or goal that the program will address, using local data to document its importance. An effective strategy is to describe the likely long-term health, social, and economic effects on the community if *no action* is taken on the problem. Even better, paint a vision of community well-being if action is taken.

- Immediately following the presentation, ask for questions and discussion. Have program staff ready to assist with the question and discussion period if necessary. Don't just be open for new ideas and criticism, ask for them!
- After the discussion, repeat the round robin, but this time ask each coalition member to share her or his responses to questions such as:
  (a) What is the primary mission of my agency, organization, or group?
  (b) What is it about this problem or program that is linked to our mission or interests?
  (c) With regard to the problem or the program envisioned, what kinds of activities would be appropriate for my agency or organization?
  (d) What *can't* my agency or organization do?
  (e) Do you know of others who ought to be a part of this coalition?
- The final task is defined in part by the extent to which the coalition reaches agreement on the overall coalition agenda or program goal. If the tone of the meeting reflects a general consensus, the next step is to begin a systematic process to delineate the major tasks that need attention and to identify coalition members willing to take on those tasks. If there is still disagreement related to some aspect of the coalition agenda, those disagreements need to be clarified and resolved before moving on.

COMBINING AND SEQUENCING COMMUNITY ELEMENTS

Figure 8.1 displays the organizational framework for a community-based program for the prevention of drug abuse in Kansas City.[50] This chart provides an example of the types of activities in a community health promotion program; it shows the first four initiating steps (problem identification, leadership training, community coordination, and training of implementors); and it reflects the continuity and the flow of relationships in the program. The training activity highlighted in Figure 8.1 reinforces the point made in Chapter 6: assessing and strengthening community capacity, readiness, confidence, and skills are part of PROCEEDing from the planning process to the organizing and implementation process. Murry Ross, generally regarded as the father of postwar community organization practice,

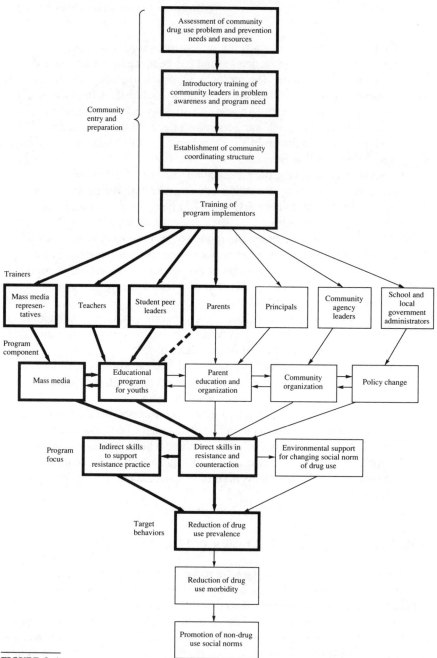

FIGURE 8.1

Organizational framework for a community program for primary prevention of
adolescent drug abuse. Training and program components progress from left to right
over a 6-year period. [From M. A. Pentz et al., *JAMA* 261 (1989, June 9): 3259–66,
with permission of the American Medical Association.]

considered increased community competence or problem-solving ability to be a defining characteristic of a community organization process.[51]

TERRITORIES: YOURS, MINE, AND OURS

Participation, coalitions, partnerships, training, technical assistance. These are the words of people working together. But they can be deceptively seductive words if they are accompanied by the illusion that close collaboration and cooperation are the automatic by-products of joining a coalition. Even with the shared goal of improving quality of life through effective disease prevention and health promotion, official agencies, voluntary and private organizations, health and other sectors compete with one another. For example, whether it is at the local, state/provincial, or national level, researchers compete with practitioners for limited resources. Likewise, although the voluntary cancer, heart, lung, diabetes, and other health organizations around the world have complementary prevention goals, they must compete with one another for donations from the community. Even within specific categorical areas of prevention, such as cancer or heart disease, organizations may be competing for prevention resources. If representatives of such competing organizations are a part of the same coalition, planners must maintain their sensitivity to the subtle, but very real, differences among those groups.[52]

MULTIPLE STRATEGIES: THE HALLMARK OF COMMUNITY INTERVENTION

Practitioners can use PRECEDE and PROCEED to untangle, understand, and develop the complex behavioral and environmental factors that influence health and quality of life. With an understanding and appreciation for the magnitude of that complexity, comes the realization that carefully planned multiple strategies, designed to influence both environmental forces and behavioral patterns at several levels within a community, are required for broad change to occur and to be sustained over time. In this section, we examine the application of multiple strategies for community interventions and call attention to some of the techniques practitioners have found helpful in selecting the most appropriate strategies for a given situation. Recognizing the growing role of mass communication in community health promotion programs, this section concludes by calling attention to key issues that practitioners need to take into account as they consider the use of mass media and social marketing.

APPLYING MULTIPLE STRATEGIES: A KENTUCKY CASE STUDY

Whether a program sets its sights on changing selected health status indicators of an entire population in a community or of some subpopulation therein, the need for using multiple strategies pertains. The literature is not wanting for examples of community-based interventions that report the use of multiple strategies; but it is comparatively lean on detailed accounts of those strategies and the principles that served as the basis for their selection and application.[53] A well-known community intervention study illustrates how these principles of selection and rationale for multiple intervention strategies have been put into action with beneficial results.

Kentucky is a rural state with high rates of mortality from cardiovascular disease and hypertension. As elsewhere, those with the least means bear a disproportionate burden of these preventable deaths. In an attempt to address this public health problem, Kotchen and her colleagues[54] carried out a community-based study in two adjacent, sparsely populated, rural Kentucky counties. The combined population of the two intervention counties was approximately 32,000; many of those residents lived in relative isolation. The population was predominantly white with adults having completed an average of 8 years of schooling. Coal mining is the major industry, but 20 percent of the men were unemployed, disabled, or retired.

Five-year results, comparing blood pressure outcomes in the intervention counties with those in a demographically similar county serving as a control, revealed significant decreases in both systolic and diastolic blood pressure in both men and women in the two intervention counties. These decreases were noted despite 5-year increases in age (increased age tends to correlate with increased blood pressure). Results showed that the intervention influenced improved medication compliance and, therefore, better control over hypertensive disease. The most striking outcome was the evidence linking the intervention effort to measurable declines in mortality. The 3-year moving averages for cardiovascular death rates, showing declines in the two intervention counties and no change in the control county, are presented in Figure 8.2.

The Program. What did Kotchen and her co-workers do to achieve such a dramatic public health success? Their activities included:

1. Hiring a full-time coordinator who was enthusiastic and energetic, and who was respected by and knew the community.
2. Establishing a Community High Blood Pressure Control Program Council with the charge to provide direction to community-wide high blood pressure control activities. Council membership included representatives from public schools, the Cooperative Agricultural Extension Service, local health departments, local medical society, businesses, and interested citizens.

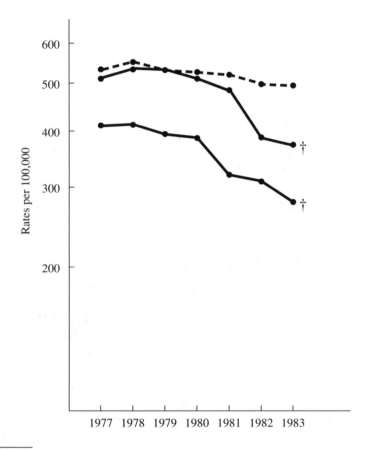

FIGURE 8.2

Three-year moving averages for cardiovascular disease death rates by year for two intervention counties and one control county (1983 rates are based on 2-year moving averages). Control county, $\cdots$; intervention counties, —— . Significant decline in mortality ($P_1.0004$), indicated by †. Mortality trend coefficient for the intervention counties is significantly different from that of the control county ($P_1.04$). [From J. M. Kotchen, H. E. McKean, S. Jackson-Thayer et al., *JAMA* 255 (1986): 2177–82, with permission of the American Medical Association.]

3. Using, wherever possible, existing resources and organizations to play a major role in the delivery and promotion of the program.
4. Expanding an existing hypertension registry within the health department to include those persons in the intervention counties identified as having high blood pressure. These individuals received periodic mailings of information on high blood pressure control, risk

reduction, and community resources and activities that might be of interest to them.

5. Using the Cooperative Extension Service Nutrition Aide Program, already established in the community, as the channel to provide cardiovascular risk reduction assistance to those identified by their physicians as being in greatest need.

6. Developing a 4-H Club cardiovascular risk reduction program in which teenagers used peer teaching techniques to present educational lessons to fifth graders.

7. Introducing a school blood pressure screening program into two high schools to identify adolescents with high blood pressure.

8. Establishing a volunteer blood pressure screening and monitoring network in the smaller churches and in businesses in the area. This network provided outreach to individuals within these organizations and to the residents in close proximity.

9. Adding a worksite high blood pressure screening program to an existing screening program provided by local health departments.

10. Securing the support of the local newspapers and radio stations as a means to reach the community as a whole with information about cardiovascular disease risk factors and benefits and the feasibility of reducing those risks. Although the project did purchase some air time, most of the media coverage was either news or was donated.

11. Promoting continuing education programs for nurses.

12. Presenting health education programs to community clubs, homemaker groups, county fairs, health fairs, and large family reunions, which are a tradition in rural Kentucky.

Implications for the Practitioner. The use of multiple activities in the Kentucky program is evident. How did they arrive at choosing that particular combination of strategies? The principal outcome the program planners wanted to affect was the blood pressure level of those at highest risk. Yet, as evident by the list of activities, their program was generally aimed at the entire community with special elements *strategically* aimed at the high-risk portion of the community. The expansion and activation of the health department hypertension registry was an especially effective method because it provided a channel through which *direct contact* could be made with those at high risk.

One of the main reasons planners need to be thorough in the behavioral and the educational/organizational diagnostic phases of PRECEDE is that such thoroughness increases the chances for detecting the critical targets for change. In the Kentucky case, the target behavior, keeping blood pressure under control, is obvious; it prevents strokes and saves lives! The more immediate targets—predisposing, enabling, and reinforcing behavior conducive to blood pressure control—become the factors that shaped the program.

Recall in Chapter 4 the discussion of the broken-appointment cycle (Fig. 4.1). The ultimate effect of the broken-appointment was a specific, problematic behavior: "not taking medications." By retracing the loops in the cycle, we see a combination of attitudinal, environmental, and behavioral barriers that would stop most of us in our tracks. The registry provided a means to make contact with known hypertensives, and to encourage and reinforce them in using their medications and practicing risk-reduction behaviors, including coming into the health department or going to their physicians for blood pressure checks. Social support for their behavior came at three levels: (1) positive reinforcement from the nurses in the health department and/or their physician, (2) messages in direct mail, and (3) the social norm endorsing risk reduction manifested by media, church activities, the cooperative extension service, school programs, community fairs, and their families. The Minnesota Heart Health Program also found that inexpensive mailouts were beneficial as a follow-up method for high blood pressure screening programs.[55]

Well-planned and grounded in sound theory, the Kentucky plan also gave thoughtful consideration to the practical implementation questions asked in the PROCEED process. This program had no "high tech," expensive program components.[56] Although there were direct costs (materials, special training, and travel) and indirect costs (volunteer time and participant time at screens), the costs for the intervention components were quite modest. Not that they could easily be replicated—good planning and intervention are anything but easy—but cost should not be a prohibitive factor for replication of this kind of program in rural areas.

The Kentucky team observed a change in the perception of hypertension by community physicians: that it was indeed an important health problem. The team also suspected that this change in perception was a precursor to the subsequent support of the program by the community physicians.[57] The project, and its multiple activities, apparently heightened physician attention to this modifiable public health problem. This, in turn, resulted in rather undramatic but influential and widespread changes in physician interactions with patients regarding hypertension and cardiovascular disease risk factors.

CROSS-CULTURAL VALIDATION OF COMMUNITY INTERVENTION

Misery loves company, but so does hope. Those who plan comprehensive community health education and health promotion programs should find comfort in the clear similarities between the intervention approach used in Kentucky and the model of community intervention used in North Karelia, Finland. Figure 8.3 presents a schema of the North Karelia model, described as follows:

COMMUNITY

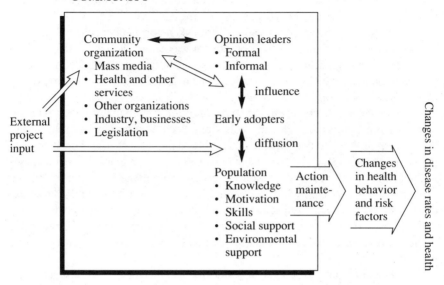

FIGURE 8.3

Model of community intervention in the North Karelia project. [From P. Puska, A. Nissinen, J. Tuomilehto et al., *Annual Reviews of Public Health* 6 (1985): 147–93, printed with permission of the publisher.]

The external input from the project affects the community both through mass media communication to the population at large (where its effect is mediated through interpersonal communication) and even more so through formal and informal opinion leaders acting as change agents to influence various aspects of community organization. This two-pronged approach is aimed at increasing knowledge, at persuasion, at teaching practical skills, and at providing the necessary social skills in the population. The acquisition and maintenance of new behaviors ultimately leads to a more favorable risk factor profile, reduced disease rates and improved health.[58]

These two intervention programs used similar approaches to planning and organizing, on opposite sides of the world in two markedly different cultures, and both produced dramatic public health benefits. The actual methods and specific messages inevitably differ from one situation to another, but the program components are similar: community participation, program management, communication, education, training, and environmental supports through policy, regulation, and organization.

Similar community health promotion models have evolved in the application of multiple strategies at multiple levels in the UCLA Prevention Research Center[59] and in the Kaiser Family Foundation Community Health Promotion Grant Program,[60] as shown by the flow chart in Figure 8.4.

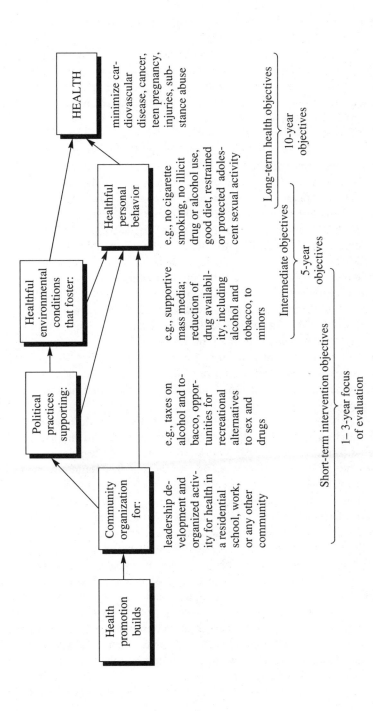

FIGURE 8.4

The sequence of relationships from community health promotion to health outcomes. [Adapted for Kaiser Family Foundation, *Stragetic Plan for Health Promotion Program* (Menlo Park, CA: Kaiser Family Foundation, 1989) from L. Breslow, *Annual Review of Public Health* 11 (1990): 20.]

TECHNIQUES FOR SELECTING MULTIPLE STRATEGIES IN THE FIELD

Since the mid-1980s, numerous efforts have been made to translate the intervention ideas developed in scientific, university-led community trials into practical community-led applications in the field. Many of those translation efforts generated practical tools to help planners in the identification and application of multiple strategies for intervention. A few of those are reviewed here.

In 1983, the Centers for Disease Control (CDC) developed a program called the Planned Approach to Community Health (PATCH).[61] PATCH is grounded in the diagnostic planning principles of PRECEDE and is designed to translate the complex methods of community intervention to communities via the state health agency. All PATCH training goes on at the community level, in vivo, and involves the collaborative efforts of health promotion staff from the local and state health departments, from CDC, and from local community participants. Within this partnership context, methods in community mobilization, community diagnosis, and intervention are covered in considerable detail. It takes about a year and a half for a PATCH community to move from the community mobilization and diagnosis process to the first intervention. In the PATCH training process, the concept of multiple strategies is introduced by using the framework shown in Figure 8.5. This technique was refined by public health specialists at the Center for Health Promotion Research and Development, University of Texas Health Science Center at Houston.[62] The health department is identified in the box to the left because it usually has the primary responsibility for coordinating intervention activity in PATCH.[63] The diagram focuses the planner's attention on three levels of strategic action: (1) governmental, (2) organizational, and (3) individual.

Suppose the health outcome of interest is a specific reduction in the number of automobile fatalities by a given time. Planners would first turn their attention to the boxes (see Fig. 8.5) under *Actions for intervention* and would translate those general activities into concrete examples, taking into account the circumstances of their locality. For example, if the community is part of a state or province that requires seat-belt use but the law is not enforced, a strategy to promote enforcement could be specified under *Governmental change*. Establishing a responsible beverage-service training program or a designated-driver program for those establishments that serve alcohol over-the-counter could be an activity in the *Organizational change* category. The immediate action under *Environmental and personal conditions* might be to have the participating establishments adopt designated-driver policies, provide incentives for adoption, and avail their employees of responsible beverage-service training programs. Working through this framework is a simple but effective way to help planners think not only in terms of multiple strategies but also in terms of the multiple levels of governmental and organizational systems that can either facilitate or impede implementation.

Once PATCH community-change agents are comfortable with the concept of three levels of change, they are introduced to another planning tool, the interven-

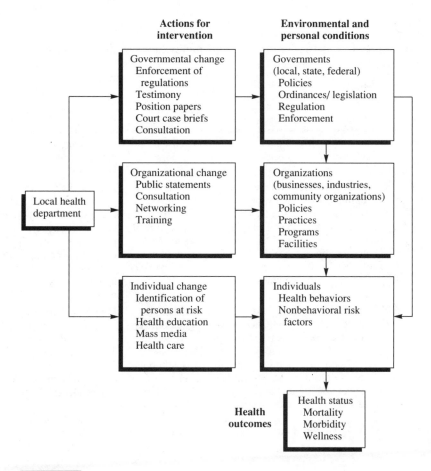

Actions for
intervention

Environmental and
personal conditions

Local health
department

Governmental change
Enforcement of
regulations
Testimony
Position papers
Court case briefs
Consultation

Governments
(local, state, federal)
Policies
Ordinances/ legislation
Regulation
Enforcement

Organizational change
Public statements
Consultation
Networking
Training

Organizations
(businesses, industries,
community organizations)
Policies
Practices
Programs
Facilities

Individual change
Identification of
persons at risk
Health education
Mass media
Health care

Individuals
Health behaviors
Nonbehavioral risk
factors

Health
outcomes

Health status
Mortality
Morbidity
Wellness

FIGURE 8.5

Local health departments' role in community-based risk reduction. (Centers for Disease Control and University of Texas Center for Health Promotion Research and Development, 1988)

tion matrix (Table 8.1). The three levels of change (government, organizational, and individual) are positioned on the vertical axis of the matrix; the general settings (school, worksite, health-care institution, and community) in which various strategies are likely to reach specific target populations are identified along the horizontal axis. The matrix was designed as a means to identify both the existing resources and the gaps for the prospective health promotion program.

Planners need to identify these settings more specifically (*which* schools, worksites, clinics, hospitals) and might expand the variety of settings depending

TABLE 8.1

Intervention planning matrix, used in the Community Intervention Handbooks
and in the CDC PATCH program

| Target | Setting | | | |
	School	Worksite	Health-care institution	Community
Individuals	Students' health behaviors	Employees' health behaviors	Patients' health behaviors	Community residents' health behaviors
Organizations	School policies, programs, practices, and facilities to foster healthful behaviors by students	Worksite policies, programs, practices, and facilities to foster healthful behaviors by employees	Institution policies, programs, practices, and facilities to foster healthful behaviors by patients	Policies, programs, practices, and facilities of community-serving organizations and institutions to foster healthful behaviors by community residents
Governments	Legislation, regulation, services, and resources affecting schools to foster healthful behaviors by students	Legislation, regulation, services, and resources affecting worksites to foster healthful behaviors by employees	Legislation, regulation, services, and resources affecting institutions to foster healthful behaviors by patients	Legislation, regulation, services, and resources affecting community sites to foster healthful behaviors by community residents

SOURCE: S. G. Brink, D. Simons-Morton, G. Parcel, and K. Tiernan, *Family and Community Health* 11 (1988): 28–35.

on the problem in question. In many areas, for example, exercise facilities,[64] religious institutions,[65] health fairs,[66] bars and restaurants,[67] and grocery stores[68] can be critical settings for health promotion activity. In rural areas, outreach to the home may be necessary.[69]

To aid in seeing the relationships between the earlier planning principles of PRECEDE and PROCEED and the selection of intervention strategies, the PATCH planners work through an exercise that leads to an integrated summary chart, similar to that in Table 8.2. In this example, the PATCH community chose the reduction of motor vehicle fatalities as the health problem and seat-belt nonuse and driving under the influence of alcohol or drugs as the primary behaviors; poorly marked and lighted streets and seat-belt laws that were unenforced were the primary environmental problems. Table 8.2 combines the intervention variables of site and actions for interventions with diagnostic information generated from

TABLE 8.2

Summary Matrix

Health Problem: To reduce motor vehicle fatalities

Behavioral Problems: Driving under the influence
                      Not using seat-belts

Environmental Problems: Poorly marked and poorly lighted streets
                         Poorly enforced seat-belt law

	Intervention factors		Diagnostic factors	
Strategies	Site	Action for intervention	Contributing factors	Adoption stage
BEHAVIORAL PROBLEMS				
Driving under the influence				
Lobby concerning state liquor laws	C	LR	E	Sk
Substance-free high-school graduation party	S	En	P/E/R	Aw/Sk/R
Poster contest in middle schools	S	Ed	P/R	Aw/R
Bartender education	W	Ed	E	Sk
Substance-free events for teens	C/S	En	P/E/R	R/Mn
Education and community work assignments for those convicted of driving under the influence	H/C	Ed	E/R	Sk/Mn
News media events	C	Ed	P/E	Aw/Mn
Not using seat-belts				
Poster contest in elementary school	S	Ed	P/R	Aw/R
Seat-belt use required in company car	W	LR	E	Sk
Buckle-up contest in high school	S	Ed	P/R	Mo/Mn
Buckle-up signs on major roads	C	Ed		Aw/R
Seat belts in school buses	C	En	E	Sk
Installation Saturday (to install seat belts on cars lacking them)	C	En	E	Sk
News media events	C	Ed	P/E	Aw/Mn
ENVIRONMENTAL PROBLEMS				
Conduct and publicize findings from study of hazards in areas of high fatality	C	En/Ed	E	Aw
Lobby local activities for improved markings and lighting	C	LR/Ed	E	Mn/Sk
Pressure local authorities to enforce seat-belt law	C	LR/Ed	E	Mn/Sk

NOTE: Letter symbols denote the following. *Site*: C=community, H=health care, W=worksite, S=school. *Action for intervention*: Ed=educational, En=environmental, LR=legislative/regulatory. *Contributing factors*: E=enabling, P=predisposing, R=reinforcing. *Adoption stage*: Aw= awareness, Mn=maintenance, Mo=motivation, Sk=skills.

the PRECEDE process and from theory – in this case, the theory of stages of self-change.[70]

These types of matrix techniques have several uses: to take an inventory of existing resources, to help set priorities for new strategies or for fund raising where resources are lacking, and to serve as heuristic devices to expand the perspective of planners who have limited experience in community work. It is not uncommon to hire a talented practitioner to coordinate a community health promotion program – a person whose prior health education experience may have been focused in a given setting, perhaps in schools or working with clinic patients. Working through and understanding the rationale of intervention matrices can call attention to the need for regulatory or media approaches that otherwise may not have come to mind.

Another useful application of the matrix approach is to apply or "test" other theoretical assumptions (e.g., in the *Adoption stage* column in Table 8.2).[71] Such an exercise of theory application can give the planner insight as to what the proposed intervention should include. Consider the following example.

Prochaska and DiClemente's "stages of change" model operates on the assumption that people do not change chronic behaviors all at once. That is, smokers don't just stop smoking, nor do sedentary persons suddenly become active; instead, they change their habitual behavior continuously through four stages: (1) *precontemplation*, a condition in which people have expressed no interest in or are not thinking about change; (2) *contemplation*, the period in which serious thought is given to change; (3) *action*, the 6-month period after an overt effort to change has been made, and (4) *maintenance*, the period from 6 months after a behavior change until the behavioral problem in question is completely terminated. By considering this model in relation to the last column of the intervention matrix, the practitioner is sensitized to the notion that different change strategies are required depending on which stage of change people are in. According to Prochaska, the vast majority of prevention programs are designed for the small minority of the people who are in the "action" stage. Using national survey data, he estimated that among those who were smokers in 1985, their 1986 "stages" were as follows:

> . . . 4% were in the maintenance stage, 12% were in action, 15% were ready for action, 34% in contemplation and 35% in the precontemplation stage. Even with a health behavior that has received the most publicity, has the greatest consensus about its deleterious consequences, and has 10,000,000 served by the National Cancer Institute intervention projects alone, nearly 70% of the smokers are not ready to take action on their own.[72]

Another way to view the stages in the psychological process of change is in relation to the major forces operating on or within the individual at the time. Diffusion and adoption theory, discussed in previous chapters, divides the process of individual change into four phases: awareness, interest, trial, and adoption.

TABLE 8.3

Features of the community supporting each phase of the psychological process of change

Phase in psychological process of change		Supporting features of the community
1 Exposure ↓	←	Social setting with acess to media
2 Attention ↓	←	Interest of family, peers, and other significant persons
3 Comprehension ↓	←	Group discussion and feedback, question-and-answer sessions
4 Belief ↓	←	Direct persuasion and social influence, actions of informal leaders
5 Decision ↓	←	Group decision making, public commitments, repeated encouragements which build self-confidence
6 Learning	←	Demonstration and guided practice with feedback and continued confidence, advice and directed assistance

SOURCE: L. W. Green and A. M. McAlister, *Health Education Quarterly* 11 (1984): 322–39, printed by permission of publisher.

These can be further refined to the six phases shown in Table 8.3, along with features of the community that can be developed or mobilized to support the individual at each phase.

Assuming the validity of the stages-of-change and stages-of-adoption models, what are the implications for the practitioner who is unaware that a substantial portion of the target population is *not ready for action*? One would be the tendency to overestimate what could realistically be achieved, especially if the interventions are directed at the stages in which the fewest people exist at the time of the program. Program failure can result from misapplication of relevant theory just as surely as from improper execution or inappropriate measurement.[73]

Acknowledging the importance of coordinating multiple intervention strategies, Preston, Baranowski, and Higginbotham[74] devised a practical scheme to aid practitioners in the selection of those strategies. Using diffusion and adoption of innovations as their primary theory base, they begin by identifying eight generic points of community intervention. Table 8.4 illustrates the eight points in the context of an example of a dietary change. The ordering of the eight points of intervention (1–8) moves from methods that are employed primarily for heightening awareness, then to those that can transmit messages about reasons for change and to potential early adopters, and eventually to skills enhancement and changes in community standards.

Major media was defined as newspapers, radio, and television intended to

TABLE 8.4
Types of intervention and segments of the community likely to be reached

Types of community intervention	Early adopters	Early majority	Late majority
1 Major media			
Newspaper	X	X	
Radio	X	X	
Cablevision and television	X	X	X
2 Minor media			
Church newsletters	X	X	X
Employer newsletters	X	X	
Customer bill inserts	X	X	
3 Institutional intervention			
(Supermarkets, grocery stores, restaurants, fast food stores)			
Point of purchase information	X	X	X
Making more food available	X	X	X
Grocery bag inserts	X	X	X
Taste testing	X	X	X
4 Special events			
Health screening events in churches, grocery stores	X	X	X
Cooking contests	X	X	
5 Existing formal social structures and networks			
Occupation-based programs	X	X	
Churches	X	X	
Community, fraternities, sororities			X
Medical care delivery	X		
Schools	X	X	X
6 Existing informal social networks			
Living room sessions (education and taste testing) with family invited participants (Tupperware Party concept)		X	X
Events in service centers, beauty and barber shops, neighborhood action committees		X	X
Training community lay health advisors		X	X
7 Center-based programs			
Test kitchen taste testing of new versions of recipes	X	X	X
8 Created social networks			
Developing a ward or block system		X	X

SOURCE: M. A. Preston et al., *International Quarterly of Community Health Education* 9 (1988–89): 11–34, printed by permission of publisher.

reach large audiences. *Minor media* included newsletters, bulletins, and other notices targeted at specific audiences because of their membership in a group. *Institutional interventions* (to affect ongoing behavior patterns) was defined as efforts to focus interventions on the institution in which a behavior is likely to take place — such as restaurant for eating, tavern or pub for drinking alcohol, grocery store for buying food. *Special events* are those designed to create heightened public awareness and attention to a problem or program; they often involve celebrities or prizes. *Formal social networks* include community organization such as churches, fraternal groups, worksites, or schools. *Informal social networks* are those characterized by informal but frequent neighborhood or friendship gatherings; *center-based* points of intervention are those where professional staff provide services or programs, as in universities, clinics, or fitness centers.

The different points of intervention have varying effects on persons at different stages of the community adoption process. Attention also must be paid to the sequencing and timing of those points of intervention. In the PROCEED process highlighted in previous chapters, time was a critical element in assessing the barriers and facilitators for program implementation. The multiple interventions of a program do not explode onto the scene all at once. Based on a variety of factors, including the theoretical underpinnings of the program, the various intervention components need to be *timed* to address the strategic objectives of the program.

In Table 8.5, Preston and her colleagues present a timeline for the implementation of interventions, again using dietary change as the example.

> The timing of the intervention strategy, therefore, takes into consideration four general purposes for the program: public awareness, the introduction of information and reasons for change into the established social system for earlier adopters, the enhancement of skills needed to make desired changes, and the modeling of new behaviors for later adopters.[75]

Note how staging intervention components in terms of their timing for intervention in part addresses the central concern raised in DiClemente and Prochaska's stages-of-change model. Working with individuals in one-to-one counseling or teaching relationships makes such staging relatively easy because the readiness of the learner can be more readily detected or inferred. But in community health promotion, generalizations must be made about where the population lies on the continuum, or more accurately, how the population distributes over the stages of change at a given time in the course of the program.

REACHING THE MASSES

It is almost impossible to find a community intervention program devoid of one or a combination of the following mass-media strategies: television, radio, newspapers, magazines, outdoor advertising, transit advertising, direct mail, tele-

TABLE 8.5
Timeline for intervention strategy

Type of intervention	Six months prior to intervention						Six months of intervention					
	1	2	3	4	5	6	1	2	3	4	5	6
Center based												
Test kitchen	P	P	P	P	P	P						
Ongoing behavior, grocery stores												
Food purchasing			P	P	P	E	E	E	E	E	E	E
Shelf labeling					P	P	I	I	I	I	I	I
Food tasting	P	P	P	P	P	P	I	I	I	I	I	I
Ongoing behavior, restaurants												
Additional menu selections	P	P	P	P	P	E	E	E	E	E	E	E
Menu labeling						I	I	I	I	I	I	I
Major media												
Newspaper						P	A	N	N	N	N	N
Radio						P	A	N	N	N	N	N
Television						P	A	N	N	N	N	N
Minor media												
Paycheck inserts						P	A	A	A			
Newsletter notices						P	A	N	N	N	N	N
Screening handouts						P	A	A				
Grocery bag stuffers						P	A	A	A	A	A	A
Special events												
Cooking contests						P	A	A				
Public health screenings						P	A	A				
Formal structures												
Group intervention	P	P	P	P	P	P	B	B	B	B		
Informal structures												
Group network intervention	P	P	P	P	P	P				B	B	B

NOTE: P=preparation, A=public awareness (media), N=notification (media), I=information dissemination, E=enabling behavior changes, B=behavior change (educational sessions).EP
SOURCE: M. A. Preston, T. Baranowski, and J. C. Higginbotham, *International Quarterly of Health Education* 9 (1988–1989): 11–34, reprinted by permission of publisher.

marketing, and special promotional events. The application of mass-media techniques is second only to the activation of community participation through community organization and coalition building as a critical element in community intervention. The literature is abundant with detailed accounts of large-scale national or regional public health applications,[76] applications at the community level,[77] and the theoretical rationale for planning and implementing mass-media strategies.[78]

This explosion of interest in mass-media techniques by health promotion practitioners is an international phenomenon, which in part confirms Richard Manoff's assumptions about the power and utility of mass media in health promotion. He identified seven beneficial characteristics of mass media[79]:

1. Mass media carry special authority—that which is seen in the cinema or on television, heard on the radio, or read in the paper has special impact.
2. Mass media assure control over the message—since the content and tone of the health messages are critical, the most desirable means of communication is the one that guarantees that whatever, whenever, and from whomever the message comes it will be the same.
3. Media lend cumulative impact to the message—the whole program is more than the arithmetic sum of the parts; mass media create a communications synergism.
4. Mass media reach the masses.
5. Mass media telescope time—they have maximum further-faster capacity.
6. Mass media influence other major audiences in important ways while directing a message to the target audience—even though a seat-belt message may be targeted at middle-aged males, others who are exposed to the message (wife, children, co-workers) can serve to reinforce the message or may themselves be influenced to consider action.
7. The mass-media campaign enhances all other methods employed in health education—it provides an umbrella for attention to the issue.

A Su Salud (To Your Health) is a mass-media health promotion program designed to reduce selected chronic-disease risks factors among Mexican Americans in southwest Texas.[80] The smoking cessation element of the mass-media program provides an excellent example of how theory and data are used in the planning process. Data generated from formative evaluation methods, especially focus groups, were combined with two theories: (1) Bandura's conceptualization of social modeling and social support[81] and (2) the previously cited stages-of-change theory.

In developing the community organization components of the program, the community supports identified earlier in Table 8.3 were mobilized through active involvement of community groups and institutions. In developing the media

TABLE 8.6

Features of communications supporting each phase of individual response to mass media

Phase in psychological process of change		Supporting features of the community
1 Exposure ↓	←	Use of most popular media of communication, program repetition
2 Attention ↓	←	Message relevance, attractiveness, novelty, drama, humor, and suspense
3 Comprehension ↓	←	Use of simple concepts with illustration and analogy
4 Belief ↓	←	Expert and trustworthy sources, counterarguments refuted
5 Decision ↓	←	Display of incentives and values of different consequences of action, messages enhancing self-confidence
6 Learning	←	Step-by-step demonstrations, guides for practice and feedback, repetition

SOURCE: L. W. Green and A. L. McAlister, *Health Education Quarterly* 11 (1984): 322–39, printed by permission of publisher.

components of *A Su Salud*, the supporting features of communications associated with each stage were developed as shown in Table 8.6.

Table 8.7 summarizes the three general stages of change, specifically for smoking cessation, and gives examples of role-model messages for each stage as developed in the mass-media component of *A Su Salud*. Residents of the Mexican-American community were recruited among those enrolled in smoking cessation programs. Scripts were developed for narrators to highlight the messages shown in the table as they were stated in the words of the community residents.

SOCIAL MARKETING: A CREDIBLE PART OF THE WHOLE

Most definitions of social marketing characterize it as a system or process, using a research base, to bring about the adoption or acceptability of ideas or practices. Lefebvre and Flora[82] accept that general description but find it useful to explain the social marketing process in terms of eight specific components.

1. Consumer orientation: A focus on the needs and interests of the target population
2. Voluntary exchanges: The assumption that adoption of new ideas or practices involves the voluntary exchange of some resource (money, services, time) for a perceived benefit

TABLE 8.7

Broad categories of the stages of change and the corresponding examples of media messages provided by role models on television in the *A Su Salud* project in southwest Texas

Three stages of smoking cessation	Examples provided by role models
I Preparation	
Information about smoking: decisional balance Dissatisfaction with dependence on cigarettes	"I decided to quit because I was pregnant. It's OK to risk my own life, but not my unborn child." "I wanted to be here [living] to see my children grown."
II Taking action	
Positive efficacy expectations Social support and reinforcement for nonsmoking Reevaluation of self	"My husband supported my decision and he joined me in the decision to stop smoking." "I physically feel better, less fatigued, less tense. I feel better."
III Maintenance	
Increasing efficacy expectations for specific situations Avoiding stimuli associated with smoking Acquisition of new coping responses General social support for stress-coping	"In social situations, I would review the reasons why I quit smoking . . ." "When nervous due to not smoking, I would talk to someone or eat a piece of candy."

SOURCE: A. G. Ramirez and A. L. McAlister, *Preventive Medicine* 17 (1988): 608–21, printed by permission of the publisher.

3. Audience analysis and segmentation: The application of qualitative research methods to obtain information on the needs and special characteristics of the target population, which has been segmented to permit greater specificity of the message

4. Formative research: Message design and pretesting of materials to be used in campaign

5. Channel analysis: The identification of the various channels of communication including media outlets, community organizations, businesses, and "life-path points"

6. Marketing mix: The process of identifying the product, price, place, and promotion characteristics of intervention planning and implementation

7. Process tracking: A system to track the delivery of the program and to assess the utilization trends; a critical evaluation tool

8. Management: A commitment to a coordinated management system to assure quality of planning, implementation, and feedback functions

Quantitative health data, so essential in measuring the severity of a problem and in assessing the effects of a program, are rarely available to give the planner insights into why a target population resists the adoption of certain actions. It is the consumer-oriented aspect of the social marketing process that makes it so complementary to epidemiologic data and, therefore, so relevant for planning an intervention. Some examples help illustrate the point.

Smith and Scammon conducted a market segment analysis to examine the beliefs and perceptions adults have that may influence their exercise behavior. They found that (1) people were generally misinformed about the frequency, intensity, and duration of activity needed to obtain a cardiovascular benefit; (2) one's doctor is the "most important" source of information regarding exercise; and (3) subjects did not perceive the health benefits of exercise to be as influential as the intrinsic psychological or emotional benefits.[83] These findings obviously have much to contribute to health promotion programs seeking to increase physical activity in the population.

Considerable attention has been paid to the creative use of social marketing methods in the major cardiovascular community-intervention trials. The effective application of social marketing to health promotion is by no means limited to affluent media markets, however. Brieger, Ramakrishna, and Adeniyi[84] made an especially creative application of social marketing research in a health promotion program aimed at controlling dracunculiasis (guinea worm) in Idere, Nigeria. They combined key principles of community participation with social marketing strategies in an attempt to increase the use of filters as a means of protection against guinea worm infection. They took steps to insure that people from the participating towns and hamlets became involved in the planning process. Based on results from qualitative research efforts, including focus groups, a program was established wherein local tailors made the cloth that was used to filter the water, other community members got involved in debating the price, and still others became salespersons. Figure 8.6 illustrates their model of integrating community involvement with the application of social marketing principles.

There are other recent examples of social marketing strategies effectively applied in developing countries. A University of South Carolina team together with Ivory Coast collaborators[85] used focus groups as a cost-effective way to obtain rich and valid information that led to improvements in controlling childhood diarrhea and malaria in sub-Saharan Africa. Another group[86] used social marketing research to increase contraceptive use in Bangladesh. Gordon[87] showed that the coordination of a national media campaign with a well-planned community intervention effort was effective in addressing the problem of dengue fever in the Dominican Republic.

Irrespective of where they are on the globe, public health workers need to

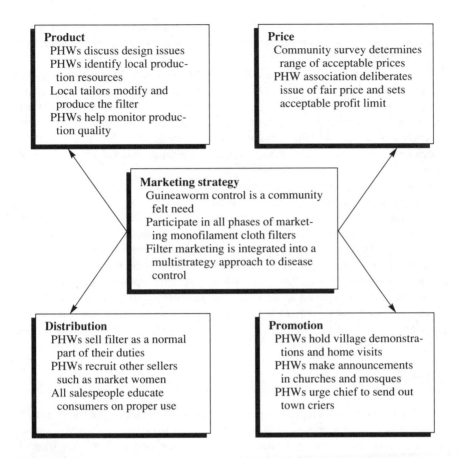

Product
PHWs discuss design issues
PHWs identify local produc-
tion resources
Local tailors modify and
produce the filter
PHWs help monitor produc-
tion quality

Price
Community survey determines
range of acceptable prices
PHW association deliberates
issue of fair price and sets
acceptable profit limit

Marketing strategy
Guineaworm control is a community
felt need
Participate in all phases of marketing monofilament cloth filters
Filter marketing is integrated into a
multistrategy approach to disease
control

Distribution
PHWs sell filter as a normal
part of their duties
PHWs recruit other sellers
such as market women
All salespeople educate
consumers on proper use

Promotion
PHWs hold village demonstrations and home visits
PHWs make announcements
in churches and mosques
PHWs urge chief to send out
town criers

FIGURE 8.6

Community involvement in social marketing of monofilament nylon-cloth water filters
for guinea worm control in Idere, Nigeria. [From W. R. Brieger, J. Ramakrishna, and
J. D. Adeniyi, *International Quarterly of Community Health Education* 8 (1987–1988):
297–316.]

become more skilled in the methods and techniques of health communications,
mass media, and social marketing. This is not to imply that such skills are a
panacea; however, increasingly consumer-oriented competition for media attention from all sectors of the market make social marketing research methods an
essential part of the practitioner's health promotion portfolio.

Developing a trusting contact with those whose culture, language, or beliefs
differ from one's own is a complex task that takes resources: time, money, and
skill. Planners must argue and budget for the first two; they must be in possession

of the third! Practitioners with competence in the application of social marketing research methods gain special insight for more precise program planning and implementation.

Yet, there remain large gaps in our ability to reach individuals at high risk who are in great need of preventive services and education. In some instances, where we are able to reach those at high risk, our methods of communications are ineffective. For the most part, these gaps continue not because of a lack of practitioners' desire and efforts to close them. They continue because of glaring deficiencies in communication and education training, cultural sensitivity, and resources available to health organizations.

As always, the literature is the primary means for responsible practitioners to stay abreast of innovations. Yet, the multidimensional complexity of the health promotion task does not lend itself to easy translation via the unidimensional written word. Even the most artful wordsmith cannot capture all of the subtleties "that make a difference." Those government and private sector institutions responsible for public health training have not kept pace with the methodological demands of the practitioner. Accessible training systems that work with trainees in the community are needed to facilitate the rapid translation of new methods, including social marketing, to those who need it most: front line prevention practitioners.

SUMMARY

This chapter has placed emphasis again on the issue of community participation. It has addressed the differences between interventions in communities and community interventions. Some guidelines are offered for engaging the realities of community politics. Some practical concepts to help practitioners in the formation of a coalition are suggested as are ideas for initially working with that coalition. The notion of multiple strategies for community intervention was examined first through a rural community intervention case study and then by reviewing some practical intervention planning techniques. Finally, this chapter considered mass media and social marketing as strategic tools for use in community-based health promotion work and offered examples and suggestions for their application.

EXERCISES

1. What is the difference between community intervention and interventions in a community? Why is it important to make that distinction?
2. Based on your interpretation of the forces of change in Mississippi, what should planners look for over the long term as a result of well-planned community-based interventions?

3. What is the paradox that major university-based community intervention trials have faced?
4. Consider any one of the following problems as the focus of a planned program effort: alcohol-related injuries and death, dracunculiasis, smoking, or AIDS. Name two political issues that planners might face if they were to try a community intervention in *your home town*. Explain how you would keep those issues from becoming a problem.
5. In terms of relevant theory, explain why the Kentucky program worked, in terms of social learning theory.
6. Apply the social marketing steps and the intervention matrix to your own program plan.
7. Suppose someone said to you: "Marketing is Madison Avenue glitz, great for selling cars and beer, but there's no place for it in health science. Besides, it just focuses on the individual, which is victim blaming!" What would your response be?

REFERENCES AND NOTES

1. B. A. Israel, "Social Networks and Social Support: Implications for Natural Helper and Community Level Interventions," *Health Education Quarterly* 12 (1985): 65–80, quotation from p. 72. *Sense of community* is defined and developed more fully in J. Allen and R. F. Allen, "A Sense of Community, a Shared Vision and a Positive Culture: Core Enabling Factors in Successful Culture-based Change," in *Community Organization: Traditional Principles and Modern Applications*, R. D. Patton and W. B. Cissel, eds. (Johnson City, TN: Latchpins Press, 1990), pp. 5–18; D. M. Chavis, J. H. Hogge, D. W. McMillan, and A. Wandersman, "Sense of Community through Brunswik's Lens: A First Look," *Journal of Community Psychology* 14 (1986): 24–40; D. M. Chavis and A. Wandersman, "Sense of Community in the Urban Environment: A Catalyst for Participation and Community Development," *American Journal of Community Psychology* 18 (1990): 55–81; D. W. McMillan and D. M. Chavis, "Sense of Community: A Definition and Theory," *Journal of Community Psychology* 14 (1986): 6–23.

2. Even though we have consciously separated community-based approaches from those carried out at the national, provincial or state levels, the positive, complementary effect that national and regional level policies and campaigns have on local efforts should not be minimized. In fact, when appropriate and feasible, community-based programs should try to time their interventions in coordination with larger population campaigns to obtain the media benefits as well as other resources that support the campaign. See, e.g., M. F. Davis and D. C. Iverson, "An Overview and Analysis of the Health Style Campaign," *Health Education Quarterly* 11 (1984): 253–72; and S. E. Samuels, "Project LEAN: A National Campaign to Reduce Dietary Fat Consumption," *American Journal of Health Promotion* 4 (1990): 435–40. Most of the principles and methods that apply to community health promotion can be applied with adaptation at the state/provincial or national level. See E. B. Arkin, "Opportunities for Improving the Nation's Health Through Collaboration with the Mass Media," *Public Health Reports* 105 (1990): 219–23; L. W. Green, P. D. Mullen, and S. Maloney, "Large-Scale Health Education Campaigns," *Health Education Quarterly* 11 (1984): issue 3.

3. E. R. Brown, "Community Organization Influence on Local Public Health Care Policy: A General Research Model and Comparative Case Study," *Health Education Quarterly* 10 (1984): 205–34. Brown's phases of development in community health care policy were later applied in the development of indicators of community action to promote "social health." See J. Rothman and E. R.

Brown, "Indicators of Societal Action to Promote Social Health," in *Health Promotion Indicators and Actions*, S. B. Kar, ed. (New York: Springer, 1989), pp. 202–20.

4. Another dimension of "community" that is important to the national and international development of health promotion is the community of interest. National advocacy organizations such as Public Voice for Food Policy, the Smoking Control Advocacy Resource Center, Americans for Non-smokers' Rights, Mothers Against Drunk Driving, and others all relate to a constituency of concerned citizens scattered around the country. Voluntary health associations and professional associations, similarly, advocate and develop health promotion initiatives through their networks of members and chapters distributed around the country. Each of these represents a community in every sense except for the locality criterion applied in this chapter. Some can support local initiatives. Much of the discussion in this chapter, however, can be applied to organizing through these interest groups on a state, national, or international scale. For more on national advocacy groups and their methods, see R. C. Paehlke, *Environmentalism and the Future of Progressive Politics* (New Haven: Yale University Press, 1989); M. Pertschuk and A. Erikson, *Smoke Fighting: A Smoking Control Movement Building Guide* (New York: American Cancer Society, 1987); M. Pertschuk and W. Schaetzel, *The People Rising: The Campaign Against the Bork Nomination* (New York: Thunder's Mouth Press, 1989); L. Wallack, "Media Advocacy: Promoting Health Through Mass Communication," in *Health Behavior and Health Education: Theory, Research, and Practice*, K. Glanz, F. M. Lewis, and B. K. Rimer, eds. (San Francisco: Jossey-Bass, 1990), chap. 16.

5. R. Cuca and C. S. Pierce, *Experiments in Family Planning: Lessons from the Developing World* (Baltimore: The Johns Hopkins University Press, for the World Bank, 1977); L. W. Green and A. L. McAlister, "Macro-intervention to Support Health Behavior: Some Theoretical Perspectives and Practical Reflections," *Health Education Quarterly* 11 (1984): 323–39.

6. See ref. 46, chap. 7; and especially, see J. W. Farquhar, S. P. Fortmann, J. A. Flora, et al., "Effects of Community-Wide Education on Cardiovascular Disease Risk Factors – The Stanford 5-City Project," *Journal of the American Medical Association* 264 (1990): 359–65; J. W. Farquhar, S. P. Fortmann, P. D. Wood, and W. L. Haskell, "Community Studies of Cardiovascular Disease Prevention," in *Prevention of Coronary Heart Disease: Practical Management of Risk Factors*, N. M. Kaplan and J. Stamler, eds. (Philadelphia: Saunders, 1983); T. Lasater, D. Abrams, L. Artz, et al., "Lay Volunteer Delivery of a Community-based Cardiovascular Risk Factor Change Program: the Pawtucket Experiment," in *Behavioral Health: A Handbook of Health Enhancement and Disease Prevention*, J. D. Matarazzo, S. M. Weiss, J. A. Herd, et al., eds. (New York: Wiley, 1984); D. Nutbeam and J. Catford, "The Welsh Heart Programme Evaluation Strategy: Progress, Plans and Possibilities," *Health Promotion* 2 (1987): 5–18.

7. N. Freudenberg, *Not in Our Backyards! Community Action for Health* (New York: Monthly Review Press, 1984); R. C. Paehlke, *Environmentalism and the Future of Progressive Politics* (New Haven: Yale University Press, 1989); C. Spretnak and F. Capra, *Green Politics* (New York: Dutton, 1984).

8. M. H. Becker and J. Joseph, "AIDS and Behavioral Change to Reduce Risk: A Review," *American Journal of Public Health* 78 (1988): 394–410; T. Coates, R. Stall, and C. Hoff, *Changes in High Risk Behavior Among Gay and Bisexual Men Since the Beginning of the AIDS Epidemic* (Washington, DC: Office of Technology Assessment, United States Congress, May 1988); L. C. Leviton and R. O. Valdiserri, "Evaluating AIDS Prevention: Outcome, Implementation, and Mediating Variables," *Evaluation and Program Planning* 13 (1990): 55–66; R. A. Winett, D. G. Altman, and A. C. King, "Conceptual and Strategic Foundations for Effective Media Campaigns for Preventing the Spread of HIV Infection," *Evaluation and Program Planning* 13 (1990): 91–104; R. E. Markland and M. L. Vincent, "Improving Resource Allocation in a Teenage Sexual Risk Reduction Program," *Socio-Economic Planning Science* 24 (1990): 35–48; H. V. McCoy, S. E. Dodds, and C. Nolan, "AIDS Intervention Design for Program Evaluation: the Miami Community Outreach Project," *Journal of Drug Issues* 20 (1990): 223–43; D. G. Ostrow, "AIDS Prevention through Effective Education," *Daedalus: Journal of the American Academy of Arts and Sciences* 118 (1989): 229–54; C. Patton, *Sex and Germs: The Politics of AIDS* (Boston: South End Press, 1985); L. S. Williams, "AIDS Risk Reduction: A Community Health Education Intervention for Minority High Risk Group Members," *Health Education Quarterly* 13 (1986):407–22.

9. R. W. Chamberlin, ed., *Beyond Individual Risk Assessment: Community Wide Approaches to*

Promoting the Health and Development of Families and Children (Washington, DC: National Center for Education in Maternal and Child Health, 1988); *Integration of Risk Factor Interventions* (Washington, DC: ODPHP Monograph Series, U.S. Department of Health and Human Services, 1986); T. E. Kottke, P. Puska, J. T. Solonen, et.al., "Projected Effects of High-risk Versus Population-based Prevention Strategies in Coronary Heart Disease," *American Journal of Epidemiology* 121 (1985):697–704.

10. B. Lewis, J. I. Mann, and M. Mancini, "Reducing the Risks of Coronary Heart Disease in Individuals and in the Population," *Lancet* 14 (1986): 956–9.

11. P. Puska, A. McAlister, J. Pekkola, and K. Koskela, "Television in Health Promotion: Evaluation of a National Programme in Finland," *International Journal of Health Education* 24 (1981): 2–14.

12. T. Dwyer, J. P. Pierce, C. D. Hannam, and N. Burke, "Evaluation of the Sydney 'Quit. For Life' Anti-smoking Campaign: Part II: Changes in Smoking Prevalence," *Medical Journal of Australia* 144 (1986): 344–7; J. P. Pierce, P. Macaskill, and D. Hill, "Long–term Effectiveness of Mass Media Led Antismoking Campaigns in Australia," *American Journal of Public Health* 80 (1990): 565–9.

13. H. A. Lando, B. Loken, B. Howard-Pitney, and T. Pechacek, "Community Impact of a Localized Smoking Cessation Contest," *American Journal of Public Health* 80 (1990): 601–3; H. A. Lando, P. G. McGovern, F. X. Barrios, and B. D. Etringer, "Comparative Evaluation of American Cancer Society and American Lung Association Smoking Cessation Clinics," *American Journal of Public Health* 80 (1990): 554–9.

14. W. J. Millar and B. E. Naegele, "Time to Quit Program," *Canadian Journal of Public Health* 78 (1987): 109–14.

15. K. E. Warner and H. A. Murt, "Premature Deaths Avoided by the Antismoking Campaign," *American Journal of Public Health* 73 (1983): 672–7.

16. M. Z. Solomon and W. DeJong, "Recent Sexually Transmitted Disease Prevention Efforts and Their Implications for AIDS Health Education," *Health Education Quarterly* 13 (1986): 301–16, quotation from p. 314.

17. R. B. Dwore and M. W. Kreuter, "Reinforcing the Case for Health Promotion," *Family and Community Health* 2 (1980): 103–19; L. W. Green, "Should Health Education Abandon Attitude-change Strategies? Perspectives from Recent Research," *Health Education Monographs* 1(30) (1970): 25–48; L. W. Green, *Status Identity and Preventive Health Behavior* (Berkeley: Pacific Health Education Reports No. 1, University of California School of Public Health, 1970); L. Green and A. McAlister, "Macro-intervention to Support Health Behavior . . . ," op. cit., *Health Education Quarterly* 11 (1984): 322–9.

18. G. Block, W. Rosenberger, B. Patterson, "Calories, Fat and Cholesterol: Intake Patterns in the U.S. Population by Race, Sex and Age," *American Journal of Public Health* 78 (1988): 1150–5; National Restaurant Association, *Foodservice Industry Forecast*, (Washington, DC: Malcolm M. Knapp Research, 1989); B. Popkin, P. Haines, and K. Reidy, "Food Consumption Trends of U.S. Women: Patterns and Determinants Between 1977 and 1985," *American Journal of Clinical Nutrition* 49 (1989): 1307–19; *Trends: Consumer Attitudes and the Supermarket* (Washington, DC: Food Marketing Institute, 1989).

19. A. Bandura, *Social Foundations of Thought and Action: A Social Cognitive Theory* (Englewood Cliffs: Prentice-Hall, 1986); N. M. Clark, "Social Learning Theory in Current Health Education Practice," in *Advances in Health Education and Promotion*, vol. 2, W. B. Ward, S. K. Simonds, P. D. Mullen, and M. H. Becker, eds. (Greenwich, CT: JAI Press, 1987), pp. 251–75; G. S. Parcel and T. Baranowski, "Social Learning Theory and Health Education," *Health Education* 12(3) (1981): 14–18.

20. For critical reviews of these debates, see L. W. Green and J. Raeburn, "Health Promotion: What Is It? What Will It Become?" *Health Promotion International* 3 (1988): 151–9; M. Minkler, "Health Education, Health Promotion and the Open Society: An Historical Perspective," *Health Education*

Quarterly 16 (1989): 17–30; B. K. Rimer, "Perspectives on Intrapersonal Theories in Health Education and Health Behavior," in *Health Behavior and Health Education: Theory, Research, and Practice*, K. Glanz, F. M. Lewis, and B. K. Rimer, eds. (San Francisco: Jossey-Bass, 1990), pp. 140–57; D. G. Simons-Morton, B. G. Simons-Morton, G. S. Parcel, and J. G. Bunker, "Influencing Personal and Environmental Conditions for Community Health: A Multilevel Intervention Model," *Family and Community Health* 11 (1988): 25–35.

21. L. W. Green, *Community Health*, 6th ed. (St. Louis: Times Mirror/Mosby, 1990), pp. 47–8; L. W. Green and A. L. McAlister, "Macro-intervention . . . ," op. cit., *Health Education Quarterly* 11 (1984): 325–9; S. E. Samuels, "Project LEAN . . . ," op. cit., *American Journal of Health Promotion* 4 (1990): 435–40. We are cognizant, however, of the limitations of this argument as it relates to the poorest segments, the unemployed and welfare-dependent. See W. J. Wilson, *The Truly Disadvantaged: The Inner City, the Underclass, and Public Policy* (Chicago: The University of Chicago Press, 1987).

22. W. J. Wilson, *The Truly Disadvantaged . . .* , op. cit., p. 124.

23. S. P. Fortmann, P. T. Williams, S. B. Hulley, et al., "Effect of Health Education on Dietary Behavior: The Stanford Three Community Study," *American Journal of Clinical Nutrition* 34 (1981): 565–71; J. W. Farquhar, S. P. Fortmann, J. A. Flora, et al., "Effects of Community-wide Education on Cardiovascular Disease Risk Factors — The Stanford 5-City Project," *Journal of the American Medical Association* 264 (1990): 359–65.

24. P. Puska, A. Nissinen, J. Tuomilehto, J. T. Salonen, et al., "The Community-based Strategy to Prevent Coronary Heart Disease: Conclusions from the Ten Years of the North Karelia Project," *Annual Review of Public Health*, 6 (1985): 147–93.

25. U.S. Department of Health and Human Services, *Surgeon General's Report on Nutrition and Health* (Washington, DC: Public Health Service, 88–50210, 1988); S. E. Samuels, "Project LEAN . . . ," op. cit., *American Journal of Health Promotion* 4 (1990): 435–40; A. R. Tarlov, B. H. Kehrer, D. P. Hall, et al., "Foundation Work: The Health Promotion Program of the Henry J. Kaiser Family Foundation," *American Journal of Health Promotion* 2 (1989): 74–80; Committee on Diet and Health, National Research Council, Food and Nutrition Board, *Diet and Health: Implications for Reducing Chronic Disease Risk* (Washington, DC: National Academy Press, 1989).

26. This estimate was based on the data presented in the Lipid Research Clinics' North American Study Population, reported in T. Gordon, M. Fisher, et al., "Relation of Diet to LDL Cholesterol, VLDL Cholesterol, and Plasma Total Cholesterol and Triglycerides in White Adults: The Lipid Research Prevalence Study," *Arteriosclerosis* 2 (1982): 502–12. More recent U.S. Department of Agriculture surveys indicate that 37 percent of calories in the American diet come from dietary fat. See U.S. Department of Health and Human Services, *Surgeon General's Report on Nutrition and Health* (Washington, DC: Public Health Service, 88–50210, 1988).

27. P. Puska, et al., 1985, op. cit.

28. R. W. Carlaw, M. Mittlemark, N. Bracht, and R. Luepker, "Organization for a Community Cardiovascular Health Program: Experiences from the Minnesota Heart Health Program," *Health Education Quarterly* 11 (1984): 243–52; L. W. Green, N. H. Gottlieb, and G. Parcel, "Diffusion Theory Extended and Applied," in *Advances in Health Education and Promotion*, vol. 3, W. Ward and F. M. Lewis, eds. (London: Jessica Kingsley Publishers, in press). An alternative view of organizational adoption of innovations sees the process as largely internal and rational or responsive to consumer demands rather than imitative or interorganizational. See, e.g., R. M. Goodman and A. B. Steckler, "Mobilizing Organizations for Health Enhancement," in *Health Behavior and Health Education*, K. Glanz, F. M. Lewis, and B. K. Rimer, eds. (San Francisco: Jossey-Bass, 1990), pp. 314–41; P. A. Schiller, A. Steckler, L. Dawson, and F. Patton, *Participatory Planning in Community Health Education: A Guide Based on the McDowell County, West Virginia, Experience* (Oakland, CA: Third Party Associates, 1987).

29. M. W. Kreuter, G. M. Christenson, and A. Divencenzo, "The Multiplier Effect of the Health

Education Risk Reduction Grants Program in 28 States and 1 Territory," *Public Health Reports* 97 (1982): 510–15.

30. D. Shimkin, "Improving Rural Health: The Lessons of Mississippi and Tanzania," *International Quarterly of Community Health Education* 7 (1986–1987): 149–65, quotation from pp. 154–5.

31. L. W. Green, "Evaluation and Measurement: Some Dilemmas for Health Education," *American Journal of Public Health* 67 (1977): 155–61.

32. L. W. Green, "The Theory of Participation: A Qualitative Analysis of Its Expression in National and International Health Policies," in *Advances in Health Education and Promotion*, vol. 1, pt. A, W. B. Ward, ed. (Greenwich, CT: JAI Press Inc., 1986), pp. 211–36. For a journalistic description of a grantmaking strategy designed to apply this model for early participation and to stimulate support to communities from the state level, see R. M. Williams, "Rx: Social Reconnaissance," *Foundation News* 31(4) (1990): 24–9.

33. L. Bozzini, "Local Community Services Centers (LCSC) in Quebec: Description, Evaluation, Perspectives," *Journal of Public Health Policy* 9 (1988): 346–75, quotation from p. 369.

34. J. Endres, "Teambuilding for Community Health Promotion," *How-To Guides on Community Health Promotion*, No. 14 (Palo Alto: Health Promotion Resource Center, Stanford Center for Research on Disease Prevention, 1990).

35. F. C. Okafor, "Basic Needs in Nigeria," *Social Indicators Research* 17 (1985): 115–25.

36. E. Nangawe, F. Shomet, E. Rowberg, et al., "Community Participation: The Maasai Health Services Project, Tanzania," *International Quarterly of Community Health Education* 7 (1986–1987): 343–51.

37. W. Farrant and A. Taft, "Building Healthy Public Policy in an Unhealthy Political Climate: A Case Study from Paddington and North Kensington," *Health Promotion* 3 (1988): 278–92.

38. P. Hanson, "Citizen Involvement in Community Health Promotion: A Rural Application of CDC's PATCH Model," *International Quarterly of Health Education* 9 (1988–1989): 177–86.

39. J. A. Fuchs, "Planning for Community Health Promotion: A Rural Example," *Health Values* 12(6) (1988): 3–8.

40. H. L. Nix, *The Community and Its Involvement in the Study Action Planning Process* (Atlanta: U.S. Department of Health, Education and Welfare, Centers for Disease Control, HEW-CDC-78-8355, 1977), quotation from pp. 5–6.

41. E. Feighery and T. Rogers, "Building and Maintaining Effective Coalitions," *How-To Guides on Community Health Promotion* (Palo Alto: Health Promotion Resource Center, Stanford Center for Research on Disease Prevention, 1990).

42. J. M. Clark, *The Social Control of Business* (New York: McGraw-Hill, 1939).

43. H. Smith, *The Power Game, How Washington Works* (New York: Random House, 1988).

44. D. Allensworth, "Building Community Support for Quality School Health Programs," *Health Education* 18 (Oct/Nov, 1987); American Medical Association Auxiliary, Inc., *Community Action: How to Work in Coalitions* (Chicago: American Medical Association Auxiliary, 1987); T. Black, "Coalition Building – Some Suggestions," *Child Welfare* 42 (1983): 264; C. Brown, *The Art of Coalition Building: A Guide for Community Leaders* (New York: The American Jewish Committee, 1984); E. Feighery and T. Rogers, "Building and Maintaining Effective Coalitions," *How-To Guides on Community Health Promotion* (Palo Alto: Health Promotion Resource Center, Stanford Center for Research on Disease Prevention, 1990); S. Miller, "Coalition Etiquette: Ground Rules for Building Unity," *Social Policy* 14(2) (1983): 49; C. L. Mulford and G. E. Klonglan, *Creating Coordination Among Organizations: An Orientation and Planning Guide* (Ames, IA: Cooperative Extension Service, Iowa State University, North Central Regional

Extension Pub. No. 80, 1982); M. Pertschuk and A. Erikson, *Smoke Fighting: A Smoking Control Movement Building Guide* (New York: American Cancer Society, 1987).

45. R. DeFrank and P. Levenson, "Ethical and Philosophical Issues in Developing a Health Promotion Consortium," *Health Education Quarterly* 14 (1987):71–7; N. Freudenberg and M. Golub, "Health Education, Public Policy and Disease Prevention: A Case History of the New York City Coalition to End Lead Poisoning," *Health Education Quarterly* 14 (1987):387–401; S. Gottlieb, "Ensuring Access to Health Care: What Communities Can Do to Make a Difference through Private Sector Coalitions," *Inquiry* 23 (1986): 322–9; R. C. Lefebvre, G. S. Peterson, S. A. McGraw, et al., "Community Intervention to Lower Blood Cholesterol: The 'Know Your Cholesterol' Campaign in Pawtucket, Rhode Island," *Health Education Quarterly* 13 (1986): 117–29, esp. p. 122; I. Miller, "Interpreneurship: A Community Coalition Approach to Health Care Reform," *Inquiry* 24 (1987): 266–75; J. Orthoefer, D. Bain, R. Empereur, and T. Nesbit, "Consortium Building among Local Health Departments in Northwest Illinois," *Public Health Reports* 103 (1988): 500–7.

46. Specificity of objectives has been addressed in previous chapters as an issue in planning and evaluation. The issue here is with specificity as a facilitator of interorganizational understanding, commitment, and cooperation in implementing a policy or common objective. See R. Elmore, "Follow Through Planned Variation," in *Social Program Implementation*, W. Williams and R. Elmore, eds. (New York: Academic Press, 1976); J. Pressman and A. Wildavsky, *Implementation*, 2nd ed. (Berkeley: University of California Press, 1973); D. Van Meter and C. Van Horn, "The Policy Implementation Process: A Conceptual Framework," *Administration and Society* 6 (1975): 445–88.

47. H. L. Nix, *The Community and Its Involvement in the Study Action Planning Process* (Atlanta: U.S. Department of Health, Education and Welfare, Centers for Disease Control, HEW-CDC-78-8355, 1977), pp. 90–1.

48. A. Steckler, K. Orville, E. Eng, and L. Dawson, *Patching It Together: A Formative Evaluation of CDC's Planned Approach To Community Health (PATCH) Program* (Chapel Hill: Department of Health Behavior and Health Education, University of North Carolina, unpublished report submitted to the Centers for Disease Control, June 1989).

49. E. Eng, J. Hatch, and A. Callan, "Institutionalizing Social Support through the Church and into the Community," *Health Education Quarterly*, 12 (1985): 81–92; J. W. Hatch and C. Jackson, "The North Carolina Baptist Church Program," *Urban Health* 10(4) (1981): 70–1; M. L. Vincent, A. F. Clearie, and C. G. Johnson, *Reducing Unintended Adolescent Pregnancy through School/ Community Education Interventions: A South Carolina Case Study* (Columbia, SC: School of Public Health, University of South Carolina, 1988); M. L. Vincent, A. F. Clearie, and M. D. Schluchter, "Reducing Adolescent Pregnancy through Schools and Community-based Education," *Journal of the American Medical Association* 257 (1987): 282–6.

50. M. A. Pentz, J. H. Dwyer, D. P. MacKinnon, et al., "A Multicommunity Trial for Primary Prevention of Drug Abuse," *Journal of the American Medical Association* 261 (1989): 3259–66.

51. M. Ross, *Community Organization: Theory and Principles* (New York: Harper & Row, 1955), cited in M. Minkler, "Improving Health Through Community Organization," in *Health Behavior and Health Education*, K. Glanz, F. M. Lewis, and B.K. Rimer, eds. (San Francisco: Jossey-Bass, 1990), p. 257.

52. For a taxonomy of community-based organizations, see R. A. Cuoto, "Promoting Health at the Grass Roots," *Health Affairs* 9 (1990): 144–51.

53. Case studies have been compiled by R. W. Carlaw, ed., *Perspectives on Community Health Education: A Series of Case Studies*, 2 vols. (Oakland, CA: Third Party Publishing, 1982); H. P. Cleary, J. M. Kichen, and P. G. Ensor, eds., *Advancing Health Through Education: A Case Study Approach* (Palo Alto, CA: Mayfield, 1985); J. Simmons, ed., "Making Health Education Work," *American Journal of Public Health* 65 (Oct. 1975 suppl.): 1–49.

54. J. M. Kotchen, H. E. McKean, S. Jackson-Thayer, et al., "Impact of a Rural High Blood Pressure

Control Program on Hypertension Control and Cardiovascular Mortality," *Journal of the American Medical Association* 225 (1986): 2177–82.

55. D. M. Murray, C. L. Kurth, J. R. Finnegan, Jr., et al., "Direct Mail as a Prompt for Follow-up Care Among Persons at Risk for Hypertension," *American Journal of Preventive Medicine* 4 (1988): 331–5.

56. There was no need for more expensive communication efforts (such as a paid media campaign) given the efficiency of existing informal communications networks and the ready cooperation of the local radio and newspaper. We hasten to point out, however, that more expensive campaigns may be cost-effective when indicated by geographic, demographic, and media characteristics.

57. Personal communication, Dr. Jane Kotchen, August 25, 1989.

58. P. Puska, A. Nissinen, J. Tuomilehto, et al., "The Community-Based Strategy to Prevent Coronary Heart Disease: Conclusions from the Ten Years of the North Karelia Project," *Annual Review of Public Health* 6 (1985): 147–93, quotation from pp. 162–3.

59. L. Breslow, "The Future of Public Health: Prospects in the United States for the 1990s," *Annual Review of Public Health* 11 (1990): 1–28.

60. Henry J. Kaiser Family Foundation, *Strategic Plan for the Health Promotion Program, 1989–1991* (Menlo Park, CA: The Foundation, 1989).

61. C. F. Nelson, M. W. Kreuter, and N. B. Watkins, "A Partnership Between the Community, State, and Federal Government: Rhetoric or Reality," *Hygie* 5(3) (1986): 27–31; C. F. Nelson, M. W. Kreuter, N. B. Watkins, and R. R. Stoddard, "Planned Approach to Community Health: The PATCH Program," in *Community-Oriented Primary Care: From Principle to Practice*, P. A. Nutting, ed. (Washington, DC: U. S. Department of Health and Human Services, Health Resources and Services Administration, HRSA-HRS-A-PE 86-1, 1986), chap. 47.

62. S. G. Brink, D. Simons-Morton, G. Parcel, and K. Tiernan, "Community Intervention Handbooks for Comprehensive Health Promotion Programming," *Family and Community Health* 11 (1988): 28–35.

63. As of September 1990, there were 50 PATCH sites in 17 states.

64. J. F. Sallis, M. F. Hovell, and C. R. Hoffstetter, et al., "Distance Between Homes and Exercise Facilities Related to Frequency of Exercise Among San Diego Residents," *Public Health Reports* 105 (1990): 179–85.

65. J. D. DePue, B. L. Wells, T. M. Lasater, and R. A. Carleton, "Volunteers as Providers of Heart Health Programs in Churches: A Report on Implementation," *American Journal of Health Promotion* 4 (1990): 361–6; E. Eng, J. Hatch, and A. Callan, "Institutionalizing Social Support through the Church and into the Community," *Health Education Quarterly* 12 (1985): 81–92; R. E. Markland and M. L. Vincent, "Improving Resource Allocation in a Teenage Sexual Risk Reduction Program," *Socio-Economic Planning Science* 24 (1990): 35–48.

66. Office of Disease Prevention and Health Promotion, *Toward a Healthy Community: Organizing Events for Community Health Promotion* (Washington, DC: U.S. Department of Health and Human Services, Pub. No. PHS 80-50113, 1981).

67. J. F. Mosher, *Community Responsible Beverage Service Programs: An Implementation Handbook* (Palo Alto, CA: The Health Promotion Research Center, Stanford Center for Research and Disease Prevention, 1990); M. O'Donnell, "Research on Drinking Locations of Alcohol-Impaired Drivers: Implication for Prevention Policies," *Journal of Public Health Policy* 6 (1985): 510–25; R. Saltz, "The Role of Bars and Restaurants in Preventing Alcohol-Impaired Driving: An Evaluation of Server Intervention," *Evaluation and Health Professions* 10 (1987): 5–27.

68. A. Cheadle, B. Psaty, E. Wagner, et al., "Evaluating Community–based Nutrition Programs: Assessing the Reliability of a Survey of Grocery Store Product Displays," *American Journal of Public Health* 80 (1990): 709–11; N. D. Ernst, M. Wu, P. Frommer, et al., "Nutrition Education at

the Point of Purchase: The Foods for Health Project Evaluated," *Preventive Medicine* 15 (1986): 60–73; M. K. Hunt, C. Lefebvre, M. L. Hixson, et al., "Pawtucket Heart Health Program Point-of-Purchase Nutrition Education Program in Supermarkets," *American Journal of Public Health* 80 (1990): 730–1; J. A. Mayer, P. M. Dubbert, and J. P. Elder, "Promoting Nutrition at the Point of Choice: A Review," *Health Education Quarterly* 16 (1989): 31–43; R. M. Mullis, M. K. Hunt, M. Foster, et al., "The Shop Smart for Your Heart Grocery Program," *Journal of Nutrition Education* 19 (1987): 225–8; J. T. Pennington, L. A. Wisniowski, and G. B. Logan, "In-Store Nutrition Information Programs," *Journal of Nutrition Education* 20 (1988): 5–10.

69. A program thoroughly applying the PRECEDE model to planning for prevention of a veterinary health problem required outreach directly to individual dairy farmers: W. B. Brown, N. B. Williamson, and R. A. Carlaw, "A Diagnostic Approach to Educating Minnesota Dairy Farmers in the Prevention and Control of Bovine Mastitis," *Preventive Veterinary Medicine* 5 (1988): 197–211. Results of the program are reported in N. B. Williamson, M. J. Burton, W. B. Brown, et al., "Changes in Mastitis Management Practices Associated with Client Education and the Effects of Adopting Recommended Mastitis Control Procedures on Herd Production," *Preventive Veterinary Medicine* 5 (1988): 213–23.

70. J. O. Prochaska and C. DiClemente, "Stages and Processes of Self-change in Smoking: Towards an Integrative Model of Change," *Journal of Consulting and Clinical Psychology* 5 (1983): 390–5.

71. See, for example, L. W. Green, "Change Process Models in Health Education," *Public Health Reviews* 5 (1976): 5–33; or L. W. Green, N. Gottlieb, and G. Parcel, "Diffusion Theory Extended and Applied," in *Advances in Health Education and Promotion* (London: Jessica Kingsley Publishers, in press).

72. J. O. Prochaska, "What Causes People To Change from Unhealthy to Health Enhancing Behavior?" paper presented at the American Cancer Society meeting on Behavioral Research in Cancer, Bloomington, Indiana, 9–10 August 1989. Quotation from p.6.

73. C. H. Weiss, *Evaluation Research: Methods of Assessing Program Effectiveness* (Engelwood Cliffs, NJ: Prentice-Hall Inc., 1972), p. 38.

74. M. A. Preston, T. Baranowski, and J. C. Higginbotham, "Orchestrating the Points of Community Intervention," *International Quarterly of Community Health Education* 9 (1988–1989): 11–34.

75. M. A. Preston, et al., op. cit., p. 31.

76. The entire issue of each of several journals have been devoted in recent years to mass media applications. See, for example, R. Blum and S. E. Samuels, eds., "Television and Teens: Health Implications," *Journal of Adolescent Health Care* 11 (1990): 1–92; L. W. Green, P. D. Mullen, and S. Maloney, eds., "Large Scale Health Education Programs," *Health Education Quarterly* 11 (1984): 221–339.

77. For example, R. Alcalay, F. Sabogal, G. Marin, et al., "Patterns of Mass Media Use Among Hispanic Smokers: Implications for Community Interventions," *International Quarterly of Community Health Education* 8 (1987–1988): 341–50; J. W. Farquhar, S. P. Fortmann, J. A. Flora, et al., "Effects of Community-Wide Education on Cardiovascular Disease Risk Factors: The Stanford 5-City Project," *Journal of the American Medical Association* 264 (1990): 359–65; R. C. Lefebvre, G. S. Peterson, S. A. McGraw, et al., "Community Intervention to Lower Blood Cholesterol: The 'Know Your Cholesterol' Campaign in Pawtucket, Rhode Island," *Health Education Quarterly*, 13 (1986): 117–29; H. V. McCoy, S. E. Dodds, and C. Nolan, "AIDS Intervention Design for Program Evaluation: The Miami Community Outreach Project," *Journal of Drug Issues* 20 (1990): 223–43: J. K. Worden, L. J. Solomon, B. S. Flynn, et al., "A Community–wide Program in Breast Self-examination Training and Maintenance," *Preventive Medicine* 19 (1990): 254–69.

78. General references include: R. Manoff, *Social Marketing: New Imperative for Public Health* (New York: Praeger, 1985); P. Kotler, *Marketing For Non-profit Organizations*, 3rd ed. (Englewood Cliffs, NJ: Prentice-Hall, 1989); For applications related to health education planning, see also,

J. A. Bonaguro and G. Miaoulis, "Marketing: A Tool for Health Education Planning," *Health Education* 14 (Jan/Feb 1983): 6–11, which specifically integrates social marketing with the PRECEDE model; G. Miaoulis and J. Bonaguro, "Marketing Strategies in Health Education," *Journal of Health Care Marketing* 1 (1980–1981): 35–44; R. De Pietro, "A Marketing Research Approach To Health Education Planning," in *Advances in Health Education and Promotion* vol. 2, W. B. Ward, ed. (Greenwich, CT: JAI Press Inc., 1987), pp. 93–118; P. Kotler and E. L. Roberto, *Social Marketing: Strategies for Changing Public Behavior* (New York: The Free Press, 1989), esp. pp. 285–94 which describes Project LEAN as a case study of planning a national social marketing program for dietary fat consumption; W. D. Novelli, "Applying Social Marketing to Health Promotion and Disease Prevention," in *Health Behavior and Health Education: Theory, Research, and Practice*, K. Glanz, F. M. Lewis, and B. K. Rimer, eds. (San Francisco, CA: Jossey-Bass, 1990), chap. 15.

79. R. K. Manoff, *Social Marketing: New Imperative for Public Health* (New York: Praeger Publishers, 1985), pp. 76–7.

80. A. G. Ramirez and A. L. McAlister, "Mass Media Campaign — *A Su Salud*," *Preventive Medicine* 17 (1988): 608–21.

81. A. Bandura, *Social Learning Theory* (New York: Prentice Hall, 1977).

82. C. R. Lefebvre and J. A. Flora, "Social Marketing and Public Health Intervention," *Health Education Quarterly* 15 (1988): 299–315.

83. J. A. Smith and D. L. Scammon, "A Market Segment Analysis of Adult Physical Activity: Exercise Beliefs, Attitudes, Intentions and Behaviors," *Advances in Nonprofit Marketing*, vol. 2 (Greenwich, CT: JAI Press, 1987).

84. W. R. Brieger, J. Ramakrishna, and J. D. Adeniyi, "Community Involvement in Social Marketing: Guineaworm Control," *International Quarterly of Community Health Education* 7 (1986–1987): 19–31.

85. D. Glik, A. Gordon, W. Ward, et al., "Focus Group Methods for Formative Research in Child Survival: An Ivoirian Example," *International Quarterly of Community Health Education* 8 (1987–1988): 297–316.

86. W. P. Schellstede and R. L. Ciszewski, "Social Marketing of Contraceptives in Bangladesh," *Studies in Family Planning* 15 (Jan/Feb 1984): 30–9.

87. A. J. Gordon, "Mixed Strategies in Health Education and Community Participation: An Evaluation of Dengue Control in the Dominican Republic," *Health Education Research, Theory and Practice* 3 (1988): 399–419.

Chapter 9

Applications in Occupational Settings

I n Chapter 1, PRECEDE was characterized as a robust model, referring to its adaptability and broad utility. The health promotion literature since the first publication of the model in 1974[1] provides numerous examples of the application of PRECEDE in planning and evaluating programs for various populations in diverse settings.[2] This chapter examines some of the unique challenges of promoting health in the worksite, and how application and adaptation of PRECEDE and PROCEED can make that task more efficient and effective.[3]

WORKSITE HEALTH PROMOTION: ITS RECENT HISTORY

The remarkable growth of worksite health promotion in industrialized nations since the late 1970s has been influenced by four phenomena: (1) changing demographic profiles in most workplaces, (2) growing concern for the burden on industry of rising medical care costs, health insurance premiums, and costs of lost productivity in unhealthy workers, (3) recognition of the greater influence of behavior and environment on health, and (4) emerging evidence that health education and health promotion strategies have been effective in altering the behavioral and environmental precursors of health.

Changing Demographic Patterns. Willie "The Actor" Sutton, the infamous American bankrobber, when asked "Why do you rob banks"? allegedly answered "Because that's where the money is"! Health promotion tends to be organized around schools for children and worksites for adults because that's where the people are. Worksites are to many adults what schools are to children and youth—places where most of

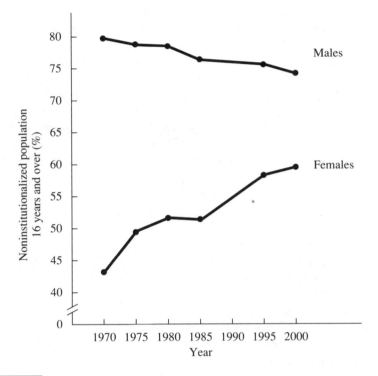

FIGURE 9.1

Civilian labor force participation rates for the U.S. population age 16 years and older, 1970–2000. [From U.S. Bureau of Labor Statistics, *Monthly Labor Review*; U.S. Bureau of the Census, *Statistical Abstract of the United States: 1990* (Washington, DC: U.S. Government Printing Office, 1989).]

the daylight hours are spent, where friendships are made, where many of the rewards that make one feel worthy are dealt, and where one can be reinforced by peers and significant others. It is also a place where one feels pressures to perform and deliver.

About three-fourths of the adult men (16 years and over) and over half of the adult women in the United States are in the labor force,[4] and 60 percent of married men who work have working wives.[5] Figure 9.1 shows the rates of participation in the U.S. labor force for men and women from 1970 to 2000. The increase in the female workforce participation rate, especially working mothers, reshaped the attitudes of employers toward employee benefits and working conditions. The workplace has replaced the neighborhood as the community of reference and social identity for many urban and suburban North Americans and Europeans.[6] These demographic and social trends — combined with the pervasive influence of occupational environments on adult health, quality of life, behavior, and life-style — make them logical if not ideal settings for health promotion programs.

Containing Health Care Costs. American business and industry took a fresh look at health promotion and disease prevention in the late 1970s as they faced alarming increases in the cost of medical care and insurance premiums for their employees.[7] In 1985, employers paid $400 billion or approximately 80 percent of private insurance premiums, which accounted for approximately one quarter of the all personal health care services in the United States.[8] The share of the burden for increases in health-care costs have fallen more heavily on industry than on individuals or governments (Fig. 9.2).[9]

Consider these dramatic expressions of health care costs by employers:

- The cost of health care added more than $480 to the price of every automobile manufactured in 1982.
- Between 1973 and 1975, high blood pressure and its complications resulted in 23,129 days of absence among 8,600 employees at New York Telephone Company. The direct costs to the company was established at $1,040,805.[10]
- Citibank reported that 7.1 percent of health care dollars were spent on cardiovascular disease, about $1 million in 1981.
- In 1980 it was estimated that the average one-pack-per-day smoker could cost an employer more than $600 per day.[11]

Recognizing the Relationships between Behavior, the Environment, and Health. The trend in adoption of health promotion programs by employers parallels the progressive steps in stages-of-change theory.[12] Except in a few innovative areas,[13] prior to the early 1980s most employers were in either a precontemplation or a not-ready-for-action stage. The earlier adopters (often chief executive officers who, because of heart attacks or other reasons, were themselves true believers in a healthful lifestyle) usually installed health promotion programs for personal more than for economic reasons. During the early 1980s employers began to initiate health promotion programs based on a growing awareness of their potential health and economic benefits.[14] Through repeated exposures to health messages via a myriad of formal and informal communication channels, the general public, including employers, began to see the relevance of the information confirming the link between health and factors they had the power to change. Tables 9.1 and 9.2 give examples of the kind of data that served as the content of those messages.

While the general public was becoming more curious about, if not committed to health promotion, business leaders were searching for ways to contain rising health care costs. They became intrigued by the potential offered by health promotion programs. One of many publications suggesting that health promotion could render cost savings was *Health Promotion Can Produce Economic Sav-*

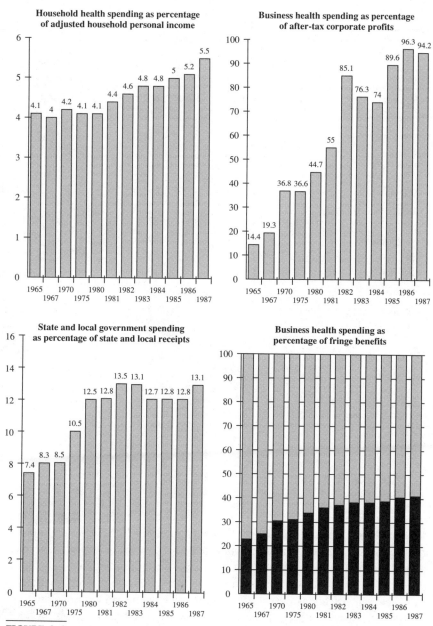

FIGURE 9.2

Burden of increased health care costs on individuals, government, and business, United States, 1965–1987. [From K. Levit et al., *Health Care Financing Review* 10 (Spring 1989): 1–11.]

TABLE 9.1

Major precursors of premature death, Unites States, 1980.

Precursor	Attributable deaths	Potential years lost before age 65	Days of hospital care
Tobacco	338,022	1,497,161	16,098,587
High blood pressure	297,162	340,752	9,781,647
Overnutrition	287,502	292,960	16,306,194
Alcohol			
total	99,247	1,795,458	3,348,354
(injury)	(53,683)	(1,497,206)	(2,229,824)
(other)	(45,564)	(298,252)	(1,118,530)
Injury risks (excluding alcohol)	64,169	1,755,720	25,470,176
Gaps in screening	56,592	172,793	3,647,729
Gaps in primary prevention	54,027	1,273,631	4,651,730
Inadequate access to care	21,974	324,709	2,141,569
Occupation	16,807	102,065	581,740
Handguns	13,365	350,683	28,514
Unintended pregnancy	8,000	520,000	n/a
Total preventable	1,258,867	8,425,932	82,056,240
(percentage)	(63.1)	(70.8)	(29.9)
Total all causes	1,995,000	11,897,174	274,508,000

SOURCE: Adapted from R. M. Amler and D. L. Eddins, "Cross-sectional Analysis of Premature Death in the U.S.," in *Closing the Gap: The Burden of Unnecessary Illness*, R. W. Amler and H. B. Dull, eds. (New York: Oxford University Press, 1987) pp. 181–7.

ings,[15] produced by the Michigan Department of Health. One of its main targets for distribution was the Michigan business community. It made the point that the rising health care costs in Michigan created the need to explore alternative approaches to restraining those costs; worksite health promotion was one of the principal alternatives. A computer model was developed to project the impact of risk-factor interventions over a lifetime for Michigan's working population over the age of 20; the model estimated the potential cost-benefit return on dollars invested for health promotion. Table 9.3 shows the estimated positive returns for interventions in seat-belt use, smoking, drinking and driving, and binge drinking. The report also projected that a combined hypertension, weight and nutrition, and physical activity risk-reduction program would yield $2.07 for every dollar spent.

TABLE 9.2

Major causes of death and associated risk factors: Michigan residents, 1985

Cause	Percentage of all deaths	Risk factors
Heart disease	38.9	Smoking[a], hypertension[a], elevated serum cholesterol[a], lack of exercise, diabetes, stress, family history
Malignant neoplasms	22.0	Smoking[a], worksite carcinogens, alcohol, diet, environmental carcinogens
Stroke	7.0	Hypertension[a], smoking[a], elevated serum cholesterol[a], stress
Motor vehicle accidents	2.1	Alcohol[a], nonuse of seat belts, speed[a], roadway design, vehicle engineering
Pneumonia and influenza	2.8	Smoking, vaccination status[a]
Accidents other than motor vehicle	2.0	Alcohol[a], drug abuse, smoking motor (fires), product design, handgun availability
Diabetes	1.8	Obesity[a]
Chronic liver disease	1.6	Alcohol[a]
Atherosclerosis	1.5	Elevated serum cholesterol[a]
Suicide	1.4	Stress[a], alcohol and drug abuse, handgun availability

[a] Major risk factor

SOURCE: *Health Promotion Can Produce Economic Savings*, Office of Health and Medical Affairs, Michigan Department of Management and Budget, and Center for Health Promotion (Lansing: Michigan Department of Public Health, Oct. 1987), p. 5.

EVIDENCE THAT HEALTH PROMOTION CAN WORK IN THE WORKSITE

Several studies have demonstrated that health and fitness programs can help contain costs and produce benefits to industry.[16] One reported a reduction of $262 in medical costs per participant in the first year of a fitness program.[17] A Canadian study showed a projected medical cost savings of $84.50 per employee one year following introduction of a fitness program in one of two financial services companies.[18]

Another study analyzed the experience of the Live for Life Program at 18 Johnson and Johnson sites with some 8,500 employees in two groups, compared with a third group of sites with 2,955 employees not receiving the Live for Life Program. Figure 9.3 shows the comparative inpatient costs incurred by the three groups, where the programs were introduced in the first two groups between January 1979 and mid–1981. These two groups showed some increases in medical costs corresponding to their increasing age and the national medical inflation rates

TABLE 9.3

Cost-benefit ratio for each of six health promotion programs, based on a prospective analysis by the Michigan Department of Health

Intervention Program	Return on dollar
Seat belts	$105.07
Smoking	15.26
Heavy drinking	2.68
Drinking/driving	1.30
Binge drinking	1.30
Combined	2.07

SOURCE: *Health Promotion Can Produce Economic Savings*, Office of Health and Medical Affairs, Department of Management and Budget, and Center for Health Promotion (Lansing: Michigan Department of Public Health, 1987).

but little increase after the program was in full swing, whereas the third group showed much greater increases after 1981.[19]

Surveys indicate progressive increases in the variety and number of health promotion programs offered in worksettings from the mid-1970s to the mid-1980s.[20] A survey of worksite health education and health promotion programs sponsored by the U.S. Department of Health and Human Services in 1986 found that nearly two-thirds of all worksites with 50 or more employees had programs of some kind.[21] Table 9.4 shows the relative prevalence of the types of programs.

TWO CAVEATS FOR HEALTH PROFESSIONALS IN THE WORKSITE

Attention to the diagnostic steps of PRECEDE can help practitioners avoid two traps that could sidetrack program efforts or undermine credibility. The first is associated with potential ethical dilemmas, the second with the tendency to be too zealous with claims of cost containment.

Watch Out for Ethical Traps. Problems can arise from (1) conflicting loyalties of health professionals, (2) focusing attention exclusively on changing the behavior of victims of worksite hazards rather than on the hazards themselves, (3) labeling and coercion of individuals, and (4) unintended consequences such as compromising of medical care benefits and discrimination in hiring practices.[22] These issues point to the need for sensitivity to issues of worker participation in planning

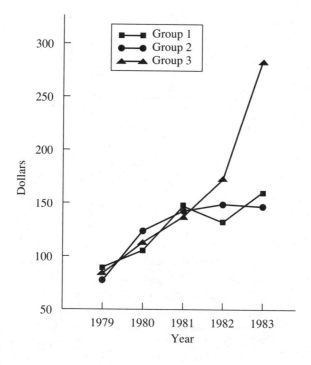

FIGURE 9.3

1979 to 1983 per capita inpatient costs, in 1979 constant dollars, following introduction of Live for Life Program in 18 sites of Johnson & Johnson Company (groups 1 and 2), between 1979 and 1981. [From J. L. Bly, R. C. Jones, and J. E. Richardson, *Journal of the American Medical Association* 256 (1986): 3235–40, reproduced with permission of the publisher. Copyright 1986, American Medical Association.]

programs, for justice, and for privacy in the implementation of health-related programs. Attention and commitment to the principle of participation highlighted in Chapter 2 is of paramount importance in helping the practitioner recognize and effectively address these critical issues.

Perhaps no worksite health promotion issue is more sensitive than one that arises when environmental problems in the workplace are ignored in favor of programs directed solely at individual responsibility for behavioral change among workers.[23] One of the greatest concerns expressed by labor groups has been the issue of "blaming the victim," particularly those workers who are exposed to potentially health-threatening working conditions such as exposure to chemicals in the work environment. The victim-blaming trap applies equally to the neglect of environmental factors that constrain or compel behavior. For example, some stress-management programs put the entire emphasis on personal coping strat-

TABLE 9.4

Most frequently reported categories of worksite health promotion activities, given as percentages of number of worksites surveyed

Type of activity	Percentage	Type of activity	Percentage
Smoking control	35.6	Exercise and fitness	22.1
Health risk assessment	29.5	Off-the-job accident prevention	19.8
Back-problem prevention and care	28.5	Nutrition education	16.8
		Blood pressure control	16.5
Stress management	26.6	Weight control	14.7

SOURCE: Adapted from J. E. Fielding and P. V. Piserchia, *American Journal of Public Health* 79 (1989): 16–20.

egies rather than on management practices and environmental conditions that create stress.[24] The concern in both instances is that employers will use the concept of behavior change and worker responsibility for health as a smokescreen to cover neglect of hazards in the work environment.[25]

The health professional negotiating a worksite health promotion program must struggle with issues of allegiance or neutrality with respect to the positions of management and workers.[26] The ideal resolution is one that *combines* behavioral and environmental approaches to health promotion, with input from *both* management and workers.[27]

Through systematic conduct of PRECEDE diagnostic steps, the practitioner in the worksite can guard against these ethical dilemmas in at least two ways: (1) The social diagnosis can promote greater collaboration between employers and employees, assuring attention to the ultimate concerns of both. (2) The epidemiological, environmental, and behavioral assessments increase the likelihood that programs will include environmental reforms to improve the working conditions, which are balanced with appropriate behavioral strategies.

The epidemiological, behavioral, and environmental assessments also help identify those circumstances where worksite hazards interact with worker behavior. Some are synergistic in their effects, such as smoking and exposure to asbestos, solvents, and other air pollutants. Some have concomitant effects on the same health problems, such as alcohol and injury exposure.[28] Some may effect worker productivity and health concomitantly but independently, such as stressful working conditions and being overweight or sedentary work and lacking physical fitness.

Recognition of these interacting relationships between working conditions and health behavior will help planners justify the application of comprehensive approaches to worksite health promotion, providing for interventions directed at (1) protecting the worker against hazardous and stressful working conditions and

(2) promoting healthful practices such as exercise, nutritional eating, and self-examination for cancer signs or symptoms.

The employers and the white collar workforce have responded well to the introduction and expansion of Employee Assistance Programs centered particularly on mental health, alcohol, and drug abuse,[29] and to health promotion programs emphasizing stress management,[30] exercise facilities, and health education offerings.[31] Blue collar workers have shown less interest in these programs and facilities except where their introduction has been through a process of collective bargaining with attention paid to perceived problems in the work environment and in the health service benefits provided by the employer.

Don't Oversell Economic Benefits. Earlier, the case was made that health promotion programs in the worksite had considerable potential for containing the costs paid by employers for their employees' health care. Although conventional wisdom may indicate that health promotion programs are good "investments" for employers, health economists and others caution practitioners to avoid exaggerating and thereby overselling the potential economic benefits to the employer's company or organization.[32]

The key to an appropriate and compelling social assessment, from the employer's perspective, is to calculate the cost per worker, or per 100 workers, of poor fitness or health outcomes and to put these costs in relation to the products or services that are the *raison d'etre* for the organization.

PHASE 1: SOCIAL DIAGNOSIS

The application of PRECEDE in the work setting, as in other organizational settings, begins with the social diagnosis. Assessments of quality-of-life concerns and potential benefits to be obtained from a health promotion program produce quite different results when viewed from the distinct perspectives of workers and management.

FROM THE PERSPECTIVE OF EMPLOYERS

If quality of life is the bottom line for the public, then productivity or profit is the corresponding bottom line for the corporate world, where the term *bottom line* was coined. The term refers to the *bottom* of the accounting balance sheet or ledger where the assets and liabilities, or credits and debits, are totaled to get the net profit or loss, surplus or deficit. If you keep asking "Why?" after each reason an employer gives for having a health promotion program for his or her employees, eventually the answer will be *profit* if it is a for-profit company, and productivity in

TABLE 9.5

Criteria used by employers in setting health promotion priorities

Direct measures of productivity (cost-benefit analysis)

Prior demonstration of benefits in comparable sites

Time frame for realization of benefits (discounting)

Relevance of the program to health costs and risks in the company, taking the benefits package into consideration

Employee interest in the program as an indication that having the program will help retain and recruit good employees

Possible negative effects of the program, such as time away from work, injuries, liability of the employer

some other terms if it is a nonprofit organization. Certainly employers want to have happier, healthier workers. But, if an employer invests in a program whose only outcome is employee "happiness," there's a good chance that the employer won't be happy very long. The day that happier, healthier workers start missing work or failing to produce because they are happier or healthier is the day that employers will begin to dismantle their worksite health promotion programs. That's the bottom line.

Various criteria can be used by employers to set bottom-line priorities among optional programs in health promotion. Some of the most commonly used criteria are listed in Table 9.5. These reflect the orientation of employers not to health as an end in itself, but to other ultimate concerns as motives to provide health promotion programs for their employees.

Two criteria—epidemiological importance and the demonstrated effectiveness of interventions—were used by the Public Health Service to establish the following national priorities in health promotion: (1) reduction of smoking, (2) reduction of alcohol and drug misuse, (3) diet and nutrition, (4) physical fitness and exercise, and (5) stress and violence control. When employers consider their own needs, resources, and potential benefits, different priorities tend to be established. For example, when immediate costs from poor employee morale, absenteeism, low productivity, and injuries are considered, alcohol abuse will be seen as the most important social problem to be addressed in the worksite. Stress management and other mental health concerns might be seen as paramount. If company image is of greatest concern to management, then exercise facilities and community-oriented activities might be given higher priority.[33]

Companies have been most concerned in recent years about the increases in cost associated with their health-care coverage of employees, as reflected in premium rates on group insurance and in benefits paid on medical claims. As in most other settings, health is not an end in itself in the worksite. Health is a resource that enables workers to perform more productively; it is an instrumental rather than terminal value. The social assessment, then, is something of a mis-nomer in the work setting as far as the employer is concerned. In its place one would begin the PRECEDE analysis with an assessment of bottom-line concerns of productivity and profitability, such as absenteeism, medical claims, sick days, workman's compensation claims, security problems, injuries and property damage caused by smokers or by alcohol- or drug-abusing employees. Other health-related concerns affecting productivity include health insurance premiums that are higher than average because of poor experience rating, turnover rates requiring more frequent hiring and training, and early retirement rates. More direct productivity measures (output per worker) are compared with competing companies who may or may not have health promotion programs.

These would be analyzed in Phase 1, not as indicators of the health or morbidity of the organization, but as meaningful consequence or morbidity. They are meaningful to the employer because they cost money, they cost time, or they represent lost productivity, any of which reduces the profit margin. They add to the cost of doing business or of maintaining the workforce. These costs must be passed on to the consumer, or they must be subtracted from the services rendered or the profit taken. The first makes the company's product or service uncompetitive; the second makes it unattractive to owners or stockholders. In the end, an unhealthy workforce can make an organization untenable.

FROM THE PERSPECTIVE OF EMPLOYEES

The workers' perspective on quality-of-life concerns makes the social assessment, for their purposes, no different from that in community programs. If the employ-ers have the final say and if they control the resources to support a program in the worksite, why would anyone bother with a social assessment on the workers? How do their social needs or their perspective matter? A community assessment carried out prior to the worksite program could serve as the social assessment from the workers' perspective. Another assessment of their quality-of-life concerns within the worksite might be redundant. It might be sufficient to concentrate the social diagnosis on the previously outlined concerns of employers.

But a unionized shop or a highly participatory management structure in a given organization makes it essential to conduct an assessment of employee perspectives on the priorities that health promotion can serve. Unions have opposed some behaviorally oriented health promotion programs because they saw them as smoke screens to divert attention from environmental problems in the worksite, or as substitutes for other benefits in the collective bargaining package. Knowing what is most important to the workers can aid in assuring that a health promotion program addresses environmental issues and appropriate other bene-fits. It can also serve to establish appropriate objectives and evaluation criteria for whatever programs are eventually offered. Finally, it can provide a baseline against which later concerns can be compared when the programs are evaluated.

PHASE 2: EPIDEMIOLOGICAL DIAGNOSIS

Although occupational health has traditionally dealt with hazards of the workplace separate from general health, there has emerged a more recent movement toward integrating health promotion into occupational health. In the early stages of occupation health, the emphasis was on the conservation of health status; more recent efforts have been directed toward the advancement of health to the optimal level, thereby improving the quality of life and performance. Work-related diseases is a concept being used to describe those diseases in which the work environment may play a partial role in causation. This definition includes health problems that may be aggravated by work conditions, thus expanding the concept of occupational health to include conditions such as high blood pressure, cardiovascular disease, ulcers, and a variety of psychological problems.

Table 9.6 lists the 10 leading work-related diseases identified by the National Institute of Occupational Safety and Health as the most frequent, severe, and of high priority. Both environmental and behavioral factors influence the work-related diseases and injuries cited in this table.

Examples of worker behavior and workplace environmental factors influencing occupational cancer are shown in Figure 9.4. These factors were identified by program personnel representing five labor unions. They participated in developing interventions designed to reduce the incidence of cancer for workers at high risk of

TABLE 9.6
Ten leading work-related diseases and injuries

1. Occupational lung disorders
2. Musculoskeletal disorders
3. Occupational cancer
4. Fractures, amputations, traumatic deaths
5. Cardiovascular disease
6. Reproductive problems
7. Neurotoxic illness
8. Noise-induced hearing loss
9. Dermatological problems
10. Psychological disorders

SOURCE: The National Institute of Occupational Safety and Health (NIOSH), *Morbidity and Mortality Weekly Report* 32 (1983): 24–26, 32.

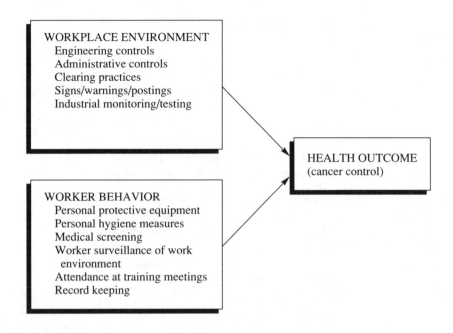

FIGURE 9.4

Epidemiological, behavioral, and environmental diagnoses of cancer risks in five industries. [From C. Y. Lovato and L. W. Green, consultation report, 1986; see ref. 34.]

cancer due to occupational exposure.[34] This assessment includes both the health factors influencing the social problem (descriptive epidemiology) as well as the behavioral and environmental causes of the priority health problems (etiological epidemiology).

Once people have identified the priorities for the health outcomes that they hope the program will influence, the final step in this phase of PRECEDE is to set objectives for each of these outcomes. These objectives might have to be long-range goals that will be unmeasurable or unachievable within the first year or more of the program. For example, the objective of a cancer control program designed by the Workers Institute for Safety and Health specified a long-range goal of reducing mortality for workers who were exposed to the bladder carcinogens used in the manufacture of textile dyes, which were later identified as carcinogens. Mortality reductions, impossible to measure directly in the short term, would be inferred (projected statistically) from an increase in lead time for treatment; that is, the program's success would reduce delay in workers' seeking diagnosis after their symptoms first appeared. Reduced mortality could also be projected from earlier treatment resulting from the program's early detection of cancer symptoms from screening.[35]

Objectives should be stated in quantitative terms so that a clear vision of the program's contribution to the organization's "bottom line" can be brought out anytime the program seems to be losing its way or its support. These objectives should state how much of what health or fitness measure (e.g., a 20% reduction of medical claims for lower back pain) might be expected in which employees (e.g., mail room workers) by when (e.g., in the second year of the program).[36]

PHASE 3: BEHAVIORAL AND ENVIRONMENTAL DIAGNOSIS

Having established the health problems of greatest importance (to employers and workers) in the given worksite and the determinants of those health problems, the third phase of the PRECEDE planning process is the further specification of the behavioral and environmental factors and assessment of their relative changeability. Using data on their importance from the epidemiological diagnosis, you can rate each of the behavioral and environmental factors on importance. Among those found to be most important, some are more amenable to change than others. Some are related to each other, which makes change in one responsive to change in another. These ratings and relationships can be used to set priorities on the behavioral and environmental factors deserving primary attention in the next phase.

Because the number of complex factors contributing to a given health indicator usually exceeds the program resources available, it is inevitable that some behavioral or environmental factors will be relegated to lower priority for action. However, by narrowing the focus of the program at this stage of analysis and assessment of needs, you save considerable effort in each of the subsequent steps in planning. Failing to rule out less important objectives or targets of change at this phase will mean wasteful analysis of their determinants in the next two phases, only to discover in the final phase of planning that you have insufficient resources to provide for these lower priority needs.

Because the environmental factors in the worksite are so much more immediate and contained than in the larger community, they deserve special attention as candidates for change in worksite health promotion planning. They also represent the factors most likely to convince workers that the commitment of the program to meaningful change is sincere. Some workers, especially those who perceive themselves at risk of environmental assaults on their health and well being in the worksite, are more likely to support and participate in the program if they see some significant attention to environmental concerns.

It seldom happens that a set of important health problems in the worksite can be attributed singularly to environmental or to behavioral causes. The choice is seldom between the two, but usually is between the numerous competing candidates for attention in both the behavioral and environmental categories.

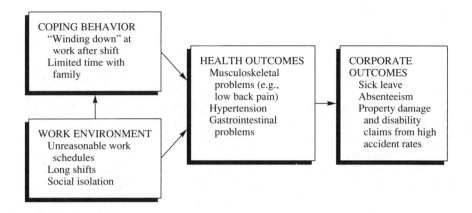

FIGURE 9.5

Behavioral and environmental diagnosis of worksite conditions related to health outcomes and corporate outcomes in the Municipal Transit Authority of San Francisco. [Based on L. W. Syme, *Preventive Medicine* 15 (1986); 492–507.]

An epidemiological diagnosis of the problems of sick leave, absenteeism, and accident rates in San Francisco bus drivers found hypertension, musculoskeletal system problems, and gastrointestinal problems at excess levels in this population of workers.[37] A traditional medical approach to this assessment might have emphasized drug treatment for the hypertension, patient education on posture for the back pain, and diet for the gastrointestinal problems. However, by simultaneously examining the potential behavioral and environmental precursors, planners found unreasonable work schedules for the bus drivers, in combination with long shifts and social isolation. A related coping behavior was the tendency for the drivers to remain at the bus yard for several hours after their shift to "wind down" before going home. This resulted in limited time with family and friends at home, which might account for some of the hostile and impatient behavior observed in the drivers. This narrowed the focus of the behavioral and environmental assessment on coping behavior of drivers and scheduling conditions of the worksite, also seeking to provide for rest stops located in or near central city areas.

This example, as shown in Figure 9.5 illustrates the interactions of environmental and behavioral factors that need to be examined in this phase of the assessment process.

The final step in this phase is to set objectives for each of the behavioral and environmental targets of change. These should state how much of what behavioral or environmental factor is expected to change by when. The changes in behavior may be expressed in the behavioral objectives as percentages of employees in a given category of the workforce (e.g., an increase of 40% of mail room workers) who will adopt a new behavior or abandon a negative health practice (e.g., practicing proper lifting techniques or not bending over when picking up heavy loads from the floor), by when (e.g., between the first week and the twelfth week of the program).

The environmental objectives might be stated in terms of the actual installation of a new facility (e.g., Waist-high conveyer belts will be installed), where (e.g., in the mail room next to each work station), by when (e.g., by the twelfth week of the program). Environmental objectives would often reflect the removal of an environmental hazard (e.g., all floor level bins for mail bags will be replaced with conveyer belts).

If the objective is to be used as the criterion of success of the program in an evaluation, this may be the time to specify the measurement procedure as part of the objective or as an operational definition of the behavior. For the behavioral objective in the foregoing example, this might be "as measured by an observer during a randomly selected one-hour work period each day for one week." For the environmental objectives, this might refer to a specific regulatory code or occupational health and safety standard (e.g., in accordance with Section 1601 of the State Safety Code), which also often provides for the inspection procedure. Alternatively, it might refer to the terms of a contract or to the contractor to be hired for the installation or removal of the facility or hazard (e.g., as specified in contract number AB21 or as specified in the standard contract of company XYZ). In the absence of codes and standards or documented specifications, the objective might need to specify the size, shape, or materials to be installed or removed (e.g., constructed with ball-bearing rollers).

PHASE 4: EDUCATIONAL AND ORGANIZATIONAL DIAGNOSIS

The task in Phase 4 is to assess the relative importance and changeability of the factors predisposing, enabling, and reinforcing the selected behavioral and environmental targets for the worksite program. These determinants of change in each of the behavioral and environmental objectives will become the immediate targets of the interventions. In a cancer-screening project for workers exposed to carcinogens, those predisposing factors determining change were identified as knowledge and awareness of the risk of bladder cancer and the advantages of early detection. Enabling factors concentrated on the development of skill in detecting symptoms and providing cancer screening. Reinforcing factors concentrated on building social support networks through the community, co-workers, and family.

In the educational and process diagnosis, you bring to bear most cogently the appropriate behavioral science and social or political science and economic theories of change. Selecting which determinants might be influencing the behavioral or environmental targets is, once again, an exercise in narrowing the field from an enormous number of possible factors to a more manageable number of important and realistic targets for change.

For example, for a complex lifestyle objective such as increasing exercise or changing dietary practices to reduce fat intake, there are dozens of component behaviors and, for each of those, dozens of possible predisposing, enabling, and reinforcing factors. The more complex the behavior, the more component parts or manifestations the behavior has. Because every component must be analyzed in Phase 4, this phase will become too complex to be practicable unless Phase 3 has been rigorous in its priority-setting step. Critical professional judgment should eliminate the least important and least changeable behaviors from further analysis. Similarly, the environmental factors identified in Phase 3 can become too complex to analyze in Phase 4 if they have not been sufficiently delineated and reduced to the most important few deserving highest priority.

Here also, the time perspective of the previously developed objectives will dictate the pace at which change in the determinants must occur to meet the behavioral and environmental objectives. The degree of urgency, in turn, will dictate some of the selection of processes of change. Educational processes are slower but often more acceptable to a population asked to make changes in its behavior than regulatory processes would be. Rules and regulations promulgated from management without first educating the workers to the need for the rules and involving them in the process of formulation sometimes results in a backlash that sets the hasty schedule back more than the gain in efficiency.[38]

The trade-offs between expediency and durability of change apply not only to the choice of emphasis between predisposing factors and enabling factors, but within educational or behavioral approaches between "internal" (cognitive) predisposing factors and "external" reinforcing factors.[39] For example, the mobilization of incentives and rewards for behavior change among employees through bonuses and competitions might stimulate more immediate participation and change,[40] but unless accompanied by or immediately followed by cognitive changes in knowledge, beliefs and attitudes, the behavioral changes are at greater risk of relapse after the incentives and external rewards are no longer offered.

The point is that a balanced approach including both learning processes and environmental change processes is almost always advisable to assure more than fleeting results and changes that are both acceptable and efficient. *Acceptability* comes with learning and associating the proposed change with values; *efficiency* comes with structural or organizational facilitation and resources for change. It is necessary in Phase 4, therefore, to assess the predisposing *and* reinforcing *and* enabling factors that influence *each* of the behavioral and environmental targets or objectives that were given high priority in Phase 3.

PREDISPOSING FACTORS

Assessing the level of commitment is the first order of business in Phase 4. This predisposing factor is the base on which all other determinants may have their effect. If the employer and worker populations have a high level of commitment or motivation for the behavioral or environmental changes identified in Phase 3, then less effort is needed on enabling and reinforcing factors. If motivation is low, then little will happen with respect to behavioral change, no matter how much emphasis is placed on enabling and reinforcing factors. Motivation or level of commitment must be at a level sufficient to obtain participation in the program.

Studies of employee participation in worksite programs indicate that the predisposing factors with the highest correlations are interest in health and knowledge of the benefits of the recommended behavior.[41] Continued participation in weight control, smoking cessation, alcohol abuse, and physical activity programs also appears to be predicted by self-efficacy.[42] High levels of perceived job stress also predict participation in exercise, weight control, and stress management programs.[43] Work stress, however, may be negatively correlated with participation in a smoking cessation program, yet positively correlated with assertiveness in asking smoking co-workers not to smoke. These effects of work stress may cancel each other out.[44]

"Loss of interest or motivation" was the most frequently cited reason for dropping out of a worksite exercise program.[45] This suggests that the predisposing factors might need to be reassessed periodically to determine changes in attitudes, beliefs, or perceptions that need to be corrected to sustain the level of participation required to achieve the behavioral or environmental objectives. This brings forth the analysis of reinforcing factors, which might be thought of as boosters to reactivate fading predisposing factors.

REINFORCING FACTORS

Motivation is a necessary but not a sufficient determinant of participation. Some of the most highly motivated workers will not continue to participate in a worksite health promotion program if they are bucking a supervisor who frowns on it or fellow workers who think it is silly or that it means more work for them. These social forces rewarding or punishing the proposed behavior are crucial determinants to be assessed in Phase 4.

Research indicates that participant satisfaction plays a major role in continued employee participation. Satisfaction increases when employees are involved actively in planning the program.[46] Employees tend to be more satisfied with programs in which health care or health promotion personnel show warmth and personal concern in their interactions.[47] The amount of contact time and the number of contacts with health-care providers have been shown to relate to higher satisfaction and blood pressure control.[48]

Overall "organizational climate" has been cited frequently as a key factor not only in reinforcing worker participation but in assuring supervisory support for worker participation as well.[49] Senior managers' attitudes and worker perception of their values with respect to the program can set up organizational norms encouraging participation and providing role models for behavioral change. But management-driven norms can also have the effect of precluding the discussion among workers that leads to stronger self-enforcement of norms and a "subtle change in the frequency and nature of workplace interactions that may no longer discourage employee smoking."[50]

Confidentiality is a reinforcing factor of importance for some behavioral and environmental objectives. Participation in a screening program, for example, is quickly discouraged if workers learn that information about their health condition or family history is shared with employers.[51] Ethical issues of confidentiality were addressed earlier in this chapter.

Boredom with a repetitive routine discourages continued participation for some, though others may find a mindless routine comforting or liberating from work stress. Fun and variety in the health promotion program activities can reinforce participation and hold the interest of some, which might account in part for the popularity of group aerobic exercise classes and worksite competitions in weight control and other areas.[52] Incentives related to competitions or in combination with other components of a program have been found effective in maintaining much higher abstinence from smoking for 6 months.[53] Caution must be exercised, however, not to substitute token rewards for the internalization of values and beliefs necessary to sustain real behavior change over time. Token reinforcements may only yield token behavior.[54]

ENABLING FACTORS

Accessibility and convenience are the key enabling factors to be assessed in Phase 4. Proximity of the program to the work stations, convenience of scheduling, and cost determine program accessibility, which represents the largest barrier to program participation.[55]

Enabling factors for environmental change in the worksite include cost of the environmental modifications, disruption of the flow or pace of work, and availability of space for new facilities or equipment.

An application of the PRECEDE model in analyzing the injury prevention behavior of construction workers is shown in Figure 9.6, illustrating the range of factors considered in Phase 4.[56]

PHASE 5: ADMINISTRATIVE AND POLICY ANALYSES

Having now identified the key determinants of the behavioral and environmental objectives, the task is to assess the resources available to influence these determinants and the organization or regulatory policies that will facilitate or hinder the

INFLUENCING FACTORS

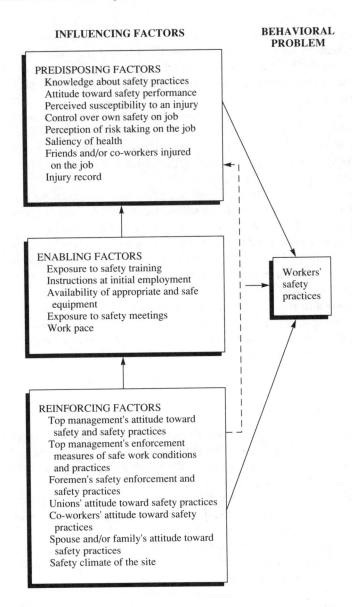

FIGURE 9.6

Predisposing, enabling and reinforcing factors in the educational assessment of construction workers' safety practices. [From N. Dedobbeleer and P. German, *Journal of Occupational Medicine* 29 (1987): 863–8; printed by permission of the publisher.]

implementation of the program. First among the resources of concern in worksite health promotion programs is time. Release time for worker participation in health programs of any kind can be a source of considerable controversy. It adds the hours of work time lost by the participants to the cost of the program. The usual solution is flex-time schedules that allow workers to participate within their workshift but to make up the time during another shift.[57]

Second among resource concerns for most worksite health promotion programs is space. Considering that the program is to be conducted within the facilities of a company or organization whose purpose is not employee health but rather some product or service production, devoting space to health promotion is not done lightly.

Policies to support or protect employee health and health behavior have become the most hotly debated subject in the worksite health promotion literature in recent years. Worksite smoking policies have been tried and evaluated in several countries with varying success.[58] Employee Assistance Programs raise similar policy issues of cost-effectiveness, ethics, employee acceptance, and civil rights.[59]

Policy, resources, and organizational support for health promotion programs in the worksite relate most directly to company profit or worker productivity issues. Experience with worker participation, satisfaction, and job performance in previous efforts to offer policies, programs, or facilities for health promotion must be reviewed within a given company to understand management attitudes toward offering new policies, programs, or facilities. Management behavior is predisposed, enabled, and reinforced just as much as everyone else's behavior. This point should lead the health promotion planner to consider applying the PRECEDE steps to an analysis of employer behavior or to the collective bargaining behavior of workers if the obstacle to starting a program for employees lies in the motivation of management.[60]

PHASES 6–9: IMPLEMENTATION AND EVALUATION

The circumstances and politics of each worksite differ, and within each worksite they will change over time. No amount of planning and policy development can anticipate each new employee's and each new day's special circumstances. Implementation must therefore adapt plans and policies to changing circumstances. The organization of advisory groups during the implementation phases should help the program stay on track with sensitivity to management and to workers' concerns. The provision for continuous feedback through supervisory lines of communication and through anonymous suggestion boxes and questionnaires can help.

Based on experience in setting up and implementing a series of worksite health promotion programs in Lycoming County, a rural area of Pennsylvania, the

County Health Improvement Program (CHIP) staff recommend the following steps in establishing and implementing programs in worksites:

1. Introduction of the program to management
2. Announcement of program to the employees
3. Recruitment and organization of a worker-management committee
4. In-house communication planning
5. Employee interest and risk-factor surveys
6. Formation of subcommittees for each risk factor
7. Exploration of community risk-factor reduction programs
8. Committee review and program selection
9. Development of a program proposal
10. Discussion of the proposal with management
11. Promotion of programs and recruitment of employees
12. Scheduling of programs
13. Program implementation, evaluation, modification, and maintenance.[61]

The details of these steps vary depending on the setting, but the logic of the implementation process described in previous chapters can be seen as having its own character in the worksite. The final step of implementation, evaluation, modification, and maintenance obviously represents a series of steps. This phase recycles through the preceding steps, beginning usually at step 5 for evaluation, and possibly as early as step 1 for program modification if the changes required are so sweeping as to require renegotiation with management.

The major issue of resource allocation arises in the implementation phase when the demand is greater than the resources to meet the needs of those interested in participating. Sometimes this is a problem of numbers, sometimes a problem of variable needs of different types of employees. Three approaches have been suggested in the literature for rationing and allocating scarce program resources during the implementation phase: (1) Screening or wait-listing employees on the basis of a procedure or set of criteria agreed upon in the planning; (2) providing self-help materials and referrals to community resources, with or without subsidies or release time; and (3) a systematic triage and stepped program of interventions based on individualized needs assessments and tailored interventions.

SCREENING AND WAIT-LISTING

The most common method of rationing health promotion resources in the worksite is simply by limiting the eligibility. Historically, worksite health promotion programs were known as executive fitness programs, or executive health examination programs, with the obvious implication of their availability to workers. Some programs screen at the other end of the hierarchy, restricting access to those with the highest risk, greatest exposure to workplace hazards, or greatest need for company subsidy or support. The use of health-risk appraisals and other screening tests to select the target groups for recruitment or admission to the program has a time-honored tradition in public health.[62]

One screening test that has particular relevance to the effectiveness of the program is a test for level of motivation. Many workers will take up space in health promotion programs without much commitment to follow through with the behavioral change recommendations. The requirement that applicants keep a diary of their behavior for a week before starting the program has served as an effective screen in some programs.[63]

SELF-CARE AND COMMUNITY REFERRALS

Much of what a company can offer through personnel and facilities provided at the worksite could be obtained through other organizations in the community, either in the form of self-help materials or in classes and facilities. The advantages of access and convenience at the worksite are obvious, and the advantages of group support among employees can be argued. But self-help materials have a good track record for the motivated.[64] Subsidy of worker participation in outside programs through direct contract with the vendor or agency, or through payment to the worker, or at least through release time to participate, can lend credence and effectiveness to the referral process.

TRIAGE AND STEPPED PROGRAM OF INTERVENTIONS

This third approach requires a more systematic process of assessing the needs of each employee, applicant, or participant in a program of interventions to determine which combination of interventions might be most needed and effective in achieving the program goals or that person's goals. The PRECEDE model can be applied in this process, especially in the educational diagnostic stage. Figure 9.7 offers an algorithm (flow chart) for the triage and stepped approach to assessing predisposing, enabling, and reinforcing factors in sequence and to intervening to strengthen those needing more attention.[65]

Evaluation can be accomplished through program records to measure implementation and process variables, through self-tests, questionnaires, and self-monitoring reports to measure impact, and through company medical or insurance records to measure health outcomes. Absenteeism, productivity, and other company bottom-line concerns can be assessed as described in the evaluation literature cited earlier in this chapter and in Chapter 7.

A CASE STUDY: SMOKING CESSATION AND CONTROL IN A STATE AGENCY

This case[66] illustrates issues concerning the planning process and the policy implementation and evaluation process in the worksite.

SOCIAL AND EPIDEMIOLOGICAL DIAGNOSES

A large state human services agency employs 14,000 persons and has its headquarters in the state capital, with field offices organized into 10 regions. In one of the regions, 1,500 employees moved into a newly constructed facility. Shortly thereafter, employees began to experience respiratory problems and allergic reactions; they associated these reactions with the recent move. They expressed their concern about these new events and the quality of air in the environment to the Building Committee, which resulted in an investigation of the building's ventilation system. It was determined that, other than systematic vigorous cleaning, there was little that could be done to improve the turnover rate of air (replacing the used air with fresh air). This finding, coupled with the efforts of employees who wanted the new building to be smoke-free, led to a concentrated approach to improvement of the air quality through reducing the ambient smoke and other pollutants in the environment and encouraging employees who smoked to stop.

BEHAVIORAL AND ENVIRONMENTAL DIAGNOSES

As seen from this description, movement from the social diagnosis to the behavioral and environmental diagnoses was as much a political process as one of professional planning. The agenda for the Building Committee was set by employee concerns, and no systematic effort was made to set priorities among quality-of-life concerns or health problems. The decision to change behavior and the environment through a policy reform was a foregone conclusion.

EDUCATIONAL AND ORGANIZATIONAL DIAGNOSES

The Building Committee, which extended its membership to include both smokers and nonsmokers, did engage in a diagnostic process to determine its strategies to address the environmental issue. It forwarded responsibility for designing the smoking cessation programs to the Wellness Committee and it assessed the options for environmental and behavioral change as follows.

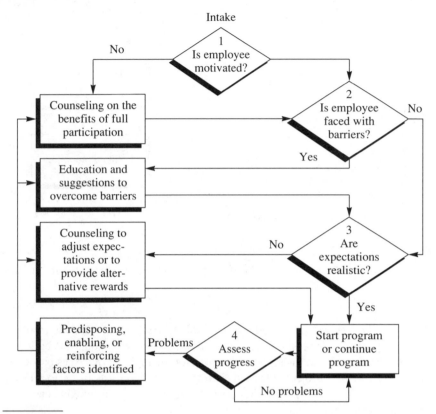

FIGURE 9.7

A flow chart or algorithm for the diagnostic procedure of assessing potential problems of adherence of employees in initiating and maintaining a behavior change. [Adapted from C. Y. Lovato and L. W. Green, *Health Education Quarterly* 17 (1990): 73–88; printed by permission of the publisher.]

The Environment. Figure 9.8 illustrates the determinants of environmental air quality. The importance and changeability of each of the enabling factors were considered:

Enabling factor	Importance	Changeability
Ventilation system improvements to increase air exchange rate	+ +	– –
Cleaning ventilation system	+	+ +
Portable smoke-eaters	–	+ +
Restrictive smoking policy	+ +	+/–

Based on this organizational and engineering analysis, it was decided to make cleaning of the ventilation system a high priority and to reduce ambient smoke in the building by recommending that a restrictive smoking policy be established.

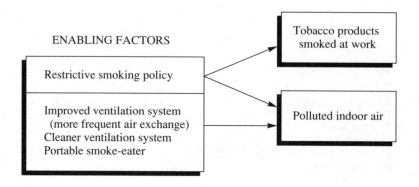

ENABLING FACTORS

Restrictive smoking policy

Improved ventilation system
(more frequent air exchange)
Cleaner ventilation system
Portable smoke-eater

Tobacco products
smoked at work

Polluted indoor air

FIGURE 9.8

Enabling factors influencing air quality in an office building with central heating and air
conditioning.

Behavior and Lifestyle. The Wellness Committee decided to conduct smoking
cessation programs for employees who smoked in the new headquarters building.
These were also offered to employees in some of the regional offices as part of an
evaluation research project. When the executive decision was made to adopt a
restrictive smoking policy, the policy was applied statewide, so smoking cessation
programs were offered statewide.

An educational and organizational diagnosis was conducted in the design of
these programs. Table 9.7 displays predisposing, reinforcing, and enabling factors for stopping smoking. This analysis flows from a behavioral perspective.

The predisposing factors are drawn primarily from the perspective of social
learning theory and the health belief model. They include the individuals' outcome
expectations of the positive and negative results of smoking, their self-efficacy for
quitting, intentions to quit, and the health beliefs of their susceptibility to and the
seriousness of smoking-related diseases. Measures of the individual's smoking
history—smoking frequency and duration (habit strength) and number and duration of cessation attempts—are also predisposing factors that have been shown to
be predictive of success in quitting. The predisposing factors vary across individuals and are useful (a) in designing interventions directed to getting persons to
decide to quit smoking and (b) in tailoring cessation programs to the target
population.

Although the cognitive factors include a motivational component of desired
outcomes from quitting, the social and material incentives provide an important
source of reinforcement for quitting. In addition, the restrictive policy brings
negative reinforcement and punishment into play. Individuals will avoid penalties
by not smoking in restricted areas, and smoking in these areas will lead to
punishment. Expectation of these reinforcements is a strong source of motivation.

TABLE 9.7

Educational and organizational diagnosis of predisposing, reinforcing, and enabling factors related to smoking cessation

Predisposing Factors

Attitudes, beliefs, and values concerning *smoking* are that it
  Increases concentration
  Decreases tension
  Provides a high
  Controls my weight
  Helps me fit in

Attitudes, beliefs, and values concerning *not smoking* are that it
  Keeps me from fitting in
  Increases my health risk
  Increases the health risks of others
  Is not compatible with my value of health
  Costs a lot
  Makes my clothes and hair smell
  Is messy

Belief in self-efficacy for quitting

Habit strength: number of years smoked

Previous cessation attempts: experience with quitting

Reinforcing factors

Social encouragement to quit and remain abstinent
  Co-worker
  Family
  Cessation group "buddy"

Material incentives
  Financial rewards for quitting

Restrictive policy violations

Enabling factors

Skills for quitting

Restrictive smoking policy

The possession of behavioral skills — including self-contracting, goal-setting, monitoring of cigarettes, identification and management of environmental cues to smoke, self-reinforcement, and techniques for coping with urges to smoke — are crucial to the individual's following through on the decision to quit. The worksite setting makes it possible to move beyond individual management of environmental cues. Cues for smoking are removed from areas in which smoking is restricted by policy. This reduces triggering of the smoking impulse in these areas. In this way, the policy restraint on one smoker becomes a support to another smoker trying to quit.

FROM ADMINISTRATIVE AND POLICY DIAGNOSES TO IMPLEMENTATION

A smoking cessation program was devised based on the educational and organizational diagnosis and the resources available in the budget and in the worksite. *Freedom from Smoking in Twenty Days*, a low-cost self-help program, was chosen to provide information and exercises designed to influence the predisposing factors (e.g., those identified by questions such as Why do you smoke? Why do you want to quit?) and the specific skills listed earlier as enabling factors.[67] The self-help manual includes forms for logging smoking patterns and analyzing cues or triggers for smoking, for making self-contracts, and for planning how one will cope with urges to smoke. Smokers, with encouragement from the manual, could select a "buddy" and find advice in the manual on how to make the most of this supportive relationship.

Additional reinforcement was mobilized at the organizational level, using two campaigns. The first was a competition between two worksites.[68] The worksite with the highest proportion of smokers recruited to the program and of non-smokers becoming "supporters" won a cold-turkey buffet the day after the Great American Smoke-Out which is sponsored by the American Cancer Society. This mobilized social reinforcement for recruitment. A second campaign, *Winning Choices*, conducted later, provided chances to win savings bonds to smokers who joined the cessation programs.[69]

The new policy restricting smoking served as an enabling factor for both the behavioral objective of smoking cessation and the environmental objective of cleaner air. The Building Committee, as part of its work in advising the agency head on how to improve air quality, carried out a survey of employees to assess opinions on whether a more restrictive policy was needed. This survey (box C in Fig. 9.9) followed the employee surveys (A and B) that had provided assessments of predisposing, enabling, and reinforcing factors.

The committee also sponsored a roundtable discussion on the smoking issue which was open to all employees at the state headquarters. Based on its findings, the committee recommended that a restrictive smoking policy be adopted. The committee, however, had only an advisory role. There was concern that top administration would not act on the recommendation. A proposed Clean Air Act, which would have required smoking policies in all worksites across the state did not pass in the state legislature that year.

At this point, an internal champion for the proposed policy emerged. A newly appointed high-level manager, who had successfully established a similar smoking policy at another agency, became an advocate for the recommended policy. The

Time

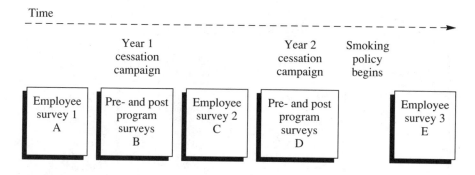

FIGURE 9.9

Quantitative data collection points in the diagnostic and evaluation phases of developing an educational and environmental approach to air quality in a state office building.

executive decision-making group developed a restrictive smoking policy for the entire agency, not just the state office.

The process of policy development and implementation always depends on the context.[70] Two of the few generalizable principles are (1) supervisors who must implement and employees who will be affected by policy should participate in the formulation of the policy and (2) the policy should be flexible enough to cover the variety of contingencies it will encounter.

A draft policy was published in the statewide employee newsletter which invited comments. Experience in smoking policy development and implementation suggests that the mere opportunity to comment, even if employees do not avail themselves of the opportunity, goes a long way toward greater acceptance of a new policy. The final policy was sent to all employees 4 months before implementation. It called for smoking to be restricted in each building, except in breakrooms designated by the regional administrator. Employee meetings held at each site served to provide advice to the regional administrator on the preferred site of the designated breakroom. Had this state agency been unionized, representation of the union would have been crucial to the development and implementation of the policy.

Figure 9.10 provides an overview of key factors in the process of policy development and implementation. The success of a smoking policy will depend on its concept or content and the process of its development (box 1), on how it fits into the context of implementation (box 2), and its implementation process (box 3). The careful planner will provide for employee ownership of the program through participation in its formulation and implementation. Anticipating variations in the worksites where the policy will be implemented helps build the necessary flexibility into the policy.

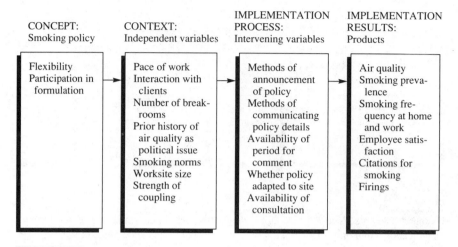

CONCEPT: Smoking policy	CONTEXT: Independent variables	IMPLEMENTATION PROCESS: Intervening variables	IMPLEMENTATION RESULTS: Products
Flexibility Participation in formulation	Pace of work Interaction with clients Number of break- rooms Prior history of air quality as political issue Smoking norms Worksite size Strength of coupling	Methods of announcement of policy Methods of communicating policy details Availability of period for comment Whether policy adapted to site Availability of consultation	Air quality Smoking preva- lence Smoking fre- quency at home and work Employee satis- faction Citations for smoking Firings

FIGURE 9.10

Smoking policy implementation in a large state agency.

The more thorough cleaning of the ventilation system, the second environmental reform, was more easily implemented. A simple regulatory directive from the agency head to the maintenance supervisor accomplished this. Bi-weekly vacuuming of external vents and monthly inspections were incorporated into the job routine of the maintenance personnel.

IMPLEMENTATION AND STRUCTURAL EVALUATION

The implementation and structural evaluation of the new smoking regulations was planned using the flow chart in Figure 9.9 and the model in Figure 9.10. Both qualitative and quantitative methods were used. The process of policy development was documented using internal records, such as newsletter articles, memoranda, minutes of committee meetings, and interviews. A survey of a random sample of employees following policy implementation ascertained their level of involvement in policy formulation and implementation (see Fig. 9.9, box E).

The new ventilation system maintenance was documented through memoranda and inspection reports.

An evaluation was also carried out for the implementation of the smoking cessation program. Records were maintained of the numbers of nonsmokers volunteering as "supporters" and smokers signing up for the program, attending the orientation, and receiving the self-help manual. The percentages of smoking and nonsmoking employees in the program were calculated using prevalence estimates from an earlier baseline survey (see Fig. 9.9, boxes A and C, respectively). This indicated the penetration of the program into the employee population.

These process evaluation reports were completed by each regional wellness coordinator and forwarded to the state coordinator. They served as the basis for making the awards in each region for the cold-turkey buffet and savings bonds drawings in the two campaigns. In addition, all media related to the campaigns were organized by date and submitted by each region to the state office. Based on this evidence, it was possible to determine the extent of implementation of the program within each region.

Process Evaluation. Changes in predisposing factors among smokers were studied using pre- and posttest questionnaires (Fig. 9.9, boxes B and D) of the beliefs and attitudes outlined in Table 9.7. Program participants were also asked what behavioral skill components in the manual they had used and, for each they had used, how helpful it had been. Items related to co-worker and family encouragement and discouragement of quitting documented the extent to which co-workers and family had provided social reinforcement for the behavior change. The extent to which the new smoking policy was perceived as a factor in the processes of quitting and maintenance of cessation was also examined.

Satisfaction with the air quality in the work area and with the smoking policy was assessed. Figure 9.11 indicates the marked differences between satisfaction of smokers and nonsmokers. Most of the change occurred in the first month following implementation of the policy.

Several approaches provided for evaluation of changes in the two enabling factors related to air quality. For smoking policy, employees were surveyed regarding their satisfaction with the policy, with how well employees abided by the policy, and with the level of enforcement at their specific worksite (Fig. 9.9, box E). The evaluation team analyzed whether these factors varied by worksite context and by individuals' smoking status. Records were maintained by the state office of employee complaints about the policy, resignations related to the policy, and policy violations and associated personnel actions. The cleaning of the ventilation system was monitored through regular inspection reports of dust accumulation before and after the policy was implemented.

Impact Evaluation. Comparison of pre- and posttest (Figure 9.9, boxes B and D) patterns of smoking indicated whether participants had reduced the number of cigarettes they smoked or quit smoking. These self-reports of quitting were validated using biochemical analysis on a sample of employees. Besides this study of program participants, a random sample of all employees was undertaken to see if the smoking prevalence had changed across the entire workforce, not just among the employees who were in the program (Figure 9.9, boxes A, C and E).

Comparisons were made also between smoking rates in worksites where smoking was allowed in restricted areas and those in which a complete ban was enforced within the buildings. Table 9.8 shows the results at 1 month and 6 months following implementation of the policies. Although the policies succeeded in

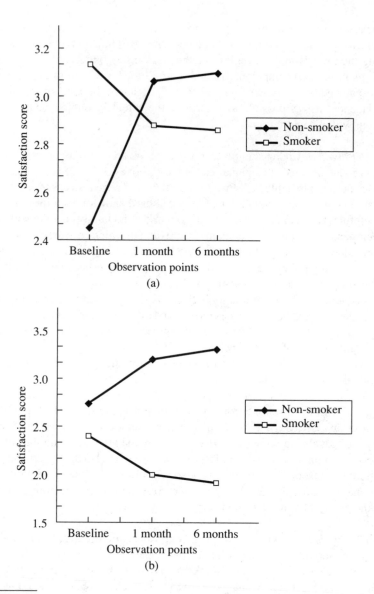

FIGURE 9.11

Satisfaction of workers with (a) air quality in their work area and (b) the smoking policy, at the time of implementation and one and six months following implementation, comparing smokers and non-smokers. [From N. H. Gottlieb, M. P. Eriksen, C. Y. Lovato, et al., *Journal of Occupational Medicine* 32 (1990): 16– 23.]

TABLE 9.8

Smoking indicators versus time in regions with restricted smoking areas and those with bans

	In restricted areas (%)			In ban areas (%)		
	Baseline	1 month	6 month	Baseline	1 month	6 month
	$n=1432$	$n=1111$	$n=967$	$n=279$	$n=238$	$n=169$
Current smokers	22.4%	21.4%	20.1%	25.1%	22.7%	16.6%
Former smokers	19.2	19.3	20.2	12.5	19.3	15.4
Never smokers	58.4	59.3	59.8	62.4	58.0	68.0
Smokers						
≥ 15 cigarettes at work	$n=313$	$n=226$	$n=190$	$n=69$	$n=49$	$n=27$
	16.9	6.6	5.8	17.4	8.2	0.0
≥ 15 cigarettes daily total	$n=314$	$n=232$	$n=194$	$n=69$	$n=51$	$n=28$
	48.7	40.9	52.1	63.8	53.8	60.7

SOURCE: N. H. Gottlieb, M. P. Eriksen, C. Y. Lovato, et al., *Journal of Occupational Medicine* 32 (1990): 16–23.

reducing smoking in the worksites, thereby achieving the program objective of improving air quality, smokers' daily total of cigarettes might have increased with more smoking at home.

Air quality was measured using self-reports of employees on pre- and post-policy surveys (Fig. 9.9, boxes C and E). In addition, an environmental engineering firm conducted an analysis of air quality before and after the policy and program were implemented.

Outcome Evaluation. It is not feasible within program resources to measure long-term health consequences of smoking cessation and air quality improvement in a situation such as this. The time lag for health effects is too long, the employee turnover is too great, and the cost of follow-up would be prohibitive for most organizations. Projections of outcome, however, can be made using risk factor equations from studies such as the Framingham Heart Study. It was possible to examine changes in self-reported respiratory symptoms before and after the program and policy were implemented in this case. Nonsmokers in smoke-free regions reported higher satisfaction with air quality and indicated they were bothered less frequently by co-workers' smoke than their peers in regions with a restrictive smoking policy allowing smoking in breakrooms.

SUMMARY

The worksite presents an opportunity and a challenge within the array of settings for the development of health promotion. The growth of the labor force with the increased participation of women may be matched in future years with a corresponding growth in the employment of older people needing or choosing to work rather than to retire. These demographic trends place new demands on employers to cope with issues of child care and employee health. Escalation of health-care costs and the increasing proportion of the burden of medical costs born by industry has brought about an explosion of alternative strategies to contain costs, with health promotion being one among many still in an experimental phase.

Whether for cost containment or other reasons, the planning, implementation, and evaluation of worksite health promotion programs can follow the PRECEDE and PROCEED phases with some adaptations described in this chapter. Particular attention to balancing the emphasis on behavioral and environmental changes can serve to assure greater support from management and employees alike. Care in the implementation process to provide for continuous monitoring and feedback through advisory and communication structures will assure continuity and sustainability of the program.

EXERCISES

1. If the counterpart of social benefits for industry are the bottom-line issues of productivity and profit, how can you express your objectives for a worksite program that will convince management to support the program?
2. Create an example in which a behavioral approach, though well-intended, may be construed as victim blaming. Then, using the appropriate steps in the PRECEDE/PROCEED model, illustrate how the accountable practitioner can avoid that criticism.

REFERENCES AND NOTES

1. L. W. Green, "Toward Cost-Benefit Evaluations of Health Education: Some Concepts, Methods and Examples," *Health Education Monographs* 2 (1974): 34–64.

2. See previous chapter notes for examples of applications in community settings. The next two chapters provide examples of applications in school and medical settings. For a bibliography of evaluations of programs based on this and other models of health education and health promotion,

see L. W. Green and F. M. Lewis, *Measurement and Evaluation in Health Education and Health Promotion* (Palo Alto, CA: Mayfield, 1986).

3. We are especially indebted to Chris Y. Lovato, Nell Gottlieb, and Michael Eriksen at the University of Texas and to Dave Ramsey at CDC for their contributions to this chapter. Dr. Lovato is now at San Diego State University.

4. U.S. Bureau of the Census, *Statistical Abstract of the United States: 1990*, 109th ed. (Washington, DC: U.S. Government Printing Office, 1989).

5. D. S. Burden and B. K. Googins, *Balancing Work Life and Homelife* (Boston: Boston University School of Social Work, 1987).

6. See, for example, L. Duhl, "The Healthy City: Its Function and Its Future," *Health Promotion* 1 (1986): 55–60; T. J. Glynn, "Psychological Sense of Community: Measurement and Application," *Human Relations* 34 (1981): 789–818; L. W. Green, "The Revival of Community and the Role of the Academic Health Center," in *The Role of the Academic Health Center in Humanizing Medicine*, R. Bulger, R. E. Bulger, and S. Reiser, eds. (Ames, Iowa: University of Iowa Press, 1990); S. Riger and P. J. Lavrakas, "Community Ties: Patterns of Attachment and Social Interaction in Urban Neighborhoods," *American Journal of Community Psychology* 9 (1981): 55–66.

7. G. H. Collings, Jr., "Perspectives of Industry Regarding Health Promotion," in R. S. Parkinson and Associates, *Managing Health Promotion in the Workplace: Guidelines for Implementation and Evaluation* (Palo Alto: Mayfield, 1982), pp. 119–26; L. W. Green, G. L. Stainbrook, and C. Y. Lovato, "The Benefits Perceived by Industry in Supporting Health Promotion Programs in the Worksite," *American Journal of Health Promotion* (in press), and in *Proceedings of the Harvard Symposium on Worksite Health Promotion* (Baltimore: Johns Hopkins University Press, in press).

8. K. E. Warner, "Selling Health Promotion to Corporate America: Uses and Abuses of the Economic Argument," *Health Education Quarterly*, 14 (1987): 39–55, data from p. 42.

9. K. R. Levit, M S. Freeland, and D. R. Waldo, "Health Spending and Ability to Pay: Business, Individuals, and Government," *Health Care Financing Review* 10 (Spring 1989): 1–11.

10. M. Alderman, L. W. Green, B. S. Flynn, "Hypertension Control Programs in Occupational Settings," *Public Health Reports* 90 (1980): 158–63; H. S. Ruchlin and M. H. Alderman, "Cost of Hypertension Control at the Workplace," *Journal of Occupational Medicine* 22 (1980): 795–800.

11. B. G. Danaher, "Smoking Cessation Programs in Occupational Settings," in *Managing Health Promotion in the Workplace: Guidelines for Implementation and Evaluation*, R. S. Parkinson and Associates, eds. (Palo Alto: Mayfield, 1982), pp. 217–32.

12. C. C. DiClemente, J. O. Prochaska, and M. Gibertine, "Self-efficacy and the Stages of Self-change of Smoking," *Cognitive Therapy and Research* 9 (1985): 181–200.

13. The "innovative" or "bellweather" states in health promotion were identified by John Naisbitt, *Megatrends: Ten New Directions Transforming Our Lives* (New York: Warner Books, 1982); see also J. Naisbitt and P. Aburdene, *Megatrends 2000: Ten New Directions for the 1990's* (New York: William Morrow, 1990). For specific accounts of the growth and diffusion of smoking control programs in the workplace, see M. P. Eriksen, "Workplace Smoking Control: Rationale and Approaches," *Advances in Health Education and Promotion*, vol. 1, pt. A (Greenwich, CT: JAI Press, 1986), pp. 65–103; D. L. Haefele, "A Survey of Non-smoking Policies in Ninety-one Large Businesses, Companies and Agencies," *Health Education* 21(4) (1990): 47–53; C. Orleans and R. Shipley, "Worksite Smoking Cessation Initiatives: Review and Recommendations," *Addictive Behaviors* 7 (1982): 1–16; R. F. Schilling, L. D. Gilchrist, and S. P. Schinke, "Smoking in the Workplace: Review of Critical Issues," *Public Health Reports* 100 (1985): 473–9; V. Todaro, J. Denard, P. Clarke, et al., "Survey of Worksite Smoking Policies," *Morbidity and Mortality Weekly Report* 36 (1987): 177–9; D. C. Walsh, "Corporate Smoking Policies: A Review and an Analysis," *Journal of Occupational Medicine* 26 (1984): 17–22. The growth trends in other worksite health promotion activities are traced in J. E. Fielding, "Health Promotion and Disease Prevention at the Worksite," *Annual Review of Public Health* 5 (1984): 237–65, and in J. E. Fielding and P. V.

Piserchia, "Frequency of Worksite Health Promotion Activities," *American Journal of Public Health* 79 (1989): 16–20.

14. J. E. Fielding, "Preventive Medicine and the Bottom Line," *Journal of Occupational Medicine* 24 (1982): 907–16; J. E. Fielding and L. Breslow, "Health Promotion Programs Sponsored by California Employers," *American Journal of Public Health* 73 (1983): 538–42; R. S. Parkinson and Associates, eds., *Managing Health Promotion in the Workplace: Guidelines for Implementation and Evaluation* (Palo Alto: Mayfield, 1982).

15. *Health Promotion Can Produce Economic Savings* (Lansing, MI: Office of Health and Medical Affairs, Department of Management and Budget and the Center for Health Promotion, Michigan Department of Health, 1987).

16. J. E. Fielding, "Worksite Health Promotion Programs in the United States: Progress, Lessons and Challenges," *Health Promotion International* 5 (1990): 75–84.

17. D. W. Bowne, M. L. Russell, J. L. Morgan, et al., "Reduced Disability and Health Care Costs in an Industrial Fitness Program," *Journal of Occupational Medicine* 26 (1984): 809–16.

18. R. J. Shephard, P. Corey, P. Renzland, et al., "The Influence of an Employee Fitness and Lifestyle Modification Program Upon Medical Care Costs," *Canadian Journal of Public Health* 73 (1982): 259–63.

19. J. L. Bly, R. C. Jones, and J. E. Richardson, "Impact of Worksite Health Promotion on Health Care Costs and Utilization," *Journal of the American Medical Association* 256 (1986): 3235–40.

20. M. F. Davis, K. Rosenberg, D. E. Iverson, et al., "Worksite Health Promotion in Colorado," *Public Health Reports* 99 (1984): 538–43; J. E. Fielding and P. V. Piserchia, "Frequency of Worksite Health Promotion Activities," *American Journal of Public Health* 79 (1989): 16–20; J. E. Fielding, "Health Promotion and Disease Prevention at the Worksite," *Annual Review of Public Health* 5 (1984): 237–65; Minnesota Department of Health, "Workplace Health Promotion Survey" (Minneapolis: Minnesota Department of Health, 1982).

21. J. E. Fielding and P. V. Piserchia, op. cit., 1989.

22. J. P. Allegrante, "Potential Uses and Misuses of Education in Health Promotion and Disease Prevention," *Teachers College Record* 86 (Winter 1984): 359–73; also *Eta Sigma Gamman* 18 (1986): 2–8; J. P. Allegrante and R. P. Sloan, "Ethical Dilemmas in Workplace Health Promotion," *Preventive Medicine* 15 (1986): 313–20; D. Beauchamp, "Public Health as Social Justice," in *Public Health and the Law*, L. Hogue, ed. (Rockville: Aspen Systems, 1980); M. H. Becker, "The Tyranny of Health Promotion," *Public Health Reviews* 14 (1986): 15–25; R. B. Hollander and J. G. Hale, "Worksite Health Promotion Programs: Ethical Issues," *American Journal of Health Promotion* 2 (Fall 1987): 37–43; T. W. O'Rourke and D. M. Macrina, "Beyond Victim Blaming: Examining the Micro-macro Issue in Health Promotion," *Wellness Perspectives: Research, Theory and Practice* 6 (1989): 7–17; J. Ratcliff and L. Wallack, "Primary Prevention in Public Health: An Analysis of Basic Assumptions," *International Quarterly of Community Health Education* 6 (1986): 215–37.

23. R. Karasek and T. Theorell, *Healthy Work: Stress, Productivity, and the Reconstruction of Working Life* (New York: Basic Books, 1990).

24. Karasek and Theorell, op. cit., 1990; K. McLeroy, L. W. Green, K. Mullen, and V. Foshee, "Assessing the Effects of Health Promotion in Worksites: A Review of the Stress Program Evaluations," *Health Education Quarterly* 11 (1984): 379–401; K. R. Pelletier and R. Lutz, "Healthy People—Healthy Business: A Critical Review of Stress Management Programs in the Workplace," *American Journal of Health Promotion* 2 (Winter 1988): 5–12.

25. R. Shipley, "Smoking Reduction Programs Help Business Snuff Out Health Problems," *Occupational Health and Safety* 56 (1987): 73–7; R. P. Sloan, J. C. Gruman, and J. P. Allegrante, *Investing in Employee Health: A Guide to Effective Health Promotion in the Workplace* (San Francisco, Jossey-Bass, 1987).

26. S. Permut, "Corporate Liability for Occupational Medicine Programs," in *Occupational Stress: Health and Performance at Work*, S. Wolf and A. Finestone, eds. (Littleton, MA: PSG Publishing Company, 1986), pp. 136–52.

27. M. A. Vojtecky, "Commentary: A Unified Approach to Health Promotion and Health Protection," *Journal of Community Health* 11 (1986): 219–21.

28. G. S. Smith and J. F. Kraus, "Alcohol and Residential, Recreational, and Occupational Injuries: A Review of the Epidemiologic Evidence," *Annual Review of Public Health* 9 (1988): 99–122.

29. B. E. Brody, "Employee Assistance Programs: An Historical and Literature Review," *American Journal of Health Promotion* 2 (Winter 1988): 13–19; D. Masi, *Designing Employee Assistance Programs* (New York: American Management Association, 1984); D. Myers, *Establishing and Building Employee Assistance Programs* (Westport, CT: Quaorum, 1985). The E.A.P.'s, however, have failed to offer primary prevention of substance abuse, just as drugs and alcohol are seldom part of other health promotion programs that do emphasize primary prevention. See R. Cook and A. Harrell, "Drug Abuse Among Working Adults: Prevalence Rates and Recommended Strategies," *Health Education Research: Theory and Practice* 2 (1987): 353–9.

30. K. R. Pelletier and R. Lutz, "Healthy People–Healthy Business: A Critical Review of Stress Management Programs in the Workplace," *American Journal of Health Promotion* 2 (Winter 1988), 5–12; R. Windom, J. M. McGinnis, and J. E. Fielding, "Examining Worksite Health Promotion Programs," *Business and Health* 4 (Sept. 1987): 26–37.

31. J. E. Fielding and P. V. Piserchia, op. cit., 1989.

32. K. E. Warner, "Selling Health Promotion to Corporate America: Uses and Abuses of the Economic Argument," *Health Education Quarterly* 14 (1987): 39–55; A. Cohen and L. Murphy, "Indicators and Measures of Health Promotion Behaviors in the Workplace," in *Health Promotion Indicators and Actions*, S. B. Kar, ed. (New York: Springer, 1989); M. Key and D. Kilian, "Counseling and Cancer Prevention Programs in Industry," in *Cancer Prevention in Clinical Medicine*, G. R. Newell, ed. (New York: Raven Press, 1983); M. A. Vojtecky, "Commentary: A Unified Approach to Health Promotion and Health Protection," *Journal of Community Health* 11(4) (1986): 219–21.

33. M. F. Cataldo, L. W. Green, J. A. Herd, et al., "Preventive Medicine and the Corporate Environment: Challenge to Behavioral Medicine," in *Health and Industry: A Behavioral Medicine Perspective*, M. F. Cataldo and T. J. Coates, eds. (New York: Wiley, 1986), pp. 399–419.

34. C. Y. Lovato and L. W. Green, "Consultation Report for National Cancer Institute's Grant to Five Unions to Develop Cancer Control Programs," Houston, University of Texas Center for Health Promotion Research and Development, paper presented at the annual meeting of the American Public Health Association, New Orleans, LA, Nov. 1986; C. Y. Lovato, L. W. Green and V. Conley, "Development and Evaluation of Occupational Health Education Programs to Reduce Exposure to Cancer Hazards," presented at the annual meeting of the American Society for Preventive Oncology, Bethesda, MD, 1986. For a discussion of data sources for epidemiological surveillance of occupational illness and injury in the United States, see E. L. Baker, J. M. Melius, and J. D. Millar, "Surveillance of Occupational Illness and Injury in the United States: Current Perspectives and Future Directions," *Journal of Public Health Policy* 9 (1988): 198–221.

35. C. Y. Lovato and L. W. Green, "Consultation Report for the Workers Institute for Safety and Health, Washington, D.C." (Houston: University of Texas Center for Health Promotion Research and Development, 1984).

36. B. D. Dunlop, P. V. Piserchia, J. E. Richardson, et al., *Evaluation of Workplace Health Enhancement Programs: A Monograph* (Research Triangle Park, NC: Research Triangle Institute, 1989); A. Cohen and L. Murphy, op. cit., 1989.

37. L. W. Syme, "Strategies for Health Promotion," *Preventive Medicine* 15 (1986): 492–507.

38. L. W. Green, A. L. Wilson, and C. Y. Lovato, "What Changes Can Health Promotion Achieve and

How Long Do These Changes Last? The Tradeoffs Between Expediency and Durability," *Preventive Medicine* 15 (1986): 508–21; W. L. Haskell and S. N. Blair, "The Physical Activity Component of Health Promotion in Occupational Settings," in *Managing Health Promotion in the Workplace: Guidelines for Implementation and Evaluation*, R. S. Parkinson and Associates, eds. (Palo Alto: Mayfield, 1982), pp. 252–71.

39. L. W. Green, "The Trade-offs Between the Expediency of Health Promotion and the Durability of Health Education," in *Topics in Health Psychology*, S. Maes, C. D. Spielberger, P. B. Defares, and I. G. Sarason, eds. (New York: Wiley, 1988), pp. 301–12.

40. K. D. Brownell and M. R. Felix, "Competitions to Facilitate Health Promotion: Review and Conceptual Analysis," *American Journal of Health Promotion* 2(1) (1987): 28–36.

41. P. Conrad, "Who Comes to Work-site Wellness Programs? A Preliminary Review," *Journal of Occupational Medicine* 29 (1987): 317–20; J. E. Fielding, "Health Promotion and Disease Prevention at the Worksite," *Annual Review of Public Health* 5 (1984): 237–65; N. B. Oldridge, "Adherence to Adult Exercise Fitness Programs," in *Behavioral Health*, J. D. Matarazzo, S. M. Weiss, J. A. Herd, et al., eds. (New York: Wiley, 1984), pp. 467–87.

42. J. G. Sallis, W. L. Haskell, S. P. Fortmann, et al., "Predictors of Adoption and Maintenance of Physical Activity in a Community Sample," *Preventive Medicine* 15 (1986): 331–41; V. J. Strecher, B. M. DeVellis, M. H. Becker, and I. M. Rosenstock, "The Role of Self-efficacy in Achieving Health Behavior Change," *Health Education Quarterly* 13 (1986): 73–91.

43. K. E. Davis, K. L. Jackson, J. J. Kronenfeld, and S. N. Blair, "Determinants of Participation in Worksite Health Promotion Activities," *Health Education Quarterly* 14 (1987): 195–205; C. Y. Lovato and L. W. Green, "Maintaining Employee Participation in Workplace Health Promotion Programs," *Health Education Quarterly* 17 (1990): 73–88; K. R. McLeroy, L. W. Green, K. D. Mullen, and V. Foshee, "Assessing the Effects of Health Promotion in Worksites: A Review of the Stress Program Evaluations," *Health Education Quarterly* 11 (1984): 379–401.

44. N. H. Gottlieb and A. Nelson, "A Systematic Effort to Reduce Smoking at the Worksite," *Health Education Quarterly* 17 (1990): 99–118.

45. L. A. Bjurstrom and N. G. Alexiou, "A Program of Heart Disease Intervention for Public Employees," *Journal of Occupational Medicine* 20 (1978): 521–31.

46. M. Alderman, L. W. Green, and B. S. Flynn, "Hypertension Control Programs in Occupational Settings," in *Managing Health Promotion in the Workplace: Guidelines for Implementation and Evaluation*, R. S. Parkinson and Associates, eds. (Palo Alto: Mayfield, 1982), pp. 162–72; G. S. Everly and R. H. Feldman, eds., *Occupational Health Promotion: Health Behavior in the Workplace* (New York: Wiley, 1985); M. P. O'Donnell and T. Ainsworth, eds., *Health Promotion in the Workplace* (New York: Wiley, 1984).

47. R. H. Feldman, "Strategies for Improving Compliance with Health Promotion Programs in Industry," *Health Education* 14(4) (1983): 21–5; R. H. Feldman, "Increasing Compliance in Worksite Health Promotion: Organizational, Educational, and Psychological Strategies," *Corporate Commentary* 1(2) (1984): 45–50.

48. M. Alderman, L. W. Green, and B. S. Flynn, op. cit., 1982.

49. G. S. Everly and R. H. Feldman, eds., *Occupational Health Promotion: Health Behavior in the Workplace* (New York: Wiley, 1985); M. Landgreen and W. Baum, "Adhering to Fitness in the Corporate Setting," *Corporate Commentary* 1 (1984): 30–5; R. Parkinson and Associates, op. cit., 1982; M. P. O'Donnell and T. Ainsworth, op. cit., 1984.

50. N. H. Gottlieb, M. P. Eriksen, C. Y. Lovato, et al., "Impact of a Restrictive Work Site Smoking Policy on Smoking Behavior, Attitudes, and Norms," *Journal of Occupational Medicine* 32 (1990): 20–3, quotation from p. 22.

51. R. H. Feldman, "Increasing Compliance in Worksite Health Promotion: Organizational, Educational, and Psychological Strategies," *Corporate Commentary* 1(2) 1984: 45–50.

52. K. D. Brownell and M. R. Felix, op. cit., 1987; K. Brownell, R. Cohen, A. Stunkard, et al., "Weight Loss Competitions at the Work Site: Impact on Weight, Morale, and Cost-Effectiveness," *American Journal of Public Health* 74 (1984): 1283–5; J. Collins, S. Wagner, and L. Weissberger, "125 Teams Lose 2,233 Pounds in a Work Site Weight Loss Competition," *Journal of the American Dietetic Association* 86 (1986): 1578–9; R. Glasgow, R. Klesges, J. Mizes, and T. Pechacek, "Quitting Smoking: Strategies Used and Variables Associated With Success in a Stop-Smoking Contest," *Journal of Consulting and Clinical Psychology* 53 (1985): 905–12.

53. L. A. Jason, S. Jayaraj, C. C. Blitz, et al., "Incentives and Competition in a Worksite Smoking Cessation Intervention," *American Journal of Public Health* 80 (1990): 205–6; R. Klesges, M. Vasey, and R. Glasgow, "A Worksite Smoking Modification Competition: Potential for Public Health Impact," *American Journal of Public Health* 76 (1986): 198–200.

54. L. W. Green, A. L. Wilson, and C. Y. Lovato, op. cit., 1986.

55. L. A. Bjurstrom and N. G. Alexiou, op. cit., 1978; W. L. Haskell and S. N. Blair, op. cit., 1982; R. Parkinson, et al., 1982.

56. N. Dedobbeleer and P. German, "Safety Practices in Construction Industry," *Journal of Occupational Medicine* 29 (1987): 863–8.

57. C. Y. Lovato and L. W. Green, "Maintaining Employee Participation in Workplace Health Promotion Programs," *Health Education Quarterly* 17 (1990): 73–88.

58. R. Borland, S. Chapman, N. Owen, and D. Hill, "Effects of Workplace Smoking Bans on Cigarette Consumption," *American Journal of Public Health* 80 (1990): 178–80; M. P. Eriksen, op. cit., 1986; N. H. Gottlieb, M. P. Eriksen, C. Y. Lovato, et al., op. cit., 1990; N. H. Gottlieb and A. Nelson, op. cit., 1990; D. C. Walsh and V. McDougall, "Current Policies Regarding Smoking in the Workplace," *American Journal of Industrial Medicine* 13 (1988): 181–90.

59. A. Colantonio, "Assessing the Effects of Employee Assistance Programs—A Review of Employee Assistance Program Evaluations," *Yale Journal of Biology and Medicine* 62 (1989): 13–22; D. C. Walsh and R. H. Egdahl, "Corporate Perspectives on Work Site Wellness Programs: A Report on the Seventh Pew Fellows Conference," *Journal of Occupational Medicine* 31 (1989): 551–6.

60. For an application of PRECEDE to the activation of workers to bring pressure on management for a policy change regarding worksite hazards, see Appendix C-1 in previous edition, L. W. Green, M. W. Kreuter, S. G. Deeds, and K. B. Partridge, *Health Education Planning: A Diagnostic Approach* (Palo Alto: Mayfield, 1980), pp. 212–24.

61. M. R. J. Felix, A. J. Stunkard, R. Y. Cohen, and N. B. Cooley, "Health Promotion at the Worksite, I. A Process for Establishing Programs," *Preventive Medicine* 14 (1985): 99–108.

62. K. J. Zavela, L. G. Davis, R. R. Cottrell, and W. E. Smith, "Do Only the Healthy Intend to Participate in Worksite Health Promotion?" *Health Education Quarterly* 15 (1988): 259–67; R. P. Sloan and J. C. Gruman, "Participation in Workplace Health Promotion Programs: The Contribution of Health and Organizational Factors," *Health Education Quarterly* 15 (1988): 269–88.

63. P. D. Mullen and D. Culjat, "Improving Attendance in Weight-Control Programs," *Health Education Quarterly* 7 (1980): 4–13.

64. D. L. Bibeau, K. D. Mullen, K. R. McLeroy, et al., "Evaluation of Workplace Smoking Cessation Programs: A Critique," *American Journal of Preventive Medicine* 4 (1988): 87–95; A. L. Davis, R. Faust, M. Ordentlich, "Self-help Smoking Cessation and Maintenance Programs: A Comparative Study With 12-Month Follow-up by the American Lung Association," *American Journal of Public Health* 74 (1984): 1212–9; T. J. Glynn, G. M. Boyd, and J. C. Gruman, "Essential Elements of Self-Help/Minimal Intervention Strategies for Smoking Cessation," *Health Education Quarterly* 17 (1990): 329–45; J. F. Sallis, R. D. Hill, P. D. Killen, et al., "Efficacy of Self-help Behavior Modification Materials in Smoking Cessation," *American Journal of Preventive Medicine* 2 (1986): 342–4; R. A. Windsor and E. E. Bartlett, "Employee Self-help Smoking Cessation Programs: A Review of the Literature," *Health Education Quarterly* 11 (1984): 349–59. For a

meta-analysis of worksite smoking cessation evaluations, see K. J. Fisher, R. E. Glasgow, and J. R. Terborg, "Work Site Smoking Cessation: A Meta-analysis of Long-term Quit Rates from Controlled Studies," *Journal of Occupational Medicine* 32 (1990): 429–39.

65. C. Y. Lovato and L. W. Green, op. cit., 1990.

66. This case description is based on work initiated at the University of Texas Center for Health Promotion Research and Development, and at U. T. Austin, with support from the Texas Affiliate of the American Heart Association, and grant K07-CA01286 from the National Cancer Institute. See N. H. Gottlieb, M. P. Eriksen, C. Y. Lovato, et al., "Impact of a Restrictive Work Site Smoking Policy on Smoking Behavior, Attitudes, and Norms," *Journal of Occupational Medicine* 32 (1990): 16–23; N. H. Gottlieb and A. Nelson, "A Systematic Effort to Reduce Smoking at the Worksite," *Health Education Quarterly* 17 (1990): 99–118. Some variations on the actual history of the case have been introduced for illustrative purposes. For another fully developed and evaluated case study of a worksite health promotion program based on the PRECEDE model, see R. L. Bertera, "Planning and Implementing Health Promotion in the Workplace: A Case Study of the DuPont Company Experience," *Health Education Quarterly* 17 (1990): 307–27. This project received the 1990 Program Excellence Award of the Society for Public Health Education.

67. For a description of the development and pilot testing of this American Lung Association Program, see V. J. Strecher, B. K. Rimer, and K. D. Monaco, "Development of a New Self-help Guide – Freedom from Smoking for You and Your Family," *Health Education Quarterly* 16 (1989): 101–12.

68. Worksite competitions have been found in several studies and reviews to have modest effectiveness in reducing smoking or weight control but substantially lower costs than classes or clinical interventions, giving them a better cost-effectiveness than other methods except self-help. See, for example, D. Altman, J. Flora, S. Fortmann, J. Farquhar, "The Cost-Effectiveness of Three Smoking Cessation Programs," *American Journal of Public Health* 77 (1987): 162–5; K. D. Brownell and M. R. Felix, op. cit., 1987. This campaign was based particularly on the experience of R. C. Klesges, M. M. Vasey, and R. E. Glasgow, "A Worksite Smoking Modification Competition: Potential for Public Health Impact," *American Journal of Public Health* 76 (1986): 198–200.

69. The lottery contest approach to recruitment was found in one worksite study to yield a 14-percent participation rate among workers in a cancer research hospital and a quit rate of 36 percent, higher than that reported in other studies of contests: K. M. Cummings, R. Hellmann, S. L. Emont, "Correlates of Participation in a Worksite Stop-Smoking Contest," *Journal of Behavioral Medicine* 11 (1988): 267–77.

70. J. M. Ottoson and L. W. Green, "Reconciling Concept and Context: A Theory of Implementation," in *Advances in Health Education and Promotion*, vol. 2, W. B. Ward, ed. (Greenwich, CT: JAI Press, 1987), pp. 339–68.

Chapter 10

Applications in
School Settings

As the social diagnosis in Chapter 2 and the educational diagnosis in Chapter 4 made clear, individuals and organizations tend to adopt healthful behaviors for reasons other than health. Important as the health benefits may be, the motivation to diet or to exercise, for example, especially for young people, is more closely linked to a desire to look good and to feel better than to improved cardiorespiratory fitness and lower risks of coronary mortality. Recognition of these motivational realities can avoid serious flaws in the health promotion planning process. This chapter, like those on applications in the worksite and community settings, will show that organizations outside the health sector also may have different reasons (motivations) for adopting and maintaining health promotion programs and policies.

SCHOOL HEALTH PROMOTION

By definition, the goal for health workers is *health*. So, it should be no surprise that health advocates enthusiastically push the health objectives of a program without much apparent attention to other needs and priorities of the intended recipients, participants, or cooperating organizations. Such single-minded tunnel vision, though well intended, calls into question one's sensitivity to the needs of individuals or populations. It often creates the feeling among the intended beneficiaries of having to cram yet one more high-priority concern into their already overburdened agenda. This leads to the feeling that the proposed activity is in competition with, rather than being complementary to, existing priorities; such sentiments do not facilitate the adoption of new actions, health promoting or not!

349

PURPOSE AND FUNCTIONS

Nowhere do the motivational differences between the health perspective and the educational perspective clash more than in school health. From the health perspective, schools represent the most valuable resource for health promotion, but they are relatively autonomous, or at least independent of the health sector. Every school day nearly 47 million students attend elementary and secondary schools in the United States; about 6 million professional and nonprofessional workers staff those schools.[1] Thus, schools constitute the center of work activity for nearly one-fifth of the U.S. population.[2] With that in mind, it is easy to see why so many health professionals believe that carefully orchestrated health promotion in schools might constitute society's most cost-effective prevention strategy.[3]

From the educator's perspective, the school has a different set of priorities, and its educational role in society should not be compromised in the pursuit of health objectives. Some argue that even behavioral objectives, including health behavior objectives, have no place in the school's mission because they detract from the primary objectives of learning critical thinking and reasoning.[4] The most acceptable basis for the justification of health promotion and health services in the school has been to assure that students would be kept healthy enough to be able to attend and benefit from school activities.

One attempt to reconcile these perspectives was a definition of the objective of school health education as assuring

> that children at each age or grade should be helped to master those health maintenance skills necessary to cope with potential threats to their health in the coming age or grade, and those additional foundation skills necessary to benefit from the instruction next year in relation to the potential health problems of the year after that.[5]

The emphasis on skills rather than behavior or health outcomes brings the health interests implicit in this definition closer to the explicit educational mission of schools. It holds schools accountable only for that which is within their range of immediate influence, is measurable in the short term, and is developmental in its perspective. The PRECEDE model was adapted for schools in accordance with this emphasis on skills as a primary objective, as discussed later in this chapter.

On the occasion of being sworn into office as assistant secretary for health in the U.S. Department of Health and Human Services, Dr. James O. Mason, former Director of the Centers for Disease Control, spelled out as the number one goal for his administration "the promotion of health and the prevention of disease and injury" and set as a goal for the year 2000 "comprehensive school health education classes from kindergarten through 12th grade in every school in the country. This is a reality that can be accomplished."[6]

Do those responsible for the stewardship of schools in the United States also share those strong sentiments? What would be your answer if you were an elementary school principal and a member of your school board asked "what is your mission?" You might expect your answer to be something like "to educate the students, to prepare them to be competent citizens capable of coping with the demands of daily living." It is unlikely that you would say "to improve the health status of students and faculty." For health institutions the mission is improved health, whereas the mission of schools is education. Though not mutually exclusive, the institutional priorities clearly differ. Health promotion planners need to be especially sensitive to those differences. Efforts to promote school health programs, whether they involve curriculum, counseling, food services, or community participation, will be problematic if they fail to be seen as contributing to the educational mission of the school.[7]

Reciprocally, school health personnel need to be more aggressive in seeking the cooperation and resources of community agencies and media in support of the school's mission. True, students spend one-third of their work-week hours in school, but they spend more than two-thirds of total hours, counting weekends, holidays, and summer vacations, outside the school. Furthermore, some of the children and youth who need health promotion the most have dropped out of school or have such high absenteeism that they will not be reached by school programs. Schools cannot solve society's health and social problems alone. They tend to sidestep the responsibility to address such problems as substance abuse and teenage pregnancy so long as they perceive their own educational performance to be threatened by the dilution of the school's resources.

The educational priorities of schools become more compelling for school personnel when budgets are tight (as they have been for decades) and when parents and employers become agitated about the decline in student performance on standardized tests in reading, writing, and arithmetic. Average SAT scores dropped by 7 percent between 1966 and 1987, from 967 to 906 (combined verbal and math). The back-to-basics pressure on schools tends to push health education, physical education, and even school nursing services into the background, signaling a perception of their diminished status.[8]

The competing priorities and diverse programs of the school setting make the comprehensive nature of the PRECEDE–PROCEED framework particularly helpful in that setting. But, before examining how the planning principles of PRECEDE and the implementation and evaluation principles of PROCEED can be applied in a school setting, it will be helpful to review the components of contemporary school health and some trends in research and policy.

COMPONENTS

The basic structure of school health programs as proffered in the literature has remained relatively unchanged for over 50 years. In a report issued by the Health Education Section of the American Physical Education Association in 1935, the school health program was described as consisting of three interdependent components: health instruction, school health services, and healthful school environment.[9] In the latest edition of their classic textbook on school health practice, Creswell and Newman continue to organize the subject around that identical structure.[10] The simplicity and comprehensiveness of that tripartite structure, coupled with its prudent logic, account for its stability over time.[11]

When characterized as a part of a larger community program, the organizational complexities of the school health program become more apparent, as indicated in Figure 10.1. The activities that make up the school health program are listed in the center box; leadership, administration, and planning input from both the community and school come from the elements delineated above the center box; and the diversity of personnel responsible for carrying out the multiple school health program activities are shown below the box. One need not hold an M.B.A. degree to see that such a complex structure requires considerable attention to planning and management.

The framework shown in Figure 10.2 expanded the traditional three–pronged structure of the school health programs.[12] In the "program components" column, the three traditional elements have been extended to include five more: integrated school and community health promotion efforts, school physical education, school food service, school counseling, and schoolsite health promotion program for faculty and staff. The vertical arrows between the program components connote the interdependence of the program activities. The remaining arrows suggest various ways in which immediate, short-term and long-term outcomes can be influenced. In both 1987 and 1990, the *Journal of School Health* dedicated an issue to the expanded concept of the comprehensive school health program.[13]

Although one may rightfully claim that the five additional components were subsumed under the three components in the earlier characterizations of the school health program, their more explicit delineation in the expanded rendition has three advantages. First, by giving greater visibility to integrated community and school programs, physical education, school food services, school counseling, and schoolsite health promotion for staff, the importance of these activities in the overall scheme of school health becomes much more salient. Salient components get attention; they become worthy of consideration, study, and support; and they are viewed as essential rather than incidental, primary rather than subsidiary. Growing scientific evidence now confirms our prior assumptions about the health and human performance benefits of good nutrition[14] and prudent physical activity.[15] These activities related to school food services (including cafeteria lunches and vending machine policies) and physical education (including curriculum, facilities, and extracurricular programs) are too important not to be given utmost attention in planning for a school health program.

The second advantage is that the expanded framework suggests the need for a team approach to school health. It identifies the important players on the team: school nurses, physicians, health educators, counselors, psychologists, food service workers, physical educators, those responsible for the school's physical

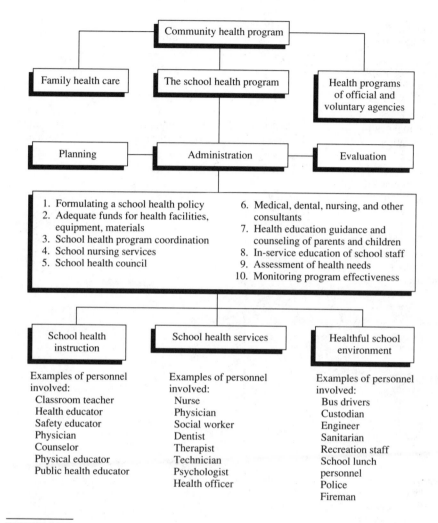

Community health program

Family health care

The school health program

Health programs
of official and
voluntary agencies

Planning

Administration

Evaluation

1. Formulating a school health policy
2. Adequate funds for health facilities, equipment, materials
3. School health program coordination
4. School nursing services
5. School health council
6. Medical, dental, nursing, and other consultants
7. Health education guidance and counseling of parents and children
8. In-service education of school staff
9. Assessment of health needs
10. Monitoring program effectiveness

School health
instruction

School health services

Healthful school
environment

Examples of personnel
involved:
  Classroom teacher
  Health educator
  Safety educator
  Physician
  Counselor
  Physical educator
  Public health educator

Examples of personnel
involved:
  Nurse
  Physician
  Social worker
  Dentist
  Therapist
  Technician
  Psychologist
  Health officer

Examples of personnel
involved:
  Bus drivers
  Custodian
  Engineer
  Sanitarian
  Recreation staff
  School lunch
  personnel
  Police
  Fireman

FIGURE 10.1

Organizational and administrative relationships of components of the school health program. [From C. Anderson and W. H. Creswell, *School Health Practice*, 8th ed. St. Louis: Times Mirror/Mosby, 1985; reprinted with permission of Mosby College Publishing.]

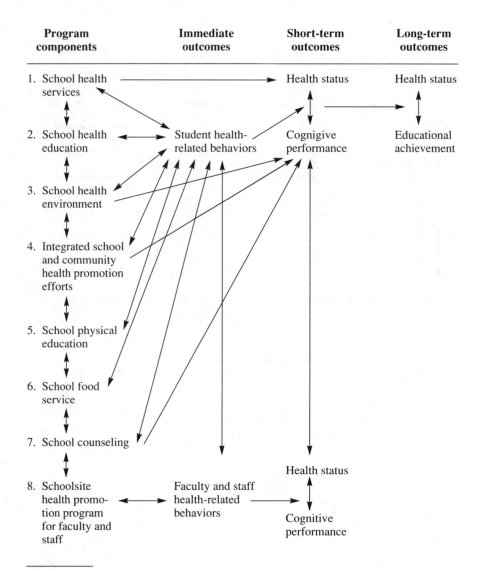

Program components	Immediate outcomes	Short-term outcomes	Long-term outcomes

1. School health services → Health status   Health status

2. School health education ↔ Student health-related behaviors   Cognigive performance   Educational achievement

3. School health environment

4. Integrated school and community health promotion efforts

5. School physical education

6. School food service

7. School counseling

Health status

8. Schoolsite health promotion program for faculty and staff ↔ Faculty and staff health-related behaviors → Health status / Cognitive performance

FIGURE 10.2

School health promotion components and outcomes. [From L. Kolbe, *Health Education* 17(5) (1986): 47–52; printed with permission of the publisher.]

and psychosocial environment, and those in the community who work in schools to improve the health of students. The third advantage of using the expanded framework is that it overtly calls attention to the fundamental mission of schools: education. In Figure 10.2, note that "cognitive performance" and "educational achievement" share equal billing with "health status" as short- and long-term outcome priorities. When health professionals lose sight of the school's raison d'etre and replace it with health priorities, a collapse of interest and support from school administrators often follows.[16]

TOWARD COMPREHENSIVENESS

Comprehensiveness, in the new framework, means more than multiple components of the school health program within the school. It also means a commitment to involving the community actively in the health affairs of the school and engaging the community, including parents, in active roles on behalf of the health of school-age children.[17]

In championing the goal of the universal availability of quality school health education for all children, Dr. J. O. Mason, assistant secretary of health, and Dr. J. Michael McGinnis, director of the Office of Disease Prevention and Health Promotion within the U.S. Department of Health and Human Services, offered this advice:[18]

> In pursuit of that goal, however, we must all maintain sensitivity to the unique educational mission of schools and the complex social and economic conditions that frequently surround them. The institutions of public health and education are complementary and, as such, they must work as partners, sharing their expertise, time, energy and resources if everyone is to realize the potential schools have in contributing to the goal of a healthier citizenry, whether that be 1990 or 2090.

PROGRESS IN SCHOOL HEALTH RESEARCH AND POLICY

Since the printing of the first edition of this book in 1980, research on health promotion in schools has virtually exploded with new and compelling evidence on the effectiveness of comprehensive approaches. Noteworthy policy advances in school health also emerged in the 1980s.

THE SCHOOL HEALTH EDUCATION EVALUATION

After decades of defending comprehensive school health on the basis of learning principles and research evidence borrowed from other fields, contemporary school health literature is suddenly laden with evaluations of well-designed school health and school health education programs. The most sweeping evidence to enter the scene in the 1980s was the nationwide evaluation of the comprehensive School Health Curriculum Project. From a handful of small-scale studies conducted before 1980 with limited controls (usually pretest-posttest designs) and with little measure of behavioral impact (usually knowledge and attitude changes only),[19] the opportunity arose in 1981 to carry out a multisite, randomized evaluation of this and several other health curricula, with support from the U.S. Office of Disease Prevention and Health Promotion and the Centers for Disease Control.

The School Health Education Evaluation was a pioneering 3-year prospective study, involving 30,000 students in grades 4–7 from 20 states. It revealed that students who were exposed to comprehensive school health education not only showed significant positive changes in their health-related knowledge and attitudes, compared with students in matched schools without such exposure, they also were considerably less likely to take up smoking. Especially relevant were those findings that clearly demonstrated that administrative support and teacher training were directly linked to the positive student outcomes detected, as were the cumulative number of hours of classroom time devoted to comprehensive school health education.[20]

THE NATIONAL INSTITUTES OF HEALTH

Following the lead of the other agencies of the Public Health Service, the National Institutes of Health (NIH) began to lend their considerable scientific prestige to the study of school health promotion. The NIH attention 10 years earlier to the development of patient education approaches to blood pressure control boosted the field of health education and health promotion into the respectability of randomized clinical trials published in the most prestigious medical journals (see Chapter 11). Now, NIH was commissioning several panels of distinguished scientists to review what had been learned about school health education. In 1986, a panel convened by the Kaiser Family Foundation concluded that drug abuse prevention programs can be most effective when implemented in the context of comprehensive school and community health promotion programs.[21]

In 1988, an expert advisory group convened by the National Cancer Institute reviewed 20 years of research on school-based efforts to prevent tobacco use. The panel found nine areas with sufficient data or experience to reach preliminary conclusions and recommendations. These areas include: program, impact, focus, context, length, ideal age for intervention, teacher training, program implementation, and need for peer and parental involvement.[22]

The National Heart, Lung and Blood Institute (NHLBI) has supported a variety of school-based research efforts, 10 of which are summarized in Table 10.1.[23] As the table indicates, these studies reflect diversity in the demographic characteristics of the populations studied, in the risk-factor focus, and in methods and channels of intervention. Several of the studies applied the PRECEDE model and emphasized the importance of a planning model to complement and organize specific theoretical models.[24] As a result, this collection of studies placed rather strong emphasis on the home to address reinforcing factors in the social environment.

COLLABORATION AND DIFFUSION BEYOND THE SCHOOL

The studies summarized in Table 10.1 are identified as school-based studies, but seven of the ten use the strategy of linking home and school as mutually reinforcing settings for the behavior of children.[25]

Efforts to expand the focus of school programs to place increasing emphasis on the home and family are supported by findings from a 1988 national school health education survey sponsored by the Metropolitan Life Foundation.[26] The survey sampled over 4,000 students from 199 public schools and 500 randomly selected parents of children attending schools. Among other things, the survey revealed that even though the majority of teachers and parents believe that parental involvement in children's health education would be of considerable help in encouraging good health habits for children, most parents (71%) report never getting involved in the process. Lack of parental involvement may in part explain why parents do not know the extent of drinking, smoking, or drug-taking by their children. Whereas 36 percent of the parents surveyed indicated that their child had had at least one alcoholic drink, 66 percent of the students said they had alcohol at least once or twice; only 14 percent of parents reported that their child had smoked a cigarette while 41 percent of students said they had smoked; 5 percent of parents said that their child had used drugs whereas 17 percent of students reported having used drugs.

International investigators have also conducted school health studies that employ close collaboration with key institutions within the community as well as the family. The North Karelia, Finland Youth Project included modifications in the school diet, health screening, mass media, comprehensive school health education, and parental support to reduce the major risk factors for noncommunicable diseases. Intended to be an ongoing program, findings after 2 years revealed significant decreases in several risk factors.[27]

The common denominators for these successful programs and others like them include: (1) a commitment to addressing specific problems or modifiable risk factors often within the context of a comprehensive approach and (2) the use of multiple intervention methods based on an assessment of the characteristics, needs, and interests of the target population. Figure 10.3 illustrates how PRECEDE was used to facilitate the application of these principles in the Bogalusa "Heart Smart" cardiovascular school health promotion program.[28]

TABLE 10.1

A summary of NHLBI school-based health promotion studies

Investigator Institution Study	Ethnicity[a] SES Grade State	Schools[b] Classes Students	Channel: Curriculum, Food service, Home	Provider	Target areas	Outcomes
Perry, Cheryl, Ph.D. Univ of Minn "Healthy Heart" "The Home Team"	W, A SES (M) Grade 3 MN, ND	24T/7C – 1405T/ 422C	Curr Home	Teachers Mail	Eating	Changes in knowledge, total fat, saturated fat, complex carbohydrate intake
Parcel, Guy, Ph.D. Univ of Texas "Go For Health"	W, H, B SES (L, M) Grades 3–4 TX	2T/2C 40 1156	Curr Food Serv	Teachers Food Workers	Eating Exercise	Changes in knowledge, self-efficacy, behavioral expectations food service, PE classes, diet
Walter, Heather, M.D. American Health Fdn "Know Your Body"	W, B, A, H SES (L, M, H) Grades 4–9 NY	22T/15C – 2075T 1313C	Curr Home	Teachers	Eating Exercise Smoking BP WT	Changes in knowledge, total fat, complex carbohydrate intake, chol, initiation of smoking
Bush, Patricia, Ph.D. Georgetown Univ "Know Your Body"	B SES (L, M, H) Grades 4–9 DC	6T/3C – 707T 334C	Home	Teachers	Eating Exercise Smoking BP WT	Changes in knowledge, smoking attitudes, BP, HDL chol, fitness, thiocyanate

				Inst		
Nader, Philip, M.D. Univ of CA/SD "Family Health Project"	H, W SES (L, M) Grades 5–6 CA	6T/6C — 163T/160C	Home	Inst	Eating Exercise	Changes in diet, chol, BP, knowledge
Cohen, Rita, Ph.D. Brownell, Kelly, Ph.D. Univ of Penn "CV Risk Reduction"	W SES (M) Grades 5–7 PA	— — 1062T 992C	Curr Home	Teachers Peers	Eating BP Smoking	Changes in knowledge, initiation of smoking, peers were equally or more effective than teachers
Fors, Stuart, Ed.D. Univ of Georgia "3R's + HBP"	W, B SES (L, M) Grade 6 GA	14T/7C 60 853T 351C	Curr Home	Teachers Students	BP	Changes in knowledge, taking BP
Ellison, R. Curtis, M.D. Univ of Mass "Food Service Project"	W, B, A SES (M, H) Grade 9 MA, NH	2 — 1100	Food Serv	Food Workers	BP Eating	Changes in BP, chol, and food service
Weinberg, Armin, Ph.D. Baylor College of Med "CV Curr/Family Tree"	W, H, B SES (L, M) Grades 9–10 TX	7 40 5787	Curr Home	Teachers	Eating Exercise BP	Changes in knowledge, attitudes, self report behavior, parents used smoking + wt + exercise
Killen, Joel, Ph.D. Farquhar, John, M.D. Stanford Univ "CV Risk Reduction"	W, H, A SES (M) Grade 10 CA	2T/2C 8 1447	Curr	Inst	Eating Exercise BP Smoking	Changes in knowledge, exercise, smoking, resting heart rate, BMI, skinfolds

a Predominant ethnic or racial group: A = Asian, B = Black, H = Hispanic, W = White
b T = treatment, C = control
SOURCE: E. J. Stone, C. L. Perry, and R. V. Luepker, *Health Education Quarterly* 16(2) (1989): 155–69.

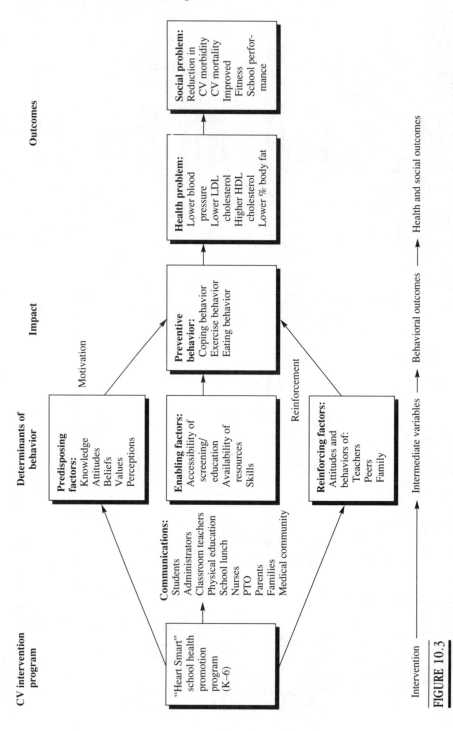

Application of the PRECEDE model in a cardiovascular health promotion program for school-age children. [From A. M. Downey, G. C. Frank, L. S. Webber, et al., *Journal of School Health* 57 (1987): 98–104; printed by permission of the publisher.]

FIGURE 10.3

POLICY ANALYSES AND ADVANCES

Partly as a result of progress in research, there has been concurrent progress in school health policy. A policy has three components: (1) the clear statement of a problem (or potential problem) that needs attention, (2) a goal to mitigate or prevent that problem and (3) a set of strategic actions to accomplish that goal. This leaves "tactics" to the implementors of policy. Well-designed regional or national surveys provide the substance and clarity that make policy credible and influence it.

The WHO cross-national survey of health behavior in school children,[29] the National Children and Youth Fitness Study,[30] and the National Adolescent Student Health Survey[31] are three examples of large surveys that have begun to influence national and international policy with regard to the health of school-aged youth. Such data require the additional effort of investigators, policy analysts, and practitioners to translate them into action or policy. Gordon Mutter of the Health Promotion Directorate, Health and Welfare Canada, clearly described how the strategic planning and systematic analysis and dissemination of the results of two national surveys in Canada resulted in documented development of policies, resources, and programs targeted to improve the health of Canadian children and youth.[32]

The document *School Health in America: An Assessment of State Policies to Protect and Improve the Health of Students*,[33] periodically updated, provides the most thorough report of state policies and program status in school health in the United States. The report presents the findings from a nationwide survey of state education agencies conducted every few years. Survey questions are organized to elicit information on seven areas akin to the expanded components of a school health program cited earlier: (1) health services, (2) health instruction, (3) a healthful school environment, (4) food services, (5) physical education, (6) guidance and counseling, and (7) school psychology. State directors for the relevant component area in each state responded to questions that explored: the nature and scope of policies, variables associated with the status of programs, and issues related to the qualifications of personnel; a 100 percent response rate was obtained.

Policy analysis of data such as those resulting from the *School Health in America* survey can provide the planner with valuable insight and justification for proposed programs. For example, in Table 10.2, the average number of hours of health education instruction per year required by each state is displayed by grade level. We can see an extremely wide variation among the states in the number of hours required for health education per year (0–150). These data are especially relevant in light of some of the findings from the School Health Education Evaluation Study, which concluded that desirable improvements in levels of students' health knowledge, attitude, and self-reported health practices occur after 50 hours of exposure to quality health education instruction.[34]

TABLE 10.2

Average number of health education hours per year in the states with a specific time requirement

State	Grade range			
	1–6	7–8	9–12	1–12
Alaska	0	0	9.00[a]	3.00[a]
Arkansas	60.00	60.00	22.50	47.50
Arizona	30.00	19.00	22.50	25.67
District of Columbia	86.00	54.00	27.00	61.00
Delaware	60.00	30.00	22.50	42.50
Florida	0	0	7.50	2.50
Georgia	30.00	30.00	18.75	26.25
Hawaii	–	45.00	22.50	15.00
Idaho	0	35.00	17.50	11.67
Illinois	–	45.00	22.50	15.00
Indiana	54.00[a]	60.00[a]	150.00[a]	87.00[a]
Kentucky	60.00	30.00	22.50	42.50
Louisiana	90.00	180.00[a]	15.00	80.00[a]
Maine	0	0	17.00	5.67
Minnesota	36.00	20.00	20.00	28.00
Montana	–	72.00[a]	36.00[a]	24.00[a]
North Carolina	–	–	22.50[a]	7.50[a]
North Dakota	0	0	30.00[a]	10.00[a]
New Hampshire	0	0	9.00	3.00
New Jersey	90.00[a]	90.00[a]	90.00[a]	90.00[a]
Nevada	–	–	22.50	7.50
New York	0	30.00	15.00	10.00
Ohio	0	48.00	22.50	15.50
Oregon	0	0	45.00	15.00
Pennsylvania	–	15.00	7.50	5.00
South Carolina	45.00	37.50	0	28.75
Tennessee	–	90.00	22.50	22.50
Texas	16.00	6.00	40.00	22.33
Utah	–	45.00	22.50	15.00
Virginia	0	72.00	36.00	24.00
Wisconsin	–	15.00	15.00	7.50
West Virginia	34.00	54.00	33.75	37.25
Total	691.00	1182.00	886.00	838.08
Mean[b]	53.154	49.271	28.597	26.190
Standard deviation	24.351	35.871	27.141	24.056

NOTE: Zero indicates no hours; dash indicates health education hours required but unable to determine how many.

[a] Hours are combined with those of physical education.

[b] Mean is based on the states that reported a requirement.

SOURCE: C. Y. Lovato and D. Allensworth, *School Health in America*, 5th ed. Kent, Ohio: American School Health Association, 1989; printed by permission of publisher.

Note in Table 10.2 that although the mean number of hours required for grades 1–6 is over 50, the mean steadily diminishes to 28 hours for grades 9–12 and 26 hours for all grades. Even though the state-level data mask the specific practices occurring at the local level, school health workers in those states with no or weak requirements would be well advised to consider how they can support advocacy efforts at the state level to correct what appears to be a problematic enabling factor.

Other policy analyses supporting or promoting school health have emerged from national commissions[35] and international study groups for the World Health Organization.[36] The voluntary health associations have published strong advocacy statements and policy analyses in support of school health promotion.[37] Professional associations also have made their voices heard.[38]

THE AIDS EPIDEMIC AS A STIMULUS TO COMPREHENSIVE SCHOOL HEALTH

History is full of examples in which breakthroughs for public good are borne out of tragedy; behind such clouds there is sometimes a silver lining. The tragic circumstances that define the global problem of AIDS (acquired immunodeficiency syndrome) have given rise to opportunities never before afforded to school health. The severity of the epidemic, the essential role of education in the world prevention strategy, together with the public demand for action, offered the perfect opportunity for a proactive response in the global fight against AIDS and for strengthening comprehensive school health education.

The *Guidelines for Effective School Health Education to Prevent the Spread of AIDS*[39] present an excellent example of the influence that strong, timely policy documents can have in focusing and implementing a nationwide health education program.[40] These guidelines legitimized the school as a credible national focal point for an important aspect of AIDS prevention. They were developed by staff at the U.S. Centers for Disease Control in close collaboration with leaders representing 16 national school and health organizations. With the support of these broad-based and influential constituencies, the guidelines were crafted such that there could be no mistake in interpreting the strategy for implementation: close collaboration among the health and education sectors, active participation and review by and with parents, and programs carried out in the context of comprehensive school health education. Specifically, "AIDS education interventions may be most effective when implemented within a more comprehensive school health education programme that establishes a foundation for understanding the relationships between personal behaviours and health."[41]

National, state, and local voices are part of a chorus of international commitment to comprehensive school health education. Irrespective of the health problems that schools may be called upon to help address, a comprehensive, skills-based, K–12 health education curriculum, taught by qualified teachers, is essential. As difficult as it may be, efforts to establish comprehensive curricula should take precedence over stop-gap efforts to address the latest health problem. The philosopher Mortimer Adler[42] viewed health education to be of secondary importance in the scheme of education. Numerous national and international bodies have since concluded the contrary, that comprehensive education about health is basic. The aim of comprehensive school health education fits the goal of education: to nurture health literate children and youth who have the competence to meet the demands of daily living. That goal is as relevant for the potential problems associated with poor nutrition and lack of exercise as it is for AIDS, drug abuse, or teen pregnancy.

USING PRECEDE AND PROCEED FOR PLANNING IN SCHOOLS

The steps for social, epidemiological, behavioral, environmental, educational, administrative, and policy diagnoses that are covered in Chapters 2–6 remain essentially the same for application in all settings. We now review some issues that require special consideration for the use of the diagnostic steps of PRECEDE in the school setting, we then present a hypothetical case study to illustrate the steps and principles of PRECEDE. Finally, PROCEED is applied to schools.

SOCIAL DIAGNOSIS

By applying the principles of the first step in the PRECEDE process, the planner will come face to face with the realities of school priorities. The following are responses one could reasonably expect from a school administrator who is asked to identify indicators that reflect "success" for his/her school:

1. Academic progress
2. Low absenteeism (students and faculty)
3. Low rates of student drop-outs
4. Competitive salary schedule
5. Minimal discipline problems
6. Parental and community support for school
7. Stable, supportive faculty and staff
8. Student pride in the school

Objective data usually available at the school level can provide insight into the kind of issues identified in items 1–5. For input on items 6–8, one could obtain valuable qualitative information through questionnaires or focus groups.[43] The latter information, often referred to as *soft data*, should not be taken as lesser in value than more objective, *hard data*. Experiences around the world have taught planners, sometimes quite painfully, this lesson: Failure to acknowledge and address the perceptions and feelings held by administrators, teachers, and parents about their schools, however difficult those sentiments may be to quantify, can stop the best-designed well-intended program dead in its tracks. So, to paraphrase the popular American Express Card slogan, "social diagnosis, don't start implementing without it!"

As in any thoughtful planning endeavor, every effort should be made to solicit participation from representative groups in the community. Attention to the broader community health issues combined with representation from people in the community will result in two benefits: (1) planning is more responsive to the needs and concerns of the population that supports the school and (2) the community gains a greater understanding and appreciation for needs of the school, thus increasing the strength of their support for programs.

In addition to documenting the subjective priorities and concerns, a social diagnosis of school health promotion needs can also draw on the now compelling evidence of the two-way cause–effect relationship between education and health.[44] As stated by the National Commission on the Role of the School and the Community in Improving Adolescent Health, "Health behaviors are an important reason why a large percentage of young people today are unable or not motivated to learn."[45] And epidemiological research has shown that no single social characteristic of people over their lifetimes correlates more consistently and determines more powerfully their health status at any subsequent age than the number of years of schooling they completed when they were adolescents.

EPIDEMIOLOGICAL DIAGNOSIS

For application in schools, planners can use one or a combination of two approaches to carry out the epidemiological diagnosis. The first approach follows the same steps as those outlined in Chapter 3 and requires analysis of local-level health data to identify the current priority health problems of the children and youth served by the school(s) in question. Sources for such data might include health records from the school (school health nurse, school-based clinic), data from the local health department, social services agency, police department, highway safety department; reports on pediatric health from local physicians or clinics; and special surveys covering the area or region. Information gathered through this procedure would enable planners to (1) increase the chances of detecting the incidence of health events occurring in excess of that which might normally be expected, (2) compare the prevalence of various health conditions in a given school population, (3) compare incidence or prevalence data of a given school population with those of the district, a neighboring region, the state, or perhaps the nation, and (4) compare the prevalence of risk factors among students in school(s) with the leading adult health problems in the community.

Because demographic characteristics, environmental conditions, and social norms all combine to shape the unique health status of a given community, it is ideal for planners to use local data. However, local data on the health of children and youth are usually limited; when they are available, these data are sometimes difficult to obtain or of dubious reliability. In such cases, planners can consider the second approach—estimating the epidemiological diagnosis by calling attention to the leading health problems for school-aged youth in the region, state, province, or nation. This approach has considerable merit despite the obvious deficiency of not being able to detect problems that may be unique or unusually high in a given school or community.

The following observation by Starfield and Budetti not only characterizes the complexities inherent in gathering health information about school-aged youth, it is a poignant justification for comprehensive approaches:[46]

> No one method is sufficient to describe the frequency of health problems in childhood. Some problems are known only to parents or families, because they are not manifested outside the home and are not brought in for medical care. Some are noticed only by teachers, who observe children under different circumstances than do their parents. Some health conditions become known only upon special questioning by qualified personnel, and some require a physician's assessment for their diagnosis. (p. 833)

Problems are a matter of degree. For example, alcohol-related motor vehicle fatalities among teens in community X may be 35 percent higher than the national average; but motor vehicle crashes remain the leading cause of death and injury for youth aged 15–24 throughout the nation. A school need not await "higher than" status to address a nation's leading cause of death for youth. The same sentiment can be expressed for other problems, including teen pregnancy, sexually transmitted diseases, alcohol and drug use, smoking, obesity, and physical inactivity. There is merit in promoting a global view of the priority problems of any country. "Think globally, act locally," as the environmental movement's slogan says. "Peace starts at home," as the child-abuse prevention slogan goes.

Such a perspective creates a spirit that the individual efforts of schools and communities are a part of a larger overall nationwide response to those health problems that threaten the health of all school-aged youth.[47]

Allensworth and Wolford,[48] Pollock,[49] and Pigg[50] are among the many school health professionals who urge the consideration of nationwide health trends as a legitimate indicator of local-level need. Data presented in Table 10.3 reflect the range of priority problems that compromise the health and performance of school-aged youth in the United States.

Note that the "health" statistics presented in Table 10.3 not only include health events like motor-vehicle-related deaths, suicide, and sexually transmitted disease, but also include behaviors like alcohol consumption, sexual activity, and levels of physical activity. This mixing of health problems and health-related behaviors is a fact of life for planners in the school setting. The temporal

TABLE 10.3

Problems of school-aged youth in the United States

The 15–24 age group was the only age group in the United States that showed an *increase* in its death rate over the past several decades.

There were roughly 400,000 cases of gonorrhea and syphilis among American teenagers in 1985, more than double the number in 1965. When all sexually transmitted diseases are added, the number is 2.5 million, which makes the rate 12 per 1,000, which is *three times* the rate in 1965.

Every year more than 1 million adolescents get pregnant. This rate—nearly one teenage girl in every ten—is at least twice as high as in other industrialized countries. This rate has nearly doubled the number of births to unmarried teens (15–19 years old) from 686 every day in 1965 to 1,298 every day in 1985.

The suicide rate for teenagers has tripled since 1959, making it the second leading cause of death among adolescents. Some 10 percent of teenage boys and nearly 20 percent of girls have attempted suicide.

Over 50 percent of high school seniors get drunk at least once a month, making drinking while driving the number one killer of adolescents. More than 21 teenagers are killed every day in alcohol-related fatalities.

The homicide rate, the fourth leading cause of death in children 1–14 and the second for youth 15–24, is almost 5 times higher for black males.

Only half of the students in grades 5–12 are meeting minimal weekly exercise requirements; both boys and girls have more body fat (based on median skinfold measures) than students 25 years ago.

SOURCE: See References and Notes 51–52 at end of chapter.

relationship between the behavior *not taking hypertensive medicine* and the health problem *stroke* is much more immediate for the 55-year-old hypertensive male than the relationship between the behavior *smoking* and the health problem *lung cancer* for a teenager. Nevertheless, there is good justification for school health planners to consider the behaviors of *smoking, chewing,* or *tobacco use* as health problems. Although the deleterious health effects of smoking, chewing, alcohol and drug abuse, high dietary fat intake, and sedentariness may not be immediate, the effects on learning and school performance may be.

However, the more traditional application of linking a behavioral problem to a health problem remains useful because not all behavioral problems manifested by school-aged youth are distant from health outcomes. The time between drinking alcohol or taking drugs and an automobile fatality is tragically and dramatically short. The highly successful alcohol-free Project Graduation program is evidence that a school and community effort to modify drinking behavior during graduation celebrations can reduce alcohol-related automobile fatalities.[53]

The PRECEDE model was never intended to be a rigid, lock-step process. Rather, it was designed as an organizing framework to enable planners to sort through the complexities inherent in addressing individual and collective health behaviors. The results of that sorting are expected to provide insights for developing or selecting effective health promotion strategies. The intermingling of health and behavioral problems for school-aged youth puts both planners and PRECEDE to the test of flexibility. As the studies cited earlier in this chapter indicate, schools do not operate in a vacuum. Schools are part of a larger community, and their programs and activities have traditionally reflected the values, interests, and expectations of that community. Accordingly, social and epidemiological diagnoses are richer if they include information about, and input from, the community as well as the school. Although amplifying the diagnosis in this way takes more time and effort, the benefits are worth it.

Earlier, this chapter extolled the value of survey data in strengthening school health policies. It emphasized the value of data in clarifying the problem the policy is aimed to mitigate and, in so doing, calling attention to and legitimizing the problem as a priority. Decision makers pay attention to important problems; the health education planner uses social and epidemiological diagnoses in combination to show the importance of the health problem.

BEHAVIORAL, ENVIRONMENTAL, AND EDUCATIONAL DIAGNOSES

Behavioral, environmental, and educational diagnoses in the school setting follow the same process described in Chapters 4 and 5. Recent school health research has confirmed the long-standing assumption that qualified teachers can have great influence on the health knowledge, attitudes, and practices of their students. But should teachers be held accountable for manifest changes in student behavior? Because schools serve communities, it is only logical to suggest that school activities and teachers are primarily accountable to community members, especially parents. Parents should reasonably expect their children to gain command of the knowledge and skill to be able to matriculate from one grade to the next. If fifth-grade pupils are supposed to be able to read at a certain rate and comprehend at a certain level, valid tests should be devised to ascertain those competencies. In health education, such tests would provide both short-range evaluation of impact and evidence that progress has been made toward enabling future behavior conducive to health.

Those who plan and implement comprehensive school health education programs that *do not* focus on specific behaviors that are determined by the epidemiological analysis to be important, should not expect to have a major impact on these behaviors in the short run. These programs are more fairly evaluated on the basis of short-term measures of student interests, comprehension, skills, and attitudes. Efforts should be made to assess whether the critical behaviors (or suitable surrogates) increase, decrease, or remain the same over time.

Unlike patient health educators, school health educators are faced with the

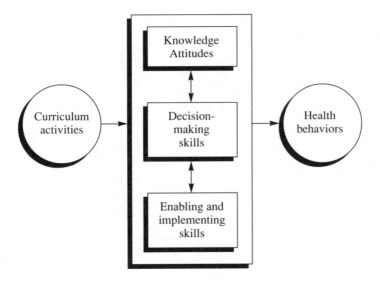

FIGURE 10.4

The elaboration of the predisposing and enabling factors targeted by a K–12 school health curriculum. [From Consultation report to BSCS, Colorado College, Colorado Springs.]

problem of linking health education activities to future behaviors, a problem confounded by the potential multitude of variables intervening over time. The PRECEDE framework can be useful in attacking this problem, with the addition of *skills* as an intervening construct between the educational constructs (predisposing, enabling, and reinforcing factors) and the behavioral construct. Since the previous edition proposed this adaptation of the PRECEDE model for school health applications, several studies have tested the model with this variation. The concept was elaborated in the development of a national curriculum by the BSCS K–8 health curriculum project of the Colorado College, as shown in Figure 10.4.

The "Know Your Body" program has been evaluated extensively applying the PRECEDE variation shown in Figure 10.5. In this 5-year study to determine the impact of the program on selected cardiovascular risk factors among students in grades 4–6 in the District of Columbia, the predisposing, enabling, and reinforcing factors were ascertained based on the skills linked to the target behaviors of smoking, drinking, weight management, and exercise. Note that the program derived from the educational diagnosis requires the participation of representative advisory boards and multiple actors, including parents.[54]

School health researchers, whose work has demonstrated positive outcomes, are unanimous in their conclusion that development of relevant cognitive skills,

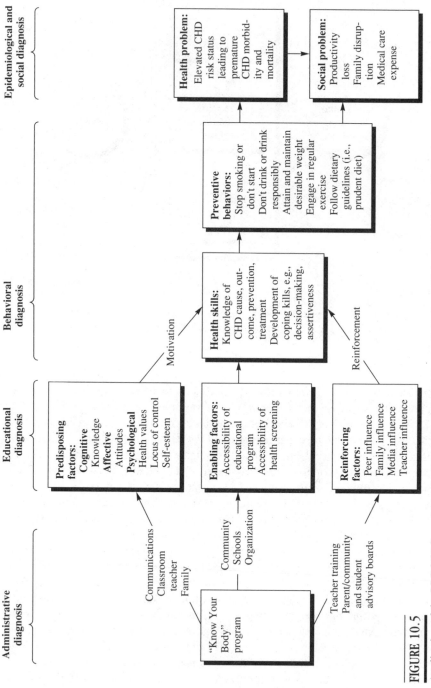

FIGURE 10.5

Application of the PRECEDE model to the "Know Your Body" Research Project. [From P. J. Bush, A. E. Zuckerman, P. K. Theiss, et al., *American Journal of Epidemiology* 129 (1989): 466–82; printed by permission of the publisher.]

resistance to peer pressure, and social competence skills, in some combination, facilitates change or resistance to change.[55] Environmental changes through regulatory and policy actions further enhance the results achieved through educational processes.

Investigations that have applied PRECEDE in the school setting include a wide range of topics from cardiovascular disease,[56] cancer,[57] and their attending risk factors, to human sexuality,[58] infectious disease control,[59] general health promotion and wellness,[60] nutrition policy,[61] seat-belt use,[62] and drunk driving.[63] Working knowledge of social, behavioral, and educational theories is essential for the expeditious identification of the predisposing, enabling, and reinforcing factors most likely to influence the skills or behaviors in question. One very practical benefit from a command of theory is that it enables planners to be precise in their selection of questions to include in a survey, thus saving precious teacher time and minimizing the burden of questionnaires. In that regard, practitioners will find Parcel's review of the major theories relevant to school health and school health education especially useful.[64]

According to the Ministry of Health in China, the smoking prevalence among adult male smokers (ages 30–50) in 1985 was nearly 75 percent.[65] To address the health problems associated with smoking in Hangzhou, Zhejiang Province, People's Republic of China, Zhang[66] and her colleagues applied PRECEDE as the basis for using school health education as a vehicle for the development and implementation of an effective smoking prevention and cessation policy and program. In 23 primary schools, 10,395 students (aged 9–12) were exposed to a curriculum with two concurrent objectives: (1) to provide students with the knowledge, attitude, and skills to resist forces that might encourage them to initiate smoking and (2) to create an effective mechanism through which students could motivate their parents (especially fathers) to quit smoking. Students became a prime vehicle for addressing the parents' knowledge of and attitudes about smoking (predisposing factors); students were also encouraged to express their feelings of concern for their parents' health (reinforcing factor).

Early results from the Hangzhou program were very encouraging. Of 10,367 quit charts that were distributed, 9,953 were completed and returned. From those charts, 6,843 (69%) were identified as smokers. Table 10.4 presents self-reported quit rates, from 1 day to over 6 months. Beyond direct educational benefits to the students, the 11.7 percent self-reported quit rate is encouraging in light of the fact that studies of smoking trends indicate that the rate of quitters is less than 5 percent among smokers in China.

To determine accurately which predisposing, enabling, and reinforcing factors require attention in an educational program, planners need data generated from valid and reliable surveys of the student population in question. School health personnel need to become familiar with and to use valid and reliable survey instruments, which are readily available. The Program Evaluation Handbooks[67] are seven practical volumes, each of which addresses a priority health behavior or problem. Each handbook contains a collection of measures for adults and for school-aged youth together with guidelines for their use. School health planners will find the data from the National Adolescent Student Health Survey (NASHS)[68] useful in preparing for an educational diagnosis. The NASHS provides a national profile of student health knowledge, attitudes, and self-reported behaviors related to AIDS, STDs, injury prevention, suicide, violence, nutrition, substance abuse, and consumer health.

A CASE EXAMPLE

Greenfield School District provides administrative support for ten elementary schools, four junior high schools, and two high schools. Greenfield is in a state that takes great pride in its system of public education and ranks in the top 15 in the nation in expenditure of state and local government resources for education as a percentage of personal income; the national percentage of adults 25 years of age and over who graduated from high school is 65 percent; the average in the state in which Greenfield lies is 71 percent. Within the state however, Greenfield ranks below the mean on all of these indicators.

The recently appointed superintendent of the Greenfield School District has established a school health committee with good representation from local health interests, key organizations in the community, and the schools, including two student representatives. The committee was charged with the mission of developing a proposal to promote and maintain health in the district, and the superintendent made the commitment to support their recommendations "within reason." As a first step, the committee elected to conduct, simultaneously, district-wide social and epidemiological diagnoses.[69] Their diagnostic data were derived from: (1) school records organized by school year and grade, (2) surveys and focus groups with school administrators, teachers, parents, students, and community gatekeepers, and (3) health statistics from school nurses, the local health department,

TABLE 10.4

Parent's self-report quit rates

Length of cessation (days)	Number of persons who quit	Percentage
1–10	6,191	90.5
11–20	4,411	64.5
21–30	3,339	48.8
31–60	2,017	30.3
61–180	800	11.7
210	800	11.7

TABLE 10.5

Student social diagnostic information from school records and survey

Problem	Greenfield	Heights
Time missed last year (per student)		
Grades K–6, mean days	4.8	7.2
Grades 7–12, mean days	5.3	8.4
10th-graders who are 1 or more years below		
expected grade level, %	17	32
Dropouts by grade 10, %	5	29
Students who "don't eat breakfast"		
Grades K–6, %	5	15
Grades 7–12, %	25	34

and selected clinics and community health centers. The information obtained from the diagnoses was voluminous, far more than the committee imagined they would get, and far more than they could handle. During the course of trying to put the information into manageable chunks, a committee member who was a pediatrician in a health center in the Greenfield neighborhood known as the Heights asked if the information collected in her service area could be compared with that from the community in general. The Heights population is primarily low-income and about 60 percent Hispanic. The committee agreed that such a comparative approach made sense and would be a good way to focus their analysis. Table 10.5 compares the information obtained from school records and some recent surveys. Table 10.6 summarizes the concerns expressed by school personnel and parents from both the Greenfield and the Heights areas. Comparative data from the epidemiological diagnosis for the students are displayed in Table 10.7 and student perceptions are summarized in Table 10.8.

The committee gathered additional information from various sources. For example, a health department report indicated that in the Greenfield area last year, there were 1,220 births to women under 20, 102 of which were out-of-wedlock births, a 19 percent increase in out-of-wedlock births in the last 5 years. (The rates were only slightly higher in the Heights.) Also, a nutritionist on the committee presented preliminary data gathered by Greenfield's Cooperative Extension Agency showing that the intake of total fat, saturated fat, and sodium among teenagers throughout Greenfield exceeded recommended levels. She said the Extension staff expressed their concern over poor nutritional habits, especially among younger students in the Heights area. They wondered if the general trend (both areas) of declining performance on aerobic fitness scores by students was related to low activity, poor nutrition, or both? Statistics from the state department of public safety indicated that there were 34 automobile fatalities among youth

TABLE 10.6

School personnel and parent response to the question: "What concerns you most about your school?"

Greenfield

Availability of drugs
Low SAT scores
Lack of parental and community support
Mass media report only the problems
Questionable competence of some school personnel
Some of the building in disrepair
Need equipment (e.g., computers, after-school recreational facilities)
Alcohol-related events (vandalism, auto crashes)

Heights

Violence and fighting
Increases in teen pregnancy
Absenteeism, truancy
Some students come to school hungry
Student apathy
Low teacher morale
Poor facilities and very limited resources

aged 14–19 in the Greenfield area. Although the data did not allow for comparison between the Heights and the rest of Greenfield, 70 percent of the fatalities occurred among white males.

It may be impossible or inappropriate in some communities to compare data in this way, but the example serves to illustrate what the data collection aspect of social and epidemiologic diagnoses is suppose to do: get planners in a position to set priorities for programmatic action based on the best information available, including input from those for whom the program is intended.

Put yourself in the place of one of the Greenfield school health committee members. What do the data tell you? They certainly confirm what we suspect that the pediatrician in the Heights already knew: The population she served bore a disproportionate burden of both social and health problems. Regardless of the setting, questions of inequities and justice must be foremost in setting our priorities.

The high rates of teen pregnancy are troubling because they trigger so many other problems: low-birth-weight babies who are vulnerable for a host of immediate and future health complications; mothers who drop out of school, severely compromising their future and significantly increasing their need for income maintenance and public assistance. Moreover, teen pregnancy implies a pattern of

TABLE 10.7

Epidemiological diagnosis: comparison of health problems in Greenfield and the Heights

Self-reported use	Greenfield, %	Heights, %
Smoking (grades 6–9)	17	22
Smoking (grades 10–12)	26	35
Alcohol (grades 6–9)	58	60
Alcohol (grades 10–12)	90	97
Drugs (grades 6–9)	29	24
Drugs (grades 10–12)	57	52
Regular seat-belt use (grades 10–12)	14	22

early sexual activity, which means a risk of contracting a sexually transmitted disease, including AIDS.

The tobacco smoking and the alcohol and drug use rates are equally troubling for some of the same reasons. The short- and long-term health effects of these addictive substances are compounded by the devastating secondary effects they mediate: absenteeism, poor academic performance, loss of part-time employment, and severe mood changes that can lead to depression, suicide, violence, arrests, fines, detention, and auto crashes. Frequently, these secondary outcomes hurt other people. Although less spectacular in the attention it gets, but very problematic nonetheless, is the recurring issue of inadequate nutrition and concurrent declines in levels of physical activity.

The committee has no shortage of problems to tackle, and it is quite likely that they now have more questions than they had at the outset. But, having completed

TABLE 10.8

Students' concerns

Greenfield	Heights
Nothing to do	Nothing to do
Not enough parking spaces	Prejudice in some teachers
Cafeteria food not good	What good is school?
Too much drinking	Drinking and drugs
	Weekends are boring

this phase of PRECEDE, they will be asking qualitatively different questions. Questions like "What should we do as a committee to address our mission?" will be replaced by questions like "Here are five documented health problems that are affecting the children in our schools, and they need attention. Which one(s) are the most important, and in which one(s) can we make a difference?"

As the committee digs into these questions and the issues associated with them, other confounding issues will surface—such as the need for more resources, the lack of community and parent involvement and support, and attitudes like "school is boring, what good is it." When planners come face to face with the interplay of these very real social, behavioral, institutional, economic, and emotional factors, the complexity can be overwhelming and, therefore, crippling. Yet it is the complexity of this challenge that plays to the ultimate strength of the PRECEDE model: its demonstrated ability to analyze complexities and use the results of that analysis to develop robust programs calling for multiple strategies from multiple sectors. One might say that attention to PRECEDE is good prevention in that it can help save the school health planner from the illusion of expecting great outcomes after making changes in only one component area.

Planners on the Greenfield school health committee were encouraged by the findings in the literature that even the most complicated problems can be effectively addressed through a well-planned school-based effort. Vincent and his co-workers[70] demonstrated that a program supported by the combined efforts of school, community, and church could be effective in reducing teen pregnancy in a predominantly African-American, low-income South Carolina county. Over a 4-year period, teen pregnancy declined over 50 percent in the intervention county; the study also demonstrated a diffusion beyond the school. There were four comparison sites: one in the same county and three in three separate counties. Pregnancy rates in the comparison site in the same county declined approximately 22 percent whereas the pregnancy rates increased in all three comparison counties. The researchers were unable to identify which element or combinations of elements accounted for the changes, including perhaps increased use of contraceptives. Nevertheless, the Greenfield planner's review of the Vincent study called attention to a subtle but important point that was common in most successful programs—that is, that credible sources *outside* of the school seemed to act as a major force for change. Perhaps it is the resources that these outside interests bring to the problem or their credibility, or some combination. As a result, the Greenfield school health committee sought consultation from both the state-education agency and the faculty with school health expertise from a nearby university.

MOVING FROM PRECEDE TO PROCEED

Have you ever heard the following rationale as the reason for a new idea or program floundering or not getting off the ground? "It was just too much ahead of its time!" The implication being that the idea or program in question was too innovative. Either the timing was off or the resources were limited; whatever the reason, the decision makers in authority were not ready to take action. The PROCEED process reviewed in Chapter 6 *assumes* that the health education or health promotion program planned in the PRECEDE process is indeed an innovation. Furthermore, PROCEED *acknowledges* the reality that matters of timing, resources, or other organizational or administrative factors, including policies, must be carefully assessed as a part of the strategic planning process; failure to take these institutional and environmental forces into account can lead to implementation delays or failure.

All of the elements of PROCEED apply to the school setting. Time constraints can be a limiting factor for all aspects of a comprehensive school health program. The school day is finite. Curricula for math, science, language, history, health, physical education, art, music, and countless other meritorious subjects or activities must compete for a part of that finite segment of time. Furthermore, school or district policies or even state codes may require that certain subjects receive a specific portion of that finite school day.

Policies can also influence program implementation. For example, the allocation of professional and support staff obviously depend on the school budget, but they also are sometimes influenced by regulations or policies that govern the personnel ceiling. So in some instances, personnel ceilings or hiring freezes can prohibit adding new personnel even if economic resources can be obtained.

It seems as if we are ever testing the validity of the aphorism: "there is no such thing as a free lunch." Whether a program is new or just a logical extension of an ongoing effort, the question of budget is inescapable. Nothing is free. All aspects of a proposed program — personnel needs, space, educational materials, health services, resources and equipment, and teacher and staff training — are inseparably tied to budget considerations. Although the health planner should not be paralyzed by budget constraints, it is important to be practical about costs when designing an intervention.

Thus, the planners' first PROCEED task is to make a careful assessment of time, personnel, materials, and resources needed for the proposed program and then to juxtapose those needs against two things: (1) the administrative and organizational realities of current operations in the school and (2) an assessment of the potential for making changes in those administrative and organizational elements that may act as barriers to program implementation. The identification of program needs should be a natural outgrowth of the PRECEDE planning process. Although the assessment of current administrative, organizational, and policy factors can by no means be taken for granted, the steps outlined in Chapter 6 can be readily applied by members of the planning group. The question of assessing the potential for influencing change in selected administrative, organizational, or policy elements merits further consideration here.

Let us return to the Greenfield scenario. Recall that the recently appointed superintendent of schools called for the formation of the school health committee, charged them with a health promotion mission and promised support "within reason." That kind of action is a signal that health is on the superintendent's agenda, and the committee would be well advised to take steps not only to keep it there but to elevate it. This is where the principles of community participation, highlighted throughout this book and incorporated in the formation of the Greenfield school health committee, are so critical.

Many things influence the decisions that school officials make. One of the more important is community opinion. The most obvious example is the loud and persistent opposition to sex education. Yet, in most cases it is not the loud outcry that most influences a decision on a program innovation, it is quiescence. Irrespective of how good a program may be, it is very easy for decision makers not to provide support if they believe that the decision makes little difference to constituents one way or another. An uninformed, quiescent community is a barrier to change. The committee should make a concerted effort to apprise parents and local leaders and to involve them in planning and implementing the proposed program.[71] This process can assure that the community committee members understand the important problems the program is designed to mitigate. Creating a ground swell of interest, and eventually support, will legitimize exploration into creative ways of obtaining resources for the program and will aid in overcoming administrative problems. One sure way to squelch an administrator's enthusiasm for school health activities is to propose programs that require large budgetary increases for personnel and materials without an accompanying plan that outlines a realistic means to meet those increases.

Policy issues also need special attention. A new health education curriculum, however creative and well-conceived it may be, by itself, will be no match for the problems in Greenfield. Lohrmann and Fors[72] are among many investigators whose work addresses this reality. In an analysis of recommendations for school-based education to prevent drug abuse, they concluded that many of the factors influencing adolescent drug use cannot be affected by exposure to a preventive curriculum. They call for greater attention to policy changes, teacher training, special programs for high-risk children, and greater participation from social institutions outside the school.

Parcel and his colleagues[73] carried out a 3-year study directed at influencing the dietary habits and exercise behaviors of third- and fourth-grade children. The program, entitled "Go For Health," incorporated classroom instruction, school food services, and physical education as intervention components and was consistent with the expanded concept of school health programs cited earlier in this chapter.

The unusual aspect of this study was not the comprehensive nature of components for intervention. Rather, it was the detailed attention paid to salient issues in the PROCEED process, that is, those organizational factors and dynamics which can act to either facilitate or hinder implementation. Parcel's group made the assumption, based on prior work done by Charters and Jones,[74] that program changes in schools generally occur sequentially in four steps: (1) institutional commitment, (2) changes in policies, (3) alterations in the roles of staff, and (4) changes in the students' learning activities. These four phases of change are illustrated in Figure 10.6. Note how looking at the change process from this organizational and policy perspective creates a very natural inventory of "change strategies" to address personnel and resource needs.

EVALUATION

In the first edition of this book, we called attention to the poverty cycle of education (Fig. 10.7), which highlights the dilemma of the 1970s: Given a sparse research base and paltry resources for programs or research it is difficult to quantify the effects of school health education. The cycle implies that diffuse educational programs lead to modest effects, which rarely yield detectable benefits. In the absence of such benefits, the probability for support of school health programs is diminished and the cycle is perpetuated. We noted then that limited resources "will dictate emphasis on process evaluation and, perhaps in sequence, impact evaluation. As resources expand, it will be possible to develop procedures for outcome evaluation."

Even though today's substantial research in school health may not have ended the poverty cycle, it has successfully fractured it. Not only can we now make a much stronger case about the relationship between many behavioral factors and health status, the evidence is strengthening on the linkages between knowledge gain, positive attitudes, health and social competence skills, and those risk behaviors. Though the need for all levels of evaluation is pressing, the responsibility for outcome studies and most impact studies, with their demands for sophisticated designs and large sample sizes, must be borne by academic researchers with grant support.

One might say that the cycle of poverty in health education has become a cycle of development in health promotion (Fig. 10.8). The increased involvement and support of other disciplines, the growing data base of descriptive and evaluative evidence, the growing policy supports, and the strengthening of professional standards all combine to make school health promotion a comprehensive and viable enterprise.

Classroom health educators should try to make process evaluation, and selected levels of impact evaluation, an integral part of their instructional program. As accountable practitioners, keeping track of the methods used in achieving educational goals and objectives provides a measure of quality assurance. One of the key findings from the School Health Education Evaluation Study was that a teacher's "fidelity" to the curriculum being taught was a critical predictor of positive student change. Administrators like to be able to tell their board about growth. Documented evidence showing increases in the number of children or

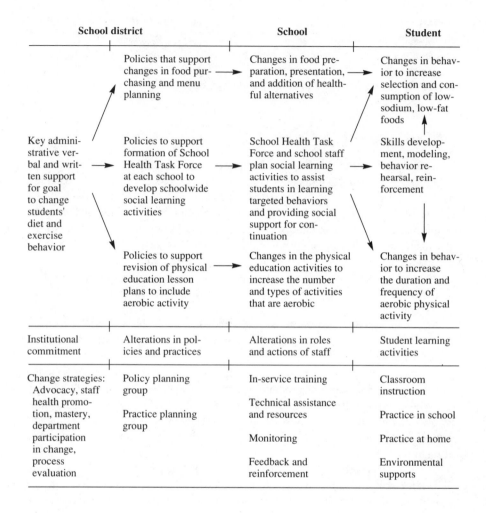

School district		School	Student
	Policies that support changes in food purchasing and menu planning →	Changes in food preparation, presentation, and addition of healthful alternatives →	Changes in behavior to increase selection and consumption of low-sodium, low-fat foods
Key administrative verbal and written support for goal to change students' diet and exercise behavior →	Policies to support formation of School Health Task Force at each school to develop schoolwide social learning activities →	School Health Task Force and school staff plan social learning activities to assist students in learning targeted behaviors and providing social support for continuation →	Skills development, modeling, behavior rehearsal, reinforcement
	Policies to support revision of physical education lesson plans to include aerobic activity →	Changes in the physical education activities to increase the number and types of activities that are aerobic	Changes in behavior to increase the duration and frequency of aerobic physical activity
Institutional commitment	Alterations in policies and practices	Alterations in roles and actions of staff	Student learning activities
Change strategies: Advocacy, staff health promotion, mastery, department participation in change, process evaluation	Policy planning group Practice planning group	In-service training Technical assistance and resources Monitoring Feedback and reinforcement	Classroom instruction Practice in school Practice at home Environmental supports

FIGURE 10.6

Model for planned change: "Go For Health." [Adapted with permission from G. Parcel, B. Simons-Morton, and L. J. Kolbe, *Health Education Quarterly* 15(4) (Winter 1988): 435–50.]

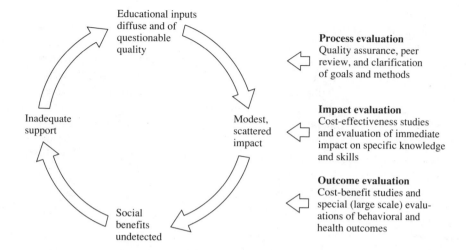

Process evaluation
Quality assurance, peer review, and clarification of goals and methods

Impact evaluation
Cost-effectiveness studies and evaluation of immediate impact on specific knowledge and skills

Outcome evaluation
Cost-benefit studies and special (large scale) evaluations of behavioral and health outcomes

FIGURE 10.7

The poverty cycle of health education.

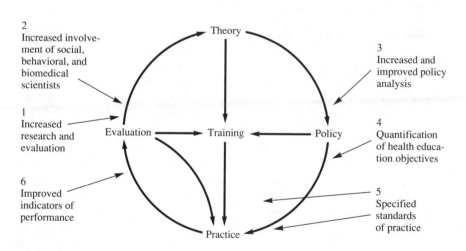

FIGURE 10.8

The cycle of development: the six points of intervention that broke the cycle of poverty in health education. [Adapted from L. W. Green, *Rev. Saude publ., San Paulo* 22(3) (1988): 217–20; printed with permission of the publisher.]

parents participating in a program, the evolution of a new school policy, or the institution of revised heart-healthy food services are examples of process changes that might well be key markers for longer range outcome measures. We strongly urge classroom teachers to make every effort to measure changes periodically in students' health knowledge, attitudes, intentions, and self-reported behaviors. With assistance and support from district or state-level health education coordinators, classroom teachers can prudently use a variety of valid and reliable measures to assess student progress and change without compromising instructional time. Using data of this kind, coupled with the results from ongoing process evaluation, effective teachers will be able to respond favorably to the ever-present question: Does the program work?

SUMMARY

This chapter tests the applicability of the PRECEDE framework to school health. A review of the current status of school health and school health education reveals a vigorous field in which the traditional innovation and diversity in the classroom have been strengthened by greater involvement with the community. Policy innovations together with remarkable research advances are beginning to give school health the national and international attention it deserves.

The value of keeping focus on the needs of the school and community when using PRECEDE and PROCEED is emphasized. Establishing a clear relationship between the quality of both community and school life, with community representatives active in the process, achieves recognition and support for the value of the role the school can play. The analytic strength of the PRECEDE process is maximized when applied within the context of the expanded concept of school health promotion. We also emphasize the importance of addressing the administrative, organizational, and policy factors inherent in schools that either can lead to severe problems or can facilitate program implementation.

Even though outcome evaluation research in school health is the job of the academic, school health personnel and teachers should attend to the critically important task of monitoring the quality of their programs, curricula, and instructional practices. Where feasible, they should also make efforts to measure the effects of their programs on students' knowledge, attitudes, intentions, and self-reported health practices.

EXERCISES

1. What is the ultimate goal of schools and how does that goal influence the school health planning process?
2. Traditionally, the school health program has been described as consisting of

three complementary components: instruction, services, and the school environment. Recently, an expanded concept of the school health program has emerged. Even though the two share commonalities, describe the advantages of the expanded model.

3. The productivity of school health researchers in the 1980s was substantial both in quality and quantity; as a result, we can now say with confidence that well-planned school health and school health education, carried out by qualified staff, make a difference. Using the summary information in Table 10.1, interpret the nature of the intervention strategies used in the NHLBI studies in light of the components and rationale of the expanded concept of school health promotion.

4. Explain how national- and state-level school health policy can be beneficial in promoting programs at the local level.

5. Review the strategy employed by CDC in the development of the national guidelines *School Health to Prevent the Spread of AIDS*. What lessons learned from that effort can be directly applied by school health planners at the local level?

6. Using the data collected by the school health committee in Greenfield:
   (a) Give an example of how a program or activity, generated by *each component* in the expanded model, could be targeted to address one or more of the problems identified.
   (b) Use PROCEED to identify potential administrative, organizational, or policy barriers and give an example of how each might be addressed.
   (c) List two process outcomes and two impact outcomes that could be assessed for each component program example you gave in (a).

REFERENCES AND NOTES

1. American Council of Life Insurance, *Wellness at the School Worksite: A Manual* (Washington, DC: Health Insurance Association of America, 1985).

2. The numbers and proportion of school-based people are larger if one includes colleges, universities, and the rapidly growing number of preschool and daycare centers. The principles discussed in this chapter apply similarly in college and in preschool health promotion. For applications of PRECEDE and related principles in the college setting, see B. G. Simons-Morton, S. G. Brink, G. S. Parcel, et al., *Preventing Alcohol-Related Health Problems Among Adolescents and Young Adults: A CDC Intervention Handbook* (Atlanta: Centers for Disease Control, 1989); B. G. Simons-Morton, S. G. Brink, D. G. Simons-Morton, et al., "An Ecological Approach to the Prevention of Injuries Due to Drinking and Driving," *Health Education Quarterly* 16 (1989): 397–411; J. G. Zapka and S. Dorfman, "Consumer Participation: Case Study of the College Health Setting," *Journal of American College Health* 30 (1982): 197–203; J. G. Zapka and J. A. Mamon, "Integration of Theory, Practitioner Standards, Literature Findings and Baseline Data: A Case Study in Planning Breast Self-examination Education," *Health Education Quarterly* 9 (1982): 330–56.

3. Carnegie Council on Adolescent Development, Task Force on Education of Young Adolescents, *Turning Points: Preparing American Youth for the 21st Century* (Washington, DC: Carnegie

Council on Adolescent Development, Carnegie Corporation of New York, 1989); National Commission on the Role of the School and the Community in Improving Adolescent Health, *Code Blue: Uniting for Healthier Youth* (Washington, DC: National Association of State Boards of Education and the American Medical Association, 1990). But these reports also note the importance of integrating and coordinating school and community approaches.

4. See the debate on this question in the *Eta Sigma Gamma Monograph Series* 4(1) (Nov., 1985): whole issue. See also L. J. Kolbe, L. W. Green, J. Foreyt, et al., "Appropriate Functions of Health Education in Schools," in *Child Health Behavior*, N. Krasnagor, J. Arasteh, and M. Cataldo, eds. (New York: Wiley, 1985), pp. 171–209; G. Stainbrook and L. W. Green, "Behavior and Behaviorism in Health Education," *Health Education* 13 (1982): 14–19. For definition and defense of the critical reasoning and higher order thinking objectives of schooling, see L. B. Resnick, *Education and Learning to Think* (Washington, DC: National Academy Press, 1987).

5. L. W. Green, P. Heit, D. C. Iverson, L. J. Kolbe, and M. Kreuter, "The School Health Curriculum Project: Its Theory, Practice, and Measurement Experience," *Health Education Quarterly* 7 (1980): 14–34, quotation from pp. 31–32.

6. J. O. Mason, "Dr. Mason Outlines Goals for Improving the Nation's Health," *Journal of School Health* 59 (1989): 289–90. For a summary of the growing federal activities in school health education in preceding years, see G. G. Gilbert, R. L. Davis, and C. L. Damberg, "Current Federal Activities in School Health Education," *Public Health Reports* 100 (1985): 499–507; D. Iverson and L. J. Kolbe, "Evaluation of the National Disease Prevention and Health Promotion Strategy: Establishing a Role for the Schools," *Journal of School Health* 53 (1983): 294–302.

7. L. W. Green, "Bridging the Gap Between Community Health and School Health," *American Journal of Public Health* 78 (1988): 1149.

8. J. F. Allanson, "School Nursing Services: Some Current Justifications and Cost-Benefit Implications," *Journal of School Health* 48 (1978): 603–7; V. Hertel, "Changing Times in School Nursing," *Journal of School Health* 52 (1982): 313–4; L. J. Kolbe, "What Can We Expect from School Health Education?" *Journal of School Health* 52 (1982): 145–50.

9. "Health Education Section, Committee Report, American Physical Education Association," *Journal of Health and Physical Education* 6 (Dec., 1935).

10. W. H. Creswell and I. M. Newman, *School Health Practice*, 9th ed. (St. Louis: Times Mirror/ Mosby, 1989).

11. Other textbooks on school health reflect similar models of the structure of school health programs. For example, H. J. Cornacchia, L. K. Olsen, and C. J. Nickerson, *Health in Elementary Schools*, 7th ed. (St. Louis: Times Mirror/Mosby, 1988); M. Pollock and K. Middleton, *Elementary School Health Instruction*, 2nd ed. (St. Louis: Times Mirror/Mosby, 1989).

12. L. Kolbe, "Increasing the Impact of School Health Promotion Programs: Emerging Research Perspectives," *Health Education* 17(5) (1986): 47–52.

13. D. Allensworth and L. J. Kolbe, eds., "The Comprehensive School Health Program: Exploring an Expanded Concept," *Journal of School Health* 57(10, whole issue) (1987): 409–73; G. H. DeFriese, C. L. Crossland, C. E. Pearson, C. J. Sullivan, eds., "Comprehensive School Health Programs: Current Status and Future Prospects," *Journal of School Health* 60(4, whole issue) (1990): 127–90.

14. L. J. Kolbe, L. W. Green, J. Foreyt, et al., "Appropriate Functions of Health Education in Schools," in *Child Health Behavior*, N. Krasnagor, J. Arasteh, and M. Cataldo, eds. (New York: Wiley, 1985), pp. 171–209. See a summary of dietary guidelines from each of five national organizations in Fig. 1 of L. Light and I. R. Contento, "Changing the Course: A School Nutrition and Cancer Education Curriculum Developed by the American Cancer Society and the National Cancer Institute," *Journal of School Health* 59 (1989): 205–9.

15. S. N. Blair, H. W. Kohl, and K. E. Powell, "Physical Activity, Physical Fitness, Exercise, and the

Public's Health," in *The Cutting Edge in Physical Education and Exercise Science Research*, M. J. Safrit and H. M. Eckert, eds. (Champaign, IL: Human Kinetics Publishers, 1987), pp. 53–69; B. G. Simons-Morton, G. S. Parcel, N. M. O'Hara, et al., "Health-Related Physical Fitness in Childhood: Status and Recommendations." *Annual Review of Public Health* 9 (1988): 403–25; K. E. Powell, C. J. Caspersen, J. P. Koplan, and E. S. Ford, "Physical Activity and Chronic Diseases," *American Journal of Clinical Nutrition* 49 (1989): 999–1006.

16. C. E. Basch, "Research on Disseminating and Implementing Health Education Programs in Schools," *Journal of School Health* 54 (1984): 57–66; C. E. Basch, J. D. Eveland, and B. Portnoy, "Diffusion Systems for Education and Learning about Health," *Family and Community Health* 9(2) (1986): 1–26; C. N. D'Onofrio, "Making the Case for Cancer Prevention in the Schools," *Journal of School Health* 59 (1989): 225–31; D. M. Murray, "Dissemination of Community Health Promotion Programs: The Fargo-Moorhead Heart Health Program," *Journal of School Health* 56 (1986): 375–81; G. S. Parcel, M. P. Eriksen, C. Y. Lovato, et al., "The Diffusion of School-Based Tobacco-Use Prevention Programs: Project Description and Baseline Data," *Health Education Research* 4 (1989): 111–24.

17. S. L. Becker, J. A. Burke, R. A. Arbogast, et al., "Community Programs to Enhance In-School Anti-tobacco Efforts," *Preventive Medicine* 18 (1989): 221–8; R. B. McKay, D. M. Levine, and L. R. Bone, "Community Organization in a School Health Education Program To Reduce Sodium Consumption," *Journal of School Health* 55 (1985): 364–6; C. L. Perry, R. V. Luepker, D. M. Murray, et al., "Parent Involvement with Children's Health Promotion: The Minnesota Home Team," *American Journal of Public Health* 78 (1988): 1156–60.

18. J. O. Mason and J. M. McGinnis, "The Role of School Health," *Journal of School Health* 55 (Oct., 1985): 299.

19. L. W. Green, P. Heit, D. Iverson, et al., "The School Health Curriculum Project: Its Theory, Practice and Measurement Experience," *Health Education Quarterly* 7 (1980): 14–34.

20. D. B. Connell, R. R. Turner, and E. F. Mason, "Summary Findings of the School Health Education Evaluation: Health Promotion Effectiveness, Implementation and Costs," *Journal of School Health* 55 (1985): 316–21. This issue of the journal is devoted to the School Health Education Evaluation.

21. C. L. Perry, ed., "Special Issue on Community Programs for Drug Abuse Prevention," *Journal of School Health* 56(9) (1986): 357–418. In this issue, the role of mass media and other community agencies in supporting school-based initiatives are analyzed: R. B. Flay, "Mass Media Linkages with School-Based Programs for Drug Abuse Preventions," *Journal of School Health* 56 (1986): 402–6; M. A. Orlandi, "Community-Based Substance Abuse Prevention: A Multicultural Perspective," *Journal of School Health* 56 (1986): 394–401; M. A. Pentz, "Community Organization and School Liaisons: How To Get Programs Started," *Journal of School Health* 56 (1986): 382–8. Pentz also shows how the PRECEDE approach to community diagnosis and planning relates to other models of community organization and school liaison.

22. T. J. Glynn, "Essential Elements of School-Based Smoking Prevention Programs," *Journal of School Health* 59 (1989): 181–8. This article describes the 15 school-based smoking prevention studies supported by the National Cancer Institute (NCI). In the same issue, eight studies of smokeless tobacco prevention trials supported by NCI are described by G. M. Boyd and E. D. Glover, "Smokeless Tobacco Use by Youth in the U.S.," *Journal of School Health* 59 (1989): 189–94. Also in this issue, the American Cancer Society's and NCI's application of the PRECEDE model to a school nutrition and cancer education curriculum is described in L. Light and I. R. Contento, "Changing the Course: A School Nutrition and Cancer Education Curriculum Developed by the American Cancer Society and the National Cancer Institute," *Journal of School Health* 59 (1989): 205–9.

23. E. J. Stone, C. L. Perry, and R. V. Luepker, "Synthesis of Cardiovascular Behavioral Research for Youth Health Promotion," *Health Education Quarterly* 16 (1989): 155–69. All work cited in Table 10.1 appears in separate articles in this issue of *Health Education Quarterly*. Another study supported by NHLBI under a separate program of grants was "Heart Smart," an extension of the

Bogalusa Heart Study in Louisiana, which applied the PRECEDE model in its design. See A. M. Downey, S. J. Virgilio, D. C. Serpas, et al., "Heart Smart—A Staff Development Model for a School-Based Cardiovascular Health Intervention," *Health Education* 19 (Oct/Nov, 1988): 64–71.

24. See commentary on the studies by J. A. Best, "Intervention Perspectives on School Health Promotion Research," *Health Education Quarterly* 16 (1989): 299–306.

25. In the Nader study the family is the primary locus of change rather than the school and its environment, which serve a supportive role. P. R. Nader, J. G. Sallis, T. L. Patterson, et al., "A Family Approach to Cardiovascular Risk Reduction: Results from the San Diego Family Health Project," *Health Education Quarterly* 16 (1989): 229–44.

26. Metropolitan Life Foundation, *An Evaluation of Comprehensive Health Education in American Public Schools* (New York: Louis Harris and Associates, for the Metropolitan Life Foundation, 1988).

27. E. Vartiainen and P. Puska, "The North Karelia Youth Project 1978–80: Effects of Two Years of Educational Intervention on Cardiovascular Risk Factors and Health Behavior in Adolescence," in *Cardiovascular Risk Factors in Childhood: Epidemiology and Prevention*, B. Hetzel and G. S. Berenson, eds. (Dublin: Elsevier, 1987), pp. 183–202.

28. A. M. Downey, G. C. Frank, L. S. Webber, et al., "Implementation of 'Heart Smart': A Cardiovascular School Health Promotion Program," *Journal of School Health* 57 (1987): 98–104.

29. L. E. Aaro, B. Wold, L. Kannas, and M. Rimpela, "Health Behavior in School Children: A WHO Cross-national Survey," *Health Promotion* 1 (1986): 17–33.

30. J. G. Ross and G. G. Gilbert, "The National Children and Youth Fitness Study," *Journal of Health, Physical Education, Recreation and Dance* 56(1) (1985): 45–50.

31. "Results from the National Adolescent Student Health Survey," *Morbidity and Mortality Weekly Report* 38 (1989): 147. See also, Children's Defense Fund, *Children 1990: A Report Card, Briefing Book, and Action Primer* (Washington, DC: Children's Defense Fund, 1990); R. Krolnick, *Adolescent Health Insurance Status: Analyses of Trends in Coverage and Preliminary Estimates of the Effects of an Employer Mandate and Medicaid Expansion on the Uninsured* (Washington, DC: U.S. Congress, Office of Technology Assessment, Government Printing Office, 1989); National Center for Children in Poverty, *Five Million Children: A Statistical Profile of Our Poorest Young Citizens* (New York: School of Public Health, Columbia University, 1990); U.S. Department of Education, Office of Educational Research and Improvement, *Youth Indicators 1988: Trends in the Well-being of American Youth* (Washington, DC: U.S. Government Printing Office, 1988); N. Zill and C. C. Rogers, "Recent Trends in the Well-being of Children in the United States and Their Implications for Public Policy," in *Family Change and Public Policy*, A. Cherlin, ed. (Washington, DC: Urban Institute Press, 1988).

32. G. Mutter, "Using Research Results as a Health Promotion Strategy: A Five-Year Case Study," *Health Promotion* 3 (1988): 393–9.

33. C. Y. Lovato and D. Allensworth, *School Health in America: An Assessment of State Policies to Protect and Improve the Health of Students*, 5th ed. (Kent, OH: American School Health Association, 1989). See also, J. J. Koshel, *An Overview of State Policies Affecting Adolescent Pregnancy and Parenting* (Washington, DC: National Governors' Association, 1990); S. R. Lovick and R. F. Stern, *School-Based Clinics—1988 Update* (Houston, TX: The Support Center for School-Based Clinics, 1988).

34. D. B. Connell, et al., "Summary Findings . . . ," op. cit., 1985.

35. State School Health Education Project, *Recommendations for School Health Education: A Handbook for State Policymakers* (Denver, CO: Education Commission of the States, 1981); Carnegie Council on Adolescent Development, *Turning Points*, op. cit., 1989; National Commission on Excellence in Education, *A Nation at Risk: The Imperative for Educational Reform* (Washington, DC: National Commission on Excellence in Education, 1983); National Commission on the Role

of the School and the Community in Improving Adolescent Health, *Code Blue: Uniting for Healthier Youth* (Washington, DC: American Medical Association and the National Association of State Boards of Education, 1990).

36. World Health Organization and United Nations Children's Fund, *Helping a Billion Children Learn About Health: Report of the WHO/UNICEF International Consultation on Health Education for School-Age Children, 1985* (Geneva: World Health Organization, 1986).

37. R. D. Corcoran and B. Portnoy, "Risk Reduction Through Comprehensive Cancer Education: The American Cancer Society Plan for Youth Education," *Journal of School Health* 59 (1989): 199–204.

38. American College Health Association, *AIDS on the College Campus* (Rockville, MD: American College Health Association, 1986); American College of Physicians, "Health Care Needs of the Adolescent," *Annals of Internal Medicine* 110 (1989): 930–5; National Professional School Health Education Organizations, "Comprehensive School Health Education," *Journal of School Health* 54 (1984): 312–5; G. S. Parcel, L. D. Muraskin, and C. M. Endert, "Community Education: Study Group Report" [of Society for Adolescent Medicine], *Journal of Adolescent Health Care* 9 (1988): 41S–5S; P. Smith, "National School Boards Association, and Center for Chronic Disease Prevention and Health Promotion, CDC, School Policies and Programs on Smoking and Health— United States, 1988," *Morbidity and Mortality Weekly Report* 38 (1989): 202–3, also in *Journal of the American Medical Association* 261 (1989): 2488.

39. Centers for Disease Control, "Guidelines for Effective School Health Education to Prevent the Spread of AIDS," *Morbidity and Mortality Weekly Report* 37 (suppl. no. S-2.) (1988): 1–14; also published in full in *Health Education* 19(3) (1988): 6–13. The President's Commission on the HIV Epidemic, in its 1988 report, also concluded that the school's contribution to AIDS education should be in the context of comprehensive school health education. *Report of the Presidential Commission on the Human Immunodeficiency Virus Epidemic* (Washington, DC: The White House, June 24, 1988).

40. L. Kolbe, J. Jones, G. Nelson, et al., "School Health Education to Prevent the Spread of AIDS: Overview of a National Programme," *Hygie* 7 (1988): 10–3.

41. Ibid., p. 11.

42. M. J. Adler, *The Paideia Problems and Possibilities* (New York, Macmillan, 1983), p. 45.

43. For indicators of these and other criteria for social, epidemiological, behavioral, environmental, organizational, and educational indicators, see L. J. Kolbe, "Indicators for Planning and Monitoring School Health Programs," in *Health Promotion Indicators and Actions*, S. B. Kar, ed. (New York: Springer, 1989), pp. 221–48.

44. L. W. Green and B. Simons-Morton, "Education and Life-style Determinants of Health and Disease," in *Oxford Textbook of Public Health*, 2nd ed., W. W. Holland, R. Detels, and G. Knox, eds. (London: Oxford University Press, in press); M. A. Winkleby, S. P. Fortmann, and D. C. Barrett, "Social Class Disparities in Risk Factors for Disease Eight-Year Prevalence Patterns by Level of Education," *Preventive Medicine* 19 (1990): 1–12.

45. National Commission on the Role..., op. cit., 1990, p. 3.

46. B. Starfield, P. Budetti, "Child Health Risk Factors," *Health Services Research* 19(6, pt. II) (1985): 817–86.

47. L. J. Kolbe and G. G. Gilbert, "Involving the School in the National Strategy to Improve the Health of Americans," in *Proceedings, Prospects for a Healthier America* (Washington, DC: U.S. Department of Health and Human Services, Office of Disease Prevention and Health Promotion, 1984).

48. D. Allensworth and C. A. Wolford, *Achieving the 1990 Objectives for the Nation's Schools* (Kent, OH: American School Health Association, 1988), pp. 4–5.

49. M. Pollock, *Health Education in Schools* (Palo Alto, CA: Mayfield, 1987), pp. 15–16.

50. R. M. Pigg, "The Contribution of School Health Programs to the Broader Goals of Public Health: The American Experience," *Journal of School Health* 59 (1989): 25–30.

51. Table 10.3 is based on various sources including D. Allensworth and C. A. Wolford, op. cit., 1988; National Center for Health Statistics, *Health United States 1989 and Prevention Profile* (Hyattsville, MD: Public Health Service, 1990); and National Commission on the Role . . . , op. cit., 1990.

52. L. J. Kolbe, L. W. Green, J. Foreyt, et al., op. cit., 1985.

53. Maine Department of Educational and Cultural Services, "Project Graduation," *Morbidity and Mortality Weekly Report* 34 (1985): 233–5.

54. P. J. Bush, A. E. Zuckerman, P. K. Theiss, et al., "Cardiovascular Risk Factor Prevention in Black School Children: Two-Year Results of the 'Know Your Body' Program," *American Journal of Epidemiology* 129 (1989): 466–82.

55. G. J. Botvin, E. Baker, N. Renick, et al., "A Cognitive-Behavioral Approach to Substance Abuse Prevention," *Addictive Behaviors* 9 (1984): 137–47; R. I. Evans and B. E. Raines, "Control and Prevention of Smoking in Adolescents: A Psychological Perspective," in *Promoting Adolescent Health: A Dialog on Research and Practice*, T. J. Coates, A. D. Peterson, and C. Perry, eds. (New York: Academic Press, 1982); B. R. Flay, "Social Psychological Approaches to Smoking Prevention: Review and Recommendations," in *Advances in Health Education and Promotion*, vol. 2, W. B. Ward and P. D. Mullen, eds. (Greenwich, CT: JAI Press, 1987), pp. 121–80; A. L. McAlister, C. Perry, J. Killen, et al., "Pilot Study of Smoking, Alcohol, and Drug Abuse Prevention," *American Journal of Public Health* 70 (1980): 719–21; D. M. Murray, C. A. Johnson, R. V. Luepker, and M. B. Mittelmark, "The Prevention of Cigarette Smoking in Children: A Comparison of Four Strategies," *Journal of Applied Social Psychology* 14 (1984): 274–88; S. P. Schinke, "A School-Based Model for Teenage Pregnancy Prevention," *Social Work in Education* 4 (1982): 34–42.

56. P. Bush, et al., op. cit., 1989; A. M. Downey, G. C. Frank, L. S. Webber, et al., "Implementation of 'Heart Smart': A Cardiovascular School Health Promotion Program," *Journal of School Health* 57 (1987): 98–104; S. W. Fors, S. Owen, W. D. Hall, et al., "Evaluation of a Diffusion Strategy for School-Based Hypertension Education," *Health Education Quarterly* 16 (1989): 255–61; G. S. Parcel, B. Simons-Morton, N. M. O'Hara, et al., "School Promotion of Healthful Diet and Physical Activity: Impact on Learning Outcomes and Self-reported Behavior," *Health Education Quarterly* 16 (1989): 181–99; H. J. Walter and E. L. Wynder, "The Development, Implementation, Evaluation, and Future Directions of a Chronic Disease Prevention Program for Children: The 'Know Your Body' Studies," *Preventive Medicine* 18 (1989): 59–71.

57. L. Light and I. R. Contento, "Changing the Course: A School Nutrition and Cancer Education Program by the American Cancer Society and the National Cancer Institute," *Journal Of School Health* 59(5) (1989): 205–9.

58. L. Rubinson and L. Baillie, "Planning School-Based Sexuality Programs Using the PRECEDE Model," *Journal of School Health* 51 (1981): 282–7.

59. H. E. Ekeh and J. D. Adeniyi, "Health Education Strategies for Tropical Disease Control in School Children," *Journal of Tropical Medicine and Hygiene* 92(2) (Apr., 1989): 55–9.

60. G. W. Simpson and B. E. Pruitt, "The Development of Health Promotion Teams as Related to Wellness Programs in Texas Schools," *Health Education* 20(1) (Feb./Mar., 1989): 26–8; M. Sutherland, C. Pittman-Sisco, T. Lacher, and N. Watkins, "The Application of a Health Education Planning Model to a School-Based Risk Reduction Model," *Health Education* 18(3) (June/July, 1987): 47–51.

61. G. C. Frank, A. Vaden, and J. Martin, "School Health Promotion: Child Nutrition," *Journal of School Health* 57 (1987): 451–60.

62. S. G. Brink, C. Y. Lovato, L. J. Kolbe, and M. E. Buoy, "Development and Evaluation of a School-Based Intervention to Increase the Use of Safety Belts by Adolescents," (submitted for publication, 1989); final report to U.S. Department of Transportation.

63. B. G. Simons-Morton, S. G. Brink, D. G. Simons-Morton, et al., "An Ecological Approach to the Prevention of Injuries Due to Drinking and Driving," *Health Education Quarterly* 16 (1989): 397–411.

64. G. S. Parcel, "Theoretical Models for Application in School Health Education Research," *Journal of School Health* 54 (1984): 39–49.

65. W. Xin-Zhi, H. Zhao-guang, and C. Dan-yang, "Smoking Prevalence in Chinese Aged 15 and Above," *Chinese Medical Journal* 100(11) (1987): 686–692.

66. Methods and preliminary results from this study were provided during a World Bank consultation with the Chinese Ministry of Health in Hangzhou, Zhejiang Province. Information is presented here with the permission of the principal investigator, Zhang De-Xiu, M.D., Center for Health Education, Zhejiang Hygiene and Epidemic Prevention Center.

67. The Program Evaluation Handbooks are a series of eight volumes which contain guidelines and questionnaire instruments designed for use in the evaluation of health education programs. Categorical topics include: drug abuse, alcohol abuse, nutrition, tobacco use, stress, physical activity, and diabetes education. Handbooks may be purchased from IOX Assessment Associates, P.O. Box 240495, Los Angeles, CA 90024-0095.

68. "National Adolescent Student Health Survey," *Health Education* 19(4) (1988): 4–8.

69. The strategy of conducting the social and epidemiological diagnoses together is often strategic and practical because it encourages those planners who typically have a strong health bias to be mindful of linking health problems to the salient social problems.

70. M. L. Vincent, A. F. Clearie, and M. D. Schluchter, "Reducing Adolescent Pregnancy Through School and Community Based Education," *Journal of the American Medical Association* 257 (1987): 3382–6.

71. A method for identifying community leadership to participate in planning and guiding the implementation of specific health programs has been developed in the context of a PRECEDE application in North Carolina: R. Michielutte and P. Beal, "Identification of Community Leadership in the Development of Public Health Education Programs," *Journal of Community Health* 15 (1990): 59–68.

72. D. K. Lohrmann and S. W. Fors, "Can School-Based Programs Really Be Expected to Solve the Adolescent Drug Problem," *Journal of Drug Education* 16(4) (1986): 327–39.

73. G. Parcel, B. Simons-Morton, and L. J. Kolbe, "Health Promotion: Integrating Organizational Change and Student Learning Strategies," *Health Education Quarterly* 15 (1988): 435–50.

74. W. Charter and J. Jones, "On the Risk of Appraising Non-events in Program Evaluation," *Educational Research* 2(11) (1973): 5–7.

Chapter 11

Applications in
Health-Care Settings

A s in schools, worksites, and other community settings, health promotion planning in hospitals, clinics, physicians' offices, pharmacies, and other health-care settings can be strengthened by the combined educational and environmental approach of PRECEDE and PROCEED. This calls for several departures from the medical model that dominates health-care planning in these settings. Each of these deviations from the medical model constitutes a section of this chapter.

First, the combined educational and environmental approach to health promotion planning in health-care settings calls for a break from the traditional medical approach of concentrating health-care diagnosis and planning on the individual patient. The PRECEDE–PROCEED model works best when applied first to a population of patients or potential patients. This population-based or epidemiological approach will be outlined in the first section.

The second departure of the educational and environmental approach from the traditional medical model as practiced in most health-care settings calls for a greater emphasis on self-care and patient-centered authority and responsibility for planning and controlling the health-care regimen. This break from medical tradition is not a break from nursing tradition. The earliest philosophies of nursing from Florence Nightingale to the present have emphasized self-care.[1] The active and informed engagement of patient decision and control from the earliest stages of seeking diagnosis to the postmedical or postsurgical self-monitoring and maintenance of lifestyle and environmental changes must be emphasized. A protocol for the application of the PRECEDE–PROCEED model to this style of health-care through self-care is offered in the second section.

The culture, environment, and professional behavior of health-care settings also must change if they are to support health promotion and self-care objectives.

The PRECEDE–PROCEED model is applied in the third section to the diagnosis of behavioral and environmental factors in the health-care setting that can be changed through educational approaches to the behavior of physicians and other health-care providers and through environmental reforms of the system itself.

AN EPIDEMIOLOGICAL AND COMMUNITY APPROACH TO HEALTH CARE

The changing epidemiology of diseases calls for a shift in medical interventions within the epidemiological triad of host-agent-environment, from a primary emphasis on the agent to a greater emphasis on the host (patient) and the environment.[2] Most efforts to maximize the benefits and to minimize the risks of medical interventions have concentrated on the regulation or control of the **agent**, the invading organism or pathology. Most medical therapies employed have emphasized technological agents such as drugs and surgical procedures. With the decline in acute communicable diseases and the increasing frequency of chronic conditions in the population, single causes in the form of a controllable pathological agent have been replaced with multiple contributing agents, many of which are embedded in normal living conditions and lifestyle. More patients must manage their own often complex, long-term regimens of drugs and lifestyle modifications. This requires a refocusing of health-care attention to environments and to more-autonomous patients outside hospitals and other clinical settings.

Most studies of patient "compliance"[3] begin with the medical-care setting as the locus of patient identification and intervention.[4] A community approach to the problems of patient adherence to medical recommendations begins with a population in which many of the potential benefactors of medical advice are in varying degrees of contact with medical practitioners, some with no contact. PRECEDE–PROCEED provides a rationale and framework for analysis of health-care issues that considers the total population at risk, including those who should be but are not receiving medical care and those who are misusing their prescribed medicines or recommended preventive or self-care practices.

The following four questions are addressed in developing the framework:

1. What groups of people in the population have illnesses, conditions, or risk factors that would benefit from medical or nursing interventions not yet received?
2. What types of patients have illnesses or conditions that would benefit from more appropriate use of the medications or self-care procedures prescribed for them?
3. What combinations of patients, conditions, medical settings, drugs, and self-care regimens are most likely to result in error and would benefit from improved education and monitoring?

4. What means of intervention for each group of patients and type of regimen appears most effective when (a) a condition is either diagnosed or undiagnosed, (b) a regimen is either prescribed or not prescribed, (c) a drug is either dispensed or not dispensed, and (d) medical regimens are either followed or not followed?

EPIDEMIOLOGY OF HEALTH-CARE ERRORS

A health-care error may be an error of commission or an error of omission. An error of *commission* occurs when a patient uses, a physician prescribes, or a pharmacist dispenses a therapeutic or preventive regimen incorrectly. It occurs also when a patient uses a drug prescribed for another patient. An error of *omission* occurs when a patient fails to receive or to apply a clinically important medication or procedure as needed. Both types of error can be attributed to failures of health-care professionals or to failures of patients, or both. The purpose of this epidemiological approach to assessing the errors is not to affix blame but to pinpoint the most strategic points for intervention.

Figure 11.1 identifies the circumstances under which patients or would-be patients might benefit from receiving health education: (A, the undiagnosed) to inform them about treatable signs and conditions; (B, the nonusers) to inform them about the risks and benefits of a preventive intervention, a drug, or alternative nonpharmacologic therapies or self-care procedures; and (C, the misusers) to inform them about the proper use of a medication or procedure. The figure identifies needs for patient education and broader public-health education to prevent errors of omission (in categories A, B, and C_2) and to prevent errors of commission (in category C).

ERRORS OF OMISSION

Potential patients can be classified into two groups, each of which could be the target of different health education programs to reduce health-care errors of omission:

1. Those who are not currently seeking or receiving medical care for their illness or condition (the undiagnosed) or for a symptom or risk factor that could warrant examination and health counseling (the unscreened).
2. Those who received a medical diagnosis but did not receive, fill, or use a prescription or recommendation for a procedure or medicine that could benefit them (the nonusers). (See Fig. 11.1.)

The Undiagnosed. The purpose of health education for people with undiagnosed conditions is to predispose and enable them to obtain screening or medical

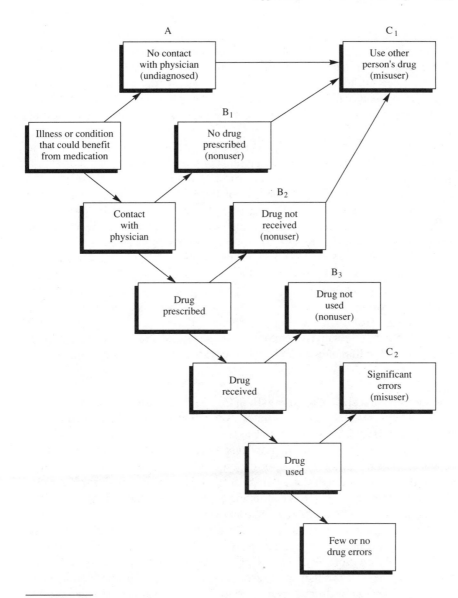

FIGURE 11.1

Flow of patients into categories of health care and health care errors. [Adapted from L. W. Green, P. D. Mullen, and R. B. Friedman, *Patient Education and Counseling* 8 (1986): 255–68; printed by permission of publisher.]

diagnosis and treatment, assuming that one or more tests, medications, or procedures would help prevent or treat their condition and would be prescribed for them.[5] General communications targeted to these people would advise them that if they have certain high-risk characteristics or are experiencing specified symptoms, they should obtain periodic screening tests or consult a physician or other health-care provider because medical or dental advice or treatment may be needed.

Health education of this kind has long been part of public health programs to induce high-risk populations to seek prenatal care, immunizations, contraceptives, blood-pressure screening, and a variety of other preventive measures.[6] The effectiveness of such efforts has been documented in primary prevention and communicable disease control[7] (accounting for the dramatic reductions in infant mortality and congenital defects and the near eradication of some childhood diseases)[8]; in high blood pressure control[9] (accounting for dramatic reductions in the incidence of strokes and cerebrovascular death rates)[10]; and in family planning,[11] cancer control,[12] mental health care,[13] and other areas of secondary prevention and early diagnosis.[14] Those suffering overt symptoms and the "worried well"[15] will be most responsive to media messages that encourage them to seek medical care to alleviate their symptoms or worries. Those with financial constraints and those with risk factors considered normal in their family, culture, or experience[16] will require more intensive case finding,[17] outreach,[18] and screening programs.[19]

Nonusers. The first class of nonusers (B_1 in Fig. 11.1) consists of patients who have preventable or treatable conditions but who do not receive self-care instruction or medical recommendations from their physicians, or who receive a prescription or recommendation for the wrong therapy or self-care regimen. These patients might benefit from some of the same information as directed to the undiagnosed even though these errors of omission are made by their health-care providers.[20] A more appropriate remedy, however, is continuing education and other improved quality-assurance activity with medical practitioners.[21]

Another category of nonusers are those patients who do not obtain recommended self-care devices (e.g., a blood pressure cuff) or medications, or who fail to fill their prescriptions (B_2). This occurs more frequently when patients cannot get to pharmacies, when they are exceptionally fearful of side effects, and when the price of devices or drugs is perceived to exceed the value of the therapy.[22]

When the medical conditions are not life-threatening, the purpose of educational communications would be to increase awareness that the patient's condition may lead to complications, may spread, or may recur if untreated. Education for patients with symptoms that cannot consistently be seen or felt, such as high blood pressure, would attempt to strengthen the belief that the conditions may nevertheless be serious.[23] For those who cannot afford the cost of drugs, information about less expensive medicines and about sources of financial aid would be most useful.

In particular, the degree of benefit from palliative regimens should be clarified so that the user is able to weigh potential benefits against financial and other costs, including possible side effects.[24]

ERRORS OF COMMISSION

Two types of possible errors of commission are (1) those made by physicians, pharmacists, or other who recommend or prescribe medications or self-care procedures and (2) those made by patients.

Professional Errors. The first type of compliance error of commission can occur when a diagnosis is applied without adequate confirmation, when drugs are prescribed in lieu of more appropriate nonpharmacological therapies, when a new drug's potential interaction with other regimens has not been evaluated, or when the proper drug is prescribed in the wrong dosage. Such errors are arguably amenable to professional media communication and continuing education or quality assurance for physicians and others who care for patients.[25] General messages to high-risk subpopulations of the public may be helpful in shaping patients' expectations.[26]

Patient Errors. Patients who are screened or diagnosed and receive self-care instructions or medications are at risk of misunderstanding and making errors in the use of procedures or drugs.[27] The amount of information provided about a particular product to prevent these errors of commission does not always correspond to the amount needed by the patient or, indeed, to what the patient can understand.[28] In the debate over patient package inserts, some proponents argued that full disclosure in a consistently available written format would at least give patients access to all the information they needed.[29] In fact, however, as with any mass medium, some patients received a great deal of unnecessary information with patient package inserts, while some others may have received but failed to notice, comprehend, or recall the specific information they needed.[30]

Uniformly distributed written or video materials for patients are to medical care what mass media are to community programs: powerful and cost-effective channels for reaching large numbers of people, especially those already motivated and eager to learn; but they are not a sufficient means of assuring the education and support of those most in need of behavioral or environmental changes. They should be designed with the average patient in mind—remembering that this average misses the people at one end of the normal curve on any particular characteristic such as reading ability, acculturation, motivation, socioeconomic status, or age. The health-care providers who use mass-produced patient education materials also must guard against the tendency to let them substitute for spending personal time with patients who have questions or concerns, and being responsive to nonverbal cues.[31]

An alternate to the universal, uniform patient information strategy, but necessarily more complicated, is to carry out systematic surveys of the behavioral and educational needs of each demographic or epidemiological grouping of patients. This should be less complicated and burdensome on practitioners than attempting to do a systematic educational diagnosis on each patient. A simplification of this approach is to develop synthetic estimates of the probabilities of drug-utilization errors in each group or subpopulation of patients and the severity of consequences associated with each potential error. A specific group's relative need for drug education or counseling can be defined mathematically and estimated from a combination of national survey data[32] and local census data. Formulas for estimating drug information need in local populations have been proposed.[33]

Nonpatient Errors. Two groups of people present special problems of compliance errors of commission, pregnant women and those persons who medicate themselves by using prescription drugs obtained for another illness or by another person. For women who are or intend to become pregnant or who are breastfeeding, more-active health education campaigns need to be launched through the mass media or through fertility clinics.[34] The campaigns need to urge these women to report fully their use of drugs, tobacco, and alcohol to their physician or to a drug information service for evaluation, even before other needs for prenatal care arise.[35] Formulas and software for synthetic estimates of women at risk of poor pregnancy outcomes due to smoking have been developed.[36]

People who use drugs obtained for previous illnesses, or from other persons, risk making a variety of mistakes, including use of an inappropriate drug, the wrong dosage of the right drug, or the right drug at the wrong time. A survey conducted by the CBS Television Network found that in 45 percent of U.S. households at least one person reported borrowing drugs or using old prescriptions to treat a medical condition.[37] Only education through nonmedical channels can reach most of these consumers to warn them about these potential hazards.[38]

PATIENT CONSIDERATIONS IN TARGETING INTERVENTIONS

Two conclusions follow from the preceding discussions: (1) Broad-scale patient educational programs must reach beyond the clinical setting; but they can be contained and targeted to demographic groups in which the prevalence of risk factors, undiagnosed conditions, or untreated illnesses is high, and (2) the remaining patient education and counseling resources can be concentrated on clinical and self-help group settings. Based on estimates of a 50-percent prevalence of compliance in patients,[39] the probability of preventing a potentially harmful error per patient per encounter could be as high as .50 if methods of patient education and counseling were 100-percent effective. To maximize their effectiveness, educational and counseling resources must be conserved and focused on those patient encounters that represent the greatest need and opportunity to improve or protect health. The first task is to determine which patients are in these target groups and which compliance errors could be prevented by effective education and counseling.

THE UNDIAGNOSED

Who are the undiagnosed? National statistics can be used to identify the groups or types of would-be patients who are most likely not to seek help or to receive care for various conditions. The prevalence of those types in a local area or population can then be estimated from census data. National statistics indicate, for instance, that women experience (or acknowledge) more symptoms than men within most broad classifications of illness,[40] and women more frequently seek diagnosis, medical care, and prescription therapy for the same symptoms than men, who are more likely to "tough it out" or to prefer home remedies.[41]

When men do seek care, they account for 40 percent of the total number of patient visits to office-based physicians and 40 percent of drug "mentions."[42] The same bias in underrepresentation of males can be found in preventive care visits as in symptomatic care.[43]

In addition, lower socioeconomic and nonwhite groups have higher incidence rates for most illnesses and lower medical and preventive care utilization rates relative to their greater need.[44] White patients tend to receive more information from physicians than do Blacks and Hispanics.[45] Low-income patients receive less information than more affluent patients.[46]

Patients over 65 years of age are more often ill and require more visits and drugs than younger people. Patients 65 years and older purchase almost 25 percent of all prescription and nonprescription drugs.[47] The elderly require more medication than younger patients for the management of acute disease,[48] and they have a higher incidence of chronic disease.[49]

Although the elderly may not make more drug-compliance errors than younger patients with the same prescriptions, the deleterious consequences of an error may be more serious,[50] less easily detected, and less easily resolved than in younger patients.[51] In addition, their complex medical regimens place the elderly at greater risk of compliance errors.[52]

The best indicators, then, for targeting broad patient education and counseling programs to reduce compliance errors of omission are male sex, lower socioeconomic status and older age. The following are the most prevalent illnesses and conditions of older men in lower socioeconomic groups (listed in order from highest to lowest): high blood pressure, respiratory, mental, nervous, digestive, skin, urinary, eye and ear conditions, arthritis, and pain in bones and joints.[53]

DIAGNOSED NONUSERS WHO RECEIVED INAPPROPRIATE MEDICAL RECOMMENDATIONS

Those patients who received no prescription or the wrong medical advice cannot be considered noncompliant, in the strictest sense, especially if they followed the wrong advice. Nevertheless, their medical-care error puts them at risk; so this class of compliance errors must be prevented or corrected. Continuing medical education of physicians and other health-care providers is expected to prevent diagnostic and prescribing errors in individual practitioners and to build a level of knowledge and skill in the medical community that might detect and correct many of the individual errors that continue. Only weak and inconsistent evidence supports this expectation of traditional forms of continuing medical education.[54] Innovative modalities of continuing education involving patients,[55] and more-comprehensive quality-assurance methods combining educational with behavioral, economic, and environmental approaches to physicians' and other professionals' practices, show greater promise but also mixed results.[56]

The evidence that prescribing can be influenced through the mass media also seems conflicted. During 1973–1981, the national media aided a campaign by the National Institute of Mental Health targeted prominently to physicians who were "overprescribing" barbiturate sedatives and minor tranquilizers. Prescriptions for these drugs declined substantially.[57] A Canadian study suggests, moreover, that some physicians have overreacted to this publicity and as a result may have underprescribed these drugs.[58] Media events such as the news of Nancy Reagan's breast cancer diagnosis tend to result in exaggerated increases in the demand for selected medical or screening procedures such as mammography.[59] Thus, it appears that certain mass communications can influence clinical behavior, prescribing patterns, and public demand for certain procedures.

NONUSERS WHO DID NOT OBTAIN DRUG OR DEVICE RECOMMENDED

For nonusers who fail to fill prescriptions, to purchase nonprescription drugs or devices, or to adopt recommended procedures, two further strategies of targeting health education and communications can be considered. One is direct-to-public advertising of the price advantage of one product or pharmacy over another. The second is patient education directed at patients in medical-care settings including pharmacies, especially for illnesses in which the cost of drugs most frequently discourages the filling or refilling of prescriptions. Such discouragement most often occurs when the illness or condition is not life-threatening, the symptoms are not very painful or noticeable, the patient is averse to taking drugs generally, or the patient simply cannot afford the cost of the drug.[60] A survey of the American Association of Retired Persons, for example, found that 20 percent of older patients never filled their prescriptions.[61]

POLICY CHANGES

As with all categories of nonusers in which financial barriers to adequate health care restrict behavior, health promotion can play a role in educating the electorate and policy makers about the need for new provisions under health insurance, Medicare, or Medicaid. Direct political organizing with influential groups such as the American Association of Retired Persons, the national medical or nursing associations, and the American Cancer Society (or Cancer Foundation in other English-speaking countries). These organizations have been powerful lobbyists and advocates on behalf of legislation and regulatory changes in support of patients.

THE MISUSERS

Misusers provide a more-efficient target for compliance-improving strategies than do nonusers for several reasons. They can be reached more readily (through providers of medical care) than the nonpatient and nonuser (B_3) groups. Patient education can be tailored more closely to their information needs and learning capacities.[62] Misusers also can be assumed to be more highly motivated, on average, to respond to drug information than nonpatients and nonusers because they have made the effort to obtain medical care and to fill their prescription or to purchase recommended nonprescription medications or devices. The cumulative evidence from 102 published evaluations of patient education directed at drug misuse indicates that patient education reduces drug errors by an average of 40–72 percent and improves clinical outcomes by 23–47 percent.[63]

The same meta-analysis of the 72 studies of patient education directed at drug compliance specifically in chronic disease treatment showed that the medium, channel, or technique of communication mattered less than the appropriate application of learning principles such as individualization, relevance, facilitation, feedback, and reinforcement.[64] These principles can be applied more efficiently, systematically, and strategically with an algorithm that sorts or "triages" patients into educational groupings according to their educational needs.[65] Such an algorithm for patient education is presented in the next section.

ALLOCATION DECISIONS

Despite the efficiencies and cost-*effectiveness* of interventions directed at patients classified as misusers or potential misusers of medical advice and prescriptions, the cost-*benefit* potential of reaching the undiagnosed and dropouts from treatment could be much greater in the long run. These nonusers represent new or lost markets for the pharmaceutical companies, who should find it beneficial to support medical and public health agencies in their efforts to reach these patients and to reduce the extent of untreated illness in the poorest populations. Recently, pharmaceutical companies, the Food and Drug Administration, consumers, and advertising firms have experimented with bringing medication information directly to the general public. Several attempts have been made by individual companies to educate consumers on signs and symptoms of certain diseases—hypertension, diabetes, and depression—without mentioning products by name. These ads are referred to as *institutional advertising* and have been applauded by both consumers and the FDA. Institutional advertising could be an efficient and profitable method of reaching the undiagnosed and nonuser groups.

Efforts to bring more of the nonusers—the undiagnosed, the dropouts, the uninsured—into the medical-care system will be frustrated if the burden on the system only makes the problems of compliance worse because of overworked staff spending too little time with patients. More widespread and more effective patient education and professional education related to the compliance problems, combined with organizational, economic, and environmental reforms of the system itself, will make the efforts to reach the nonusers worthwhile.

This has been the philosophy and developing strategy of a movement within the health services professions called Community-Oriented Primary Care (COPC), which has developed methods and procedures for practicing "denominator medicine" through community analysis of the population served by the health-care institution or practice. It seeks to apply the types of PRECEDE and PROCEED diagnoses of community perceptions and epidemiological distributions of health problems and risk factors described in this chapter. COPC has been adopted variously within the community health centers and migrant health centers funded by the Health Services and Resources Administration, the Indian Health Service, and various foundations.[66]

APPLICATION OF EDUCATIONAL DIAGNOSIS TO INDIVIDUAL PATIENTS

The PRECEDE–PROCEED concepts can be applied with some adaptation to the health-care or counseling setting, including patient education, nutrition counseling, smoking cessation, and other self-care or self-help programs.[67] It suggests a protocol for the stepped education and support of patients and the continuing education of health-care workers.

All too often physicians arrive at a correct medical diagnosis and nurses or dieticians devise appropriate management plans, only to be frustrated by unsatisfactory outcomes resulting from the patient's not understanding instructions or, in many instances, choosing to ignore them. What sustains an outpatient's adherence to a prescribed medical or dietary regimen between visits? The answer, apparently, is that not enough sustains their behavior. Patient-adherence failure, often called noncompliance, is reflected most clearly in relapse rates ranging from 20 to 80 percent, not only in nonadherence to medications but even more in ignoring advice on lifestyle modifications.[68] Reviews of patient education studies and epidemiological models suggest that more-effective interaction between health-care providers and patients could reduce drug errors by as much as 72 percent and improve clinical outcomes by as much as 47 percent over conventional treatment.[69] Improved interaction results not only in correcting many of the errors of patients but also those attributable to the health-care providers who become more conscious of the patient's specific needs.

THE RELAPSE CURVE

Figure 11.2 shows the typical relapse pattern in a variety of practices recommended to patients, especially those practices relating to addiction, compulsive behavior, pleasures, comforts, unpleasant side effects, inconveniences, costs, and even simple habits. Assuming that 100 percent of the patients who leave a medical-care encounter are committed to adopting the prescribed practice, there is a characteristic drop of 40–80 percent in actual maintenance behavior during the first 6 weeks.[70]

Though the shape of the curve is highly predictable, the drop in percentage before it levels off is not. More-effective intervention for selected self-care practices can alter the curve's slope and plateau levels.[71] For example, physicians can reduce a male patient's daily consumption of cigarettes by simply giving advice, as shown in a randomized clinical trial that also documented lower mortality in lung cancer compared with the control group.[72] Figure 11.3 shows how three smoking-cessation clinics achieved relapse curves of identical shape but different levels of plateau depending on their effectiveness in applying educational and behavioral principles.[73]

A long-term follow-up of Johns Hopkins ambulatory patients in a randomized controlled trial using the PRECEDE model to tailor health education for hypertension found lower relapse rates, greater sustained improvement in blood pressure control, and half as many deaths among those who had received some combination of three patient education methods than in those who received the usual medical care.[74] In another study using PRECEDE in a family planning clinic, women smoked less when they were exposed to a combination of a physician's advice and waiting room media than when they were exposed only to waiting room media.[75] Dozens of other studies have shown the effectiveness of well-designed patient-education and self-care education programs.

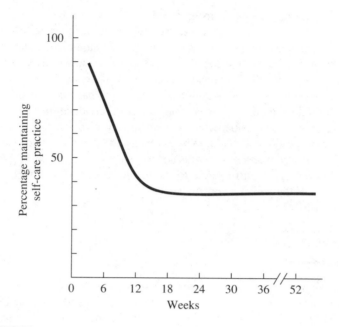

FIGURE 11.2

Relapse curve typical of self-care practices. [Adapted from L. W. Green, *West. J. Med.* 147 (1987): 346–9; printed by permission of the publisher.]

A more positive way of interpreting the relapse curve is to note that as much as 40–60 percent of the population *does* maintain its self-care practices. This fact indicates that any *global* intervention program designed to prevent relapse may be unnecessary and probably wasteful for a large portion of patients entering health-care programs. Furthermore, the interventions designed to prevent relapse range from simple, inexpensive methods effective for only a few patients to complex, obtrusive, and costly methods effective for most but needed by few.

A HIERARCHY OF FACTORS AFFECTING SELF-CARE BEHAVIOR

Considerable study has been devoted to identifying the characteristics of patients or participants in medical care and health programs who typically drop out or fail to sustain the recommended behavioral changes. Comparative and prospective studies have identified four sets of correlates that predict adherence or relapse: (1) demographic and socioeconomic characteristics; (2) motivational characteristics; (3) physical, manual, or economic facilitators and barriers; and (4) circumstantial rewards and penalties associated with the behavior, especially in the social environment.

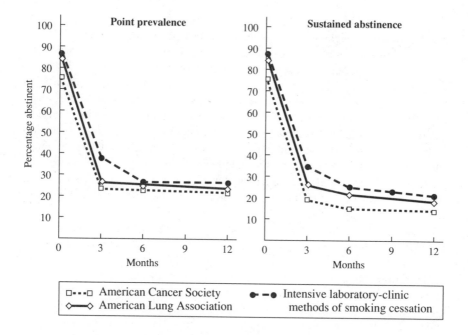

FIGURE 11.3

Three smoking-cessation clinics achieved identical patterns of quitting or relapse but slightly different levels of effectiveness depending on their populations and success in applying educational and behavioral principles. [From H. A. Lando, P. G. McGovern, F. X. Barrios, and B. D. Etringer, *American Journal of Public Health* 80 (1990): 554–9; printed by permission of the publisher.]

The first set, demographic and socioeconomic characteristics, cannot be easily changed, especially in the clinical setting; the other three sets of factors can. These modifiable factors are the predisposing, enabling, and reinforcing factors of the PRECEDE–PROCEED model. Predisposing factors need to change before enabling factors; that is, a patient will not devote effort to learning skills or pursuing resources if he or she has little motivation or commitment to the goal of the behavior. Enabling factors need to change before the reinforcing factors; that is, efforts to reward a behavior that has not yet been enabled would be wasted. This hierarchy of factors that influence adherence and relapse suggests a logical order of intervention that should maximize the support to a patient while conserving the energy and time of health-care staff. The logic would dictate the concentration of educational resources on patients according to which of the three changeable characteristics they possess.[76] It would further dictate that if a patient possesses more than one of the changeable characteristics predicting relapse, a combination of interventions designed to change the characteristics should be applied.[77]

The three sets of changeable characteristics predicting adherence or relapse reflect a natural hierarchy of action from wanting to do, being able to do, and being rewarded for doing. This hierarchy produces a logical flow of intervention from strengthening motivation, to enabling, and then to reinforcing the self-care behavior. A need to conserve resources, however, dictates skipping those interventions not required if a patient is already motivated, enabled, or reinforced. The skip pattern can be guided by a minimum of questions designed to detect the motivational state, the barriers, and the potential rewards and side effects for the patient. The skip pattern can also include assessments, decision nodes, and recursive loops in an algorithm for patient education, diagnosis, and intervention, as suggested in Figure 11.4.

The recommended procedure entails assessing a patient's educational needs by asking a sequence of "diagnostic" questions to assure relevance of the intervention to the patient's motivation, skill, and resources and to reinforce adherence to the prescribed medical regimen or lifestyle modifications. The sequence of questions and interventions minimizes the time required by staff and patients and maximizes the probability of medical benefit to the patient. The protocol can be applied by physicians, nurses, dieticians, pharmacists, counselors, and others who work with patients on a one-to-one relationship. It can also be adapted for use with self-help groups and counseling for behavior change in well individuals.

The principles of relevance (predisposing factors), facilitating (enabling factors), and feedback combined with social support (reinforcing factors) were tested prospectively in a patient education study.[78] The combined interventions yielded significant improvements in compliance and blood pressure control after 3 years[79] and a 50 percent reduction in mortality after 5 years.[80]

A more refined model of patient decisions in accepting influenza vaccination has been derived from patient questionnaires and tested prospectively with correct prediction of vaccination behavior for 82 percent of high-risk patients.[81] This hierarchical utility model questionnaire could provide the source of more specific answers to the initial questions in Figure 11.4.

PHASE 1: INITIAL TRIAGE OF PATIENTS ACCORDING TO MOTIVATION

The first question a physician or other clinical staff needs to answer is whether a patient cares enough about the problem to bother with the prescribed regimen. This can be answered on three levels, according to the health belief model.[82]

1. Does the patient believe there may be continuing problems if the recommended behavior is not adopted?
2. Does the patient believe the problems associated with failure to comply with the recommended behavior are severe?

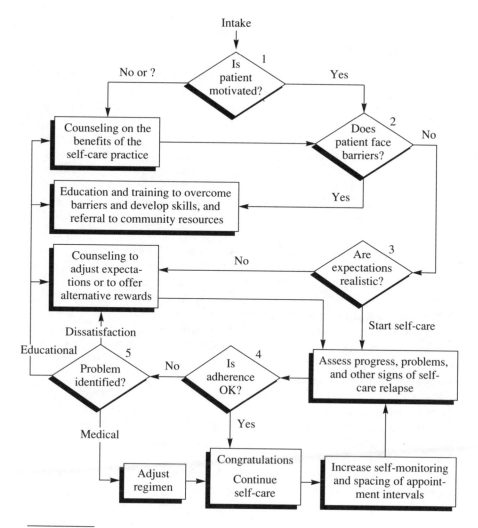

FIGURE 11.4

A triage algorithm for assessing predisposing, enabling, and reinforcing factors in
patient education for self-care. [Adapted from L. W. Green, *West J. Med.* 147 (1987):
346–9; printed by permission of publisher.]

3. Does the patient perceive the benefits of adopting the recommended behavior to be greater than the perceived risks, costs, side effects, barriers, and hassles?

If the answer to all three questions is yes, the patient is likely to be willing to try the recommended behavior. The clinical staff need not lecture this patient nor strive to convince the patient of the importance of following the prescribed regimen. The patient has sufficient motivation.

If a patient is already willing, considerable time and energy otherwise spent on persuasion can be conserved for training or support. If a patient is not motivated according to these three criteria, then it would be premature to train the patient in skills or to counsel the patient to overcome barriers in the home environment. The time and resources of the health-care worker should be spent first on educating the patient on the importance and benefits of the recommended practice. The purpose of this initial education is to strengthen the preceding three beliefs in the patient.

In this situation, written materials are no substitute for face-to-face, two-way communication. In our systematic assessment of 102 controlled studies of patient education related to prescription drugs, the factors that predicted the magnitude of change in patient knowledge and beliefs, as well as in drug errors and clinical effects, were not the media or channels of communication, but rather the individual attention, relevance, and feedback provided in the communication.[83]

If a patient's motivation cannot be assessed after a few direct questions, the best predictor of the need for patient education and counseling at this first level is the years of school completed by the patient. Less formal education means a greater need for patient education.[84] This might seem too obvious to warrant mention, but an irony of medical practice is that physicians tend to talk more to patients who ask more questions—typically those of higher educational achievement—than to those who ask fewer questions but probably need more answers.[85] Cultural and language barriers similarly impede effective interaction between health-care providers and patients. Regardless of the patient's level of education or the provider's level of cultural sensitivity, a health-care provider can easily probe for a patient's level of understanding by asking the patient to repeat the instructions he or she is to follow.

PHASE 2: STEPS IN TRIAGE ACCORDING TO ENABLING FACTORS

Once the interaction between staff and patient establishes that a patient is motivated, the next diagnostic step is to assure that the patient is able to carry out the prescribed behavior. Problems that need to be investigated are the skills, resources, and barriers in the home or work environment that the patient needs help to develop or overcome. If the patient is highly motivated and willing to try the regimen prescribed by the physician but faces inability, lack of needed resources, or barriers that cannot be overcome alone, the patient will be frustrated and ultimately discouraged. Skill deficiencies are most common in young children; arthritic patients who cannot open certain containers; illiterate, low-literate, or non-English-speaking patients who cannot read or understand directions; old patients whose poor eyesight or lack of mobility makes adherence to certain regimens impossible; and other disabled or poor patients who cannot obtain or afford the necessary resources to follow the recommended practices.

If any of these enabling factors is found to be deficient in the patients, those persons recommending the unattainable regimen have some obligation to help the patient find ways to overcome the deficiency. Some training of the patient in the necessary skills, or modification of the regimen to fit the patient's circumstances, is the minimal intervention expected of the physician. At the very least, the health-care worker owes it to the patient to provide systematic referral to other agencies or resources in the community to help deal with these enabling factors.

PHASE 3: ASSESSING REINFORCING FACTORS NECESSARY TO PATIENTS' COMPLIANCE

Even with the predisposing and enabling factors in place, there remains one more level of possible breakdown in a patient's compliance with a prescribed regimen. If the recommended behavior is met with side effects, inconvenience, derision by family or friends, criticism by employer or teacher or other sources of discouragement, the patient is likely to discontinue the practice prescribed or recommended. The opposite of these discouraging factors are reinforcing factors. The health-care staff can help build reinforcement of patient compliance in two ways.

First, the physician can provide reinforcement by ensuring that the patient's expectations are realistic, so that nothing that happens during the course of the treatment comes as a shock. Side effects should be anticipated. Counseling can help prevent the relapse that is typically associated with the first signs of side effects.[86] Difficulties in following a diet or in stopping smoking should be described in advance and the patient ecouraged to expect and cope with troubles rather than give up at the first discouraging experience or event. If a patient has unrealistic expectations about the smooth course of recovery, weight loss, abstention, or adoption of a new health practice, the physician needs to correct these misperceptions before they become an excuse for giving up.

The second way that health-care professionals can reinforce the adoption of a complex regimen requiring behavioral change at home or at work is to communicate directly or indirectly with family members or others in a patient's immediate circle of daily contacts. Family members can be invited to accompany the patient in discussing the prescribed regimen with the physician. Often family members are left sitting in the waiting room when they could be participating in the discussion of home strategies to support the patient in adapting the prescribed regimen to daily routines. If the important parties cannot be influenced in the physician's office, a written message to them from the physician, taken by the patient or mailed or phoned to them with the patient's permission, could carry as much weight. The power of involving family members in reinforcing support of patients has been well established.[87]

PHASE 4: SELF-MONITORING

Once the patient is motivated and the provider has addressed the enabling and reinforcing factors as well as the counseling, referrals, and support necessary to make the patient's self-care possible, return appointments can be spaced at increasing intervals. With each subsequent visit, some of the signs, symptoms, risk factors, or problems that the physician looks for can be made the responsibility of the patient to self-monitor. Transferring increasing responsibility for self-care to the patient should be accompanied by the patient's increasing self-monitoring skills.

Health-care providers miss a powerful educational tool when they hoard data and methods of observation that would make patients capable of obtaining their own feedback on progress and success in self-management. By transferring these skills and tools—such as self-monitoring blood pressure devices—to patients, providers enable the patients to obtain more immediate feedback on adjustments they are making in their lifestyle or in a dietary or medication regimen. Feedback from self-monitoring can, over time, become the most powerful source of reinforcement for positive behavior. If a patient continues to depend on the health-care professional for this reinforcement, the patient can fail to make the conversion to self-reliance that is so essential to long-term maintenance and control coincident with chronic or compulsive disorders.

CHANGING THE BEHAVIOR OF HEALTH-CARE STAFF

Why do physicians, nurses, and other health-care workers behave as they do with respect to prevention and health promotion? Although medical education and training have not emphasized either prevention or health promotion, physicians and allied health professionals are showing a growing interest in enhancing their prevention practices. Nursing education and the professional preparation of dieticians, pharmacists, and other health-care workers have given greater emphasis to patient counseling, but their working circumstances often conspire against enabling and reinforcing their preventive practices. Some principles of behavioral change that apply to the continuing education and support of health-care workers to become more effective in counseling their patients to change lifestyles and environments are presented in the concluding sections of this chapter.

BEHAVIORAL AND EDUCATIONAL DIAGNOSES OF PHYSICIAN BEHAVIOR

The following discussion could apply to any of the health-care professions, but let us take the physician as the example. Other health-care professionals may want to contemplate how the PRECEDE and PROCEED concepts might be applied to behavior changes of decision makers and policy changes in the health-care system. Until recently, most people assumed that physicians routinely carried out preventive measures and patient counseling as part of their practice. They probably did until specialization and technology, along with rapidly expanding medical information and new economic circumstances, began to crowd these elements out of medical care. Now, even primary care physicians have difficulty devoting much time, attention, or effort to the education of their patients about behavioral risk factors and ways to modify them.[88] Recent studies have found large discrepancies among physician initiatives, patient expectations, and published guidelines.[89]

In attempting to understand the practices of physicians, the three categories of behavioral influence (predisposing, enabling, and reinforcing factors) represent a convenient classification because they group the more specific influences, such as knowledge, attitudes and beliefs, skills, incentives, and rewards under broader rubrics according to the measures that might be used to change behavior.[90] This classification provides a useful conceptual framework, even though the three domains are not mutually independent for health professionals any more than they are for patients, students, consumers, or others.

PREDISPOSING FACTORS

The problem is partly attitudinal. Physicians and others trained in the medical tradition appear to doubt the importance of some behavioral risk factors.[91] In a survey of primary care physicians, less than half agreed that moderating or eliminating alcohol use, decreasing salt consumption, avoiding saturated fats, engaging in regular exercise, avoiding cholesterol, and minimizing sugar intake are very important for health promotion. Most of these physicians, however, agreed that reducing cigarette smoking is important. This suggests that physicians' attitudes are determined in part by the weight and general acceptance of scientific evidence.[92]

Some studies indicate large differences between medical specialties in their rates of patient counseling.[93] The preventive roles of physicians thus appear to be partly determined by their specialty; other researchers find little difference between general and family practitioners when the year of graduation from medical school is controlled for.[94]

Recent surveys indicate that health-care personnel are becoming more interested in the health behavior of their patients. This probably reflects societal trends and interests, to which health professionals generally subscribe and respond. A statewide survey of primary care physicians in Texas found that most of them considered health promotion a challenging and enjoyable part of their practice. They considered smoking the most important risk factor.[95] A survey on nutrition counseling in private practices in Minnesota reported that physicians believe it is important to educate their patients about health risks, but they devote little time to it because they do not think patients want or will follow their advice.[96] A survey of primary care physicians found that most believe they should modify patient behavior to minimize risk factors, but only a small percentage report success in helping patients achieve behavioral change.[97]

The predisposing attitudinal factors, then, seem to be shifting toward a greater appreciation of the importance of behavioral risk factors and the importance of intervening to modify those factors. The problem now appears to center on the physician's diffidence in carrying out the intervention.[98] This, in turn, appears to relate to a justifiable lack of self-confidence in knowing how to intervene effectively and a perception that the patients are not receptive to advice or willing to change. On the other side of the same coin, patients often perceive their physicians to be uninterested in their efforts to change, such as to quit smoking.[99]

Physicians who believe the patient does not want to quit or is unable to do so are less likely to provide advice.[100] Physicians consider this pessimism to be the greatest barrier to their preventive counseling.[101]

These cognitive, attitudinal, and perceptual problems can be classified as the predisposing factors influencing professional behavior. Depending on a health-care provider's degree of self-confidence and his or her perception of the patient's willingness and ability to change, the provider will be more or less predisposed to take action to support the patient in making behavioral changes. Predisposing factors include the professional's values, beliefs, attitudes, and perceptions. Values include more basic orientations, such as the role of the professional, the patient's autonomy, and the issues of privacy of patient behavior or lifestyle outside the immediate medical realm. These are very important but have not been well studied. They can potentially predispose health-care workers to pursue or avoid counseling and encouraging patients to pursue healthful lifestyles.

Beliefs include the more immediate and changeable viewpoints of the professional on matters such as patients' willingness to change their lifestyles or their ability to change their health practices. Related to the professional's beliefs about the patient's ability is the professional's belief in his or her own ability. This is referred to in social learning theory as a *self-efficacy* belief. Many physicians apparently feel unprepared to counsel patients about their lifestyles and consequently tend to avoid doing do.[102] In large measure this probably reflects the training experience of physicians. Studies suggest that recent graduates of family practice residencies have greater confidence in their counseling effectiveness.[103] The need for attention to these matters at the undergraduate and graduate levels of medical education should be apparent.[104]

ENABLING FACTORS

The foregoing predisposing factors account for the motivation and confidence of health-care professionals, but even with motivation, they sometimes fail to take the appropriate action because they lack the necessary skills or resources to do so. The combination of low self-efficacy and a lack of fiscal and other resources to offer smoking cessation services may account for most of the missed counseling opportunities reported by physicians and patients.[105] When preventive services are not reimbursed, a physician may be discouraged from learning new skills as well as from applying them. Predisposing factors must be quite strong to offset the disincentive of cost. In addition, though many practices might determine that preventive services could best be provided by someone other than the physician, there may not be another person available.

In a survey of 120 randomly selected primary care physicians in New York City, 87 percent agreed that physicians should practice more preventive medicine. However, the physicians cited lack of time, inadequate reimbursement, and unclear recommendations as the main obstacles to preventive care.[106] These obstacles represent a second class of factors influencing behavior—factors that enable the behavior.

The lack of staff and space and the paucity of tested educational materials are major barriers to preventive services.[107] A computerized health maintenance prompting system was gladly accepted by physicians in one study and seemed to improve their attitudes toward health promotion.[108] In another study, a twofold increase in preventive care measures was found among a group of physicians using computer-prompted reminders.[109]

Actual skills in the practice of patient counseling represent another set of enabling factors. Skills that are lacking, usually because of education, differ from a poor "perceived self-efficacy" in that they are real deficits, not just a lack of confidence. Perceptions of skill predispose; competence enables.

Enabling factors, then, can be as simple as available space, materials, or reminders. They often take a more substantial form in the minds of professionals themselves. Adequate reimbursement functions as an enabling factor by promising the resources that enable the health-care professional to invest time and effort in patient education and preventive medicine.

REINFORCING FACTORS

Reimbursement that has actually been received functions later as a reinforcing factor. It rewards behavior and therefore increases the probability that the behavior will recur at the next opportunity.

Reinforcing factors also include visible results, support from colleagues, and feedback from patients.[110] Colleague behavior is both reinforcing and predisposing.

Curative treatment yields visible, usually short-term results that are satisfying to the patient and therefore rewarding to the health-care professional. Preventive measures often yield no palpable results, at least in the short term, so there is no positive feedback and reinforcement. Treatment failures, or the absence of visible results, are more common in preventive care than in acute care. Because much illness is self-limited, the efficacy of treatment and the natural history of the illness combine to create the perception of efficacy. Preventive care has a longer time frame and its effect — a change in prospective health status — is delayed or may never be evident to the patient or the professional care provider.

PRINCIPLES OF HEALTH EDUCATION AND THE BEHAVIOR OF HEALTH-CARE PROFESSIONALS AND PATIENTS

If the determinants of the preventive and health promotion practices of health workers can be distilled from the wide range of studies into three broad categories, how can one proceed to use these categories to organize interventions to enhance preventive practices? A study of the cancer prevention practices of primary care physicians found variables that could be classified as predisposing, enabling, and reinforcing, but the specific mix of determinants varied with the cancer site.[111] This suggests that attempts to alter physician behavior should follow an assessment of the factors that require primary attention and modification.

PRINCIPLE OF EDUCATIONAL DIAGNOSIS

The first task in changing behavior is to determine its causes. We refer to this as the diagnostic principle of changing behavior. Just as the physician must diagnose an illness before it can be properly treated, a behavior must be diagnosed before it can be properly changed. *Properly* in this context means interventions that are essentially educational rather than coercive or manipulative. If the causes of a behavior can be understood, professionals can intervene with the most appropriate and efficient combination of education, training, resource development, and rewards to influence the factors that predispose, enable, or reinforce the behavior.

Until it is possible to diagnose each health professional, all we can know is that insufficient preventive care is being provided. If there are insufficient diagnostic data, some analogies from medical practice may apply: (1) Treating the symptom, (2) treating presumptively using broadly effective therapy, and (3) treating the specific etiological or underlying problem. In symptomatic treatment, we recognize the lack of preventive care and choose one level (e.g., predisposing, enabling, or reinforcing) at which to intervene.

Treating the problem with broad-based intervention, working at multiple levels simultaneously, is more likely to be effective. However, as with medication, there are potential adverse consequences. First, this approach is likely to cost more. Secondly, it may elicit an "allergic" reaction. If health professionals consider an educational intervention inappropriate or redundant, they may perceive it as criticism and become hypersensitive. Should this occur, they will be unlikely to cooperate with efforts to change their behavior. Educational interventions that consistently elicit this response could make the professional relatively resistant to further efforts. Because of these risks, broad-based efforts to change behavior should focus on predisposing factors; if enabling or reinforcing factors are addressed, the intervention should be individualized for each health-care worker.

Finally, an intervention linked to a diagnosed problem has the greatest chance of success. A program based on the PRECEDE model to help physicians in rural western Pennsylvania assess their own learning needs was developed at Johns Hopkins University. Experimental groups of primary care physicians participated in audiovisual self-study programs tailored to their own assessments of their educational needs. The course's impact was measured using questionnaires to gauge gains in knowledge and using simulated patient visits to observe performance with patients with chronic obstructive pulmonary disease. The experimental groups retained significantly greater amounts of information 9 months after the program and used more program material in counseling patients than did the control group.[112]

HIERARCHICAL PRINCIPLE

The second principle of behavioral change, which can be called the hierarchical principle, states that there is a natural precedence in the sequence of factors influencing behavior: You ensure that predisposing factors are in place before intervening in the enabling factors and that enabling factors have been addressed before intervening in the reinforcing factors. In reality, the opportunities for intervention are usually fleeting; so, in most circumstances, all three types of factors must be addressed simultaneously. In addition, a single intervention can address several factors at once. The hierarchical principle aligns the interventions (education, counseling, training, resources, feedback, rewards) so that they are expended or deployed in the most efficient and logical order.

It is inefficient and sometimes ineffective to train someone in skills to enable a behavior when that person lacks prior motivation. We have seen evidence that many physicians lack confidence in the efficacy or importance of some preventive maneuvers; of those who accept the value of the procedures, many doubt their own competence or the ability of the patient to make changes. Unless these beliefs are dealt with first, there is little point in training physicians in preventive or health promotion skills.

Similarly, reinforcement designed to reward a behavior for which a health-care professional was not predisposed is useless. There is little point in setting up a reward system for physicians who perform sigmoidoscopies if the physicians have not been educated to understand the need for them or trained to perform them.[113]

PRINCIPLE OF CUMULATIVE LEARNING

Related to the hierarchical principle is the principle of cumulative learning. To affect the behavior of professionals or patients, a set of learning experiences must be planned in a sequence that takes into account the prior learning experiences and concurrent incidental experiences to which the learners are exposed. Learning does not occur in a vacuum. Behavior responds to the cumulative learning experiences of the individual, including those that preceded and those that were incidental to the planned educational or behavioral change program. Physician behavior is a product not only of medical education but of all prior education, formal and informal; of concurrent life experiences; and of the society in which the physician was raised, educated, and trained, and in which he or she practices. In gathering data, physicians first learn a fairly rote and uniform approach. They need an equally circumscribed, basic approach to preventive medicine and patient education.

Clearly, the medical curriculum of the past has not given physicians a base of learning that would predispose or enable them to take maximum advantage of new educational opportunities in preventive medicine, much less practice it effec-tively.[114] Preventive medicine remains one of the "orphan" areas of medical education.[115] However, postgraduate training appears to be changing, and new medical graduates are demanding more behavioral medicine and patient education in their residencies.[116] Federal programs in the United States that support physi-cian training, advisory committees, certifying and accrediting organizations, and employers of physicians are all broadening their expectations of physician ca-pabilities and responsibilities in this regard.

PRINCIPLE OF PARTICIPATION

The prospects for success in any attempt to change professional behavior will be greater if the professionals have helped identify their own need for change and have selected the method that will enable them to make the change.[117] No principle of behavioral change has greater generalizability than the principle of participation.[118]

The principle of participation allows packaged behavioral change programs to adapt to the diversity of prior learning experiences and concurrent circumstances in a population of health-care professionals. Physicians who adapt education materials to their own needs, for example, are more committed to using the materials.[119]

PRINCIPLE OF SITUATIONAL SPECIFICITY

The principle of situational specificity holds that there is nothing inherently superior or inferior about any method of intervention to achieve behavioral change. It always depends on the circumstances, the target audience, the timing, and the enthusiasm and commitment of the instructor or other agent of change. New methods of education or intervention often appear to have an advantage over "traditional" methods in randomized trials, but this advantage typically fades when the method loses its novelty. This "novelty effect" makes some methods seem superior, but the long history of educational research is strewn with new educational technologies that prove in the long run to be no better than the older technologies except in their strategic application to the right audience, at the right time, with enthusiasm and commitment. Thus, efforts to change behavior must rely more on the diagnostic principle and the principle of participation.[120]

PRINCIPLE OF MULTIPLE METHODS

The principle of multiple methods also follows from the diagnostic principle, insofar as multiple causes are invariably found for any given behavior. For each of the multiple predisposing, enabling, and reinforcing factors identified, a different method or component of a comprehensive behavioral change program must be provided.

Primary care physicians attempting to promote health or offer preventive services often use methods that are ineffective. Only one fourth of those who give advice regularly offer a systematic behavioral or educational intervention.[121] Physicians tend to use the same multiplicity of approaches in preventive medicine as they use to obtain information for therapeutic decisions.[122]

PRINCIPLE OF INDIVIDUALIZATION

The tailoring or individualization of learning essentially applies the principles of cumulative learning, participation, and situational specificity. *Tailoring* refers to the adaptation of learning experiences to each individual. This becomes impossible for large-scale programs, which is one reason why reading continues to be rated by physicians as a preferred information source for preventive medicine decisions.[123] The physician can control the selection, pace, repetition, skipping pattern, and other aspects of the learning experience better with reading material than with any other learning method. But reading fails to provide the practice and feedback necessary for successful behavior change. This leads us to the final principle.

FEEDBACK PRINCIPLE

The principle of feedback is critical. It ensures that individuals whose behavior is expected to change obtain direct and immediate feedback on the progress and effects of their behavior. This ensures that learners are able to adapt to both the learning process and the behavioral responses within their own situation and pace. As with other principles, the feedback principle applies to both professionals and patients.

One of the reasons physicians rely on reading for their primary source of information on prevention is because there is little feedback from patients or colleagues on preventive practice. Peer comparison feedback on physician performance in colorectal screening was found to improve compliance with recommended standards of care and played an important role in quality assurance.[124]

One study demonstrated that physicians trained to give antismoking advice to their patients did so following their training but did so less frequently without feedback. A subsequent intervention in which the advice-giving rates of the physicians were monitored monthly and physicians were given immediate corrective feedback resulted in sustained antismoking advice-giving by the physicians.[125]

SUMMARY

Factors predisposing, enabling, and reinforcing patients and the health-care professionals who provide preventive care and education to their patients about lifestyle changes have been identified in various recent studies. The organization of these findings within a framework for planning educational and behavioral change interventions suggests a series of learning principles that can be applied with greater effect than the standard continuing education format. Essentially the same PRECEDE–PROCEED steps and principles that apply to patients and populations apply to health-care professionals.

The opportunities and needs for patient education and counseling exceed the current supply, not so much in quantity available as in quality, willingness, and distribution. Much of the available energy devoted to patient education and counseling fails to reach the patients who need it most, when they need it, and in ways that would be most helpful to them. This chapter describes compliance problems in terms of errors of omission and errors of commission. An epidemiological assessment of needs for intervention on the various categories of compliance errors would segment the potential patient population into five high-risk groups: (1) nonusers who are not under medical care but have a condition that would benefit from use of a prescription or other medical or lifestyle regimen; (2) nonuser patients whose medical-care provider has not recommended or prescribed a needed drug, device, or lifestyle regimen; (3) nonuser patients who did not purchase a recommended drug or device or adopt a recommended lifestyle modification; (4) misusers who are using someone else's drug or a medication or procedure previously recommended or prescribed for another problem; and (5) misusers who are not following the schedule or dosage recommended. The environments, channels, and methods for communicating effectively with each of these groups vary systematically in ways that recommend new strategies for the support of public health education, professional education, and patient education.

Pharmaceutical companies and third-party payers could play a more active role in direct mass communications to the public about the risk factors, signs, and symptoms of diseases and conditions for which medical or self-care measures are available. Encouraging and enabling patients who have such risk factors, signs, or symptoms to seek screening or medical advice would improve the public health more in the long run than increased efforts to eliminate noncompliance for those already under care. On the other hand, burdening the medical system with more patients when it is failing to deal effectively with patient compliance problems because staff have too little time to spend understanding and interacting with patients will only make the problems worse.

The efficiency of patient education for those under care could be improved by systematic analyses of compliance error rates in various subpopulations of patients. This would lead in most settings to a greater allocation of patient education and counseling effort directed at males, lower socioeconomic, and older patients relative to females, higher income, and younger patients. A similar epidemiological analysis of relative rates of compliance error for specific pathologies or symptomatologies could segment the patient population for effective educational triage within demographic groups.

Medical schools and other continuing education and quality assurance resources could be targeted more sharply to those physicians who are prescribing drugs incorrectly or who are unconvinced about the efficacy or benefit-risk ratio of underused drugs or procedures. Physicians, for example, do not have as much conviction and belief in their ability to modify dietary practices in their patients as they do to control blood pressure. Similarly, these educational resources could give greater emphasis to patient education and counseling skills required by physicians in educating and strengthening the motivation of their patients to fill prescriptions and to adhere to the prescribed regimens. Such an investment, according to the net results of 102 published evaluations of patient education related to errors with drug regimens, would reduce drug errors by 40 percent to 72 percent and would improve clinical outcomes such as blood pressure control and fewer emergency room visits by 23–47 percent.

Sufficient knowledge has now accumulated to enable health-care professionals to approach the problem of patient compliance with greater confidence, effectiveness, and efficiency. Greater confidence should come from the accumulated evidence from studies of teaching and counseling patients on self-medication and more complex lifestyle changes. Greater effectiveness should come from the increased awareness among health professionals that basic principles of learning have been instrumental in transferring knowledge, skills, and responsibility to patients. Greater efficiency should come from the stepped-care approach to patient education and counseling outlined above. By concentrating their time and effort at the level of help needed by each patient, health professionals can bypass needless motivational appeals and skill development for some patients and can target their counseling for other patients who most need these levels of help.

A final maneuver in consigning greater responsibility to patients for their own care and health maintenance is to transfer self-monitoring skills and tools to them. These become both the enabling and the reinforcing factors in patients' long-term maintenance of behaviors conducive to health. They enable people, in the final analysis, to take ownership and control of their own lives and the determinants of their own health and quality of life.

EXERCISES

1. For a given clinical setting, describe the distribution of health problems presented by patients and justify the selection of a particular problem as the first priority for health education planning.
2. For the priority health problem, show the procedures you would follow in conducting a behavioral diagnosis and write a behavioral objective for the highest priority behavior to be addressed in this population of patients.
3. For the chosen behavior, develop a inventory of predisposing, enabling, and reinforcing factors, set priorities on one or two of each, and write education objectives for these.

REFERENCES AND NOTES

1. For a history that traces the evolution of the concept of self-care from Nightingale's "helping the helpless" and her distinction between "sick nursing and health nursing," through Shaw and Harmer's textbooks of nursing at the turn of the century, to current nursing concepts of self-care,

see Nursing Development Conference Group, *Concept Formalization in Nursing: Process and Product* (Boston: Little, Brown, 1973); D. E. Orem, *Nursing: Concepts of Practice* (New York: McGraw-Hill, 1971). For a broader history of the concept of self-care in contrast to the medical model, and its relationship to parallel movements such as consumer participation, see L. W. Green, S. H. Werlin, H. H. Schauffler, and C. H. Avery, "Research and Demonstration Issues in Self-care: Measuring the Decline of Medicocentrism," *Health Education Monographs* 5 (1977): 161–89; L. S. Levin and E. L. Idler, "Self-care in Health," *Annual Review of Public Health* 4 (1983): 181–201; E. M. Russell and E. L. Iljonforeman, "Self-care in Illness — A Review," *Family Practice* 2 (1985): 108–21.

2. This section is based on an adaptation of L. W. Green, P. D. Mullen, and R. B. Friedman, "An Epidemiological Approach to Targeting Drug Information," *Patient Education and Counseling* 8 (1986): 255–68. The environmental focus of this chapter is on the environment of patients, including the home, the workplace, and the health-care setting itself. For consideration of the role of hospitals and health-care workers in community health, school health, or worksite health promotion, we refer the reader to the respective previous chapters. For current resources on hospital-based community health promotion planning, contact the American Hospital Association, 840 N. Lake Shore Drive, Chicago, IL 60611. For an application of PRECEDE, see E. Malo and L. C. Leviton, "Decision Points for Hospital-Based Health Promotion," *Hospital and Health Services Administration* 32 (1987): 49–61.

3. We use the term *compliance* and *patient* for convenience and convention, even though several of the types of error we discuss are not patient errors of failing to follow physicians' directions, but rather are errors of physicians, nurses, or pharmacists themselves, or of patients who have not yet received appropriate directions from a physician or other health-care provider. We introduce the term *health-care error* to encompass the wider range of behavioral and environmental sources of medical or health-care problems that PRECEDE–PROCEED attempts to address.

4. S. Cohen, ed., *New Directions in Patient Compliance* (Lexington, MA: Lexington Books, D.C. Heath, 1979); M. D. Goldbloom and R. B. Lawrence, eds., *Preventing Disease: Beyond the Rhetoric* (New York: Springer-Verlag, 1990); L. W. Green, "The Revival of Community and the Obligation of Academic Health Centers to the Public," in *Institutional Values and Human Environments for Teaching, Inquiry and Practice*, R. J. Bulger, S. J. Reiser, and R. E. Bulger, eds. (Des Moines: University of Iowa Press, 1990); R. B. Haynes, D. W. Taylor, and D. M. Sackett, eds., *Compliance in Health Care* (Baltimore: Johns Hopkins University Press, 1979); S. Maes, C. D. Spielberger, P. B. Defares, and I. G. Sarason, eds., *Topics in Health Psychology* (New York: Wiley, 1988); D. Schmidt and I. E. Leppik, eds., *Compliance in Epilepsy* (Amsterdam: Elsevier Science Publishers B.V., 1988); S. A. Shumaker, S. Parker, and J. Wolle, eds., *The Handbook of Health Behavior Change* (New York: Springer, 1990); S. Weiss, A. Herd, and B. Fox, eds., *Perspectives on Behavioral Medicine* (New York: Academic Press, 1981).

5. R. Goldbloom and R. N. Battista, "The Periodic Health Examination: 1. Introduction," *Canadian Medical Association Journal* 134 (1986): 721–3; M. D. Goldbloom and R. B. Lawrence, op. cit., 1990; U.S. Preventive Services Task Force, *Guide to Clinical Preventive Services: An Assessment of the Effectiveness of 169 Interventions* (Baltimore: William & Wilkens, 1989).

6. R. Anderson, *A Behavioral Model of Families' Use of Health Services* (Chicago: University of Chicago Center for Health Administration Studies Research Series, no. 25, University of Chicago Press, 1968); L. W. Green, *Community Health*, 6th ed. (St. Louis: Mosby, 1990); L. W. Green and B. J. Roberts, "The Research Literature on Why Women Delay in Seeking Medical Care for Breast Symptoms," *Health Education Monographs* 2 (1974): 129–77; J. G. Zapka, A. M. Stoddard, M. E. Costanza, and H. L. Greene, "Breast Cancer Screening by Mammography: Utilization and Associated Factors," *American Journal of Public Health* 79 (1989): 1499–1502.

7. U.S. Preventive Services Task Force, *Guide to Clinical Preventive Services: An Assessment of the Effectiveness of 169 Interventions* (Baltimore: Williams & Wilkins, 1989).

8. *Health, United States, and Prevention Profile, 1989* (Hyattsville, MD: National Center for Health Statistics, DHHS Pub. No. (PHS) 90–1232, 1990).

9. C. Lenfant and E. J. Roccella, "Trends in Hypertension Control in the United States," *Chest* 86 (1984): 459–62. A specific application of the PRECEDE model for increased use of health services for high blood pressure control was D. M. Levine, D. E. Morisky, L. R. Bone, et al., "Data-based Planning for Educational Interventions Through Hypertension Control Programs for Urban and Rural Populations in Maryland," *Public Health Reports* 97 (1982): 107–12.

10. W. M. Garraway and J. P. Whisnant, "The Changing Pattern of Hypertension and the Declining Incidence of Stroke," *Journal of the American Medical Association* 258 (1987): 214–7.

11. R. Cuca and C. S. Pierce, *Experiments in Family Planning: Lessons from the Developing World* (Baltimore, MD: Johns Hopkins University Press, for the World Bank, 1977); D. A. Dawson, "The Effects of Sex Education on Adolescent Behavior," *Family Planning Perspectives* 18 (1986): 162–70; J. Udry, L. Clark, C. Chase, et al., "Can Mass Media Advertising Increase Contraceptive Use?" *Family Planning Perspectives* 4 (1972): 37–44; M. Zelnik and Y. J. Kim, "Sex Education and Its Association with Teenage Sexual Activity," *Family Planning Perspectives* 14 (1982): 117–26.

12. M. Butler and W. Paisley, "Communicating Cancer Control to the Public," *Health Education Monographs* 5 (1977): 5–24; J. Cullen, B. Fox, and R. Isom, eds., *Cancer: The Behavioral Dimensions* (New York: Raven Press, 1976); L. W. Green, B. Rimer, and T. W. Elwood, "Public Education," in *Cancer Epidemiology and Prevention*, D. Shottenfeld and J. Fraumeni, Jr., eds. (Philadelphia, PA: W. B. Saunders, 1982), pp. 1100–10. This last review uses the PRECEDE model to assess strengths and gaps in the cancer prevention and screening efforts of the 1970s. Subsequent studies of cancer education and screening efforts that applied the PRECEDE model include L. J. Brailey, "Effects of Health Teaching in the Workplace on Women's Knowledge, Beliefs, and Practices Regarding Breast Self-examination," *Research in Nursing and Health* 9 (1986): 223–31; M. K. Keintz, B. K. Rimer, L. Fleisher, and P. Engstrom, "Educating Older Adults About Their Increased Cancer Risk," *Gerontologist* 28 (1988): 487–90; B. K. Rimer, S. W. Davis, P. F. Engstrom, et al., "Some Reasons for Compliance and Noncompliance in a Health Maintenance Organization Breast Cancer Screening Program," *Journal of Compliance in Health Care* 3 (1988): 103–14; B. K. Rimer, W. Jones, C. Wilson, et al., "Planning a Cancer Control Program for Older Citizens," *Gerontologist* 23 (1983): 384–9; J. Shamian and L. Edgar, "Nurses as Agents for Change in Teaching Breast Self-examination," *Public Health Nursing* 4 (1987): 29–34; J. K. Worden, L. J. Solomon, B. S. Flynn, et al., "A Community-wide Program in Breast Self-examination Training and Maintenance," *Preventive Medicine* 19 (1990): 254–69; J. G. Zapka and J. A. Mamon, "Integration of Theory, Practitioner Standards, Literature Findings, and Baseline Data: A Case Study in Planning Breast Self-examination Education," *Health Education Quarterly* 9 (1982): 332–56.

13. J. C. Hersey, L. S. Klibanoff, D. J. Lam, and R. L. Taylor, "Promoting Social Support: The Impact of California's 'Friends Can Be Good Medicine' Campaign," *Health Education Quarterly* 11 (1984): 293–311.

14. M. B. Bakdash, "The Use of Mass Media in Community Periodontal Education," *Journal of Public Health Dentistry* 43 (1983): 128–31; M. B. Bakdash, A. L. Lange, and D. G. McMillan, "The Effect of a Televised Periodontal Campaign on Public Periodontal Awareness," *Journal of Periodontology* 54 (1983): 666–70; D. P. Kraft, "The Prevention and Treatment of Alcohol Problems on a College Campus," *Journal of Alcohol and Drug Education* 34 (1988): 37–51; R. Lau, R. Kane, S. Berry, et al., "Channeling Health: A Review of the Evaluation of Televised Health Campaigns," *Health Education Quarterly* 7 (1980): 56–89; S. Redman, E. A. Spencer, and R. W. Sanson-Fisher, "The Role of Mass Media in Changing Health-Related Behaviour: A Critical Appraisal of Two Models," *Health Promotion International* 5 (1990): 85–101.

15. S. R. Garfield, "The Delivery of Medical Care," *Scientific American* 222 (1970): 15–18.

16. J. G. Zapka, A. Stoddard, R. Barth, et al., "Breast Cancer Screening Utilization by Latina Community Health Center Clients," *Health Education Research* 4 (1989): 461–8.

17. P. S. German, S. Shapiro, E. A. Skinner, et al., "Detection and Management of Mental-

health Problems of Older Patients by Primary Care Providers," *Journal of the American Medical Association* 257 (1987): 489–93.

18. E. M. Bertera and R. L. Bertera, "The Cost-Effectiveness of Telephone vs. Clinic Counseling for Hypertensive Patients: A Pilot Study," *American Journal of Public Health* 71 (1981): 626–9; R. Brimberry, "Vaccination of High-Risk Patients for Influenza: A Comparison of Telephone and Mail Reminder Methods," *Journal of Family Practice* 26 (1988): 397–400; J. A. Earp, M. G. Ory, and D. S. Strogatz, "The Effects of Family Involvement and Practitioner Home Visits on the Control of Hypertension," *American Journal of Public Health* 72 (1982): 1146–54; R. Fink and S. Shapiro, "Significance of Increased Efforts to Gain Participation in Screening for Breast Cancer," *American Journal of Preventive Medicine* 6 (1990): 34–41; M. Hindi-Alexander and G. J. Cropp, "Community and Family Programs for Children with Asthma," *Annals of Allergy* 46 (1981): 143–8.

19. L. P. Fried and T. L. Bush, "Morbidity as the Focus of Prevention in the Elderly," *Epidemiological Review* 103 (1988): 48–64; R. S. Thompson, S. Taplin, A. P. Carter, et al., "A Risk Based Breast Cancer Screening Program," *HMO Practice* 2 (1988): 177–91.

20. C. E. Lewis, "Disease Prevention and Health Promotion Practices of Primary Care Physicians in the United States," *American Journal of Preventive Medicine* 4(4) (suppl., 1988): 9–16; I. J. Silvers, M. F. Hovell, M. H. Weisman, and M. R. Mueller, "Assessing Physician-Patient Perceptions in Rheumatoid Arthritis – A Vital Component in Patient Education," *Arthritis and Rheumatism* 28 (1985): 300–7.

21. S. A. Eraker and P. Politser, "How Decisions Are Reached – Physican and Patient," *Annals of Internal Medicine* 97 (1982): 262–8; D. O. Fedder, "Managing Medication and Compliance: Physician-Pharmacist-Patient Interactions," *Journal American Geriatric Society* 11 (suppl., 1982): 113–7; R. J. Pels, D. H. Bor, and R. S. Lawrence, "Decision Making for Introducing Clinical Preventive Services," *Annual Review of Public Health* 10 (1989): 363–83.

22. *Patient Information and Prescription Drugs: Parallel Surveys of Physicians and Pharmacists* (New York: Louis Harris and Associates, 1983).

23. J. G. Bruhn, "The Application of Theory in Childhood Asthma Self-help Programs," *Journal of Allergy and Clinical Immunology* 5 (pt 2, 1983): 561–77; A. C. King, J. E. Martin, E. M. Morrell, et al., "Highlighting Specific Patient Education Needs in an Aging Cardiac Population," *Health Education Quarterly* 13 (1986): 29–38; T. Korhonen, J. K. Huttunen, A. Aro, et al., "A Controlled Trial on the Effects of Patient Education in Treatment of Insulin-Dependent Diabetes," *Diabetes Care* 6 (1983): 256–61; G. B. Landman, M. D. Levine, L. Rappaport, "A Study of Treatment Resistance Among Children Referred for Encopresis," *Clinical Pediatrics* 8 (1984): 449–52; L. L. Pederson and J. C. Baskerville, "Multivariate Prediction of Smoking Cessation Following Physician Advice To Quit Smoking: A Validation Study," *Preventive Medicine* 12 (1983): 430–6.

24. P. S. German, L. E. Klein, S. J. McPhee, and C. R. Smith, "Knowledge of and Compliance with Drug Regimens in the Elderly," *Journal of the American Geriatric Society* 30 (1982): 568–71; L. E. Klein, P. S. German, and D. M. Levine, "Adverse Drug Reactions Among the Elderly: A Reassessment," *Journal of the American Geriatric Society* 29 (1981): 525–30; P. L. DeTullio, S. A. Eraker, and C. Jepson, et al., "Patient Medication Instruction and Provider Interactions: Effects on Knowledge and Attitudes," *Health Education Quarterly* 13 (1986): 51–60.

25. M. P. Eriksen, L. W. Green, and F. G. Fultz, "Principles of Changing Health Behavior," *Cancer* 62 (1988): 1768–75; R. D. France, J. L. Houpt, C. S. Orleans, and P. J. Trent, "Teaching Psychotherapy Interventions to Family Practice Residents: A Controlled Study," *American Journal of Psychiatry* 136 (1979): 1596–7; J. Lomas and R. B. Haynes, "A Taxonomy and Critical Review of Tested Strategies for the Application of Clinical Practice Recommendations: From 'Official' to 'Individual' Clinical Policy," *American Journal of Preventive Medicine* 4(4) (suppl., 1988): 77–94.

26. *Prescription Drug Information for Patients and Direct-to-Consumer Advertising* (Boston: Medicine in the Public Interest, Inc., 1984).

27. D. L. Roter, J. A. Hall, and N. R. Katz, "Patient-Physician Communication: A Descriptive Summary of the Literature," *Patient Education & Counseling* 12 (1988): 99–119; D. M. Vickery and J. F. Fries, "Effect of Self-care Book," *Journal of the American Medical Association* 245 (1981): 341–2; D. M. Vickery, H. Kalmer, D. Lowry, et al., "Effect of a Self-care Education Program on Medical Visits," *Journal of the American Medical Association* 250 (1983): 2952–6.

28. F. M. Gregor, "Factors Affecting the Use of Self-instructional Material by Patients with Ischemic Heart Disease," *Patient Education and Counseling* 6 (1984): 155–9; K. V. Mann and P. L. Sullivan, "Effect of Task-Centered Instructional Programs on Hypertensives' Ability to Achieve and Maintain Reduced Dietary Sodium Intake," *Patient Education and Counseling* 10 (1987): 53–72; D. A. Tuckett, M. Boulton, and M. Olson, "A New Approach to the Measurement of Patients' Understanding of What They Are Told in Medical Consultations," *Journal of Health and Social Behavior* 26 (1985): 27–38.

29. L. W. Green and R. Faden, "Potential Effects of Patient Package Inserts on Patients and Drug Consumers," *Drug Information Journal* 2 (suppl., 1977): 64–70.

30. S. Fisher, B. Mansbridge, and D. A. Lankford, "Public Judgments of Information in a Diazepam Patient Package Insert," *Archives of General Psychiatry* 39 (1982): 707–11.

31. A. Esdale and H. L. Harris, "Evaluation of a Closed-Circuit Television Patient Education Program: Structure, Process and Outcome," *Patient Education and Counseling* 7 (1985): 193–215; L. A. Maiman, L. W. Green, G. Gibson, and E. J. MacKenzie, "Education for Self-treatment by Adult Asthmatics," *Journal of the American Medical Association* 241 (1979): 1919–22.

32. L. Lawrence and T. McLemore, "National Ambulatory Medical Care Survey," *Vital and Health Statistics Series* 88 (Washington, DC: National Center for Health Statistics, 1983).

33. L. W. Green, P. D. Mullen, and R. B. Friedman, "An Epidemiological Approach to Targeting Drug Information," *Patient Education and Counseling* 8 (1986): 255–68.

34. I. T. Hill, *Reaching Women Who Need Prenatal Care* (Washington, DC: National Governors Association, 1988).

35. Committee to Study Outreach for Prenatal Care, Institute of Medicine, *Prenatal Care: Reaching Infants* (Washington, DC: National Academy Press, 1988).

36. L. W. Green, P. Hogan, and M. Deutsch, *Estimating Need: Manual for Estimating Prevalence of Women at Risk of Poor Pregnancy Outcomes Due to Smoking,* (Houston: Center for Health Promotion Research and Development, University of Texas Health Science Center, 1987).

37. CBS Television Network, *A Study of Attitudes, Concerns and Information Needs for Prescription Drugs and Related Illnesses* (New York: CBS Television Network, 1984).

38. National Research Council, *Improving Risk Communication* (Washington, DC: National Academy Press, 1989).

39. D. L. Sackett and J. C. Snow, "The Magnitude of Compliance and Noncompliance," in *Compliance in Health Care*, R. B. Haynes, D. W. Taylor, and D. L. Sackett, eds. (Baltimore, MD: The Johns Hopkins University Press, 1979).

40. T. J. Glynn, ed., *Women and Drugs: Research Issues* 31 (Washington, DC: Govt. Printing Office, DHHS Pub. No. 271-80-3720, 1983).

41. G. J. Povar, M. Mantell, and L. A. Morris, "Patients' Therapeutic Preferences in an Ambulatory Care Setting," *American Journal of Public Health* 74 (1984): 1395–7.

42. C. Baum, D. L. Kennedy, M. B. Forbes, and J. K. Jones, *Drug Utilization in the U.S.* (Rockville, MD: Food and Drug Administration, 1983). By convention, the National Disease and Therapeutic Index employs the term *mentions* (including refills and renewal of prescriptions) to reflect drug usage. The term should not be interpreted as equivalent to number of patients or prescriptions.

43. T. Stephens and C. A. Schoenborn, "Adult Health Practices in the United States and Canada," in National Center for Health Statistics, *Vital and Health Statistics* series 5, no. 3 (Washington, DC: Govt. Printing Office, DHHS-PHS 88-1479, 1988).

44. S. Woolhandler and D. U. Himmelstein, "Reverse Targeting of Preventive Care Due to Lack of Health Insurance," *Journal of the American Medical Association* 259 (1988): 2872–4.

45. J. A. Hall, D. L. Roter, and N. R. Katz, "Meta-analysis of Correlates of Provider Behavior in Medical Encounters," *Medical Care* 26 (1988): 657–75.

46. H. Waitzkin, "Information Giving in Medical Care," *Journal of Health & Social Behavior* 26 (1985): 81–101.

47. R. Kayne, ed., *Drugs and the Elderly* (Los Angeles: Univ. Southern California Press, 1984).

48. P. German, L. Klein, S. McPhee, and C. Smith, "Knowledge of and Compliance with Drug Regimens in the Elderly," *Journal of the American Geriatric Society* 9 (1982): 568–71.

49. National Center for Health Statistics, A. J. Moss and V. L. Parsons, "Current Estimates from the National Health Interview Survey, United States, 1985," *Vital and Health Statistics,* series 10, no. 160 (Washington, DC: Govt. Printing Office, DHHS-PHS 86-1588, 1986).

50. P. Lamy and R. S. Beardsley, "The Older Adult and the Pharmacist Educator," *American Pharmacist* 22(5) (1982): 40.

51. J. Williamson and J. M. Chapin, "Adverse Reactions to Prescribed Drugs in the Elderly: A Multicare Investigation," *Age and Aging* 9 (1980): 73–80.

52. L. W. Green, P. D. Mullen, and G. L. Stainbrook, "Programs To Reduce Drug Errors in the Elderly: Direct and Indirect Evidence from Patient Education," *Journal of Geriatric Drug Therapy* 1 (1986): 3–16.

53. National Center for Health Statistics, T. McLemore and J. DeLozier, "1985 Summary: National Ambulatory Medical Care Survey," *Advance Data from Vital and Health Statistics*, no. 128 (Washington, DC: DHHS-PHS 87-1250, Govt. Printing Office, 1987).

54. R. B. Haynes, D. A. Davis, A. McKibbon, and A. P. Tugwell, "A Critical Appraisal of the Efficacy of Continuing Medical Education," *Journal of the American Medical Association* 251 (1984): 61–4.

55. J. Avorn and S. B. Soumerai, "Improving Drug-Therapy Decisions Through Educational Outreach: A Randomized Controlled Trial of Academically Based Detailing," *New England Journal of Medicine* 308 (1983): 1457–63.

56. D. A. Davis, R. B. Haynes, L. W. Chambers, et al., "The Impact of CME: A Methodologic Review of the Continuing Medical Education Literature," *Evaluation and the Health Professions* 7 (1984): 251–83.

57. C. Baum, D. L. Kennedy, M. B. Forbes, and J. K. Jones, *Drug Utilization in the U.S. – 1981: Third Annual Report* (Rockville, MD: Food and Drug Administration, 1982).

58. W. W. Rosser, "Benzodiapazine Use in a Family Medicine Center," *Drug Protocol* 2(10) (1987): 9–15.

59. *Morbidity and Mortality Weekly Report* 38 (1989): 137.

60. L. W. Green and D. Fedder, "Drug Information: The Pharmacist and the Community," *American Journal of Pharmaceutical Education* 41 (1977): 444–8.

61. L. W. Green, "Some Challenges to Health Services Research on Children and Elderly," *Health Service Research* 19 (1985): 793–815.

62. T. S. Inui, W. B. Carter, R. E. Pecoraro, et al., "Variations in Patient Compliance with Common Long-term Drugs," *Medical Care* 17 (1980): 986–93.

63. P. D. Mullen and L. W. Green, "Educating Patients about Drugs," *Promoting Health* 6(6) (1985): 6–8.

64. P. D. Mullen, L. W. Green, and G. S. Persinger, "Clinical Trials of Patient Education for Chronic Conditions: A Comparative Meta-analysis of Intervention Types," *Preventive Medicine* 14 (1985): 753–81.

65. L. W. Green, "How Physicians Can Improve Patients' Participation and Maintenance in Self-care," *Western Journal of Medicine* 147 (1987): 346–9.

66. D. R. Garr, "Community-Oriented Primary Care," *Journal of Family Practice* 28 (1989): 654; F. Mullan, "Community-Oriented Primary Care: An Agenda for the '80s," *New England Journal of Medicine* 307 (1982): 1076–8; P. A. Nutting, ed., *Community-Oriented Primary Care: From Principle to Practice.* (Washington, DC: U.S. Department of Health and Human Services, Health Resources and Services Administration, HRS-A-PE 86-1, 1987); P. A. Nutting, "Community-Oriented Primary Care: A Critical Area of Research for Primary Care," *Primary Care Research: An Agenda for the 90s* (Washington, DC: U.S. Department of Health and Human Services, Agency for Health Care Policy and Research, 1990).

67. L. W. Green, "How Physicians Can Improve Patients' Participation and Maintenance of Patients in Self-Care," *Western Journal of Medicine* 147 (1987): 346–9.

68. R. B. Haynes, D. W. Taylor, and D. L. Sackett, eds., *Compliance in Health Care* (Baltimore, Johns Hopkins University Press, 1979).

69. P. D. Mullen and L. W. Green, "Educating Parents about Drugs," *Promoting Health* 6(6): 6–8.

70. G. A. Marlatt and J. R. Gordon, eds., *Relapse Prevention: Maintenance Strategies in the Treatment of Addictive Behaviors* (New York, Guilford Press, 1985).

71. S. A. Brunton, "Physicians as Patient Teachers," in Personal Health Maintenance (Special Issue), *Western Journal of Medicine*, 131 (Dec, 1984): 855–60.

72. G. Rose, P. J. Hamilton, L. Colwell, et al., "A Randomized Controlled Trial of Anti-smoking Advice: 10-Year Results," *Journal of Epidemiology and Community Health* 36 (1982): 102–8.

73. H. A. Lando, P. G. McGovern, F. X. Barrios, and B. D. Etringer, "Comparative Evaluation of American Cancer Society and American Lung Association Smoking Clinics," *American Journal of Public Health* 80 (1990): 554–9.

74. D. E. Morisky, D. M. Levine, L. W. Green, et al., "Five-Year Blood Pressure Control and Mortality Following Health Education for Hypertensive Patients," *American Journal of Public Health* 73 (1983): 153–62.

75. V. C. Li, T. J. Coates, L. A. Spielberg, et al., "Smoking Cessation with Young Women in Public Family Planning Clinics: The Impact of Physician Messages and Waiting Room Media," *Preventive Medicine* 13 (1984): 477–89.

76. J. C. Cantor, D. E. Morisky, L. W. Green, et al., "Cost-Effectiveness of Educational Intervention to Improve Patient Outcomes in Blood Pressure Control," *Preventive Medicine* 14 (1984): 782–800.

77. E. E. Bartlett, "Eight Principles from Patient Education Research," *Preventive Medicine* (14) 1985: 667–9.

78. L. W. Green, D. M. Levine, and S. G. Deeds, "Clinical Trials of Health Education for Hypertensive Outpatients: Design and Baseline Data," *Preventive Medicine* 4 (1975): 417–25.

79. D. M. Levine, L. W. Green, S. G. Deeds, et al., "Health Education for Hypertensive Outpatients," *Journal of the American Medical Association* 241 (1979): 1700–3.

80. D. E. Morisky, D. M. Levine, L. W. Green, et al., "Five-Year Blood Pressure Control and Mortality Following Health Education for Hypertensive Patients," *American Journal of Public Health* 73 (1983): 153–62.

81. W. B. Carter, L. R. Beach, T. S. Inui, et al., "Developing and Testing a Decision Model for Predicting Influenza Vaccination Compliance," *Health Service Research* 20 (1986): 897–932.

82. N. K. Janz and M. H. Becker, "The Health Belief Model: A Decade Later," *Health Education Quarterly* 11 (1984): 1–47. See Chapter 5 for detailed discussion of the Health Belief Model.

83. P. D. Mullen, L. W. Green, and G. Persinger, "Clinical Trials of Patient Education for Chronic Conditions: A Comparative Meta-analysis of Intervention Types," *Preventive Medicine* (14) 1985: 753–81.

84. M. E. Hatcher, L. W. Green, D. M. Levine, et al., "Validation of a Decision Model for Triaging Hypertensive Patients to Alternate Health Education Interventions," *Social Science & Medicine* 22 (1986): 813–19.

85. D. L. Roter, "Patient Participation in the Patient-Provider Interaction: The Effects of Patient Question Asking on the Quality of Interaction, Satisfaction and Compliance," *Health Education Monographs* 5 (1977): 281–315.

86. C. Jacobs, R. Ross, I. M. Walker, et al., "Behavior of Cancer Patients: A Randomized Study of the Effects of Education and Peer Support Groups," *American Journal of Clinical Oncology* 6 (1983): 347–50.

87. D. E. Morisky, N. M. Demuth, M. Field-Fass, et al., "Evaluation of Family Health Education to Build Social Support for Long-term Control of High Blood Pressure," *Health Education Quarterly* 12 (1985): 35–50; and J. L. Earp, M. G. Ory, and D. S. Strogatz, "The Effects of Family Involvement and Practitioner Home Visits on the Control of Hypertension," *American Journal of Public Health* 72 (1982): 1146–54.

88. H. Wechsler, S. Levine, R. K. Idelson, M. Rothman, and J. O. Taylor, "The Physician's Role in Health Promotion: Survey of Primary Care Practitioners," *New England Journal of Medicine* 308 (1983): 97–100; A. McAlister, P. D. Mullen, S. A. Nixon, et al., "Health Promotion Among Primary Care Physicians in Texas," *Texas Medicine* 81 (1985): 55–8; P. A. Nutting, "Health Promotion in Primary Medical Care: Problems and Potential," *Preventive Medicine* 15 (1986): 537–48; N. H. Gottlieb, P. D. Mullen, and A. L. McAlister, "Patients' Substance Abuse and the Primary Care Physician: Patterns of Practice," *Addictive Behavior* (1987): 1223–32.

89. R. F. Anda, P. L. Remington, D. G. Sienko, and R. M. Davis, "Are Physicians Advising Smokers To Quit: The Patient's Perspective," *Journal of the American Medical Association* 257 (1987): 1916–19; S. J. McPhee, R. J. Richard, and S. N. Solkowitz, "Performance of Cancer Screening in a University General Internal Medicine Practice," *Journal of General Internal Medicine* 1 (1986): 275–81; R. J. Romm, S. W. Fletcher, and B. S. Hulka, "The Periodic Health Examination: Comparison of Recommendations and Internists' Performance," *Southern Medical Journal* 74 (1981): 265–71; K. B. Welles, C. E. Lewis, B. Leake, M. K. Schleiter, and R. H. Brook, "The Practices of General and Subspecialty Internists in Counseling About Smoking and Exercise," *American Journal of Public Health* 76 (1986): 1009–13; B. Woo, B. Woo, F. Cook, M. Weisberg, and L. Goldman, "Screening Procedures in the Asymptomatic Adult: Comparison of Physicians' Recommendations, Patients' Desires, Published Guidelines, and Actual Practice," *Journal of the American Medical Association* 254 (1985): 1480–4.

90. L. W. Green, "How the Physician Can Improve Participation and Maintenance in Self-care," *Western Journal of Medicine* 147 (1987): 346–9.

91. R. N. Battista, "Adult Cancer Prevention in Primary Care: Patterns of Practice in Quebec," *American Journal of Public Health* 73 (1983): 1036–9; J. Sobal, C. M. Valente, H. L. Muncie, Jr., D. M. Levine, and B. R. Deforge, "Physicians' Beliefs about the Importance of 25 Health Promoting Behaviors," *American Journal of Public Health* 75 (1986): 1427–8.

92. H. Wechsler, et al., op. cit., 1983.

93. S. E. Radecki and R. C. Mandenhall, "Patient Counseling by Primary Care Physicians: Results of a Nationwide Survey," *Patient Education and Counseling* 8 (1986): 165–77.

94. L. Attarian, M. Fleming, P. Barron, and V. Strecher, "A Comparison of Health Promotion Practices of General Practitioners and Residency-Trained Family Physicians," *Journal of Community Health* 8 (1987): 31–9.

95. A. McAlister, et al., op. cit., 1985.

96. T. Kottke, J. Foels, C. Hill, T. Choi, and D. Fendersonet, "Nutrition Counseling in Private Practice: Attitudes and Activities of Family Physicians," *Preventive Medicine* 13 (1984): 219–25.

97. C. M. Valente, J. Sobal, H. L. Muncie, Jr., D. M. Levine, and A. M. Antilitz, "Health Promotion: Physicians' Beliefs, Attitudes, and Practices," *American Journal of Preventive Medicine* 2 (1986): 82–8.

98. K. M. Cummings, G. Giovino, S. L. Emont, R. Sciandra, and M. Koenigsberg, "Factors Influencing Success in Counseling Patients to Stop Smoking," *Patient Education and Counseling* 8 (1986): 189–200; C. T. Orleans, L. K. George, J. L. Houpt, and K. H. Brodie, "Health Promotion in Primary Care: A Survey of U.S. Family Practitioners," *Preventive Medicine* 14 (1985): 636–47; K. B. Wells, J. E. Ware, and C. E. Lewis, "Physicians' Attitudes in Counseling Patients about Smoking," *Medical Care* 22 (1984): 360–5.

99. R. F. Anda, et al., op. cit., 1987.

100. K. M. Cummings, G. Giovino, R. Sciandra, M. Koenigsberg, and S. L. Emont, "Physician Advice To Quit Smoking: Who Gets It and Who Doesn't," *American Journal of Preventitive Medicine* 3 (1987): 69–75.

101. B. Maheux, R. Pineault, and F. Beland, "Factors Influencing Physicians' Orientation Toward Prevention," *American Journal of Preventive Medicine* 3 (1987): 12–18.

102. H. Wechsler, et al., op. cit., 1983; C. T. Orleans, et al., 1985.

103. B. Goldstein, P. M. Fischer, J. W. Richards, A. Goldstein, and J. C. Shank, "Smoking Counseling Practices of Recently Trained Family Physicians," *Journal of Family Practice* 24 (1987): 195–7.

104. General Professional Education of Physicians Panel, *Physicians for the Twenty-first Century: the GPEP Report* (Washington, DC: Association of American Medical Colleges, 1984).

105. R. F. Anda, et al., op. cit., 1987.

106. D. H. Gemson and J. Elinson, "Prevention in Primary Care: Variability in Physician Practice Patterns in New York City," *American Journal of Preventive Medicine* 2 (1986): 226–34.

107. W. B. Carter, D. W. Belcher, and T. S. Inui, "Implementing Preventive Care in Clinical Practice. II. Problems for Manager, Clinicians and Patients," *Medical Care Review* 38 (1981): 19–24.

108. B. P. Knight, M. S. O'Malley, and S. W. Fletcher, "Physician Acceptance of a Computerized Health Maintenance Prompting Program," *American Journal of Preventive Medicine* 3 (1987): 19–24.

109. C. J. McDonald, S. L. Hui, D. M. Smith, et al., "Reminders to Physicians from an Introspective Computer Medical Record: A Two-Year Randomized Trial," *Annals of Internal Medicine* 100 (1984): 130–8.

110. M. A. Orlandi, "Promoting Health and Preventing Disease in Health Care Settings: An Analysis of Barriers," *Preventive Medicine* 16 (1987): 119–30; R. N. Winickoff, K. L. Coltin,

M. M. Morgan, R. C. Busbaum, and G. O. Barnett, "Improving Physician Performance through Peer Comparison," *Medical Care* 22 (1984): 527–34.

111. R. N. Battista, J. L. Williams, and L. A. MacFarlane, "Determinants of Primary Medical Practice in Adult Cancer Prevention," *Medical Care* 24 (1986): 216–24.

112. P. B. Terry, V. L. Wang, B. S. Flynn, et al., "A Continuing Medical Education Program in Chronic Obstructive Pulmonary Diseases: Design and Outcome," *American Review of Respiratory Distress* 123 (1981): 41–6; V. L. Wang, P. Terry, B. S. Flynn, J. Williamson, L. W. Green, and R. Faden, "Multiple Indicators of Continuing Medical Education Priorities for Chronic Lung Diseases in Appalachia," *Journal of Medical Education* 54 (1979): 803–11.

113. D. R. Perera, J. P. LoGerfo, E. Shulenberger, J. T. Ylvisaker, and H. L. Kirz, "Teaching Sigmoidoscopy to Primary Care Physicians: A Controlled Study of Continuing Medical Education." *Journal of Family Practice* 16 (1983): 785–99.

114. A. Pokorny, P. Putnam, and J. E. Fryer, "Drug Abuse and Alcoholism Teaching in U.S. Medical and Osteopathic Schools, 1975–77," in M. Galantes, ed. *Alcohol and Drug Abuse in Medical Education* (Washington, DC: U.S. Government Printing Office, DHEW Pub. no. (ADM) 79–81, 1980).

115. A. R. Somers, "Four 'Orphan' Areas in Current Medical Education: What Hope for Adoption?" *Family Medicine* 19 (1987): 137–40.

116. D. M. Cassatta and B. L. Kirkman-Liff, "Mental Health Activities of Family Physicians," *Journal of Family Practice* 12 (1981): 683–92; S. G. Kosch and J. J. Dallman, "Essential Areas for Behavioral Science Training: A Needs Assessment Approach," *Journal of Medical Education* 58 (1983): 619–26.

117. J. Westberg, "Gaining Physician Support for Effective Patient Education," *Patient Education and Counseling* 8 (1986): 407–14.

118. L. W. Green, "The Theory of Participation: A Qualitative Analysis of Its Expression in National and International Policies," *Adv. Health Education and Promotion* 1(A) (1986): 407–14.

119. P. B. Terry, et al., op. cit., 1981.

120. P. Mullen and L. W. Green, "Meta-analysis Points Way Toward More Effective Medication Teaching," *Promotion of Health* 6 (Nov–Dec., 1985): 6–8.

121. C. T. Orleans, et al., op. cit., 1985.

122. M. Weinberger, S. A. Mazzuca, S. J. Cohen, and C. J. McDonald, "Physicians' Ratings of Information Sources About their Preventive Medicine Decisions," *Preventive Medicine* 11 (1982): 717–23.

123. Ibid.

124. R. N. Winickoff, et al., op. cit., 1984.

125. C. K. Ewart, V. C. Li, and T. J. Coates, "Increasing Physicians' Antismoking Influence by Applying an Inexpensive Feedback Technique," *Journal of Medical Education* 58 (1983): 468–73.

Glossary

action Conduct of individuals, families, groups, community decision makers and administrators, government or industrial policy makers, health professionals and others who might influence the health of themselves or others.

administrative diagnosis An analysis of the policies, resources and circumstances prevailing in an organizational situation to facilitate or hinder the development of the health promotion program.

advocacy Working for political, regulatory, or organizational change on behalf of a particular interest group or population.

age-adjusted rate The total rate for a population, adjusted to ignore the age distribution of the specific population by multiplying each of its age-specific rates by the proportion of a standard population (usually national) in that age group, and then adding up the products.

agent An epidemiological term referring to the organism or object that transmits a disease from the environment to the host.

age-specific rate The incidence (number of events during a specified period) for an age group, divided by the total number of people in that age group.

allocation A distribution of resources to specific categories of expenditure or to specific organizations or subpopulations.

assessment Estimation of the relative magnitude, importance, or value of objects observed.

attitude A relatively constant feeling, predisposition, or set of beliefs directed toward an object, person, or situation.

authorization A step in the legislative process in which the maximum amount of money to be allocated and the assignment of authority to spend it are decided.

behavior An action that has a specific frequency, duration, and purpose, whether conscious or unconscious.

behavioral diagnosis Delineation of the specific health-related actions that most likely effect, or could effect, a health outcome.

behavioral intention   A mental state in which the individual expects to take a specified action at some time in the future.

behavioral objective   A statement of desired outcome that indicates who is to demonstrate how much of what action by when.

belief   A statement or proposition, declared or implied, that is emotionally and/or intellectually accepted as true by a person or group.

benefits   Valued health outcomes or improvements in quality of life or social conditions having some known relationship to health promotion or health-care interventions.

central location intercept   A survey procedure that seeks interviews with an unsystematic sample of people on the street or in a shopping center to represent the opinions of those likely to be the target of a program.

coalition   A group of organizations or representatives of groups within a community joined to pursue a common objective.

coercive strategies   Preventive methods that bypass the motivation and decisions of people by dictating or precluding choices.

community   A collective of people identified by common values and mutual concern for the development and well-being of their group or geographical area.

community organization   The set of procedures and processes by which a population and its institutions mobilize and coordinate resources to solve a mutual problem or to pursue mutual goals.

compliance   Adherence to a prescribed therapeutic or preventive regimen.

conditions of living   The combination of behavioral and environmental circumstances that make up one's lifestyle and health-related social situation.

construct   The representation of concepts within a causal explanation or theoretical framework. For example, predisposing, enabling, and reinforcing factors are constructs for the representation of more specific concepts or variables such as health beliefs, attitudes, skills, and rewards.

cost-benefit   A measure of the cost of an intervention relative to the benefits it yields, usually expressed as a ratio of dollars saved or gained for every dollar spent on the program.

cost-effectiveness   A measure of the cost of an intervention relative to its impact, usually expressed in dollars per unit of effect.

delphi technique   A method of sampling the opinions or preferences of a small number of experts, opinion leaders, or informants, whereby successive questionnaires are sent by mail and the results (rankings or value estimates) are summarized for further refinement on subsequent mailings.

diagnosis   Health or behavioral information that designates the "problem" or need; its status, distribution, or frequency in the person or population; and the probable causes or risk factors associated with the problem or need.

disability   The inability to perform specific functions resulting from disease, injury or birth defects.

dose-response relationship   A term borrowed from clinical trials of drugs; when applied to health promotion, it refers to the increases in outcome measures associated with proportionate increases in the program resources expended or intervention effort.

early adopters   Those in the population who accept a new idea or practice soon after the innovators (but before the middle majority) who tend to be opinion leaders for the middle majority.

economy of scale The point in the growth of a program or service at which each additional element of service costs less to produce.

education of the electorate A process of political change in which those affected by policies are educated so that they will be more likely to vote for candidates or referenda that are in their best interests.

educational diagnosis The delineation of factors that predispose, enable, and reinforce a specific behavior.

educational tool Any material or method designed to aid learning and teaching through sight and sound.

effectiveness The extent to which the intended effect or benefits that could be achieved under optimal conditions are achieved in practice.

efficacy The extent to which an intervention can be shown to be beneficial under optimal conditions.

efficiency The proportion of total costs (e.g., money, resources, time) that can be related to the number of people served or benefits achieved in practice.

empowerment education A process of encouraging a community to take control of its own education, assess its own needs, set its own priorities, develop its own self-help programs, and, if necessary, challenge the power structure to provide resources.

enabling factor Any characteristic of the environment that facilitates action and any skill or resource required to attain a specific behavior. (Absence of the resource blocks the behavior; barriers to the behavior are included in lists of enabling factors to be developed. Skills are sometimes listed separately as predisposing factors or intermediate outcomes of education.)

environment The totality of social, biological, and physical circumstances surrounding a defined quality of life, health, or behavioral goal or problem.

environmental diagnosis A systematic assessment of factors in the social and physical environment that interact with behavior to produce health effects or quality-of-life outcomes. Also referred to as ecological assessment.

environmental factor One of the specific elements or components of the social, biological, or physical environment determined during the environmental diagnosis to be causally linked to health or quality of life goals or problems identified in the social or epidemiological diagnosis.

epidemiology The study of the distribution and causes of health problems in populations.

epidemiological diagnosis The delineation of the extent, distribution, and causes of a health problem in a defined population.

etiology The origins or causes of a disease or condition under study; the first steps in the natural history of a disease.

evaluation The comparison of an object of interest against a standard of acceptability.

excise tax A tax on the manufacture, sale, or use of certain products such as alcohol or tobacco to generate revenue for a government or to control consumption, or both.

expansionist An approach to diagnosis that seeks explanation or causes beyond the immediate determinants at hand; the opposite of reductionist.

external validity Assurance that the results of an evaluation can be generalized to other populations or settings.

fear A mental state that motivates problem-solving behavior if an action (fight or flight) is immediately available; if not, it motivates other defense mechanisms such as denial or suppression.

focus group method   Used in testing the perception and receptivity of a target population to an idea or method by recording the reactions of a sample of eight to ten people discussing it with each other.

formative evaluation   Any combination of measurements obtained and judgments made before or during the implementation of materials, methods, activities, or programs to control, assure, or improve the quality of performance or delivery. (Measurements *during* implementation are sometimes called process evaluation.)

Gannt chart   A timetable showing each activity in a program plan as a horizontal line that extends from the start to the finish date so that at any given time a program manager can see what activities should be underway, about to begin, or due to be completed.

habituation   The incorporation of a pattern of behavior into one's lifestyle to the degree that it is performed virtually without thought, but does not necessarily entail physical or psychological dependence.

Health Belief Model   A paradigm used to predict and explain health behavior, based on value-expectancy theory.

health-directed behavior   The conscious pursuit of actions for the protection or improvement of health.

health education   Any planned combination of learning experiences designed to predispose, enable, and reinforce voluntary behavior conducive to health in individuals, groups, or communities.

health enhancement   A dimension of health promotion pertaining to its goal of reaching higher levels of wellness beyond the mere absence of disease or infirmity.

health field concept   The notion that the factors influencing health can be subsumed under four categories: environment, human biology, behavior, and health-care organization.

health outcome   Any medically or epidemiologically defined characteristic of a patient or health problem in a population that results from health promotion or care provided or required as measured at one point in time.

health promotion   Any planned combination of educational, political, regulatory, and organizational supports for actions and conditions of living conducive to the health of individuals, groups, or communities.

health protection   A strategy parallel to health promotion in some national policies; the focus is on environmental rather than behavioral determinants of health, and the methods are more like those of engineers and regulatory agencies than those of educational and social or health service agencies.

health-related behavior   Those actions undertaken for reasons other than the protection or improvement of health, but which have health effects.

host   A concept from epidemiology referring to an individual who harbors or is at risk of harboring a disease or condition.

impact evaluation   The assessment of program effects on intermediate objectives including changes in predisposing, enabling, and reinforcing factors, and behavioral and environmental changes.

implementation   The act of converting program objectives into actions through policy changes, regulation, and organization.

internal validity   Assurance that the results of an evaluation can be attributed to the object (method or program) evaluated.

incidence   A measure of the frequency of occurrence of a disease or health problem in a population based on the number of new cases over a given period of time (usually one year). An incidence *rate* is obtained by dividing this number by the midyear population and multiplying the quotient by 1,000 or 100,000.

informed consent   A medical-legal doctrine that holds providers responsible for ensuring that consumers or patients understand the risks and benefits of a procedure or medicine before it is administered.

innovators   Those in a population who are first to adopt a new idea or practice, usually based on information from sources outside the community.

intervention   The part of a strategy, incorporating method and technique, that actually reaches a person or population.

late majority   The segment of the population most difficult to reach through mass communication channels or to convince of the need to adopt a new idea or practice, either because they cannot afford it or cannot get to the source or because of cultural and language differences or other difficulty.

leveraging   The use of initial investments in a program to draw larger investments.

lifestyle   The culturally, socially, economically, and environmentally conditioned complex of actions characteristic of an individual, group, or community as a pattern of habituated behavior over time that is health related but not necessarily health directed.

market testing   The placement of a message or product in a commercial context to determine how it influences consumer behavior.

morbidity   The existence or rate of disease or infirmity.

mortality   The event or rate of death.

middle majority   The segment of the population who adopt a new idea or practice after the innovators and early adopters but before the late adopters, usually influenced by a combination of mass media, interpersonal communication, and endorsements by famous personalities or organizations of which they are members.

need   (1) Whatever is required for health or comfort, or (2) an estimation of the interventions required based on a diagnosis of the problem and, in populations, the number of people eligible to benefit from the intervention(s).

nominal group process   An interactive group method for assessing community needs by having opinions listed without critique from the group and then rated by secret ballot, thereby minimizing the influence of interpersonal dynamics and status on the ratings.

normative effect   The influence of perceived social patterns of and expectations for behavior on the actions taken by individuals and groups.

objective   A defined result of specific activity to be achieved in a finite period of time by a specified person or number of people. Objectives state *who* will experience *what* change or benefit by *how much* and by *when*.

organization   The act of marshalling and coordinating the resources necessary to implement a program.

outcome evaluation   Assessment of the effects of a program on the ultimate objectives, including changes in health and social benefits or quality of life.

planning   The process of defining needs, establishing priorities, diagnosing causes of problems, assessing resources and barriers, and allocating resources to achieve objectives.

policy   The set of objectives and rules guiding the activities of an organization or an administration, and providing authority for allocation of resources.

PRECEDE   Acronym for the diagnostic planning and evaluation model outlined in this book, emphasizing *p*redisposing, *r*einforcing, and *e*nabling *c*onstructs in *e*ducational (and *e*nvironmental) *d*iagnosis and *e*valuation.

predisposing factor   Any characteristic of a person or population that motivates behavior prior to the occurrence of the behavior.

prevalence   A measure of the extent of a disease or health problem in a population based on the number of cases (old and new) existing in the population at a given time. See also *incidence*.

priority   Alternatives ranked according to feasibility or value (importance) or both.

PROCEED   Acronym for *p*olicy, *r*egulatory, and *o*rganizational *c*onstructs in *e*ducational and *e*nvironmental *d*evelopment, the phases of resource mobilization, implementation, and evaluation following the diagnostic planning phases of PRECEDE.

process evaluation   The assessment of policies, materials, personnel, performance, quality of practice or services, and other inputs and implementation experiences.

program   A set of planned activities over time designed to achieve specified objectives.

quality assessment   Measurement of professional or technical practice or service for comparison with accepted standards to determine the degree of excellence.

quality assurance   Formal process of implementing quality assessment and quality improvement in programs to assure stakeholders that professional activities have been performed appropriately.

quality of life   The perception of individuals or groups that their needs are being satisfied and that they are not being denied opportunities to achieve happiness and fulfillment.

reach   The number of people attending or exposed to an intervention or program.

reductionist   The approach to diagnosis that seeks to explain the cause of a problem or event within the person having the problem or within the immediate environment of the event.

relative risk   The ratio of mortality or incidence of a disease or condition in those exposed to a given risk factor (e.g., smokers) to the mortality or incidence in those not exposed (e.g., nonsmokers). A relative risk (RR) ratio of 1.0 indicates no greater risk in those exposed than in those not exposed.

regulation   The act of enforcing policies, rules, or laws.

reinforcing factor   Any reward or punishment following or anticipated as a consequence of a behavior, serving to strengthen the motivation for the behavior after it occurs.

risk factors   Characteristics of individuals (genetic, behavioral, environmental exposures, and sociocultural living conditions) that increase the probability that they will experience a disease or specific cause of death as measured by population relative risk ratios.

risk ratio   The mortality or incidence of a disease or condition in those exposed to a given risk factor divided by the mortality or incidence in those not exposed. See also *relative risk*.

self-efficacy   A construct from social learning theory referring to the belief an individual holds that he or she is capable of performing a specific behavior.

sensitivity   The ability of a test to identify all people who have a particular characteristic or condition, that is, the ability to avoid missing cases in a population screening. See also *specificity*.

social diagnosis   The assessment in both objective and subjective terms of high-priority problems, defined for a population by economic and social indicators and by individuals in terms of their quality of life.

social indicator   A quality having a numerical value whose change is expected to reflect a change in the quality of life for a population.

socialization   A process of developing behavioral patterns or lifestyle through modeling or imitating socially important persons including parents, peers, and media personalities.

social problem   A situation that a significant number of people believe to be a source of difficulty or unhappiness. A social problem consists of objective circumstances as well as a social interpretation of its unacceptability.

social reconnaissance   Diagnostic procedures applied to a large geographic area with the active participation of people having various levels of authority and resources, including government officials and professionals in health and other sectors, and potential recipients of new programs or services.

specificity   The ability of a test to rule out cases not possessing a particular characteristic or condition—that is, to avoid false-positive results in a population screening. See also *sensitivity*.

specific rates   Morbidity, mortality, fertility, or other rates calculated for specific age, gender, race, or other demographic groupings.

stakeholders   People who have an investment or a stake in the outcome of a program and therefore have reasons to be interested in the evaluation of the program.

stepped approach   A method of intervention following triage, in which minimal resources or effort are expended on the first group or level, more intensive effort on the second level, and most intensive on the third.

strategy   A plan of action that anticipates barriers and resources in relation to achieving a specific objective.

surveys   Methods of polling a group or population to estimate the norms and distribution of characteristics from a sample, using direct observations, questionnaires or interviews.

tactic   A method or approach employed as a part of a strategy.

triage   A method of sorting people into (usually three) groups for purposes of setting priorities on allocation of resources.

value   A preference shared and transmitted within a community.

wellness   A dimension of health beyond the absence of disease or infirmity, including social, emotional, and spiritual aspects of health.

Bibliography

Aaro, L. E., D. Wold, L. Kannas, and M. Rimpela (1986). "Health Behavior in School Children: A WHO Cross-National Survey," *Health Promotion* 1: 17–33.

Abelin, T. (1988). "Getting Health Promotion Off the Ground in Switzerland," *Journal of Public Health Policy* 9: 284–85.

Abelin, T., Z. J. Brzezinski, and V. D. Carstairs, eds. (1987). *Measurement in Health Promotion and Protection* (Copenhagen: World Health Organization Regional Publications, European Series No. 22).

Abelson, R. P., E. Aronson, W. J. McGuire et al. (1968). *Theories of Cognitive Consistency: A Sourcebook* (Chicago: Rand McNally College).

Abramson, J. H., R. Gofin, J. Habib et al. (1982). "Indicators of Social Class: A Comparative Appraisal of Measures for Use in Epidemiological Studies," *Social Science and Medicine* 16: 1739–46.

Ackerman, A. and H. Kalmer (1977). "Health Education and a Baccalaureate Nursing Curriculum— Myth or Reality" (paper presented at the 105th annual meeting of the American Public Health Association, Washington, DC, 1 Nov).

Adamson, T. E. and D. S. Gullion (1986). "Assessment of Diabetes Continuing Medical Education," *Diabetes Care* 9: 11–16.

Aday, L. A., R. Andersen, and G. V. Fleming (1980). *Health Care in the U.S.: Equitable for Whom?* (Beverly Hills: Sage).

Aday, L. A. and R. Eichhorn (1973). *The Utilization of Health Services: Indices and Correlates* (Washington, DC: National Center for Health Services Research, DHEW Pub. No. HSM 73-3003).

Aday, L. A., C. Sellers, and R. Andersen (1981). "Potentials of Local Health Surveys: A State-of-the-Art Summary," *American Journal of Public Health* 71: 835–40.

Adler, M. J. (1983). *The Paideia Problems and Possibilities* (New York: McMillan).

Aho, W. (1979). "Smoking, Dieting, and Exercise: Age Differences in Attitudes and Behavior Relevant to Selected Health Belief Model Variables. The Perceived Seriousness Is an Important Factor Influencing Behavior," *Rhode Island Medical Journal* 62: 85–92.

Ajzen, I. and M. Fishbein (1980). *Understanding Attitudes and Predicting Social Behavior* (Englewood Cliffs, NJ: Prentice-Hall).

437

Ajzen, I. and J. T. Madden (1986). "Prediction of Goal-Directed Behavior: Attitudes, Intentions, and Perceived Behavioral Control," *Journal of Experimental Social Psychology* 22: 453–74.

Alcalay, R., F. Sabogal, G. Marin et al. (1987–88). "Patterns of Mass Media Use Among Hispanic Smokers: Implications for Community Interventions," *International Quarterly of Community Health Education* 8: 341–50.

Alderman, M., L. W. Green, and B. S. Flynn (1980). "Hypertension Control Programs in Occupational Settings," *Public Health Reports* 90(1980); also in *Managing Health Promotion in the Workplace: Guidelines for Implementation and Evaluation*, R. S. Parkinson and Associates, eds. (Palo Alto, CA: Mayfield), pp. 162–72.

Algona, M. (1980). "Perception of Severity of Disease and Health Locus of Control in Compliant and Noncompliant Diabetic Patients," *Diabetes Care* 3: 533–34.

Alinsky, S. D. (1972). *Rules for Radicals: A Pragmatic Primer for Realistic Radicals* (New York: Vintage Books).

Alkin, M. C., R. Daillak, and P. White (1979). *Using Evaluations: Does Evaluation Make a Difference?* (Beverly Hills: Sage Library of Social Research, vol. 76).

Allanson, J. F. (1978). "School Nursing Services: Some Current Justifications and Cost-Benefit Implications," *Journal of School Health* 48: 603–07.

Allegrante, J. P. (1984). "Potential Uses and Misuses of Education in Health Promotion and Disease Prevention," *Teachers College Record* 86: 359–73; also in *Eta Sigma Gamman* 18(1986): 2–8.

Allegrante, J. P. and L. W. Green (1981). "When Health Policy Becomes Victim Blaming," *New England Journal of Medicine* 305: 1528–29.

Allegrante, J. P. and R. P. Sloan (1986). "Ethical Dilemmas in Workplace Health Promotion," *Preventive Medicine* 15: 313–20.

Allen, J. and R. F. Allen (1986). "Achieving Health Promotion Objectives Through Cultural Change Systems," *American Journal of Health Promotion* 1: 42–49.

Allen, J. and R. F. Allen (1990). "A Sense of Community, a Shared Vision and a Positive Culture: Core Enabling Factors in Successful Culture-Based Change," in *Community Organization: Traditional Principles and Modern Applications*, R. D. Patton and W. B. Cissel, eds. (Johnson City, TN: Latchpins Press), pp. 5–18.

Allensworth, D. (1987). "Building Community Support for Quality School Health Programs," *Health Education* 18(Oct/Nov): 32–38.

Allensworth, D. and L. J. Kolbe, eds. (1987). "The Comprehensive School Health Program: Exploring an Expanded Concept," *Journal of School Health* 57(10): 409–73, whole issue.

Allensworth, D. and C. A. Wolford (1988). *Achieving the 1990 Objectives for the Nation's Schools* (Kent, OH: American School Health Association).

Allison, G. (1971). *Essence of Decision* (Boston: Little, Brown).

Altman, D. G. and L. W. Green (1988). "Area Review: Education and Training in Behavioral Medicine," *Annals of Behavioral Medicine* 10: 4–7.

American College Health Association (1986). *AIDS on the College Campus* (Rockville, MD: American College Health Association).

American College of Physicians (1989). "Health Care Needs of the Adolescent," *Annals of Internal Medicine* 110: 930–35.

American College of Preventive Medicine and Fogarty Center (1976). *Preventive Medicine USA* (New York: Prodist).

American Council of Life Insurance (1985). *Wellness at the School Worksite: A Manual* (Washington, DC: Health Insurance Association of America).

American Medical Association Auxiliary, Inc. (1987). *Community Action: How to Work in Coalitions* (Chicago: American Medical Association Auxiliary).

American Physical Education Association (1935). "Health Education Section, Committee Report, American Physical Education Association," *Journal of Health and Physical Education* 6: 204–09.

Amler, R. W. and H. B. Dull (1987). *Closing the Gap: The Burden of Unnecessary Illness* (New York: Oxford University Press).

Anda, R. F., P. L. Remington, D. G. Sienko, and R. M. Davis (1987). "Are Physicians Advising Smokers to Quit?: The Patient's Perspective," *Journal of the American Medical Association* 257: 1916–19.

Andersen, R. (1968). *A Behavioral Model of Families' Use of Health Services* (Chicago: University of Chicago, Center for Health Administration Studies, Research Series No. 25, University of Chicago Press).

Andersen, R., M. Chen, L. A. Aday, and L. Cornelius (1987). "Health Status and Medical Care Utilization," *Health Affairs* 6: 136–56.

Andersen, R. and R. Mullner (1990). "Assessing the Health Objectives of the Nation," *Health Affairs* 9: 152–62.

Andersson, R. (1985). "Health Education at Local Level," in *Vigor* (Intl. Ed.), N. Ostby, ed. (Stockholm: Division for Health Education, National Board of Health and Welfare).

Andrews, F. M. and S. B. Withey (1976). *Social Indicators of Well-Being: Americans' Perceptions of Life Quality* (New York: Plenum).

Aneshensel, C. R., R. Frerichs, V. A. Clark et al. (1982). "Telephone Versus In-Person Surveys of Community Health Status," *American Journal of Public Health* 72: 1017–21.

Argyris, C. (1964). *Integrating the Individual and the Organization* (New York: Wiley).

Arkin, E. B. (1989). *Making Health Communication Programs Work: A Planner's Guide* (Bethesda, MD: Office of Cancer Communications, National Cancer Institute, NIH-89-1493).

Arkin, E. B. (1990). "Opportunities for Improving the Nation's Health Through Collaboration with the Mass Media," *Public Health Reports* 105: 219–23.

Arnstein, S. R. (1969). "A Ladder of Citizen Participation," *Journal of the American Institute of Planners* 35: 216–24.

Arsham, G. M. (1980). "Behavioral Diagnosis for Patient Education," in *Patient Education in the Primary Care Setting: 1979 Proceedings*, P. LaVigne, ed. (Minneapolis: University of Minnesota).

Attarian, L., M. Fleming, P. Barron, and V. Strecher (1987). "A Comparison of Health Promotion Practices of General Practitioners and Residency-Trained Family Physicians," *Journal of Community Health* 8: 31–39.

Atwater, J. B. (1974). "Adapting the Venereal Disease Clinic to Today's Problem," *American Journal of Public Health* 64: 433–37.

Australia, Department of Transport and Communication (1987). *Road Crash Statistics Australia* (Canberra: Department of Transport and Communication).

Australian Bureau of Statistics (1986). *Deaths Australia* (Canberra: Australian Bureau of Statistics Cat. No. 3302.0).

Avorn, J. and S. B. Soumerai (1983). "Improving Drug-Therapy Decisions Through Educational Outreach: A Randomized Controlled Trial of Academically Based Detailing," *New England Journal of Medicine* 308: 1457–63.

Awani, A. O. (1983). *Project Management Techniques* (New York: Petrocelli Books).

Bailey, J. (1973). "An Evaluative Look at a Family Planning Radio Campaign in Latin America," *Studies in Family Planning* 4: 275–78.

Bailey, J. and M. C. Zambrano (1974). "Contraceptive Pamphlets in Colombian Drugstores," *Studies in Family Planning* 5: 178–82.

Bailey, S. L. and R. L. Hubbard (1990). "Developmental Variation in the Context of Marijuana Initiation Among Adolescents," *Journal of Health and Social Behavior* 31: 58–70.

Bakdash, M. B. (1983). "The Use of Mass Media in Community Periodontal Education," *Journal of Public Health Dentistry* 43: 128–31.

Bakdash, M. B., A. L. Lange, and D. G. McMillan (1983). "The Effect of a Televised Periodontal Campaign on Public Periodontal Awareness," *Journal of Periodontology* 54: 666–70.

Baker, E. L., J. M. Melius, and J. D. Millar (1988). "Surveillance of Occupational Illness and Injury in the United States: Current Perspectives and Future Directions," *Journal of Public Health Policy* 9: 198–221.

Bandura, A. (1977). *Social Learning Theory* (Englewood Cliffs, NJ: Prentice-Hall).

Bandura, A. (1982). "Self-Efficacy Mechanisms in Human Agency," *American Psychologist* 37: 122–47.

Bandura, A. (1986). *Social Foundations of Thought and Action: A Social Cognitive Theory* (Englewood Cliffs, NJ: Prentice-Hall).

Bardach, E. (1977). *The Implementation Game: What Happens After a Bill Becomes a Law* (Cambridge: MIT Press).

Bartlett, E. E. (1982). "Behavioral Diagnosis: A Practical Approach to Patient Education," *Patient Counseling and Health Education* 4: 29–35.

Bartlett, E. E. (1985). "Eight Principles from Patient Education Research," *Preventive Medicine* 14: 667–69.

Basch, C. E. (1984). "Research on Disseminating and Implementing Health Education Programs in Schools," *Journal of School Health* 54: 57–66.

Basch, C. E. (1987). "Assessing Health Education Needs: A Multidimensional-Multimethod Approach," in *Handbook of Health Education*, 2nd ed., P. M. Lazes, L. H. Kaplan, and K. A. Gordon, eds. (Rockville, MD: Aspen), chap. 3.

Basch, C. E. (1987). "Focus Group Interview: An Underutilized Research Technique for Improving Theory and Practice in Health Education," *Health Education Quarterly* 14: 411–48.

Basch, C. E. (1989). "Preventing AIDS Through Education: Concepts, Strategies, and Research Priorities," *Journal of School Health* 59: 296–300.

Basch, C. E., J. D. Eveland, and B. Portnoy (1986). "Diffusion Systems for Education and Learning About Health," *Family and Community Health* 9(2): 1–26.

Basch, C. E., E. M. Sliepcevich, R. S. Gold et al. (1985). "Avoiding Type III Errors in Health Education Program Evaluations: A Case Study," *Health Education Quarterly* 12: 315–31.

Bates, I. J. and A. E. Winder (1984). *Introduction to Health Education* (Palo Alto, CA: Mayfield).

Battista, R. N. (1983). "Adult Cancer Prevention in Primary Care: Patterns of Practice in Quebec," *American Journal of Public Health* 73: 1036–39.

Battista, R. N., J. L. Williams, and L. A. MacFarlane (1986). "Determinants of Primary Medical Practice in Adult Cancer Prevention," *Medical Care* 24: 216–24.

Bauer, R. A., ed. (1966). *Social Indicators* (Cambridge: MIT Press).

Baum, C., D. L. Kennedy, M. B. Forbes, and J. K. Jones (1982). *Drug Utilization in the U.S. – 1981: Third Annual Report* (Rockville, MD: Food and Drug Administration).

Baum, C., D. L. Kennedy, M. B. Forbes, and J. K. Jones (1983). *Drug Utilization in the U.S.* (Rockville, MD: Food and Drug Administration).

Bauman, K. E. and R. L. Chenoweth (1984). "The Relationship Between the Consequences Adolescents Expect from Smoking and Their Behavior: A Factor Analysis with Panel Data," *Journal of Social Psychology* 14: 28–41.

Bausell, R. B., ed. (1983). "Quality Assurance: Methods," *Evaluation and the Health Professions* 6(3): whole issue.

Beauchamp, D. (1980). "Public Health as Social Justice," in *Public Health and the Law*, L. Hogue, ed. (Rockville, MD: Aspen Systems).

Beauchamp, G. K. and M. Moran (1982). "Dietary Experience and Sweet Taste Preference in Human Infants," *Appetite: Journal for Intake Research* 3: 139–52.

Beck, K. H. (1981). "Driving While Under the Influence of Alcohol: Relationship to Attitudes and Beliefs in a College Population," *American Journal of Drug and Alcohol Abuse* 8: 377–88.

Becker, M. H., ed. (1974). "The Health Belief Model and Personal Health Behavior," *Health Education Monographs* 2: 324–473, whole issue.

Becker, M. H. (1986). "The Tyranny of Health Promotion," *Public Health Reviews* 14: 15–25.

Becker, M. H., D. Haefner, S. Kasl et al. (1977). "Selected Psychosocial Models and Correlates of Individual Health-Related Behaviors," *Medical Care* 15(Suppl, 1977): 27–46.

Becker, M. H. and J. Joseph (1988). "AIDS and Behavioral Change to Reduce Risk: A Review," *American Journal of Public Health* 78: 394–410.

Becker, M. H., M. M. Kaback, and I. M. Rosenstock (1975). "Some Influences on Public Participation in a Genetic Screening Program," *Journal of Community Health* 1: 3–14.

Becker, M. H., L. Maiman, J. Kirscht et al. (1977). "The Health Belief Model and Prediction of Dietary Compliance: A Field Experiment," *Journal of Health and Social Behavior* 18: 348–66.

Becker, M. H., C. A. Nathanson, M. D. Drachman, and J. P. Kirscht (1977). "Mothers' Health Beliefs and Children's Clinic Visits: A Prospective Study," *Journal of Community Health* 3: 125–33.

Becker, M. H., S. Radius, I. Rosenstock et al. (1978). "Compliance with a Medical Regimen for Asthma: A Test of the Health Belief Model," *Public Health Reports* 93: 268–77.

Becker, S. L., J. A. Burke, R. A. Arbogast et al. (1989). "Community Programs to Enhance In-School Anti-Tobacco Efforts," *Preventive Medicine* 18: 221–28.

Bell, W. (1958). "Social Choice, Life Styles, and Suburban Residence," in *The Suburban Community*, W. Dobriner, ed. (New York: Putnam), pp. 225–42.

Belloc, N. B. (1973). "Relationship of Health Practices and Mortality," *Preventive Medicine* 3: 125–35.

Belloc, N. B. and L. Breslow (1972). "Relationship of Physical Health Status and Health Practices," *Preventive Medicine* 1: 409–21.

Bennett, B. I. (1977). "A Model for Teaching Health Education Skills to Primary Care Practitioners," *International Journal of Health Education* 20: 232–39.

Berger, P. L. and R. J. Neuhaus (1977). *To Empower People: The Role of Mediating Structures in Public Policy* (Washington, DC: American Enterprise Institute for Public Policy Research).

Bergner, M. (1985). "Measurement of Health Status," *Medical Care* 23: 696–704.

Bergner, M. and M. L. Rothman (1987). "Health Status Measures: An Overview and Guide for Selection," *Annual Review of Public Health* 8: 191–210.

Berkanovic, E., C. Telesky, and S. Reeder (1981). "Structural and Social Psychological Factors in the Decision to Seek Medical Care for Symptoms," *Medical Care* 19: 693–709.

Berkman, L. F. and L. Breslow (1983). *Health and Ways of Living: The Alameda County Study* (New York: Oxford University Press).

Berman, P. and M. McLaughlin (1976). "Implementation of Educational Innovation," *The Educational Forum* 40: 347–70.

Berman, S. H. and A. Wandersman (1990). "Fear of Cancer and Knowledge of Cancer — A Review and Proposed Relevance to Hazardous Waste Sites," *Social Science and Medicine* 31: 81–90.

Bernier, M. and J. Avard (1986). "Self-Efficacy, Outcome, and Attrition in a Weight-Reduction Program," *Cognitive Therapy and Research* 10: 319–38.

Bertera, E. M. and R. L. Bertera (1981). "The Cost-Effectiveness of Telephone vs. Clinic Counseling for Hypertensive Patients: A Pilot Study," *American Journal of Public Health* 71: 626–29.

Bertera, R. L. (1990). "The Effects of Workplace Health Promotion on Absenteeism and Employment Costs in a Large Industrial Population," *American Journal of Public Health* 80: 1101–05.

Bertera, R. L. (1990). "Planning and Implementing Health Promotion in the Workplace: A Case Study of the Du Pont Company Experience," *Health Education Quarterly* 17: 307–27.

Bertera, R. L. and J. C. Cuthie (1984). "Blood Pressure Self-Monitoring in the Workplace," *Journal of Occupational Medicine* 26: 183–88.

Bertera, R. and L. W. Green (1979). "Cost-Effectiveness of a Home Visiting Triage Program for Family Planning in Turkey," *American Journal of Public Health* 69: 950–53.

Bertera, R. L., L. K. Oehl, and J. M. Telepchak (1990). "Self-Help Versus Group Approaches to Smoking Cessation in the Workplace: Eighteen-Month Follow-Up and Cost Analysis," *American Journal of Health Promotion* 4: 187–92.

Bertram, D. A. and P. A. Brooks-Bertram (1977). "The Evaluation of Continuing Medical Education: A Literature Review," *Health Education Monographs* 5: 330–62.

Best, J. A. (1989). "Intervention Perspectives on School Health Promotion Research," *Health Education Quarterly* 16: 299–306.

Best, J. A., S. J. Thomson, S. M. Santi et al. (1988). "Preventing Cigarette Smoking Among School Children," *Annual Review of Public Health* 9: 161–201.

Better Health Commission (1986). *Looking Forward to Better Health* (Canberra: Australian Government Printing Service, vols. 1–3).

Bettes, W. A. (1976). "A Method of Allocating Resources for Health Education Services by the Indian Health Service," *Public Health Reports* 91: 256–60.

Bibeau, D. L., K. D. Mullen, K. R. McLeroy et al. (1988). "Evaluations of Workplace Smoking Cessation Programs: A Critique," *American Journal of Preventive Medicine* 4: 87–95.

Bivens, E. C. (1979). "Community Organization: An Old but Reliable Health Education Technique," in *The Handbook of Health Education*, P. M. Lazes, ed. (Germantown, MD: Aspen).

Bjurstrom, L. A. and N. G. Alexiou (1978). "A Program of Heart Disease Intervention for Public Employees," *Journal of Occupational Medicine* 20: 521–31.

Black, R. (1980). "Support for Genetic Services: A Survey," *Health and Social Work* 5: 27–34.

Black, T. (1983). "Coalition Building—Some Suggestions," *Child Welfare* 42: 264.

Blackburn, H. (1987). "Research and Demonstration Projects in Community Cardiovascular Disease Prevention," *Journal of Public Health Policy* 4: 398–421.

Blair, S. N., H. W. Kohl, and K. E. Powell (1987). "Physical Activity, Physical Fitness, Exercise, and the Public's Health," in *The Cutting Edge in Physical Education and Exercise Science Research*, M. J. Safrit and H. M. Eckert, eds. (Champaign, IL: Human Kinetics Publishers), pp. 53–69.

Blake, S. M., R. W. Jeffrey, J. R. Finnegan et al. (1987). "Process Evaluation of a Community-Based Physical Activity Campaign: The Minnesota Heart Health Experience," *Health Education Research* 2: 115–21.

Block, G., W. Rosenberger, and B. Patterson (1988). "Calories, Fat, and Cholesterol: Intake Patterns in the U.S. Population by Race, Sex, and Age," *American Journal of Public Health* 78: 1150–55.

Bloom, B. S. and G. H. DeFriese, eds. (1983). *Cost-Benefits, Cost-Effectiveness, and Other Decision-Making Techniques in Health Resource Allocation* (New York: Biomedical Information).

Blum, R. and S. E. Samuels, eds. (1990). "Television and Teens: Health Implications," *Journal of Adolescent Health Care* 11: 1–92, whole issue no. 1.

Bly, J. L., R. C. Jones, and J. E. Richardson (1986). "Impact of Worksite Health Promotion on Health Care Costs and Utilization," *Journal of the American Medical Association* 256: 3235–40.

Bogue, D. J., R. Burs, and J. Mayo (1979). *Communicating to Combat VD: The Los Angeles Experiment* (Chicago: Community and Family Study Center Monographs, University of Chicago).

Bolman, L. and T. Deal (1979). *The Political Frame* (Cambridge: Harvard Graduate School of Education).

Bonaguro, J. A. and G. Miaoulis (1983). "Marketing: A Tool for Health Education Planning," *Health Education* 14(Jan/Feb): 6–11.

Botvin, G. J., E. Baker, N. Renick et al. (1984). "A Cognitive-Behavioral Approach to Substance Abuse Prevention," *Addictive Behaviors* 9: 137–47.

Botvin, G. J. and A. Eng (1980). "A Comprehensive School-Based Smoking Prevention Program," *Journal of School Health* 50: 209–13.

Botvin, G. J. and A. Eng (1982). "The Efficacy of a Multicomponent Approach to the Prevention of Cigarette Smoking," *Preventive Medicine* 11: 199–211.

Botvin, G. J. and A. McAlister (1982). "Cigarette Smoking Among Children and Adolescents: Causes and Prevention," in *Annual Review of Disease Prevention*, C. B. Arnold, ed. (New York: Springer).

Bourne, P. G. (1974). "Approaches to Drug Abuse Prevention and Treatment in Rural Areas," *Journal of Psychedelic Drugs* 6: 285–89.

Bowler, M. H. and D. E. Morisky (1983). "Small Group Strategy for Improving Compliance Behavior and Blood Pressure Control," *Health Education Quarterly* 10: 57–69.

Bowne, D. W., M. L. Russell, J. L. Morgan et al. (1984). "Reduced Disability and Health Care Costs in an Industrial Fitness Program," *Journal of Occupational Medicine* 26: 809–16.

Boyd, G. M. and E. D. Glover (1989). "Smokeless Tobacco Use by Youth in the U.S.," *Journal of School Health* 59: 189–94.

Boyte, H. C. (1984). *Community Is Possible: Repairing America's Roots* (New York: Harper & Row).

Bozzini, L. (1988). "Local Community Services Centers (LCSC) in Quebec: Description, Evaluation, Perspectives," *Journal of Public Health Policy* 9: 346–75.

Bracht, N., ed. (1990). *Community Organization Strategies for Health Promotion* (New York: Sage).

Bradburn, N. M. (1969). *The Structure of Psychological Well-Being* (Chicago: Aldine).

Brailey, L. J. (1986). "Effects of Health Teaching in the Workplace on Women's Knowledge, Beliefs, and Practices Regarding Breast Self-Examination," *Research in Nursing and Health* 9: 223–31.

Braithwaite, R. L. and N. Lythcott (1989). "Community Empowerment as a Strategy for Health Promotion for Blacks and Other Minorities," *Journal of the American Medical Association* 261: 282–83.

Braverman, M. T., ed. (1989). *Health Promotion Programs* (San Francisco: Jossey-Bass).

Breckon, D. J. (1982). *Hospital Health Education: A Guide to Program Development* (Rockville, MD: Aspen).

Breckon, D. J., J. R. Harvey, and R. B. Lancaster (1989). *Community Health Education: Settings, Roles, and Skills*, 2nd ed. (Rockville, MD: Aspen).

Brennan, A. J. (1982). "Health Promotion: What's In It for Business and Industry?" *Health Education Quarterly* 9(Suppl, Fall): 9–19.

Breslow, L. (1990). "The Future of Public Health: Prospects in the United States for the 1990s," *Annual Review of Public Health* 11: 1–28.

Breslow, L. and J. D. Egstrom (1980). "Persistence of Health Habits and Their Relationship to Mortality," *Preventive Medicine* 9: 469–83.

Brieger, W. R., J. Ramakrishna, and J. D. Adeniyi (1986–87). "Community Involvement in Social Marketing: Guineaworm Control," *International Quarterly of Community Health Education* 7: 19–31.

Brimberry, R. (1988). "Vaccination of High-Risk Patients for Influenza: A Comparison of Telephone and Mail Reminder Methods," *Journal of Family Practice* 26: 397–400.

Brink, S. G., C. Y. Lovato, L. J. Kolbe, and M. E. Buoy (submitted for publication, 1989). "Development and Evaluation of a School-Based Intervention to Increase the Use of Safety Belts by Adolescents."

Brink, S. G., B. Simons-Morton, and D. Zane (1989). "A Hospital-Based Infant Safety Seat Program for Low-Income Families: Assessment of Population Needs and Provider Practices," *Health Education Quarterly* 16: 45–56.

Brink, S. G., D. Simons-Morton, G. Parcel, and K. Tiernan (1988). "Community Intervention Handbooks for Comprehensive Health Promotion Programming," *Family and Community Health* 11: 28–35.

Brody, B. E. (1988). "Employee Assistance Programs: An Historical and Literature Review," *American Journal of Health Promotion* 2: 13–19.

Brown, C. (1984). *The Art of Coalition Building: A Guide for Community Leaders* (New York: The American Jewish Committee).

Brown, E. R. (1984). "Community Organization Influence on Local Public Health Care Policy: A General Research Model and Comparative Case Study," *Health Education Quarterly* 10: 205–34.

Brown, W. B., N. B. Williamson, and R. A. Carlaw (1988). "A Diagnostic Approach to Educating Minnesota Dairy Farmers in the Prevention and Control of Bovine Mastitis," *Preventive Veterinary Medicine* 5: 197–211.

Brownell, K., R. Cohen, A. Stunkard et al. (1984). "Weight Loss Competitions at the Work Site: Impact on Weight, Morale, and Cost-Effectiveness," *American Journal of Public Health* 74: 1283–85.

Brownell, K. D. and M. R. J. Felix (1987). "Competitions to Facilitate Health Promotion: Review and Conceptual Analysis," *American Journal of Health Promotion* 2(1): 28–36.

Bruhn, J. B. (1983). "The Application of Theory in Childhood Asthma Self-Help Programs," *Journal of Allergy and Clinical Immunology* 72(Suppl, Nov, Pt 2): 561–77.

Brunk, S. E. and J. Goeppinger (1990). "Process Evaluation: Assessing Re-Invention of Community-Based Interventions," *Evaluation and the Health Professions* 13: 186–203.

Brunton, S. A. (1984). "Physicians as Patient Teachers," in "Personal Health Maintenance" (Special Issue), *Western Journal of Medicine* 131: 855–60.

Bryant, N. H., W. Stender, V. Frist, and A. R. Somers (1976). "VD Hotline: An Evaluation," *Public Health Reports* 91: 231–35.

Bryk, A. S., ed. (1983). *Stakeholder-Based Evaluation* (San Francisco, Jossey-Bass).

Buck, C. (1986). "Beyond Lalonde; Creating Health," *Journal of Public Health Policy* 20: 444–57.

Budd, R., S. Bleiner, and C. Spencer (1983). "Exploring the Use and Non-Use of Marijuana as Reasoned Actions: An Application of Fishbein and Ajzen's Methodology," *Drug and Alcohol Dependence* 11: 217–24.

Budd, R., D. North, and C. Spencer (1984). "Understanding Seat-Belt Use: A Test of Bentler and Speckart's Extension of the 'Theory of Reasoned Action,'" *European Journal of Social Psychology* 14: 69–78.

Bunker, J. P., D. S. Gomby, and B. H. Kehrer (1989). *Pathways to Health: The Role of Social Factors* (Menlo Park, CA: Kaiser Family Foundation).

Burden, D. S. and B. K. Googins (1987). *Balancing Work Life and Homelife* (Boston: Boston University School of Social Work).

Burnham, J. C. (1984). "Change in the Popularization of Health in the United States," *Bulletin of the History of Medicine* 58(Summer): 183–97.

Bush, J. W. (1984). "Relative Preferences Versus Relative Frequencies in Health-Related Quality of Life Evaluations," in *Assessment of Quality of Life in Clinical Trials of Cardiovascular Therapies*, N. K. Wenger, M. E. Mattson, C. D. Furber, and J. Elinson, eds. (New York: Le Jacq), pp. 118–39.

Bush, P. J. and R. J. Iannotti (1990). "A Children's Health Belief Model," *Medical Care* 28: 69–86.

Bush, P. J., A. E. Zuckerman, P. K. Theiss et al. (1989). "Cardiovascular Risk Factor Prevention in Black School Children — Two-year Results of the Know Your Body Program," *American Journal of Epidemiology* 129: 466–82.

Butler, M. and W. Paisley (1977). "Communicating Cancer Control to the Public," *Health Education Monographs* 5: 5–24.

Calnan, M. (1984). "The Health Belief Model and Participation in Programmes for the Early Detection of Breast Cancer: A Comparative Analysis," *Social Science and Medicine* 19: 823–30.

Calnan, M. and S. Moss (1984). "The Health Belief Model and Compliance with Education Given at a Class in Breast Self-Examination" *Journal of Health and Social Behavior* 25: 198–210.

Campbell, D. T. (1969). "Reforms as Experiments," *American Psychologist* 24: 409–29.

Campbell, R. and B. Chenoweth (1981). "Health Education as a Basis for Social Support," *The Gerontologist* 21: 619–27.

Cantor, J. C., D. E. Morisky, L. W. Green et al. (1985). "Cost-Effectiveness of Educational Interventions to Improve Patient Outcomes in Blood Pressure Control," *Preventive Medicine* 14: 782–800.

Carlaw, R. W., ed. (1982). *Perspectives on Community Health Education: A Series of Case Studies*, 2 vols. (Oakland, CA: Third Party Publishing).

Carlaw, R. W., M. Mittlemark, N. Bracht, and R. Luepker (1984). "Organization for a Community Cardiovascular Health Program: Experiences from the Minnesota Heart Health Program," *Health Education Quarterly* 11: 243–52.

Carlton, B. and M. Carlton (1978). "Defining a Role for the Health Educator in the Primary Care Setting," *Health Education* 9(Mar/Apr): 22–23.

Carnegie Council on Adolescent Development, Task Force on Education of Young Adolescents (1989). *Turning Points: Preparing American Youth for the 21st Century* (Washington, DC: Carnegie Council on Adolescent Development, Carnegie Corporation of New York).

Carter, W. B., L. R. Beach, and T. S. Inui et al. (1986). "Developing and Testing a Decision Model for Predicting Influenza Vaccination Compliance," *Health Service Research* 20: 897–932.

Carter, W. B., D. W. Belcher, and T. S. Inui (1981). "Implementing Preventive Care in Clinical Practice. II. Problems for Managers, Clinicians, and Patients," *Medical Care Review* 38: 19–24.

Cartwright, D. (1949). "Some Principles of Mass Persuasion: Selected Findings from Research on the Sale of United States War Bonds," *Human Relations* 2: 53–69.

Cassatta, D. M. and B. L. Kirkman-Liff (1981). "Mental Health Activities of Family Physicians," *Journal of Family Practice* 12: 683–92.

Casswell, S., L. Stewart, and P. Duignan (1989). "The Struggle Against the Broadcast of Anti-Health Messages: Regulation of Alcohol Advertising in New Zealand 1980–87," *Health Promotion* 4: 287–96.

Cataldo, M. F. and T. J. Coates, eds. (1986). *Health and Industry: A Behavioral Medicine Perspective* (New York: Wiley).

Cataldo, M. F., L. W. Green, J. A. Herd et al. (1986). "Preventive Medicine and the Corporate Environment: Challenge to Behavioral Medicine," in *Health and Industry: A Behavioral Medicine Perspective*, M. F. Cataldo and T. J. Coates, eds. (New York: Wiley), pp. 399–419.

Catford, J. C. (1983). "Positive Health Indicators – Toward a New Information Base for Health Promotion," *Community Medicine* 5: 125–32.

CBS Television Network (1984). *A Study of Attitudes, Concerns, and Information Needs for Prescription Drugs and Related Illnesses*. (New York: CBS Television Network).

Celentano, D. D. and D. Holtzman (1983). "Breast Self-Examination Competency: An Analysis of Self-Reported Practice and Associated Characteristics," *American Journal of Public Health* 73: 1321–23.

Centers for Disease Control (1978). *The Ten Leading Causes of Death* (Atlanta: Centers for Disease Control).

Centers for Disease Control (1986). "Premature Mortality in the United States: Public Health Issues in the Use of Years of Potential Life Lost," *Morbidity and Mortality Weekly Report* 35(Suppl): 2S.

Centers for Disease Control (1988). "Guidelines for Effective School Health Education to Prevent the Spread of AIDS," *Morbidity and Mortality Weekly Report* 37(Suppl No. S-2): 1–14, also in *Health Education* 19(3): 6–13.

Cerkoney, K. A. and L. K. Hart (1980). "The Relationship Between the Health Belief Model and Compliance of Persons with Diabetes Mellitus," *Diabetes Care* 3: 594–98.

Cernada, E. C., Y. J. Lee, and M. Y. Lin (1974). "Family Planning Telephone Services in Two Asian Cities," *Studies in Family Planning* 5: 111–14.

Cernada, G. P. (1974). "The Case of the Unplanned Child," *Human Organization* 33: 106–09.

Cernada, G. P. (1982). *Knowledge Into Action* (New York: Baywood).

Chamberlin, R.W., ed. (1988). *Beyond Individual Risk Assessment: Community-Wide Approaches to Promoting the Health and Development of Families and Children* (Washington, DC: National Center for Education in Maternal and Child Health).

Champion, V. (1984). "Instrument Development for Health Belief Model Constructs," *Advances in Nursing Science* 6: 73–85.

Chapman, S. (1990). "Intersectoral Action to Improve Nutrition: The Roles of the State and the Private Sector. A Case Study from Australia," *Health Promotion International* 5: 35–44.

Charter, W. and J. Jones (1973). "On the Risk of Appraising Non-Events in Program Evaluation," *Educational Research* 2(11): 5–47.

Chase, G. (1979). "Implementing a Human Services Program: How Hard Can It Be?" *Public Policy* 27: 385–435.

Chassin, L., E. Corty, C. Presson et al. (1984). "Cognitive and Social Influence Factors in Adolescent Smoking Cessation," *Addictive Behaviors* 9: 383–90.

Chassin, L., L. Mann, and K. Sher (1988). "Self-Awareness Theory, Family History of Alcoholism, and Adolescent Alcohol Involvement," *Journal of Abnormal Psychology* 97: 206–17.

Chassin, L., C. C. Presson, M. Bensenberg, E. Corty, R. W. Olshavsky, and S. J. Sherman (1984). "Predicting Adolescents' Intentions to Smoke Cigarettes," *Journal of Health and Social Behavior* 22: 445–55.

Chavis, D. M., J. H. Hogge, D. W. McMillan, and A. Wandersman (1986). "Sense of Community Through Brunswik's Lens: A First Look," *Journal of Community Psychology* 14: 24–40.

Chavis, D. M. and A. Wandersman (1990). "Sense of Community in the Urban Environment: A Catalyst for Participation and Community Development," *American Journal of Community Psychology* 18: 55–81.

Cheadle, A., B. Psaty, E. Wagner et al. (1990). "Evaluating Community-Based Nutrition Programs: Assessing the Reliability of a Survey of Grocery Store Product Displays," *American Journal of Public Health* 80: 709–11.

Checkoway, B. (1989). "Community Participation for Health Promotion: Prescription for Public Policy?" *Wellness Perspectives: Research, Theory, and Practice* 6: 18–26.

Chen, M. K. (1979). "The Gross National Health Product: A Proposed Population Health Index," *Public Health Reports* 94: 119–23.

Chen, M. S., Jr. and D. Bill (1983). "Statewide Survey of Risk Factor Prevalence: The Ohio Experience," *Public Health Reports* 98: 443–48.

Chen, T. L. and G. P. Cernada (1985). *Recommended Health Education Readings: An Annotated Bibliography* (Taipei: Maplewood Press).

Children's Defense Fund (1990). *Children 1990: A Report Card, Briefing Book, and Action Primer* (Washington, DC: Children's Defense Fund).

Chin, R. (1976). "The Utility of System Models and Developmental Models for Practitioners," in *The Planning of Change*, 3rd ed., W. B. Bennis, K. D. Benne, R. Chin, and K. E. Corey, eds. (New York: Holt, Rinehart and Winston), pp. 90–102.

Chwalow, A. J., L. W. Green, D. M. Levine, and S. G. Deeds (1978). "Effects of the Multiplicity of Interventions on the Compliance of Hypertensive Patients with Medical Regimens in an Inner-City Population," *Preventive Medicine* 7: 51.

City of Toronto Department of Public Health (1984). *The City of Toronto Community Health Survey: A Description of the Health Status of Toronto Residents* (Toronto: City of Toronto Department of Public Health, July).

Clark, J. M. (1939). *The Social Control of Business* (New York: McGraw-Hill).

Clark, N. M. (1987). "Social Learning Theory in Current Health Education Practice," in *Advances in Health Education and Promotion*, vol. 2, W. B. Ward, S. K. Simonds, P. D. Mullen, and M. H. Becker, eds., (Greenwich, CT: JAI Press), pp. 251–75.

Cleary, H. P. (1986). "Issues in the Credentialing of Health Education Specialists: A Review of the State of the Art," in *Advances in Health Education and Promotion*, vol. 1, pt A, W. Ward and Z. Salisbury (Greenwich, CT: JAI Press), pp. 129–54.

Cleary, H. P., J. M. Kichen, and P. G. Ensor (1985). *Advancing Health Through Education: A Case Study Approach* (Palo Alto, CA: Mayfield).

Cleary, P. D., T. F. Rogers, E. Singer et al. (1986). "Health Education About AIDS Among Seropositive Blood Donors," *Health Education Quarterly* 13: 317–30.

Coates, T., R. Stall, and C. Hoff (1988). *Changes in High Risk Behavior Among Gay and Bisexual Men Since the Beginning of the AIDS Epidemic* (Washington, DC: Office of Technology Assessment, United States Congress, May).

Cohen, A. and L. Murphy (1989). "Indicators and Measures of Health Promotion Behaviors in the Workplace," in *Health Promotion Indicators and Actions*, S. B. Kar, ed. (New York: Springer).

Cohen, H., C. Harris, and L. W. Green (1979). "Cost-Benefit Analysis of Asthma Self-Management Educational Programs in Children," *Journal of Allergy and Clinical Immunology* 64: 155–56.

Cohen, J. M. and N. T. Uphoff (1980). "Participation's Place in Rural Development: Seeking Clarity Through Specificity," *World Development* 8: 213–35.

Cohen, R. Y., M. R. J. Felix, and K. D. Brownell (1989). "The Role of Parents and Older Peers in School-Based Cardiovascular Prevention Programs: Implications for Program Development," *Health Education Quarterly* 16: 245–53.

Cohen, S., ed. (1979). *New Directions in Patient Compliance* (Lexington, MA: Lexington Books, D.C. Heath).

Cohen, W. J. (1968). "Social Indicators: Statistics of Public Policy," *American Statistician* 22: 14–16.

Collin, D. F. (1982–83). "Health Educators: Change Agents or Techno/Peasants?" *International Quarterly of Community Health Education* 3: 131–44.

Collings, G. H., Jr. (1982). "Perspectives of Industry Regarding Health Promotion," in *Managing Health Promotion in the Workplace: Guidelines for Implementation and Evaluation*, R. S. Parkinson and Associates, eds. (Palo Alto, CA: Mayfield), pp. 119–26.

Collins, J., S. Wagner, L. Weissberger (1986). "125 Teams Lose 2,233 Pounds in a Work Site Weight Loss Competition," *Journal of the American Dietetic Association* 86: 1578–79.

Committee on Diet and Health, National Research Council, Food and Nutrition Board (1989). *Diet and Health: Implications for Reducing Chronic Disease Risk* (Washington, DC: National Academy Press).

Committee on Risk Perception and Communication, National Research Council (1989). *Improving Risk Communication* (Washington, DC: National Academy Press).

Committee on Trauma Research (1989). *Injury in America: A Continuing Public Health Problem* (Washington, DC: National Academy Press).

Committee to Study Outreach for Prenatal Care, Institute of Medicine (1988). *Prenatal Care: Reaching Infants* (Washington, DC: National Academy Press).

Condiotte, M. M. and E. Lichtenstein (1981). "Self-Efficacy and Relapse in Smoking Cessation Programs," *Journal of Consulting and Clinical Psychology* 49: 648–58.

Conn, R. H., and D. Anderson (1971). "D.C. Mounts Unfunded Program of Screening for Lead Poisoning," *HSMHA Health Report* (now *Public Health Reports*) 86: 409–13.

Connell, D. B., R. R. Turner, and E. F. Mason (1985). "Summary of Findings of the School Health Education Evaluation: Health Promotion Effectiveness, Implementation, and Costs," *Journal of School Health* 55: 316–21.

Conrad, P. (1987). "Who Comes to Work-Site Wellness Programs? A Preliminary Review," *Journal of Occupational Medicine* 29: 317–20.

Consumer Self-Care in Health (Rockville, MD: National Center for Health Services Research Proceeding Series, DHEW Publication No. HRA 77-3181, 1977).

Cook, R. and A. Harrell (1987). "Drug Abuse Among Working Adults: Prevalence Rates and Recommended Strategies," *Health Education Research: Theory and Practice* 2: 353–59.

Corcoran, R. D. and B. Portnoy (1989). "Risk Reduction Through Comprehensive Cancer Education: The American Cancer Society Plan for Youth Education," *Journal of School Health* 59: 199–204.

Coreil, J. and J. S. Levin (1985). "A Critique of the Life Style Concept in Public Health Education," *International Quarterly of Community Health Education* 5: 103–14.

Cornacchia, H. J., L. K. Olsen, and C. J. Nickerson (1988). *Health in Elementary Schools*, 7th ed. (St. Louis: Times Mirror/Mosby).

Cottrell, L. S. (1976). "The Competent Community," in *Further Exploration in Social Psychiatry*, B. H. Kaplan, R. N. Wilson, and A. H. Leighton, eds. (New York: Basic Books), pp. 195–209.

Covello, V. T., D. von Winterfeldt, and P. Slovic (1986). "Risk Communication: A Review of the Literature," *Risk Abstracts* 3(Oct): 171–82.

Cox, C. (1979). "A Pilot Study: Using the Elderly as Community Health Educators," *International Journal of Health Education* 22: 49–52.

Crawford, R. (1977). "You Are Dangerous to Your Health: The Ideology and Politics of Victim Blaming," *International Journal of Health Services* 7: 663–80.

Creswell, W. H. and I. M. Newman (1989). *School Health Practice*, 9th ed. (St. Louis: Times Mirror/ Mosby).

Crow, R., H. Blackburn, D. Jacobs et al. (1986). "Population Strategies to Enhance Physical Activity: The Minnesota Heart Health Program," *Acta Medica Scandinavica* 711(Suppl): 93–112.

Cuca, R. and C. S. Pierce (1977). *Experiments in Family Planning: Lessons from the Developing World* (Baltimore: Johns Hopkins University Press, for the World Bank).

Cullen, J., B. Fox, and R. Isom, eds. (1976). *Cancer: The Behavioral Dimensions* (New York: Raven Press).

Cummings, K., M. Becker, J. Kirscht, and N. Levin (1982). "Psychosocial Factors Affecting Adherence to Medical Regimens in a Group of Hemodialysis Patients," *Medical Care* 20: 567–80.

Cummings, K. M., G. Giovino, S. L. Emont et al. (1986). "Factors Influencing Success in Counseling Patients to Stop Smoking," *Patient Education and Counseling* 8: 189–200.

Cummings, K. M., G. Giovino, R. Sciandra et al. (1987). "Physician Advice to Quit Smoking: Who Gets It and Who Doesn't," *American Journal of Preventive Medicine* 3: 69–75.

Cummings, K. M., A. M. Jette, B. Brock, and D. Haefner (1979). "Psychosocial Determinants of Immunization Behavior in a Swine Influenza Campaign," *Medical Care* 17: 639–49.

Cummings, K. M., A. M. Jette, and I. M. Rosenstock (1979). "Construct Validation of the Health Belief Model," *Health Education Monographs* 6: 394–405.

Cummings, O. W., J. R. Nowakowski, T. A. Schwandt et al. (1988). "Business Perspectives on Internal/External Evaluation," in *Evaluation Utilization*, J. A. McLaughlin, L. J. Weber, R. W. Covert, and R. B. Ingle, eds. (San Francisco: Jossey-Bass).

Cuoto, R. A. (1990). "Promoting Health at the Grass Roots," *Health Affairs* 9: 144–151.

Cwikel, J. M. B., T. E. Dielman, J. P. Kirscht, and B. A. Israel (1988). "Mechanisms of Psychosocial Effects on Health: The Role of Social Integration, Coping Style, and Health Behavior," *Health Education Quarterly* 15: 151–73.

Danaher, B. G. (1982). "Smoking Cessation Programs in Occupational Settings," in *Managing Health Promotion in the Workplace: Guidelines for Implementation and Evaluation*, R. S. Parkinson and Associates, eds. (Palo Alto, CA: Mayfield), pp. 217–32.

Danforth, N. and B. Swaboda (1978). *Agency for International Development Health Education Study* (Washington, DC: Westinghouse Health Systems, 17 Mar).

Davidson, A. R. and J. J. Jaccard (1975). "Population Psychology: A New Look at an Old Problem," *Journal of Personality and Social Psychology*, cited by J. Jaccard, op. cit., p. 158.

Davidson, L., S. Chapman, and C. Hull (1979). *Health Promotion in Australia 1978–1979* (Canberra: Commonwealth of Australia).

Davis, D. A., R. B. Haynes, and L. W. Chambers et al. (1984). "The Impact of CME: A Methodologic Review of the Continuing Medical Education Literature," *Evaluation and the Health Professions* 7: 251–83.

Davis, K. E., K. L. Jackson, J. J. Kronenfeld, and S. N. Blair (1987). "Determinants of Participation in Worksite Health Promotion Activities," *Health Education Quarterly* 14: 195–205.

Davis, M. F. and D. C. Iverson (1984). "An Overview and Analysis of the HealthStyle Campaign," *Health Education Quarterly* 11: 253–72.

Davis, M. F., K. Rosenberg, D. E. Iverson et al. (1984). "Worksite Health Promotion in Colorado," *Public Health Reports* 99: 538–43.

Dawson, D. A. (1986). "The Effects of Sex Education on Adolescent Behavior," *Family Planning Perspectives* 18: 162–70.

Deeds, S. G. and P. D. Mullen (1982). "Managing Health Education in HMOs: Part II," *Health Education Quarterly* 9: 3–95.

DeFrank, R. S. and P. M. Levenson (1987). "Ethical and Philosophical Issues in Developing a Health Promotion Consortium," *Health Education Quarterly* 14: 71–77.

DeFriese, G. H. (1986). "Cost Effectiveness as a Basis for Assessing the Policy Significance of Health Promotion," *Advances in Health Education and Health Promotion*, vol. 1, pt A, W. B. Ward, ed. (Greenwich, CT: JAI Press), pp. 7–21.

DeFriese, G. H. (1989). *Promoting Health in America: Breakthroughs and Harbingers* (Battle Creek, MI: W. K. Kellogg Foundation).

DeFriese, G. H., C. L. Crossland, C. E. Pearson, and C. J. Sullivan, eds. (1990). "Comprehensive School Health Programs: Current Status and Future Prospects," *Journal of School Health* 60(4): 127–90, whole issue.

DeJong, W. and J. A. Winsten (1990). "The Use of Mass Media in Substance Abuse Prevention," *Health Affairs* 9: 30–46.

de Kadt, E. (1982). "Community Participation for Health: The Case of Latin America," *World Development* 10: 573–84.

Delbecq, A. L. (1983). "The Nominal Group as a Technique for Understanding the Qualitative Dimensions of Client Needs," in *Assessing Health and Human Service Needs*, R. A. Bell et al., eds. (New York: Human Sciences Press), pp. 191–209.

deLeeuw, E. J. J. (1989). *Health Promotion: The Sane Revolution* (Maastricht, The Netherlands: Van Gorcum).

De Pietro, R. (1987). "A Marketing Research Approach to Health Education Planning," in *Advances in Health Education and Promotion*, vol. 2, W. B. Ward and S. K. Simonds, eds. (Greenwich, CT: JAI Press), pp. 93–118.

DePue, J. D., B. L. Wells, T. M. Lasater, and R. A. Carleton (1990). "Volunteers as Providers of Heart Health Programs in Churches: A Report on Implementation," *American Journal of Health Promotion* 4: 361–66.

Dershewitz, R. A. and J. W. Williamson (1977). "Prevention of Childhood Household Injuries: A Controlled Clinical Trial," *American Journal of Public Health* 67: 1148–53.

DeTullio, P. L., S. A. Eraker, and C. Jepson et al. (1986). "Patient Medication Instruction and Provider Interactions: Effects on Knowledge and Attitudes," *Health Education Quarterly* 13: 51–60.

Dever, G. E. (1976). "An Epidemiological Model for Health Policy Analysis," *Social Indicators Research* 2: 453–66.

Devine, E. C. and T. D. Cook (1983). "A Meta-Analytic Analysis of Effects of Psycho-Educational Interventions on Length of Postsurgical Hospital Stay," *Nursing Research* 32: 267–74.

DeVries, H., M. Dijkstra, and P. Kuhlman (1988). "Self-Efficacy: The Third Factor Besides Attitude and Subjective Norm as a Predictor of Behavioral Intentions," *Health Education Research* 3: 273–82.

DeVries, H. and G. J. Kok (1986). "From Determinants of Smoking Behaviour to the Implications for a Prevention Programme," *Health Education Research* 1: 85–94.

Dewey, J. (1909). *Moral Principles in Education* (Boston: Houghton Mifflin).

Dewey, J. (1938). *Logic: The Theory of Inquiry* (New York: Henry Holt).

Dewey, J. (1946). *The Public and Its Problems: An Essay in Political Inquiry* (Chicago: Gateway Books).

DiClemente, C. C. and J. O. Prochaska (1982). "Self-Change and Therapy Change of Smoking Behavior: A Comparison of Process of Change in Cessation and Maintenance," *Addictive Behaviors* 7: 133–42.

DiClemente, C. C., J. O. Prochaska, and M. Gibertine (1985). "Self-Efficacy and the Stages of Self-Change of Smoking," *Cognitive Therapy and Research* 9: 181–200.

Dielman, T. E., S. L. Leech, M. H. Becker et al. (1980). "Dimensions of Children's Health Beliefs," *Health Education Quarterly* 7: 219–38.

Dietz, T., P. C. Stern, and R. W. Rycroft (1989). "Definitions of Conflict and the Legitimation of Resources: The Case of Environmental Risk," *Sociological Forum* 4(1): 47–70.

Dignan, M. B. (1986). *Measurement and Evaluation of Health Education* (Springfield, IL: Charles C. Thomas).

Dignan, M. B. and P. A. Carr (1981). *Introduction to Program Planning: A Basic Text for Community Health Education* (Philadelphia: Lea & Febiger).

Division of Health Education, Center for Health Promotion and Education, Centers for Disease Control (1988). *Reference Manuals: Planned Approach to Community Health* (Atlanta: Centers for Disease Control).

Dobson, D. and T. J. Cook (1980). "Avoiding Type III Error in Program Evaluation: Results from a Field Experiment," *Evaluation and Program Planning* 3: 269–76.

Doherty, W., H. Schrott, L. Metcalf, and V. Iasiello (1983). "Effect of Spouse Support and Health Beliefs on Medical Adherence," *Journal of Family Practice* 17: 837–41.

Donald, C. A. and J. E. Ware, Jr. (1982). *The Quantification of Social Contacts and Resources* (Santa Monica, CA: Rand).

D'Onofrio, C. N. (1989). "Making the Case for Cancer Prevention in the Schools," *Journal of School Health* 59: 225–31.

Dore, R. and Z. Mars (1981). *Community Development* (London: Croom Helm and UNESCO).

Douglas, B., B. Wertley, and S. Chaffee (1970). "An Information Campaign That Changed Community Attitudes," *Journalism Quarterly* 47: 220–27.

Downey, A. M., G. C. Frank, L. S. Webber et al. (1987). "Implementation of 'Heart Smart': A Cardiovascular School Health Promotion Program," *Journal of School Health* 57: 98–104.

Downey, A. M., S. J. Virgilio, D. C. Serpas et al. (1988). "Heart Smart—A Staff Development Model for a School-Based Cardiovascular Health Intervention," *Health Education* 19(5): 64–71.

Doyle, E., C. A. Smith, and M. C. Hosokawa (1989). "A Process Evaluation of a Community-Based Health Promotion Program for a Minority Target Population," *Health Education* 20(5): 61–64.

Drazen, M., J. S. Nevid, N. Pace, and R. M. O'Brien (1982). "Worksite-Based Behavioral Treatment of Mild Hypertension," *Journal of Occupational Medicine* 24: 511–64.

Duhl, L. (1986). "The Healthy City: Its Function and Its Future," *Health Promotion* 1: 55–60.

Duncan, D. F. and R. S. Gold (1986). "Reflections: Health Promotion—What Is It?" *Health Values* 10(May/June): 47–48.

Dunlop, B. D., P. V. Piserchia, and J. E. Richardson et al. (1989). *Evaluation of Workplace Health Enhancement Programs: A Monograph* (Research Triangle Park, NC: Research Triangle Institute).

Dunn, H. L. (1977). *High Level Wellness* (Thorofare, NJ: Charles B. Slack).

Dupuy, H. J. (1984). "The Psychological General Well-Being Index," in *Assessment of Quality of Life in Clinical Trials of Cardiovascular Therapies*, N. K. Wenger et al., eds. (New York: Le Jacq), pp. 170–83.

Dwore, R. B. and M. W. Kreuter (1980). "Update: Reinforcing the Case for Health Promotion," *Family and Community Health* 2: 103–19.

Dwyer, T., J. P. Pierce, C. D. Hannam, and N. Burke (1986). "Evaluation of the Sydney 'Quit. For Life' Anti-Smoking Campaign: Part II: Changes in Smoking Prevalence," *Medical Journal of Australia* 144: 344–47.

Earp, J., M. G. Ory, and D. S. Strogatz (1982). "The Effects of Family Involvement and Practitioners Home Visits on the Control of Hypertension," *American Journal of Public Health* 72(1982): 1146–54.

Eiser, J. R., S. R. Sutton, and M. Wober (1979). "Smoking, Seat-Belts, and Beliefs About Health," *Addictive Behavior* 4: 331–38.

Ekeh, H. E. and J. D. Adeniyi (1989). "Health Education Strategies for Tropical Disease Control in School Children," *Journal of Tropical Medicine and Hygiene* 92(2): 55–59.

Eklundh, B. and B. Pettersson (1987). "Health Promotion Policy in Sweden: Means and Methods in Intersectoral Action," *Health Promotion* 2: 177–94.

Elinson, J. (1977). "Have We Narrowed the Gap Between the Poor and the Nonpoor?" *Medical Care* 15: 675–77.

Ellickson, P. L. and R. M. Bell (1990). "Drug Prevention in Junior High: A Multi-Site Longitudinal Test," *Science* 247: 1299–305.

Ellickson, P. L. and R. M. Bell (1990). *Prospects for Preventing Drug Use Among Young Adolescents* (Santa Monica, CA: RAND, R-3896-CHF).

Ellison, R. C., A. L. Capper, R. J. Goldberg et al. (1989). "The Environmental Component: Changing School Food Service to Promote Cardiovascular Health," *Health Education Quarterly* 16: 285–97.

Elmore, R. (1976). "Follow Through Planned Variation," in *Social Program Implementation*, W. Williams and R. Elmore, eds. (New York: Academic Press).

Elwood, T. W., E. Ericson, and S. Lieberman (1978). "Comparative Educational Approaches to Screening for Colorectal Cancer," *American Journal of Public Health* 68: 135–38.

Emmons, C. A., J. G. Joseph, R. C. Kessler et al. (1986). "Psychosocial Predictors of Reported Behavior Change in Homosexual Men at Risk for AIDS," *Health Education Quarterly* 13: 331–45.

Endres, J. (1990). "Teambuilding for Community Health Promotion," *How-To Guides on Community Health Promotion*, No. 14 (Palo Alto, CA: Health Promotion Resource Center, Stanford Center for Research on Disease Prevention).

Enelow, A. J. and J. B. Henderson, eds. (1975). *Applying Behavioral Science to Cardiovascular Risk* (New York: American Heart Association).

Eng, E., J. Hatch, and A. Callan (1985). "Institutionalizing Social Support Through the Church and into the Community," *Health Education Quarterly* 12: 81–92.

Epp, J. (1986). "Achieving Health for All: A Framework for Health Promotion," *Health Promotion* 1: 419–28.

Epstein, S. (1979). "The Stability of Behavior: I. On Predicting Most of the People Much of the Time," *Journal of Personality and Social Psychology* 37: 1097–126.

Eraker, S., M. Becker, V. Strecher, and J. Kirscht (1985). "Smoking Behavior, Cessation Techniques, and the Health Decision Model," *American Journal of Medicine* 78: 817–25.

Eraker, S. A. and P. Politser (1982). "How Decisions Are Reached—Physician and Patient," *Annals of Internal Medicine* 97: 262–68.

Eriksen, M. P. (1986). "Workplace Smoking Control: Rationale and Approaches," *Advances in Health Education and Promotion*, vol. 1, pt A (Greenwich, CT: JAI Press), pp. 65–103.

Eriksen, M. P. and A. C. Gielen (1983). "The Application of Health Education Principles to Automobile Child Restraint Programs," *Health Education Quarterly* 10: 30–55.

Eriksen, M. P., L. W. Green, and F. G. Fultz (1988). "Principles of Changing Health Behavior," *Cancer* 62: 1768–75.

Ernst, N. D., M. Wu, P. Frommer et al. (1986). "Nutrition Education at the Point of Purchase: The Foods for Health Project Evaluated," *Preventive Medicine* 15: 60–73.

Esdale, A. and H. L. Harris (1985). "Evaluation of a Closed-Circuit Television Patient Education Program: Structure, Process, and Outcome," *Patient Education and Counseling* 7: 193–215.

Eta Sigma Gamma Monograph Series (1985). 4(1 Nov): whole issue.

Evans, R. I. and B. E. Raines (1982). "Control and Prevention of Smoking in Adolescents: A Psychological Perspective," in *Promoting Adolescent Health: A Dialog on Research and Practice*, T. J. Coates, A. D. Peterson, and C. Perry, eds. (New York: Academic Press).

Evans, R. I., R. M. Rozelle, S. E. Maxwell et al. (1981). "Social Modeling Films to Deter Smoking in Adolescents: Results of a Three-Year Field Investigation," *Journal of Applied Psychology* 66: 399–414.

Everly, G. S. and R. H. Feldman, eds. (1985). *Occupational Health Promotion: Health Behavior in the Workplace* (New York: Wiley).

Evers, A. (1989) "Promoting Health – Localizing Support Structures for Community Health Projects," *Health Promotion* 4: 183–88.

Ewart, C. K., V. C. Li, and T. J. Coates (1983). "Increasing Physicians' Antismoking Influence by Applying an Inexpensive Feedback Technique," *Journal of Medical Education* 58: 468–73.

Ewles, L. and I. Simnett (1985). *Promoting Health: A Practical Guide to Health Education* (New York: Wiley).

Faden, R. R. (1987). "Ethical Issues in Government Sponsored Public Health Campaigns," *Health Education Quarterly* 14: 27–37.

Farquhar, J. W. (1978). "The Community-Based Model of Life Style Intervention Trials," *American Journal of Epidemiology* 108: 103–11.

Farquhar, J. W., S. P. Fortmann, J. A. Flora et al. (1990). "Effects of Community-Wide Education on Cardiovascular Disease Risk Factors – the Stanford Five-City Project," *Journal of the American Medical Association* 264: 359–65.

Farquhar, J. W., S. Fortmann, N. Maccoby et al. (1984). "The Stanford Five City Project: An Overview," in *Behavioral Health: A Handbook of Health Enhancement and Disease Prevention*, J. D. Matarazzo, S. M. Weiss, J. A. Herd et al., eds. (New York: Wiley), pp. 1154–65.

Farquhar, J. W., S. P. Fortman, P. D. Wood, and W. L. Haskell (1983). "Community Studies of Cardiovascular Disease Prevention," in *Prevention of Coronary Heart Disease: Practical Management of Risk Factors*, N. M. Kaplan and J. Stamler, eds. (Philadelphia: W. B. Saunders).

Farquhar, J. W., N. Maccoby, and P. D. Wood (1977). "Community Education for Cardiovascular Health," *Lancet* 1(8023) June: 1192–95.

Farrant, W. and A. Taft (1988). "Building Healthy Public Policy in an Unhealthy Political Climate: A Case Study from Paddington and North Kensington," *Health Promotion International* 3: 287–92.

Fedder, D. O. (1982). "Managing Medication and Compliance: Physician-Pharmacist-Patient Interactions," *Journal American Geriatric Society* 11(Suppl): 113–17.

Fedder, D. and R. Beardsley (1979). "Preparing Pharmacy Patient Educators," *American Journal of Pharmacy Education* 43(2): 127–29.

Feighery, E. and T. Rogers (1990). "Building and Maintaining Effective Coalitions," *How-To Guides on Community Health Promotion* (Palo Alto, CA: Health Promotion Resource Center, Stanford Center for Research on Disease Prevention).

Feldman, R. H. (1983). "Strategies for Improving Compliance with Health Promotion Programs in Industry," *Health Education* 14(4): 21–25.

Feldman, R. H. (1984). "Increasing Compliance in Worksite Health Promotion: Organizational, Educational, and Psychological Strategies," *Corporate Commentary* 1(2): 45–50.

Fellman, C. and M. Fellman (1981). *Making Sense of Self: Medical Advice Literature in Late Nineteenth-Century America* (Philadelphia: University of Pennsylvania Press).

Fielding, J. E. (1982). "Effectiveness of Employee Health Improvement Programs," *Journal of Occupational Medicine* 24: 907–16.

Fielding, J. E. (1982). "Preventive Medicine and the Bottom Line," *Journal of Occupational Medicine* 24: 907–16.

Fielding, J. E. (1984). "Health Promotion and Disease Prevention at the Worksite," *Annual Review of Public Health* 5: 237–65.

Fielding, J. E. (1990). "Worksite Health Promotion Programs in the United States: Progress, Lessons, and Challenges," *Health Promotion International* 5: 75–84.

Fielding, J. E. and L. Breslow (1983). "Health Promotion Programs Sponsored by California Employers," *American Journal of Public Health* 73: 538–42.

Fielding, J. E. and Nelson, S. (1976). "Health Education for Job Corps Enrollees," *Public Health Reports* 91: 243–48.

Fielding, J. E. and P. V. Piserchia (1989). "Frequency of Worksite Health Promotion Activities," *American Journal of Public Health* 79: 16–20.

Figa-Talamanca, I. (1975). "Problems in the Evaluation of Training of Health Personnel," *Health Education Monographs* 3(Fall): 232–50.

Fincham, J. and A. Wertheimer (1985). "Using the Health Belief Model to Predict Initial Drug Therapy Defaulting," *Social Science and Medicine* 20: 101–05.

Fink, R. and S. Shapiro (1990). "Significance of Increased Efforts to Gain Participation in Screening for Breast Cancer," *American Journal of Preventive Medicine* 6: 34–41.

Finnegan, J. R., Jr., D. M. Murray, C. Kurth, and P. McCarthy (1989). "Measuring and Tracking Education Program Implementation: The Minnesota Heart Health Program Experience," *Health Education Quarterly* 16: 77–90.

Fiori, F. B., M. de la Vega, and M. J. Vacarro (1974). "Health Education in a Hospital Setting: Report of a Public Health Service Project in Newark, New Jersey," *Health Education Monographs* 2(1): 11–29.

First International Conference on Health Promotion (1986). "The Ottawa Charter for Health Promotion," *Health Promotion* 1(4): iii–v.

Fisher, A. A. (1978). "The Health Belief Model and Contraceptive Behavior: Limits to the Application of a Conceptual Framework," *Health Education Monographs* 5: 244–48.

Fisher, A., L. W. Green, A. McCrae, and C. Cochran (1976). "Training Teachers in Population Education Institutes in Baltimore," *Journal of School Health* 46: 357–60.

Fisher, A., J. Laign, and J. Stoeckel (1983). *Handbook for Family Planning Research Design* (New York: Population Council).

Fisher, S., B. Mansbridge, and D. A. Lankford (1982). "Public Judgments of Information in a Diazepam Patient Package Insert," *Archives of General Psychiatry* 39: 707–11.

Flay, B. R. (1985). "Psychosocial Approaches to Smoking Prevention: A Review of Findings," *Health Psychology* 4: 449–88.

Flay, B. R. (1986). "Efficacy and Effectiveness Trials in the Development of Health Promotion Programs," *Preventive Medicine* 15: 451–74.

Flay, B. R. (1986). "Mass Media Linkages with School-Based Programs for Drug Abuse Preventions," *Journal of School Health* 56: 402–6.

Flay, B. R. (1987). "Social Psychological Approaches to Smoking Prevention: Review and Recommendations," in *Advances in Health Education and Promotion*, vol. 2, W. B. Ward and P. D. Mullen, eds. (Greenwich, CT: JAI Press), pp. 121–80.

Flay, B. R. and T. D. Cook (1981). "Evaluation of Mass Media Prevention Campaigns," in *Public Communication Campaigns*, R. E. Rice and W. J. Paisley, eds. (London: Sage), pp. 239–64.

Fletcher, S. W., T. M. Morgan, M. S. O'Malley et al. (1989). "Is Breast Self-Examination Predicted by Knowledge, Attitudes, Beliefs, or Sociodemographic Characteristics?" *American Journal of Preventive Medicine* 5: 207–16.

Focal Points (Atlanta: Bureau of Health Education, Centers for Disease Control, U.S. Department of Health, Education, and Welfare, July 1977).

Folch-Lyon, E. and J. F. Trost (1981). "Conducting Focus Group Sessions," *Studies in Family Planning* 12: 443–49.

Fonaroff, A. (1983). *Community Involvement in Health Systems for Primary Health Care* (Geneva: World Health Organization SHS/83.6).

Food and Nutrition Board, National Research Council (1989). *Diet and Health* (Washington, DC: National Academy Press).

Fors, S. W., S. Owen, W. D. Hall et al. (1989). "Evaluation of a Diffusion Strategy for School-Based Hypertension Education," *Health Education Quarterly* 16: 255–61.

Fortmann, S. P., P. T. Williams, S. B. Hulley et al. (1981). "Effect of Health Education on Dietary Behavior: The Stanford Three-Community Study," *American Journal of Clinical Nutrition* 34: 565–71.

France, R. D., J. L. Houpt, C. S. Orleans, and P. J. Trent (1979). "Teaching Psychotherapy Interventions to Family Practice Residents: A Controlled Study," *American Journal of Psychiatry* 136: 1596–97.

Frank, G. C., A. Vaden, and J. Martin (1987). "School Health Promotion: Child Nutrition," *Journal of School Health* 57: 451–60.

Franz, J. C. and R. J. Weisser, Jr. (1978). "Venereal Disease Education in West Virginia, USA," *British Journal of Venereal Diseases* 54: 269–73.

Franz, M., A. Kresnick, B. Maschak-Carey et al. (1986). *Goals for Diabetes Education* (Alexandria, VA: American Diabetes Association).

Frederiksen, L. W., L. J. Solomon, and K. A. Brehony, eds. (1984). *Marketing Health Behavior: Principles, Techniques, and Applications* (New York: Plenum).

Freeman, H. P. (1989). "Cancer in the Economically Disadvantaged," *Cancer* 64(Suppl): 324–34.

Freire, P. (1970). *Pedagogy of the Oppressed* (New York: The Seabury Press).

Freudenberg, N. (1978). "Shaping the Future of Health Education: From Behavior Change to Social Change," *Health Education Monographs* 6: 372–77.

Freudenberg, N. (1984). "Citizen Action for Environmental Health: Report on a Survey of Community Organizations," *American Journal of Public Health* 74(1984): 444–48.

Freudenberg, N. (1984). *Not in Our Backyards! Community Action for Health and the Environment* (New York: Monthly Review Press).

Freudenberg, N. (1984–85). "Training Health Educators for Social Change," *International Quarterly of Community Health Education* 5: 37–52.

Freudenberg, N. and M. Golub (1987). "Health Education, Public Policy, and Disease Prevention: A Case History of the New York City Coalition to End Lead Poisoning," *Health Education Quarterly* 14: 387–401.

Fried, L. P. and T. L. Bush (1988). "Morbidity as the Focus of Prevention in the Elderly," *Epidemiological Review* 103: 48–64.

Friedman, L., E. Lichtenstein, and A. Biglan (1985). "Smoking Onset Among Teens: An Empirical Analysis of Initial Situations," *Addictive Behaviors* 10: 1–13.

Fries, J., L. W. Green, and S. Levine (1989). "Health Promotion and the Compression of Morbidity," *Lancet* 1: 481–84.

Fuchs, J. A. (1988). "Planning for Community Health Promotion: A Rural Example," *Health Values* 12(6): 3–8.

Garfield, S. R. (1970). "The Delivery of Medical Care," *Scientific American* 222: 15–18.

Garr, D. R. (1989). "Community-Oriented Primary Care," *Journal of Family Practice* 28: 654.

Garraway, W. M. and J. P. Whisnant (1987). "The Changing Pattern of Hypertension and the Declining Incidence of Stroke," *Journal of the American Medical Association* 258: 214–17.

Geiger, H. J. (1984). "Community Health Centers: Health Care as an Instrument of Social Change," in *Reforming Medicine: Lessons of the Last Quarter Century*, V. Sidel and R. Sidel, eds. (New York: Pantheon).

Gemson, D. H. and J. Elinson (1986). "Prevention in Primary Care: Variability in Physician Practice Patterns in New York City," *American Journal of Preventive Medicine* 2: 226–34.

General Professional Education of Physicians Panel (1984). *Physicians for the Twenty-First Century: The GPEP Report* (Washington, DC: Association of American Medical Colleges).

George, L. K. (1981). "Subjective Well-Being: Conceptual and Methodological Issues," in *Annual Review of Gerontology and Geriatrics*, vol. 2, C. Eisdorfer, ed. (New York: Springer), pp. 345–82.

German, P. S., L. E. Klein, S. J. McPhee, and C. R. Smith (1982). "Knowledge of and Compliance with Drug Regimens in the Elderly," *Journal of the American Geriatric Society* 30: 568–71.

German, P. S., S. Shapiro, and E. A. Skinner et al. (1987). "Detection and Management of Mental-Health Problems of Older Patients by Primary Care Providers," *Journal of the American Medical Association* 257: 489–93.

Gerstein, D., ed. (1984). *Toward the Prevention of Alcohol Problems* (Washington, DC: National Academy Press).

Giannetti, V., J. Reynolds, and T. Rihn (1985). "Factors Which Differentiate Smokers from Ex-Smokers Among Cardiovascular Patients: A Discriminant Analysis," *Social Science and Medicine* 20: 241–45.

Gielen, A. C. and S. Radius (1984). "Project KISS (Kids in Safety Belts): Educational Approaches and Evaluation Measures," *Health Education* 15(Aug/Sept): 43–47.

Gilbert, G. G., R. L. Davis, and C. L. Damberg (1985). "Current Federal Activities in School Health Education," *Public Health Reports* 100: 499–507.

Gilmore, G. D. (1977). "Needs Assessment Processes for Community Health Education," *International Journal of Health Education* 20: 164–73.

Gilmore, G. D., M. D. Campbell, and B. L. Becker (1989). *Needs Assessment Strategies for Health Education and Health Promotion* (Indianapolis: Benchmark Press).

Gittenberg, J. (1974). "Adapting Health Care to a Cultural Setting," *American Journal of Nursing* 74: 2218–21.

Glanz, K., F. M. Lewis, and B. K. Rimer, eds. (1990). *Health Behavior and Health Education: Theory, Research, and Practice* (San Francisco: Jossey-Bass).

Glasgow, R., R. Klesges, J. Mizes, and T. Pechacek (1985). "Quitting Smoking: Strategies Used and Variables Associated with Success in a Stop-Smoking Contest," *Journal of Consulting and Clinical Psychology* 53: 905–12.

Glasgow, R. E., L. Schafer, and H. K. O'Neill, (1981). "Self-Help Books and Amount of Therapist Contact in Smoking Cessation Programs," *Journal of Consulting and Clinical Psychology* 49: 659–67.

Glik, D., A. Gordon, W. Ward et al. (1987–88). "Focus Group Methods for Formative Research in Child Survival: An Ivoirian Example," *International Quarterly of Community Health Education* 8: 297–316.

Glynn, S. M., C. L. Gruder, J. A. Jerski (1986). "Effects on Treatment Success and on Mis-Reporting Abstinence," *Health Psychology* 5(2): 125–36.

Glynn, S. M. and A. J. Ruderman (1986). "The Development and Validation of an Eating Self-Efficacy Scale," *Cognitive Therapy and Research* 10: 403–20.

Glynn, T. J. (1981). "Psychological Sense of Community: Measurement and Application," *Human Relations* 34: 789–818.

Glynn, T. J., ed. (1983). *Women and Drugs: Research Issues* 31, (Washington, DC: U.S. Government Printing Office, DHHS Pub. No. 271–80–3720).

Glynn, T. J. (1989). "Essential Elements of School-Based Smoking Prevention Programs," *Journal of School Health* 59: 181–88.

Gochman, D. S. and G. S. Parcel, eds. (1982). "Children's Health Beliefs and Health Behaviors," *Health Education Quarterly* 9: 104–270 (whole issue).

Godin, G. and R. J. Shephard (1990). "An Evaluation of the Potential Role of the Physician in Influencing Community Exercise Behavior," *American Journal of Health Promotion* 4: 255–59.

Goeppinger, J. and A. J. Baglioni (1985). "Community Competence: A Positive Approach to Needs Assessment," *American Journal of Community Psychology* 13: 507–23.

Goldbloom, R. B. and R. N. Battista (1986). "The Periodic Health Examination: 1. Introduction," *Canadian Medical Association Journal* 134: 721–23.

Goldbloom, R. B. and R. S. Lawrence, eds. (1990). *Preventing Disease: Beyond the Rhetoric* (New York: Springer-Verlag).

Goldsmith, F. and L. E. Kerr (1983). "Worker Participation in Job Safety and Health," *Journal of Public Health Policy* 4: 447–66.

Goldstein, B., P. M. Fischer, J. W. Richards et al. (1987). "Smoking Counseling Practices of Recently Trained Family Physicians," *Journal of Family Practice* 24: 195–97.

Goldstein, M., S. Greenwald, T. Nathan et al. (1977). "Health Behavior and Genetic Screening for Carriers of Tay-Sachs Disease: A Prospective Study," *Social Science and Medicine* 11: 515–20.

Goldston, S. E., R. H. Ojemann, and R. H. Nelson (1975). "Primary Prevention and Health Promotion," in E. J. Lieberman, ed., *Mental Health: The Public Health Challenge* (Washington, DC: American Public Health Association).

Goodman, L. E. and M. J. Goodman (1986). "Prevention—How Misuse of a Concept Can Undercut Its Worth," *Hastings Center Report* 3: 26–38.

Goodman, R. M. and A. B. Steckler (1987–88). "The Life and Death of a Health Promotion Program: An Institutionalization Case Study," *International Quarterly of Community Health Education* 8: 5–21.

Goodman, R. M. and A. Steckler (1989). "A Framework for Assessing Program Institutionalization," *Knowledge in Society* 2: 57–71.

Goodman, R. M. and A. B. Steckler (1989). "A Model for the Institutionalization of Health Promotion Programs," *Family and Community Health* 11(4): 63–78.

Goodman, R. M. and A. B. Steckler (1990). "Mobilizing Organizations for Health Enhancement," in *Health Behavior and Health Education*, K. Glanz, F. M. Lewis, and B. K. Rimer, eds. (San Francisco: Jossey-Bass), pp. 314–41.

Goodstadt, M., R. I. Simpson, and P. O. Loranger (1987). "Health Promotion: A Conceptual Integration," *American Journal of Health Promotion* 1: 58–63.

Gordon, A. J. (1988). "Mixed Strategies in Health Education and Community Participation: An Evaluation of Dengue Control in the Dominican Republic," *Health Education Research Theory and Practice* 3: 399–419.

Gordon, N. (1986). "Never Smokers, Triers, and Current Smokers: Three Distinct Target Groups for School-Based Antismoking Programs," *Health Education Quarterly* 13: 163–80.

Gordon, T., M. Fisher, N. Ernst, and B. M. Rifkind (1982). "Relation of Diet to LDL Cholesterol, VLDL Cholesterol, and Plasma Total Cholesterol and Triglycerides in White Adults: The Lipid Research Clinics Prevalence Study," *Arteriosclerosis* 2: 502–12.

Gottlieb, N. (1983). "The Effect of Health Beliefs on the Smoking of College Women," *Journal of American College Health* 31: 214–21.

Gottlieb, N. H., M. P. Eriksen, and C. Y. Lovato et al. (1990). "Impact of a Restrictive Work Site Smoking Policy on Smoking Behavior, Attitudes, and Norms," *Journal of Occupational Medicine* 32: 20–23.

Gottlieb, N. H. and L. W. Green (1984). "Life Events, Social Network, Life-Style, and Health: An Analysis of the 1979 National Survey of Personal Health Practices and Consequences," *Health Education Quarterly* 11: 91–105.

Gottlieb, N. H. and L. W. Green (1987). "Ethnicity and Lifestyle Health Risk: Some Possible Mechanisms," *American Journal of Health Promotion* 2: 37–45.

Gottlieb, N. H., C. Y. Lovato, M. P. Eriksen, and L. W. Green (1990). "The Implementation of a Restrictive Worksite Smoking Policy in a Large Decentralized Agency," (unpublished).

Gottlieb, N. H., P. D. Mullen, and A. L. McAlister (1987). "Patients' Substance Abuse and the Primary Care Physician: Patterns of Practice," *Addictive Behavior* 12: 32–33.

Gottlieb, N. H. and A. Nelson (1990). "A Systematic Effort to Reduce Smoking at the Worksite," *Health Education Quarterly* 17: 99–118.

Gottlieb, S. (1986). "Ensuring Access to Health Care: What Communities Can Do to Make a Difference Through Private Sector Coalitions," *Inquiry* 23: 322–29.

Governor of Mississippi (1980). *Social Reconnaissance: State of Mississippi* (Jackson, MS: Office of the Governor).

Great Britain Expenditures Committee (1977). *First Report from the Expenditures Committee. Session 1976–1977: Preventive Medicine* (London: Her Majesty's Stationery Office).

Green, L. W. (1970). "Should Health Education Abandon Attitude-Change Strategies? Perspectives from Recent Research," *Health Education Monographs* 1(30): 25–48.

Green, L. W. (1970). *Status Identity and Preventive Health Behavior* (Berkeley: Pacific Health Education Reports No. 1, University of California School of Public Health).

Green, L. W. (1974). "Toward Cost-Benefit Evaluations of Health Education: Some Concepts, Methods, and Examples," *Health Education Monographs* 2(Suppl 1): 34–64.

Green, L. W. (1975). "Diffusion and Adoption of Innovations Related to Cardiovascular Risk Behavior in the Public," in *Applying Behavioral Sciences to Cardiovascular Risk*, A. Enelow and J. B. Henderson, eds. (New York: American Heart Association).

Green, L. W. (1976). "Change Process Models in Health Education," *Public Health Reviews* 5: 5–33.

Green, L. W. (1976). "Site- and Symptom-Related Factors in Secondary Prevention of Cancer," in *Cancer: The Behavioral Dimensions*, J. Cullen, B. Fox, and R. Isom, eds. (New York: Raven Press), pp. 45–61.

Green, L. W. (1977). "Evaluation and Measurement: Some Dilemmas for Health Education," *American Journal of Public Health* 67: 155–61.

Green, L. W. (1978). "Determining the Impact and Effectiveness of Health Education as It Relates to Federal Policy," *Health Education Monographs* 6: 28–66.

Green, L. W. (1978). "The Oversimplification of Policy Issues in Prevention," *American Journal of Public Health* 68: 953–54.

Green, L. W. (1979). "Health Promotion Policy and the Placement of Responsibility for Personal Health Care," *Family and Community Health* 2: 51–64.

Green, L. W. (1979). "National Policy in the Promotion of Health," *International Journal of Health Education* 22: 161–68.

Green, L. W. (1979). "Toward National Policy for Health Education," in *Alcohol, Youth, and Social Policy*, H. Blane and M. E. Chafetz, eds. (New York: Plenum), pp. 283–305.

Green, L. W. (1980). "Current Report: Office of Health Information, Health Promotion, and Physical Fitness and Sports Medicine," *Health Education* 11: 28.

Green, L. W. (1980). "Healthy People: The Surgeon General's Report and the Prospects," in *Working for a Healthier America*, W. J. McNerney, ed. (Cambridge: Ballinger), pp. 95–110.

Green, L. W. (1980). "To Educate or Not to Educate: Is That the Question?" *American Journal of Public Health* 70(1980): 625–26.

Green, L. W. (1980). *Toward a Healthy Community: Organizing Events for Community Health Promotion* (Washington, DC: U.S. Department of Health and Human Services, Public Health Service, Office of Disease Prevention and Health Promotion, 80-50113).

Green, L. W. (1981). "Emerging Federal Perspectives on Health Promotion," in *Health Promotion Monographs*, no. 1, J. P. Allegrante, ed. (New York: Teachers College, Columbia University).

Green, L. W. (1982). "Reconciling Policy in Health Education and Primary Health Care," *International Journal of Health Education* 24(Suppl 3): 1–11.

Green, L. W. (1983). "New Policies in Education for Health," *World Health* (April/May): 13–17.

Green, L. W. (1984). "A Participant-Observer During a Period of Professional Change," in *Advancing Health Through Education: A Case Study Approach*, H. P. Cleary, J. M. Kichen, and P. G. Ensor, eds. (Palo Alto, CA: Mayfield), pp. 374–81.

Green, L. W. (1984). "Health Education Models," in *Behavioral Health: A Handbook of Health Enhancement and Disease Prevention*, J. D. Matarazzo, S. M. Weiss, J. A. Herd et al., eds. (New York: Wiley), pp. 181–98.

Green, L. W. (1984). "Modifying and Developing Health Behavior," *Annual Review of Public Health* 5: 215–36.

Green, L. W. (1984). "A Triage and Stepped Approach to Self-Care Education," *Medical Times* 111: 75–80.

Green, L. W. (1985). "Some Challenges to Health Services Research on Children and Elderly," *Health Service Research* 19: 793–815.

Green, L. W. (1986). "Evaluation Model: A Framework for the Design of Rigorous Evaluation of Efforts in Health Promotion," *American Journal of Health Promotion* 1(1): 77–79.

Green, L. W. (1986). "Individuals vs. Systems: An Artificial Classification That Divides and Distorts," *Health Link* (National Center for Health Education) 2: 29–30.

Green, L. W. (1986). "Models of Health Education," in *Behavioral Health: A Handbook of Health Enhancement and Disease Prevention*, J. Matarazzo, S. M. Weiss, J. A. Herd et al., eds. (New York: Wiley).

Green, L. W. (1986). *New Policies for Health Education in Primary Health Care* (Geneva: World Health Organization).

Green, L. W. (1986). "Research Agenda: Building a Consensus on Research Questions," *American Journal of Health Promotion* 1(2): 70–72.

Green, L. W. (1986). "The Theory of Participation: A Qualitative Analysis of Its Expression in National and International Health Policies," in *Advances in Health Education and Promotion*, vol. 1, pt A, W. B. Ward, ed. (Greenwich, CT: JAI Press), pp. 211–36.

Green, L. W. (1987). "How Physicians Can Improve Patients' Participation and Maintenance in Self-Care," *Western Journal of Medicine* 147: 346–49.

Green, L. W. (1987). *Program Planning and Evaluation Guide for Lung Associations* (New York: American Lung Association).

Green, L. W. (1987). "Three Ways Research Influences Policy and Practice: The Public's Right to Know and the Scientist's Responsibility to Educate," *Health Education* 18(Aug/Sept): 44–49.

Green, L. W. (1988). "Bridging the Gap Between Community Health and School Health," *American Journal of Public Health* 78: 1149.

Green, L. W. (1988). "Policies for Decentralization and Development of Health Education," *Revue Saude Publica* (Sao Paulo, Brazil) 22: 217–20.

Green, L. W. (1988). "Promoting the One-Child Policy of China," *Journal of Public Health Policy* 9: 273–83.

Green, L. W. (1988). "The Trade-Offs Between the Expediency of Health Promotion and the Durability of Health Education," in *Topics in Health Psychology*, S. Maes, C. D. Spielberger, P. B. Defares, and I. G. Sarason, eds. (New York: Wiley), pp. 301–12.

Green, L. W. (1989). "Comment: Is Institutionalization the Proper Goal of Grantmaking?" *American Journal of Health Promotion* 3: 44.

Green, L. W. (1990). *Community Health*, 6th ed. (St. Louis: Times Mirror/Mosby).

Green, L. W. (1990). "The Revival of Community and the Obligation of Academic Health Centers to the Public," in *Institutional Values and Human Environments for Teaching, Inquiry, and Practice*, R. J. Bulger, S. J. Reiser, and R. E. Bulger, eds. (Des Moines: University of Iowa Press).

Green, L. W., R. Blakenbaker, F. Trevino et al. (1987). "Report of the Subcommittee on Data Gaps in Disease Prevention and Health Promotion," *Annual Report of the U.S. National Committee on Vital and Health Statistics* (Washington, DC: National Center for Health Statistics).

Green, L. W. and P. Brooks-Bertram (1978). "Peer Review and Quality Control in Health Education," *Health Values* 2: 191–97.

Green, L. W., M. P. Eriksen, and E. L. Schor (1988). "Preventive Practices by Physicians: Behavioral Determinants and Potential Interventions," *American Journal of Preventive Medicine* 4(Suppl 4, 1988): 101–17, reprinted in R. N. Battista and R. S. Lawrence, eds., *Implementing Preventive Services* (New York: Oxford University Press), pp. 101–17.

Green, L. W. and R. Faden (1977). "Potential Effects of Patient Package Inserts on Patients and Drug Consumers," *Drug Information Journal* 2(Suppl): 64–70.

Green, L. W. and D. Fedder (1977). "Drug Information: The Pharmacist and the Community," *American Journal of Pharmaceutical Education* 41: 444–48.

Green, L. W. and I. Figa-Talamanca (1974). "Suggested Designs for Evaluation of Patient Education Programs," *Health Education Monographs* 2: 54–71.

Green, L. W., A. Fisher, R. Amin, and A. B. M. Shafiullah (1975). "Paths to the Adoption of Family Planning: A Time-Lagged Correlation Analysis of the Dacca Experiment in Bangladesh," *International Journal of Health Education* 18: 85–96.

Green, L. W., R. A. Goldstein, and S. R. Parker, eds. (1983). "Research on Self-Management of Childhood Asthma," *Journal of Allergy and Clinical Immunology* 72: 519–629.

Green, L. W. and N. Gordon (1982). "Productive Research Designs for Health Education Investigations," *Health Education* 13(May/June): 4–10.

Green, L. W., N. H. Gottlieb, and G. S. Parcel (in press). "Diffusion Theory Extended and Applied," in *Advances in Health Education and Promotion*, vol. 3, W. Ward and F. M. Lewis, eds. (London: Jessica Kingsley Publishers).

Green, L. W., P. Heit, D. C. Iverson, L. J. Kolbe, and M. Kreuter (1980). "The School Health Curriculum Project: Its Theory, Practice, and Measurement Experience," *Health Education Quarterly* 7: 14–34.

Green, L. W., P. Hogan, and M. Deutsch (1987). *Estimating Need: Manual for Estimating Prevalence of Women at Risk of Poor Pregnancy Outcomes Due to Smoking* (Houston: Center for Health Promotion Research and Development, University of Texas Health Science Center).

Green, L. W. and M. W. Kreuter. (1990). "Health Promotion as a Public Health Strategy for the 1990s," *Annual Review of Public Health*, vol. 11, L. Breslow, ed. (Palo Alto, CA: Annual Reviews Inc.), pp. 319–34.

Green, L. W., M. W. Kreuter, S. G. Deeds, and K. B. Partridge (1980). *Health Education Planning: A Diagnostic Approach* (Palo Alto, CA: Mayfield).

Green, L. W. and K. J. Krotki (1968). "Class and Parity Biases in Family Planning Programs: The Case of Karachi," *Social Biology* 15: 235–51.

Green, L. W., D. M. Levine, and S. G. Deeds (1975). "Clinical Trials of Health Education for Hypertensive Outpatients: Design and Baseline Data," *Preventive Medicine* 4: 417–25.

Green, L. W., D. M. Levine, J. Wolle, and S. G. Deeds (1979). "Development of Randomized Patient Education Experiments with Urban Poor Hypertensives," *Patient Counseling and Health Education* 1: 106–11.

Green, L. W. and F. M. Lewis (1986). *Measurement and Evaluation in Health Education and Health Promotion* (Palo Alto, CA: Mayfield).

Green, L. W., F. M. Lewis, and D. M. Levine (1980). "Balancing Statistical Data and Clinician Judgments in the Diagnosis of Patient Educational Needs," *Journal of Community Health* 6: 79–91.

Green, L. W. and A. L. McAlister (1984). "Macro-Intervention to Support Health Behavior: Some Theoretical Perspectives and Practical Reflections," *Health Education Quarterly* 11: 323–39.

Green, L. W., P. D. Mullen, and R. Friedman (1986). "An Epidemiological Approach to Targeting Drug Information," *Patient Education and Counseling* 8: 255–68.

Green, L. W., P. D. Mullen, and S. Maloney, eds. (1984). "Large-Scale Health Education Campaigns," *Health Education Quarterly* 11: 221–339.

Green, L. W., P. D. Mullen, and G. L. Stainbrook (1986). "Programs to Reduce Drug Errors in the Elderly: Direct and Indirect Evidence from Patient Education," *Journal of Geriatric Drug Therapy* 1: 3–16.

Green, L. W. and J. Raeburn (1988). "Health Promotion: What Is It? What Will It Become?" *Health Promotion International* 3: 151–59.

Green, L. W., B. Rimer, T. W. Elwood (1981). "Biobehavioral Approaches to Cancer Prevention and Detection," in *Perspectives on Behavioral Medicine*, S. Weiss, A. Herd, and B. Fox, eds. (New York: Academic Press), pp. 215–34.

Green, L. W., B. Rimer, and T. W. Elwood (1982). "Public Education," in *Cancer Epidemiology and Prevention*, D. Shottenfeld and J. Fraumeni, Jr., eds. (Philadelphia: W. B. Saunders), pp. 1100–10.

Green, L. W. and B. J. Roberts (1974). "The Research Literature on Why Women Delay in Seeking Medical Care for Breast Symptoms," *Health Education Monographs* 2: 129–77.

Green, L. W. and D. G. Simons-Morton (1990). "Education and Life-Style Determinants of Health and Disease," in *Oxford Textbook of Public Health*, 2nd ed., W. W. Holland, R. Detels, and G. Knox, eds. (London: Oxford University Press).

Green, L. W., G. L. Stainbrook, and C. Y. Lovato (in press). "The Benefits Perceived by Industry in Supporting Health Promotion Programs in the Worksite," in *Proceedings of the Harvard Symposium on Worksite Health Promotion* (Baltimore: Johns Hopkins University Press).

Green, L. W., V. L. Wang, S. G. Deeds et al. (1978). "Guidelines for Health Education in Maternal and Child Health Programs," *International Journal of Health Education* 21(Suppl): 1–33.

Green, L. W., V. L. Wang, and P. Ephross (1974). "A Three-Year Longitudinal Study of The Effectiveness of Nutrition Aides on Rural Poor Homemakers," *American Journal of Public Health* 64: 722–24.

Green, L. W., S. H. Werlin, H. H. Shauffler, and C. H. Avery (1977). "Research and Demonstration Issues In Self-Care: Measuring the Decline of Medicocentrism," *Health Education Monographs* 5: 161–89; also in *The SOPHE Heritage Collection of Health Education Monographs*, vol. 3, J. G. Zapka, ed. (Oakland, CA: Third Party Publishing), pp. 40–69.

Green, L. W., A. L. Wilson, and C. Y. Lovato (1986). "What Changes Can Health Promotion Achieve and How Long Do These Changes Last? The Tradeoffs Between Expediency and Durability," *Preventive Medicine* 15: 508–21.

Green, L. W., R. W. Wilson, and K. G. Bauer (1983). "Data Required to Measure Progress on the Objectives for the Nation in Disease Prevention and Health Promotion," *American Journal of Public Health* 73: 18–24.

Greenberg, J. S. (1987). *Health Education: Learner Centered Instructional Strategies* (Dubuque: Wm. C. Brown).

Gregor, F. M. (1984). "Factors Affecting the Use of Self-Instructional Material by Patients with Ischemic Heart Disease," *Patient Education and Counseling* 6: 155–59.

Grundy, S. M., P. Greenland, J. A. Herd et al. (1987). "Cardiovascular and Risk Factor Evaluation of Healthy American Adults: A Statement for Physicians by an Ad Hoc Committee Appointed by the Steering Committee, American Heart Association," *Circulation* 97: 1340A–62A.

Guba, E. G. and Y. S. Lincoln (1989). *Fourth Generation Evaluation* (Newbury Park, CA: Sage).

Guild, P. A. (1990). "Goal-Oriented Evaluation as a Program Management Tool," *American Journal of Health Promotion* 4: 296–301.

Gustafson, D. (1979). *An Approach to Predicting the Implementation Potential of Recommended Actions in Health Planning* (Madison, WI: The Institute for Health Planning).

Haefele, D. L. (1990). "A Survey of Non-Smoking Policies in Ninety-One Large Businesses, Companies, and Agencies," *Health Education* 21(4): 47–53.

Hall, J. A., D. L. Roter, and N. R. Katz (1988). "Meta-Analysis of Correlates of Provider Behavior in Medical Encounters," *Medical Care* 26: 657–75.

Hallal, J. (1979). "The Relationship of Health Beliefs, Health Locus of Control, and Self Concept to the Practice of Breast Self-Examination in Adult Women," *Nursing Research* 20: 17–29.

Hammond, E. C. and L. Garfinkel (1969). "Coronary Heart Disease, Stroke, and Aortic Aneurysm: Factors in the Etiology," *Archives of Environmental Health* 19: 167–82.

Hancock, T. (1985). "Beyond Health Care: From Public Health Policy to Healthy Public Policy," *Canadian Journal of Public Health* 76: 9–11.

Handbook for Evaluating Drug Abuse and Alcohol Prevention Programs (1987). (Rockville, MD: Office of Substance Abuse Prevention, U.S. Department of Health and Human Services, DHHS (ADM) 87-1512).

Handel, G. and L. Rainwater (1964). "Persistence and Change in Working-Class Life Style," in *Blue-Collar World*, A. B. Shostack and W. Gomberg, eds. (Englewood Cliffs, NJ: Prentice-Hall), pp. 36–41.

Hanson, P. (1988–89). "Citizen Involvement in Community Health Promotion: A Rural Application of CDC's PATCH Model," *International Quarterly of Health Education* 9: 177–86.

Hardin, G. (1968). "The Tragedy of the Commons," *Science* 143: 1243–46.

Hargrove, E. (1975). *The Missing Link: The Study of the Implementation of Social Policy* (Washington, DC: The Urban Institute, paper 797–801).

Harris, R., M. W. Linn, and L. Pollack (1984). "Relationship Between Health Beliefs and Psychological Variables in Diabetic Patients," *British Journal of Medical Psychology* 57: 253–59.

Harris, R., J. Skyler, M. W. Linn et al. (1982). "Relationship Between the Health Belief Model and Compliance as a Basis for Intervention in Diabetes Mellitus," in *Pediatric and Adolescent Endocrinology: Vol 10 Psychological Aspects of Diabetes in Children and Adolescents*, Z. Loron and A. Galatzer, eds. (Basel, Switzerland: Karger), pp. 123–32.

Harrison, J. and S. Carlsson (1984). "Methodological Issues in Process and Outcome Studies: Psychophysiology, Systematic Desensitization, and Dental Fear," *Scandinavian Journal of Behaviour Therapy* 13: 97–116.

Harrison, J. A., P. D. Mullen, and L. W. Green (1990). "A Meta-Analysis of Studies of the Health Belief Model," *Health Education Research* 5(1990): in press.

Harrison, M. I. (1987). *Diagnosing Organizations: Methods, Models, and Processes* (Beverly Hills: Sage).

Hartman, P. and M. H. Becker (1978). "Non-Compliance with Prescribed Regime Among Chronic Hemodialysis Patients: A Method of Prediction and Educational Diagnosis," *Dialysis and Transplantation* 7: 978–89.

Harvard Total Project Manager II (1986). (Mountain View, CA: Software Publishing).

Haskell, W. L. and S. N. Blair (1982). "The Physical Activity Component of Health Promotion in Occupational Settings," in *Managing Health Promotion in the Workplace: Guidelines for Implementation and Evaluation*, R. S. Parkinson and Associates, eds. (Palo Alto, CA: Mayfield), pp. 252–71.

Hatch, J. W. and C. Jackson (1981). "The North Carolina Baptist Church Program," *Urban Health* 10(4): 70–71.

Hatcher, M. E., L. W. Green, D. M. Levine, and C. E. Flagle (1986). "Validation of a Decision Model for Triaging Hypertensive Patients to Alternate Health Education Interventions," *Social Science and Medicine* 22: 813–19.

Haughton, B. (1987). "Developing Local Food Policies: One City's Experiences," *Journal of Public Health Policy* 8: 180–91.

Hawthorne, V. M., G. Pohl, and G. V. Amburg (1984). *Smoking Is Killing Your Constituents: Deaths Due to Smoking by Michigan State Senate Districts* (Lansing, MI: Division of Health Education, Michigan Department of Public Health, Nov).

Haynes, R. B., D. A. Davis, A. McKibbon, and A. P. Tugwell (1984). "A Critical Appraisal of the Efficacy of Continuing Medical Education," *Journal of the American Medical Association* 251: 61–64.

Haynes, R. B., D. W. Taylor, and D. L. Sackett, eds. (1979). *Compliance in Health Care* (Baltimore: Johns Hopkins University Press).

Health and Welfare Canada (1988). *Canada's Health Promotion Survey: Technical Report* (Ottawa: Minister of Supply and Services Canada).

Health Education Center (1977). *Strategies for Health Education in Local Health Departments* (Baltimore: Maryland State Department of Health and Mental Hygiene).

Health Education Unit, Regional Office of Education, WHO Regional Office for Europe (1986). "Life-Styles and Health," *Social Science and Medicine* 22: 117–24.

Health Promotion: A Discussion Document on the Concept and Principles (Copenhagen: World Health Organization Regional Office for Europe, ICP/HSR 602, Sept 1984), reprinted in *Health Promotion* 1(1986): 73–76.

Healthy Communities 2000: Model Standards (1991). 3rd ed. (Washington, DC: American Public Health Association).

Healthy People 2000: National Health Promotion and Disease Prevention Objectives (1990). Conference ed. (Washington, DC: Public Health Service, U.S. Department of Health and Human Services).

Henderson, A. C. (1987). "Developing a Credentialing System for Health Educators," in *Advances in Health Education and Health Promotion*, vol. 2, W. B. Ward and S. K. Simonds, eds. (Greenwich, CT: JAI Press), pp. 59–91.

Henderson, A. C., J. M. Wolle, P. A. Cortese, and D. I. McIntosh (1981). "The Future of the Health Education Profession: Implications for Preparation and Practice," *Public Health Reports* 96: 555–60.

Hersey, J. C., L. S. Klibanoff, D. J. Lam, and R. L. Taylor (1984). "Promoting Social Support: The Impact of California's 'Friends Can Be Good Medicine' Campaign," *Health Education Quarterly* 11: 293–311.

Hershey, J., B. Morton, J. Davis, and M. Reichgott (1980). "Patient Compliance with Antihypertensive Medication," *American Journal of Public Health* 70: 1081–89.

Hertel, V. (1982). "Changing Times in School Nursing," *Journal of School Health* 52: 313–14.

Hill, I. T. (1988). *Reaching Women Who Need Prenatal Care* (Washington, DC: National Governors Association).

Hindi-Alexander, M. and G. J. Cropp (1981). "Community and Family Programs for Children with Asthma," *Annals of Allergy* 46: 143–48.

Hinthorne, R. A. and R. Jones (1978). "Coordinating Patient Education in the Hospital," *Hospitals* 52: 85–88.

Hochbaum, G. M. (1956). "Why People Seek Diagnostic X-Rays," *Public Health Reports* 71: 377–80.

Hochbaum, G. M. (1959). *Public Participation in Medical Screening Programs: A Social-Psychological Study* (Washington, DC: Public Health Service, PHS-572).

Hoffman, L. M. (1989). *The Politics of Knowledge: Activist Movements in Medicine and Planning* (Albany: State University of New York Press).

Hoffman, S. B. (1983). "Peer Counselor Training with the Elderly," *The Gerontologist* 23: 358–60.

Hollander, R. B. and J. G. Hale (1987). "Worksite Health Promotion Programs: Ethical Issues," *American Journal of Health Promotion* 2(2): 37–43.

Hollis, J., G. Sexton, S. Connors et al. (1984). "The Family Heart Dietary Intervention Program: Community Response and Characteristics of Joining and Nonjoining Families," *Preventive Medicine* 13: 276–85.

Holtzman, N. (1979). "Prevention: Rhetoric or Reality," *International Journal of Health Services* 9: 25–39.

Huberman, A. M. and M. B. Miles (1984). *Innovation Up Close: How School Improvement Works* (New York: Plenum Press).

Hunt, M. K., C. Lefebvre, M. L. Hixson et al. (1990). "Pawtucket Heart Health Program Point-of-Purchase Nutrition Education Program in Supermarkets," *American Journal of Public Health* 80: 730–31.

Hunt, S. M. (1988). "Subjective Health Indicators and Health Promotion," *Health Promotion* 3: 23–34.

Ingledew, D. (1989). "Target Setting for the Health of Populations: Some Observations," *Health Promotion* 4: 357–69.

Integration of Risk Factor Interventions (1986). (Washington, DC: ODPHP Monograph Series, U.S. Department of Health and Human Services).

Inui, T. S., W. B. Carter, R. E. Pecoraro et al. (1980). "Variations in Patient Compliance with Common Long-Term Drugs," *Medical Care* 17: 986–93.

Inui, T. S., E. Yourtee, and J. Williamson (1976). "Improved Outcomes in Hypertension After Physician Tutorials: A Controlled Trial," *Annals of Internal Medicine* 84: 646–51.

IOX Assessment Associates (1988). *Program Evaluation Handbook: Diabetes Education, ...Drug Abuse Education, ...Nutrition Education, ...Alcohol Abuse Education, ...Physical Fitness Programs, ...Stress Management* (Los Angeles: IOX Assessment Associates).

Isely, R. B. (1977). "The Village Health Committee: Starting Point for Rural Development," *WHO Chronical* 31: 307–15.

Israel, B. A. (1985). "Social Networks and Social Support: Implications for Natural Helper and Community Level Interventions," *Health Education Quarterly* 12: 65–80.

Iverson, D. C. and L. W. Green (1981). "Drug Abuse Prevention from a Public Health Perspective – A Proposal for the 1980s," in *NIDA Drug Abuse Prevention Monograph*, W. Bukowski, ed. (Washington, DC: National Institute of Drug Abuse).

Iverson, D. C. and L. J. Kolbe (1983). "Evaluation of the National Disease Prevention and Health Promotion Strategy: Establishing a Role for the Schools," *Journal of School Health* 53: 294–302.

Jaccard, J. (1975). "A Theoretical Analysis of Selected Factors Important to Health Education Strategies," *Health Education Monographs* 3: 152–67.

Jacobs, C., R. Ross, I. M. Walker et al. (1983). "Behavior of Cancer Patients: A Randomized Study of the Effects of Education and Peer Support Groups," *American Journal of Clinical Oncology* 6: 347–50.

Janis, I., ed. (1982). *Counseling on Personal Decisions* (New Haven: Yale University Press).

Janz, N. K. and M. H. Becker (1984). "The Health Belief Model: A Decade Later," *Health Education Quarterly* 11: 1–47.

Jasnoski, M. L. and G. E. Schwartz (1985). "A Synchronous Systems Model for Health," *American Behavioral Scientist* 28: 468–85.

Jenkins, C. D. (1966). "Group Differences in Perception: A Study of Community Beliefs and Feelings About Tuberculosis," *American Journal of Sociology* 71: 417–29.

Jenkins, C. D. (1979). "An Approach to the Diagnosis and Treatment of Problems of Health-Related Behavior," *International Journal of Health Education* 22(Suppl): 1–24.

Jette, A. M., K. M. Cummings, B. Brock et al. (1981). "The Structure and Reliability of Health Belief Indices," *Health Services Research* 16: 81–98.

Joseph, J., S. Montgomery, C. A. Emmons et al. (1987). "Magnitude and Determinants of Behavior Risk Reduction: Longitudinal Analysis of a Cohort at Risk for AIDS," *Psychology and Health* 1: 73–96.

Kaiser Family Foundation (1989). *Strategic Plan for the Health Promotion Program, 1989–1991* (Menlo Park, CA: The Henry J. Kaiser Family Foundation).

Kaiser Family Foundation (1990). *The Health Promotion Program of the Henry J. Kaiser Family Foundation* (Menlo Park, CA: The Henry J. Kaiser Family Foundation).

Kaluzny, A. D., A. Schenck, and T. Ricketts (1986). "Cancer Prevention in the Workplace: An Organizational Innovation," *Health Promotion* 1: 293–99.

Kanfer, F. H. and G. Saslow (1969). "Behavioral Diagnosis," in *Behavior Therapy: Appraisal and Status*, C. M. Franks, ed. (New York: McGraw-Hill).

Kannas, L. (1982). "The Dimensions of Health Behavior Among Young Men in Finland," *International Journal of Health Education* 24: 146–55.

Kantor, R. (1983). *The Change Masters* (New York: Simon and Schuster).

Kaplan, R. M. (1988). "Health-Related Quality of Life in Cardiovascular Disease," *Journal of Consulting and Clinical Psychology* 56: 382–92.

Kar, S. B. (1986). "Communication for Health Promotion: A Model for Research and Action," in *Advances in Health Education and Promotion*, vol. 1, pt A, W. B. Ward and S. B. Kar, eds. (Greenwich, CT: JAI Press), pp. 267–302.

Kar, S. B., ed. (1989). *Health Promotion Indicators and Actions* (New York: Springer).

Karasek, R. and T. Theorell (1990). *Healthy Work: Stress, Productivity, and the Reconstruction of Working Life* (New York: Basic Books).

Katatsky, M. E. (1977). "The Health Belief Model as a Conceptual Framework for Explaining Contraceptive Compliance," *Health Education Monographs* 5: 232–42.

Katz, S. ed. (1987). "The Portugal Conference: Measuring Quality of Life and Functional Status in Clinical Practice and Epidemiological Research," *Journal of Chronic Diseases* 40: whole issue 6.

Kegeles, S. S. (1963). "Why People Seek Dental Care: A Test of a Conceptual Formulation," *Journal of Health and Human Behavior* 4: 166–73.

Kegeles, S. S. (1969). "A Field Experiment Attempt to Change Beliefs and Behavior of Women in an Urban Ghetto," *Journal of Health and Social Behavior* 10: 115–24.

Keil, J. E. (1984). "Incidence of Coronary Heart Disease in Blacks in Charleston, South Carolina," *American Heart Journal* 108: 779.

Keintz, M. K., B. K. Rimer, L. Fleisher, and P. Engstrom (1988). "Educating Older Adults About Their Increased Cancer Risk," *Gerontologist* 28: 487–90.

Kemper, D. (1986). "The Healthwise Program: Growing Younger," in *Wellness and Health Promotion for the Elderly*, K. Dychtwald, ed. (Rockville, MD: Aspen), pp. 263–273.

Kernaghan, S. G. and R. E. Giloth (1988). *Tracking the Impact of Health Promotion on Organizations: A Key to Program Survival* (Chicago: American Hospital Association).

Key, M. and D. Kilian (1983). "Counseling and Cancer Prevention Programs in Industry," in *Cancer Prevention in Clinical Medicine*, G. R. Newell, ed. (New York: Raven Press).

Kickbusch, I. (1986). "Health Promotion: A Global Perspective," *Canadian Journal of Public Health* 77: 321–26.

Kickbusch, I. (1986). "Lifestyle and Health," *Social Science and Medicine* 22: 117–24.

Kickbusch, I. (1989). "Approaches to an Ecological Base for Public Health," *Health Promotion* 4: 265–68.

Kielhofner, G. and C. Nelson (1983). "A Study of Patient Motivation and Cooperation/Participation in Occupational Therapy," *Occupational Therapy Journal of Research* 3: 35–46.

King, A. C., J. E. Martin, E. M. Morrell et al. (1986). "Highlighting Specific Patient Education Needs in an Aging Cardiac Population," *Health Education Quarterly* 13: 29–38.

King, A. J. C. et al. (1986). *Canada Health Attitudes and Behaviors Survey: 9-, 12-, and 15-Year Olds, 1984–85* (Ottawa: Health and Welfare Canada, Health Promotion Directorate).

King, J. B. (1982). "The Impact of Patients' Perceptions of High Blood Pressure on Attendance at Screening: An Extension of the Health Belief Model," *Social Science and Medicine* 16: 1079–91.

King, J. B. (1984). "Psychology in Nursing, II. The Health Belief Model," *Nursing Times* 80(43): 53–55.

Kingsley, R. G. and J. Shapiro (1977). "A Comparison of Three Behavioral Programs for the Control of Obesity in Children," *Behavioral Theory* 8: 30–33.

Kirscht, J. P. (1974). "The Health Belief Model and Illness Behavior," *Health Education Monographs* 2: 387–408.

Kirscht, J., M. Becker, and J. Eveland (1976). "Psychological and Social Factors as Predictors of Medical Behavior," *Medical Care* 14: 422–31.

Kirscht, J. and I. Rosenstock (1977). "Patient Adherence to Antihypertensive Medical Regimens," *Journal of Community Health* 3: 115–24.

Klein, L. E., P. S. German, and D. M. Levine (1981). "Adverse Drug Reactions Among the Elderly: A Reassessment," *Journal of the American Geriatric Society* 29: 525–30.

Knight, B. P., M. S. O'Malley, and S. W. Fletcher (1987). "Physician Acceptance of a Computerized Health Maintenance Prompting Program," *American Journal of Preventive Medicine* 3: 19–24.

Knox, S. R., B. Mandel, and R. Lazarowicz (1981). "Profile of Callers to the VD National Hotline," *Sexually Transmitted Diseases* 8: 245–54.

Kok, G. J. and S. Siero (1985). "Tin-Recycling: Awareness, Comprehension, Attitude, Intention, and Behavior," *Journal of Economic Psychology* 6: 157–73.

Kolbe, L. J. (1982). "What Can We Expect from School Health Education?" *Journal of School Health* 52: 145–50.

Kolbe, L. J. (1984). "Improving the Health of Children and Youth: Frameworks for Behavioral Research and Development," in *Health Education and Youth: A Review of Research and Development*, G. Campbell, ed. (Philadelphia: Falmer Press), pp. 7–32.

Kolbe, L. J. (1986). "Increasing the Impact of School Health Promotion Programs: Emerging Research Perspectives," *Health Education* 17(5): 47–52.

Kolbe, L. J. (1989). "Indicators for Planning and Monitoring School Health Programs," in *Health Promotion Indicators and Actions*, S. B. Kar, ed. (New York: Springer), pp. 221–48.

Kolbe, L. J. and G. G. Gilbert (1984). "Involving the School in the National Strategy to Improve the Health of Americans," in *Proceedings, Prospects for a Healthier America* (Washington, DC: U.S. Department of Health and Human Services, Office of Disease Prevention and Health Promotion).

Kolbe, L. J., L. W. Green, J. Foreyt et al. (1985). "Appropriate Function of Health Education in Schools," in *Child Health Behavior*, N. Krasnagor, J. Arasteh, and M. Cataldo, eds. (New York: Wiley), pp. 171–209.

Kolbe, L., D. C. Iverson, M. W. Kreuter et al. (1981). "Propositions for an Alternate and Complementary Health Education Paradigm," *Health Education* 12(May/June): 24–30.

Kolbe, L., J. Jones, G. Nelson et al. (1988). "School Health Education to Prevent the Spread of AIDS: Overview of a National Programme," *Hygiene* 7: 10–13.

Korhonen, T., J. K. Huttunen, A. Aro et al. (1983). "A Controlled Trial on the Effects of Patient Education in Treatment of Insulin-Dependent Diabetes," *Diabetes Care* 6: 256–61.

Kosch, S. G. and J. J. Dallman (1983). "Essential Areas for Behavioral Science Training: A Needs Assessment Approach," *Journal of Medical Education* 58: 619–26.

Koshel, J. J. (1990). *An Overview of State Policies Affecting Adolescent Pregnancy and Parenting* (Washington, DC: National Governors' Association, 1990).

Kotchen, J. M., H. E. McKean, S. Jackson-Thayer et al. (1986). "Impact of a Rural High Blood Pressure Control Program on Hypertension Control and Cardiovascular Mortality," *Journal of the American Medical Association* 255: 2177–82.

Kotler, P. (1989). *Marketing for Non-Profit Organizations*, 3rd ed. (Englewood Cliffs, NJ: Prentice-Hall).

Kotler P. and E. L. Roberto (1989). *Social Marketing: Strategies for Changing Public Behavior* (New York: Free Press).

Kottke, T., J. Foels, C. Hill et al. (1984). "Nutrition Counseling in Private Practice: Attitudes and Activities of Family Physicians," *Preventive Medicine* 13: 219–25.

Kottke, T. E., P. Puska, J. T. Solonen et al. (1985). "Projected Effects of High-Risk Versus Population-Based Prevention Strategies in Coronary Heart Disease," *American Journal of Epidemiology* 121: 697–704.

Kraft, D. P. (1988). "The Prevention and Treatment of Alcohol Problems on a College Campus," *Journal of Alcohol and Drug Education* 34: 37–51.

Kreuter, M. W. (1984). "Health Promotion: The Public Health Role in the Community of Free Exchange," *Health Promotion Monographs*, no. 4, J. M. Dodds, ed. (New York: Teachers College, Columbia University).

Kreuter, M. W., ed. (1985). "Results of the School Health Education Evaluation," *Journal of School Health* 55(Oct): whole issue no. 8.

Kreuter, M. W. (1985). "Statement to the Michigan Senate Health Committee on Senate Bills 4 and 5," (Atlanta: Centers for Disease Control, 5 Feb), unpublished.

Kreuter, M. W. (1989). "Activity, Health, and the Public," in *Academy Papers* (Reston, VA: Academy of Physical Education, Alliance for Health, Physical Education, Recreation, and Dance), chap. 15.

Kreuter, M. W., G. M. Christensen, and R. Davis (1984). "School Health Education Research: Future Uses and Challenges," *Journal of School Health* 54: 27–32.

Kreuter, M. W., G. M. Christensen, and A. DiVincenzo (1982). "The Multiplier Effect of the Health Education-Risk Reduction Grants Program in 28 States and 1 Territory," *Public Health Reports* 97: 510–15.

Kreuter, M. W., G. M. Christiansen, M. Freston, and G. Nelson (1981). "In Search of a Baseline: The Need for Risk Prevalence Surveys," *Proceedings of the Annual National Risk Reduction Conference* (Atlanta: Centers for Disease Control).

Kreuter, M. W. and L. W. Green (1978). "Evaluation of School Health Education: Identifying Purpose, Keeping Perspective," *Journal of School Health* 48(Apr): 228–35.

Krieger, N. and J. C. Lashof (1988). "AIDS, Policy Analysis, and the Electorate: The Role of Schools of Public Health," *American Journal of Public Health* 78: 411–15.

Krolnick, R. (1989). *Adolescent Health Insurance Status: Analyses of Trends in Coverage and Preliminary Estimates of the Effects of an Employer Mandate and Medicaid Expansion on the Uninsured* (Washington, DC: U.S. Congress, Office of Technology Assessment, U.S. Government Printing Office).

Kronenfeld, J. J. (1986). "Self-Help and Self-Care as Social Movements," in *Advances in Health Education and Promotion*, vol. 1, pt A, W. B. Ward and Z. Salisbury, eds. (Greenwich, CT: JAI Press), pp. 105–27.

Kwon, E. H. (1971). "Use of the Agent System in Seoul," *Studies in Family Planning* 2: 237–340.

Lacy, W. B. (1981). "The Influence of Attitudes and Current Friends on Drug Use Intentions," *Journal of Social Psychology* 113: 65–76.

LaLonde, M. A. (1974). *A New Perspective on the Health of Canadians* (Ottawa, Canada: Ministry of National Health and Welfare).

Land, K. C. and S. Spilerman, eds. (1975). *Social Indicator Models* (New York: Russell Sage Foundation).

Landgreen, M. and W. Baum (1984). "Adhering to Fitness in the Corporate Setting," *Corporate Commentary* 1: 30–35.

Landman, G. B., M. D. Levine, L. Rappaport (1984). "A Study of Treatment Resistance Among Children Referred for Encopresis," *Clinical Pediatrics* 8: 449–52.

Lando, H. A., B. Loken, B. Howard-Pitney, and T. Pechacek (1990). "Community Impact of a Localized Smoking Cessation Contest," *American Journal of Public Health* 80: 601–03.

Lando, H. A., P. G. McGovern, F. X. Barrios, and B. D. Etringer (1990). "Comparative Evaluation of American Cancer Society and American Lung Association Smoking Cessation Clinics," *American Journal of Public Health* 80: 554–59.

Landry, F. ed. (1983). *Health Risk Estimation, Risk Reduction, and Health Promotion* (Ottawa: Canadian Public Health Association).

Lane, D. (1983). "Compliance with Referrals from a Cancer Screening Project," *Journal of Family Practice* 17: 811–17.

Langlie, J. (1977). "Social Networks, Health Beliefs, and Preventive Health Behavior," *Journal of Health and Social Behavior* 18: 244–60.

LaPorte, R. E., L. L. Adams, D. D. Savage et al. (1984). "The Spectrum of Physical Activity, Cardiovascular, and Health: An Epidemiologic Perspective," *American Journal of Epidemiology* 120: 507–17.

LaPorte, R. E., H. J. Montoye, and C. J. Caspersen (1985). "Assessment of Physical Activity in Epidemiologic Research: Problems and Prospects," *Public Health Reports* 100: 131–46.

Larson, E., E. Olsen, W. Cole, and S. Shortell (1979). "The Relationship of Health Beliefs and a Postcard Reminder to Influenza Vaccination," *Journal of Family Practice* 8: 1207–11.

Lasater, T., D. Abrams, L. Artz et al. (1984). "Lay Volunteer Delivery of a Community-Based Cardiovascular Risk Factor Change Program: The Pawtucket Experiment," in *Behavioral Health: A Handbook of Health Enhancement and Disease Prevention*, J. D. Matarazzo, S. M. Weiss, J. A. Herd et al., eds. (New York: Wiley).

Lau, R., R. Kane, S. Berry et al. (1980). "Channeling Health: A Review of the Evaluation of Televised Health Campaigns," *Health Education Quarterly* 7: 56–89.

Lawrence, L. and T. McLemore (1983). "National Ambulatory Medical Care Survey," *Vital and Health Statistics Series* 88 (Washington, DC: National Center for Health Statistics).

Lawrence, R. S. (1988). "Summary of Workshop Sessions of the International Symposium on Preventive Services in Primary Care: Issues and Strategies," *American Journal of Preventive Medicine* 4 (Suppl 4): 188–89.

Leavitt, F. (1979). "The Health Belief Model and Utilization of Ambulatory Care Services," *Social Science and Medicine* 13A: 105–12.

Lefebvre, R. C. and J. A. Flora (1988). "Social Marketing and Public Health Intervention," *Health Education Quarterly* 15: 299–315.

Lefebvre, R. C., G. S. Peterson, S. A. McGraw et al. (1986). "Community Intervention to Lower Blood Cholesterol: The 'Know Your Cholesterol' Campaign in Pawtucket, Rhode Island," *Health Education Quarterly* 13: 117–29.

Lenfant, C. and E. J. Roccella (1984). "Trends in Hypertension Control in the United States," *Chest* 86: 459–62.

Leppo, K. and T. Melkas (1988). "Toward Healthy Public Policy: Experiences in Finland 1972–1987," *Health Promotion* 3: 195–203.

Leupker, R. V., V. E. Pallonen, D. M. Murray, and P. L. Pirie (1989). "Validity of Telephone Surveys in Assessing Cigarette Smoking in Young Adults," *American Journal of Public Health* 79: 202–04.

Levin, L. S. (1971). "Consumer Participation in Health Services," *Journal of the Institute of Health Education* (London) 9: 19–24.

Levin, L. S. (1982). "Forces and Issues in the Revival of Interest in Self-Care: Impetus for Redirection in Health," in *The SOPHE Heritage Collection of Health Education Monographs, Vol. 2: The*

Practice of Health Education, B. P. Mathews, ed. (Oakland, CA: Third Party Publishing), pp. 268–73.

Levin, L. S. (1983). "Lay Health Care: The Hidden Resource in Health Promotion," in *Health Promotion Monographs*, no. 3, K. A. Gordon, ed. (New York: Teachers College, Columbia University).

Levin, L. S. and E. L. Idler (1983). "Self-Care in Health," *Annual Review of Public Health* 4: 181–201.

Levin, L. S., A. Katz, and E. Holst (1978). *Self-Care: Lay Initiatives in Health* (New York: Prodist).

Levine, D. M. and L. W. Green (1981). "Cardiovascular Risk Reduction: An Interdisciplinary Approach to Research Training," *International Journal of Health Education* 24: 20–25.

Levine, D. M. and L. W. Green (1983). "Behavioral Change Through Health Education," in *Prevention of Coronary Heart Disease: Practical Management of the Risk Factors*, N. M. Kaplan and J. Stamler, eds. (Philadelphia: W. B. Saunders), pp. 161–69.

Levine, D. M. and L. W. Green (1985). "Patient Education: State of the Art in Research and Evaluation," *Bulletin of the New York Academy of Medicine* 61: 135–43.

Levine, D. M., L. W. Green, S. G. Deeds et al. (1979). "Health Education for Hypertensive Patients," *Journal of the American Medical Association* 241: 1700–03.

Levine, D. M., D. E. Morisky, L. R. Bone et al. (1982). "Data-Based Planning for Educational Interventions Through Hypertension Control Programs for Urban and Rural Populations in Maryland," *Public Health Reports* 97: 107–12.

Levine, S., P. White, and N. Scotch (1963). "Community Interorganizational Problems in Providing Medical Care and Social Services," *American Journal of Public Health* 53: 1183–95.

Levit, K. R., M. S. Freeland, and D. R. Waldo (1989). "Health Spending and Ability to Pay: Business, Individuals, and Government," *Health Care Financing Review* 10(2): 1–11.

Leviton, L. C. and R. O. Valdiserri (1990). "Evaluating AIDS Prevention: Outcome, Implementation, and Mediating Variables," *Evaluation and Program Planning* 13: 55–66.

Lewis, B., J. I. Mann, and M. Mancini (1986). "Reducing the Risks of Coronary Heart Disease in Individuals and in the Population," *Lancet* 14: 956–59.

Lewis, C. E. (1988). "Disease Prevention and Health Promotion Practices of Primary Care Physicians in the United States," *American Journal of Preventive Medicine* 4(4, Suppl): 9–16.

Lewis, F. M. (1987). "The Concept of Control: A Typology and Health-Related Variables," in *Advances in Health Education and Promotion*, vol. 2, W. Ward and M. H. Becker, eds. (Greenwich, CT: JAI Press), pp. 277–309.

Lewis, F. M. and M. V. Batey (1982). "Clarifying Autonomy and Accountability in Nursing Service: Part 2," *Journal of Nursing Administration* 12(Oct): 10–15.

Li, F. P., N. Y. Schlief, C. J. Chang, and A. C. Gaw (1972). "Health Care for the Chinese Community in Boston," *American Journal of Public Health* 62: 536–39.

Li, V. C., T. J. Coates, L. A. Spielberg et al. (1984). "Smoking Cessation with Young Women in Public Family Planning Clinics: The Impact of Physician Messages and Waiting Room Media," *Preventive Medicine* 13: 477–89.

Liburd, L. C. and J. V. Bowie (1989). "Intentional Teenage Pregnancy: A Community Diagnosis and Action Plan," *Health Education* 20(5): 33–38.

Lichter, M., P. L. Arens, N. Reinstein et al. (1986). "Oakwood Hospital Community Health Promotion Program," *Health Care Management Review* 11: 75–87.

Light, L. and I. R. Contento (1989). "Changing the Course: A School Nutrition and Cancer Education Program by the American Cancer Society and the National Cancer Institute," *Journal of School Health* 59: 205–09.

Lightner, M. D. (1976). "The Health Education Coordinating Council," *Health Education* 7(Nov/Dec): 25–26.

Linstone, H. A. and M. Turoff (1975). *The Delphi Method: Techniques and Applications* (Reading, MA: Addison-Wesley).

Lippitt, G. L., P. Langseth, and J. Mossop (1985). *Implementing Organizational Change* (San Francisco: Jossey-Bass).

Lohr, K. N., ed. (1989). "Advances in Health Status Assessment: Conference Proceedings," *Medical Care* 27(Suppl): whole issue no. 3.

Lohrmann, D. K. and S. W. Fors (1986). "Can School-Based Programs Really Be Expected to Solve the Adolescent Drug Problem?" *Journal of Drug Education* 16(4): 327–39.

Lomas, J. and R. B. Haynes (1988). "A Taxonomy and Critical Review of Tested Strategies for the Application of Clinical Practice Recommendations: From 'Official' to 'Individual' Clinical Policy," *American Journal of Preventive Medicine* 4(4, Suppl): 77–94.

London, F. B. (1982). "Attitudinal and Social Normative Factors as Predictors of Intended Alcohol Abuse Among Fifth- and Seventh-Grade Students," *Journal of School Health* 52: 244–49.

Longe, M. (1985). *Innovative Hospital-Based Health Promotion* (Chicago: American Hospital Association).

Lorig, K. and J. Laurin (1985). "Some Notions About Assumptions Underlying Health Education," *Health Education Quarterly* 12: 231–43.

Lovato, C. Y. and D. Allensworth (1989). *School Health in America: An Assessment of State Policies To Protect and Improve the Health of Students*, 5th ed. (Kent, OH: American School Health Association).

Lovato, C. Y. and L. W. Green (1984). "Consultation Report for the Workers Institute for Safety and Health, Washington, DC" (Houston: University of Texas Center for Health Promotion Research and Development).

Lovato, C. Y. and L. W. Green (1986). "Consultation Report for National Cancer Institute's Grant to Five Unions to Develop Cancer Control Programs" (Houston: University of Texas Center for Health Promotion Research and Development), paper presented at the annual meeting of the American Public Health Association, New Orleans, LA.

Lovato, C. Y. and L. W. Green (1990). "Maintaining Employee Participation in Workplace Health Promotion Programs," *Health Education Quarterly* 17: 73–88.

Lovato, C. Y., L. W. Green, and V. Conley, (1986). "Development and Evaluation of Occupational Health Education Programs to Reduce Exposure to Cancer Hazards," presented at the annual meeting of the American Society for Preventive Oncology, Bethesda, MD.

Lovick, S. R. and R. F. Stern (1988). *School-Based Clinics—1988 Update* (Houston: The Support Center for School-Based Clinics).

Luke, R. D. and R. E. Modrow (1982). "Professionalism, Accountability, and Peer Review," *Health Services Research* 17: 113–23.

Maccoby, N., J. W. Farquahr, and P. D. Wood (1977). "Reducing the Risk of Cardiovascular Disease: Effects of a Community-Based Campaign on Knowledge and Behavior," *Journal of Community Health* 23: 100–14.

Macrina, D. M. and T. W. O'Rourke (1986–87). "Citizen Participation in Health Planning in the U.S. and the U.K.: Implications for Health Education Strategies," *International Quarterly of Community Health Education* 7: 225–39.

Maes, S., C. D. Spielberger, P. B. Defares, and I. G. Sarason, eds. (1988). *Topics in Health Psychology* (New York: Wiley).

Mahaffey, M. and J. W. Hanks, eds. (1982). *Practical Politics: Social Work and Political Responsibility* (Silver Springs, MD: National Association of Social Workers).

Maheux, B., R. Pineault, and F. Beland (1987). "Factors Influencing Physicians' Orientation Toward Prevention," *American Journal of Preventive Medicine* 3: 12–18.

Maiman, L. A., M. H. Becker, J. P. Kirscht et al. (1977). "Scales for Measuring Health Belief Model Dimensions: A Test of Predictive Value, Internal Consistency, and Relationships Among Beliefs," *Health Education Monographs* 5: 215–30.

Maiman, L. A., L. W. Green, G. Gibson, and E. J. MacKenzie (1979). "Education for Self-Treatment by Adult Asthmatics," *Journal of the American Medical Association* 241: 1919–22.

Maine Department of Educational and Cultural Services (1985). "Project Graduation," *Morbidity and Mortality Weekly Report* 34: 233–35.

Malo, E. and L. C. Leviton (1987). "Decision Points for Hospital-Based Health Promotion," *Hospital and Health Services Administration* 32: 49–61.

Mamon, J. A. and J. G. Zapka (1986). "Breast Self-Examination by Young Women. I. Characteristics Associated with Frequency," *American Journal of Preventive Medicine* 2: 61–69.

Mann, K. V. and P. L. Sullivan (1987). "Effect of Task-Centered Instructional Programs on Hypertensives' Ability to Achieve and Maintain Reduced Dietary Sodium Intake," *Patient Education and Counseling* 10: 53–72.

Manoff, R. K. (1985). *Social Marketing: New Imperative for Public Health* (New York: Praeger).

Marcus, A. C., L. G. Reeder, L. A. Jordan, and T. E. Seeman (1980). "Monitoring Health Status, Access to Health Care, and Compliance Behavior in a Large Urban Community," *Medical Care* 18: 253–65.

Markland, R. E. and M. L. Vincent (1990). "Improving Resource Allocation in a Teenage Sexual Risk Reduction Program," *Socio-Economic Planning Science* 24: 35–48.

Marlatt, G. A. and J. R. Gordon, eds. (1985). *Relapse Prevention: Maintenance Strategies in the Treatment of Addictive Behaviors* (New York: Guilford Press).

Marsick, V. J. (1987). "Designing Health Education Programs," in *Handbook of Health Education*, 2nd ed., P. M. Lazes, L. H. Kaplan, and K. A. Gordon, eds. (Rockville, MD: Aspen), chap. 1.

Masi, D. (1984). *Designing Employee Assistance Programs* (New York: American Management Association).

Mason, J. O. (1984). "Health Promotion and Disease Prevention: The Federal and State Roles," *Focal Points* 1: 1–2.

Mason, J. O. (1989). "Dr. Mason Outlines Goals for Improving the Nation's Health," *Journal of School Health* 59: 289–90.

Mason, J. O. (1990). "A Prevention Policy Framework for the Nation," *Health Affairs* 9: 22–29.

Mason, J. O. and J. M. McGinnis (1985). "The Role of School Health," *Journal of School Health* 55: 299.

Mattarazzo, J. D. (1984). "Behavioral Health: A 1990 Challenge for the Health Sciences Professions," in *Behavioral Health: A Handbook of Health Enhancement and Disease Prevention*, J. D. Mattarazzo, S. M. Weiss, J. A. Herd et al., eds. (New York: Wiley).

Mattarazzo, J. D., S. M. Weiss, J. A. Herd et al., eds. (1984). *Behavioral Health: A Handbook of Health Enhancement and Disease Prevention* (New York: Wiley).

Mayer, J. A., P. M. Dubbert, and J. P. Elder (1989). "Promoting Nutrition at the Point of Choice: A Review," *Health Education Quarterly* 16: 31–43.

Mazmanian, D. and P. Sabatier (1983). *Implementation and Public Policy* (Glenview, IL: Scott, Foresman).

Mazzuca, S. A. (1982). "Does Patient Education in Chronic Disease Have Therapeutic Value?" *Journal of Chronic Disease* 35: 521–29.

McAlister, A., P. D. Mullen, and S. A. Nixon et al. (1985). "Health Promotion Among Primary Care Physicians in Texas," *Texas Medicine* 81: 55–58.

McAlister, A. L., C. Perry, J. Killen et al. (1980). "Pilot Study of Smoking, Alcohol, and Drug Abuse Prevention," *American Journal of Public Health* 70: 719–21.

McAlister, A., P. Puska, J. T. Salonen et al. (1982). "Theory and Action for Health Promotion — Illustrations from the North Karelia Project," *American Journal of Public Health* 72: 43–50.

McCarty, D., S. Morrison, and K. C. Mills (1983). "Attitudes, Beliefs, and Alcohol Use: An Analysis of Relationships," *Journal of Studies on Alcohol* 2: 328–41.

McCaul, K. D. and R. E. Glasgow (1985). "Preventing Adolescent Smoking: What Have We Learned About Treatment Construct Validity?" *Health Psychology* 4: 361–87.

McCaul, K., R. Glasgow, H. O'Neill et al. (1982). "Predicting Adolescent Smoking," *Journal of School Health* 52: 342–46.

McCoy, H. V., S. E. Dodds, and C. Nolan (1990). "AIDS Intervention Design for Program Evaluation: The Miami Community Outreach Project," *Journal of Drug Issues* 20: 223–43.

McCuan, R. and L. W. Green (1991). "Multivariate Statistical Methods for Evaluation of Health Education and Health Promotion Programs," in *Advances in Health Education and Promotion*, vol. 3, W. Ward and F. M. Lewis, eds. (London: Jessica Kingsley, in press).

McDonald, C. J., S. L. Hui, D. M. Smith et al. (1984). "Reminders to Physicians from an Introspective Computer Medical Record: A Two-Year Randomized Trial," *Annals of Internal Medicine* 100: 130–38.

McGinnis, J. M. (1980). "Trends in Disease Prevention: Assessing the Benefits of Prevention," *Bulletin of the New York Academy of Medicine* 56: 38–44.

McGinnis, J. M. (1982). "Targeting Progress in Health," *Public Health Reports* 97: 295–307.

McGinnis, J. M. (1990). "Setting Objectives for Public Health in the 1990s: Experience and Prospects," *Annual Review of Public Health* 11: 231–49.

McGuire, A. (1987). "There's Death on the Block, There's Hope in Congress," *Journal of Public Health Policy* 8: 451–54.

McKay, R. B., D. M. Levine, and L. R. Bone (1985). "Community Organization in a School Health Education Program to Reduce Sodium Consumption," *Journal of School Health* 55: 364–66.

McKeown, T. (1979). *The Role of Medicine: Dream, Mirage, or Nemesis*, 2nd ed. (Princeton, NJ: Princeton University Press).

McKinlay, J. B. (1975). "A Case for Refocusing Upstream—The Political Economy of Illness," in *Applying Behavioral Science to Cardiovascular Risk*, A. J. Enelow and J. B. Henderson, eds. (New York: American Heart Association), pp. 7–17.

McLemore, T. and J. DeLozier (1987). "1985 Summary: National Ambulatory Medical Care Survey," in *Advance Data From Vital and Health Statistics*, no. 128 (National Center for Health Statistics, Washington, DC: DHHS-PHS 87-1250, U.S. Government Printing Office).

McLeroy, K. R., D. Bibeau, A. Steckler, and K. Glanz (1988). "An Ecological Perspective on Health Promotion Programs," *Health Education Quarterly* 15: 351–77.

McLeroy, K. R., N. H. Gottlieb, and J. N. Burdine (1987). "The Business of Health Promotion: Ethical Issues and Professional Responsibilities," *Health Education Quarterly* 14: 91–109.

McLeroy, K. R., L. W. Green, K. Mullen, and V. Foshee (1984). "Assessing the Effects of Health Promotion in Worksites: A Review of the Stress Program Evaluations," *Health Education Quarterly* 11: 379–401.

McLeroy, K. R., A. Steckler, and D. Bibeau, eds. (1988). "The Social Ecology of Health Promotion Interventions," *Health Education Quarterly* 15: 351–486.

McMillan, D. W. and D. M. Chavis (1986). "Sense of Community: A Definition and Theory," *Journal of Community Psychology* 14: 6–23.

McPhee, S. J., R. J. Richard, and S. N. Solkowitz (1986). "Performance of Cancer Screening in a University General Internal Medicine Practice," *Journal of General Internal Medicine* 1: 275–81.

Mechanic, D. (1979). "The Stability of Health and Illness Behavior: Results from a 16-Year Follow-Up," *American Journal of Public Health* 69: 1142–45.

Mendelsohn, H. (1973). "Some Reasons Why Information Campaigns Can Succeed," *Public Opinion Quarterly* 39: 50–61.

Metropolitan Life Foundation (1988). *An Evaluation of Comprehensive Health Education in American Public Schools* (New York: Louis Harris and Associates, for the Metropolitan Life Foundation).

Miaoulis, G. and J. Bonaguro (1980–81). "Marketing Strategies in Health Education," *Journal of Health Care Marketing* 1: 35–44.

Michaels, J. M. (1982). "The Second Revolution in Health: Health Promotion and Its Environmental Base," *American Psychologist* 37: 936–41.

Michielutte, R. and P. Beal (1990). "Identification of Community Leadership in the Development of Public Health Education Programs," *Journal of Community Health* 15: 59–68.

Mico, P. R. (1965). "Community Self-Study: Is There a Method to the Madness?" *Adult Leadership* 13: 288–92.

Milio, N. (1976). "A Framework for Prevention: Changing Health-Damaging to Health-Generating Life Patterns," *American Journal of Public Health* 66: 435–39.

Milio, N. (1983). *Promoting Health Through Public Policy* (Philadelphia: F. A. Davis), reprinted by the Canadian Public Health Association, 1987.

Millar, W. J. and B. E. Naegele (1987). "Time to Quit Program," *Canadian Journal of Public Health* 78: 109–14.

Miller, I. (1987). "Interpreneurship: A Community Coalition Approach to Health Care Reform," *Inquiry* 24: 266–75.

Miller, J. R. (1984). "Liaisons: Using Health Education Resources Effectively," in *Advancing Health Through Education: A Case Study Approach*, H. P. Cleary, J. M. Kichen, and P. G. Ensor, eds. (Palo Alto, CA: Mayfield), pp. 112–14.

Miller, L. V. and J. Goldstein (1972). "More Efficient Care of Diabetic Patients in a County-Hospital Setting," *New England Journal of Medicine* 286: 1383–91.

Miller, N. E. (1984). "Learning: Some Facts and Needed Research Relevant to Maintaining Health," in *Behavioral Health: A Handbook of Health Enhancement and Disease Prevention*, J. D. Matarazzo, S. M. Weiss, J. A. Herd et al., eds. (New York: Wiley), pp. 199–208.

Miller, S. (1983). "Coalition Etiquette: Ground Rules for Building Unity," *Social Policy* 14(2): 49.

Minkler, M. (1980–81). "Citizen Participation in Health in the Republic of Cuba," *International Quarterly of Community Health Education* 1: 65–78.

Minkler, M. (1985). "Building Supportive Ties and Sense of Community Among the Inner-City Elderly: The Tenderloin Senior Outreach Project," *Health Education Quarterly* 12: 303–14.

Minkler, M. (1986). "The Social Component of Health," *American Journal of Health Promotion* 1: 33–38.

Minkler, M. (1989). "Health Education, Health Promotion, and the Open Society: An Historical Perspective," *Health Education Quarterly* 16: 17–30.

Minkler, M. (1990). "Improving Health Through Community Organization," in *Health Behavior and Health Education*, K. Glanz, F. M. Lewis, and B. K. Rimer, eds. (San Francisco: Jossey-Bass), p. 257.

Minkler, M. and B. Checkoway (1988). "Ten Principles for Geriatric Health Promotion," *Health Promotion International* 3: 277–86.

Minkler, M. and C. Cox (1980–81). "Creating Critical Consciousness in Health: Applications of Freire's Philosophy and Methods to the Health Care Setting," *International Journal of Health Services* 20: 311–22.

Minkler, M., S. Frantz, and R. Wechsler (1982–83). "Social Support and Social Action Organizing in a 'Grey Ghetto': The Tenderloin Experience," *International Quarterly of Community Health Education* 3: 3–15.

Minnesota Department of Health (1982). "Workplace Health Promotion Survey," (Minneapolis: Minnesota Department of Health).

Model Standards: A Guide for Community Preventive Health Services (1985). 2nd ed. (Washington, DC: American Public Health Association).

Mootz, M. (1988). "Health (Promotion) Indicators: Realistic and Unrealistic Expectations," *Health Promotion* 3: 79–84.

Morbidity and Mortality Weekly Report (1989). 38: 147–50.

Morbidity and Mortality Weekly Report (1989). 38: 137.

Morgan, P. A. (1988). "Power, Politics, and Public Health: The Political Power of the Alcohol Beverage Industry," *Journal of Public Health Policy* 9: 177–97.

Morisky, D. E., N. M. DeMuth, M. Field-Fass et al. (1985). "Evaluation of Family Health Education to Build Social Support for Long-Term Control of High Blood Pressure," *Health Education Quarterly* 12: 35–50.

Morisky, D. E., D. M. Levine, L. W. Green et al. (1980). "The Relative Impact of Health Education for Low- and High-Risk Patients with Hypertension," *Preventive Medicine* 9: 550–58.

Morisky, D. E., D. M. Levine, L. W. Green et al. (1983). "Five-Year Blood-Pressure Control and Mortality Following Health Education for Hypertensive Patients," *American Journal of Public Health* 73: 153–62.

Morisky, D. E., D. M. Levine, L. W. Green, and C. Smith (1982). "Health Education Program Effects on the Management of Hypertension in the Elderly," *Archives of Internal Medicine* 142: 1935–38.

Morisky, D. E., D. M. Levine, J. C. Wood et al. (1981). "Systems Approach for the Planning, Diagnosis, Implementation, and Evaluation of Community Health Education Approaches in the Control of High Blood Pressure," *Journal of Operations Research* 50: 625–34.

Mosher, J. F. (1990). *Community Responsible Beverage Service Programs: An Implementation Handbook* (Palo Alto, CA: The Health Promotion Resource Center, Stanford Center for Research in Disease Prevention).

Mosher, J. F. and D. H. Jernigan (1988). "Public Action and Awareness to Reduce Alcohol-Related Problems: A Plan of Action," *Journal of Public Health Policy* 9: 17–41.

Mosher, J. F. and D. H. Jernigan (1989). "New Directions in Alcohol Policy," *Annual Review of Public Health* 10: 245–79.

Mowatt, C., J. Isaly, and M. Thayer (1985). "Project Graduation—Maine," *Morbidity and Mortality Weekly Report* 34: 233–35.

Moynihan, D. P. (1969). *Maximum Feasible Misunderstanding: Community Action in the War on Poverty* (New York: Free Press).

Mucchielli, R. (1970). *Introduction to Structural Psychology* (New York: Funk & Wagnalls).

Mulford, C. L. and G. E. Klonglan (1982). *Creating Coordination Among Organizations: An Orientation and Planning Guide* (Ames, IA: Cooperative Extension Service, Iowa State University, North Central Regional Extension Pub. No. 80).

Mullan, F. (1982). "Community-Oriented Primary Care: An Agenda for the '80s, *New England Journal of Medicine* 307: 1076–78.

Mullen, P. D. and L. W. Green (1985). "Meta-Analysis Points Way Toward More Effective Medication Teaching," *Promoting Health* 6(6): 6–8.

Mullen, P. D., L. W. Green, and G. Persinger (1985). "Clinical Trials of Patient Education for Chronic Conditions: A Comparative Meta-Analysis of Intervention Types," *Preventive Medicine* 14: 753–81.

Mullen, P. D., J. Hersey, and D. C. Iverson (1987). "Health Behavior Models Compared," *Social Science and Medicine* 24: 973–81.

Mullen, P. D. and D. C. Iverson (1982). "Qualitative Methods for Evaluative Research in Health Education Programs," *Health Education* 13(3): 11–18.

Mullen, P., K. Kukowski, and S. Mazelis (1979). "Health Education in Health Maintenance Organizations," in *Handbook of Health Education*, P. Lazes, ed. (Germantown, MD: Aspen Systems), pp. 53–76.

Mullen, P. D. and J. G. Zapka (1981). "Health Education and Promotion in HMOs: The Recent Evidence," *Health Education Quarterly* 8: 292–315.

Mullen, P. D. and J. G. Zapka (1982). *Guidelines for Health Promotion and Education Services in HMOs* (Washington, DC: U.S. Government Printing Office).

Mullen, P. D. and J. G. Zapka (1989). "Assessing the Quality of Health Promotion Programs," *HMO Practice* 3: 98–103.

Mullis, R. M., M. K. Hunt, M. Foster, et al. (1987). "The Shop Smart for Your Heart Grocery Program," *Journal of Nutrition Education* 19: 225–28.

Mumford, E., H. J. Schlesinger, and G. V. Glass (1982). "The Effects of Psychological Intervention on Recovery from Surgery and Heart Attacks: An Analysis of the Literature," *American Journal of Public Health* 72: 141–51.

Murray, D. M. (1986). "Dissemination of Community Health Promotion Programs: The Fargo-Moorhead Heart Health Program," *Journal of School Health* 56: 375–81.

Murray, D. M., C. A. Johnson, R. V. Luepker, and M. B. Mittelmark (1984). "The Prevention of Cigarette Smoking in Children: A Comparison of Four Strategies," *Journal of Applied Social Psychology* 14: 274–88.

Murray, D. M., C. L. Kurth, J. R. Finnegan, Jr. et al. (1988). "Direct Mail as a Prompt for Follow-Up Care Among Persons at Risk for Hypertension," *American Journal of Preventive Medicine*, 4: 331–35.

Murray, D. M. and C. L. Perry (1987). "The Measurement of Substance Use Among Adolescents: When Is the 'Bogus Pipeline' Method Needed?" *Addictive Behaviors* 12: 225–33.

Mutter, G. (1988). "Using Research Results as a Health Promotion Strategy: A Five-Year Case Study," *Health Promotion* 3: 393–99.

Myers, D. (1985). *Establishing and Building Employee Assistance Programs* (Westport, CT: Quorum).

Nader, P. R., J. G. Sallis, T. L. Patterson et al. (1989). "A Family Approach to Cardiovascular Risk Reduction: Results from the San Diego Family Health Project," *Health Education Quarterly* 16: 229–44.

Nagy, V. and G. Wolfe (1984). "Cognitive Predictors of Compliance in Chronic Disease Patients," *Medical Care* 22: 912–21.

Naisbitt, J. (1982). *Megatrends: Ten New Directions Transforming Our Lives* (New York: Warner Books).

Naisbitt, J. and P. Aburdene (1990). *Megatrends 2000: Ten New Directions for the 1990's* (New York: William Morrow).

Nangawe, E., F. Shomet, E. Rowberg et al. (1986–87). "Community Participation: The Maasai Health Services Project, Tanzania," *International Quarterly of Community Health Education,* 7: 343–51.

"National Adolescent Student Health Survey" (1988). *Health Education* 19(4): 4–8.

National Center for Children in Poverty (1990). *Five Million Children: A Statistical Profile of Our Poorest Young Citizens* (New York: School of Public Health, Columbia University, 1990).

National Center for Health Statistics (1989). *Health, United States, 1988* (Washington, DC: U.S. Government Printing Office, DHHS-PHS-89-1232).

National Center for Health Statistics (1990). *Health, United States, 1989 and Prevention Profile* (Hyattsville, MD: Public Health Service, DHHS-PHS-90-1232).

National Commission on Excellence in Education (1983). *A Nation at Risk: The Imperative for Educational Reform* (Washington, DC: National Commission on Excellence in Education, 1983).

National Commission on the Role of the School and the Community in Improving Adolescent Health (1990). *Code Blue: Uniting for Healthier Youth* (Washington, DC: National Association of State Boards of Education and the American Medical Association).

National Committee for Injury Prevention and Control (1989). *Injury Prevention: Meeting the Challenge* (New York: Oxford University Press), as a supplement to the *American Journal of Preventive Medicine*, vol. 5, no. 3.

National Professional School Health Education Organizations (1984). "Comprehensive School Health Education," *Journal of School Health* 54: 312–15.

National Research Council (1989). *Improving Risk Communication* (Washington, DC: National Academy Press).

National Restaurant Association (1989). *Foodservice Industry Forecast* (Washington, DC: Malcolm M. Knapp Research).

National Survey of Worksite Health Promotion Activities: A Summary (1987). (Washington, DC: U.S. Department of Health and Human Services, Public Health Service, Office of Disease Prevention and Health Promotion).

Neill, J. S. and J. O. Bond (1964). *Hillsborough County Oral Polio Vaccine Program* (Jacksonville: Florida State Board of Health Monograph No. 6).

Nelkin, D. (1987). "AIDS and the Social Sciences: Review of Useful Knowledge and Research Needs," *Reviews of Infectious Diseases* 9: 980–86.

Nelson, C. F., M. W. Kreuter, and N. B. Watkins (1986). "A Partnership Between the Community, State, and Federal Government: Rhetoric or Reality," *Hygie* (Paris) 5(3): 27–31.

Nelson, C. F., M. W. Kreuter, N. B. Watkins, and R. R. Stoddard (1987). "Planned Approach to Community Health: The PATCH Program," in *Community-Oriented Primary Care: From Principle to Practice*, P. A. Nutting, ed. (Washington, DC: U.S. Government Printing Office, U.S. Department of Health and Human Services, HRS-A-PE 86-1), chap. 47.

Nelson, E., W. Stason, R. Neutra et al. (1978). "Impact of Patient Perceptions of Compliance with Treatment for Hypertension," *Medical Care* 16: 893–906.

Neufeld, V. R. and G. R. Norman, eds. (1985). *Assessing Clinical Competence* (New York: Springer).

New Approaches to Health Education in Primary Health Care: Report of a WHO Expert Committee (1983). (Geneva: World Health Organization, Technical Report Series 690).

Newman, I. M. and G. L. Martin (1982). "Attitudinal and Normative Factors Associated with Adolescent Cigarette Smoking in Australia and the USA: A Methodology to Assist Health Education Planning," *Community Health Studies* 6: 47–56.

Newman, I. M., G. L. Martin, and K. A. Farrell, (1978). "Changing Health Values Through Public Television," *Health Values* 2(2): 92–95.

Newman, I. M., G. L. Martin, and R. Weppner (1982). "A Conceptual Model for Developing Prevention Programs," *The International Journal of the Addictions* 17: 493–504.

Nichols, W. H. and C. J. Stewart (1983). "Assessment of the Client-Centered Planning Approach in Continuing Education for Public Health Professionals," *Mobius* 3(3): 12–21.

Nickens, H. W. (1990). "Health Promotion and Disease Prevention Among Minorities," *Health Affairs* 9: 133–43.

Nix, H. L. (1969). "Concepts of Community and Community Leadership," *Sociology and Social Research* 53: 500–10.

Nix, H. L. (1970). *Identification of Leaders and Their Involvement in the Planning Process* (Washington, DC: U.S. Public Health Service, Pub. No. 1998).

Nix, H. L. (1977). *The Community and Its Involvement in the Study Action Planning Process* (Atlanta: U.S. Department of Health, Education and Welfare, Centers for Disease Control, HEW-CDC-78-8355).

Nix, H. L. and N. R. Seerly (1971). "Community Reconnaissance Method: A Synthesis of Functions," *Journal of Community Development Society* 11(Fall): 62–69.

Nix, H. L. and N. R. Seerly (1973). "Comparative Views and Actions of Community Leaders and Nonleaders," *Rural Sociology* 38: 427–28.

Noack, H. and D. McQueen (1988). "Towards Health Promotion Indicators," *Health Promotion* 3: 73–78.

Norman, S. A., R. Greenberg, K. Marconi et al. (1990). "A Process Evaluation of a Two-Year Community Cardiovascular Risk Reduction Program: What Was Done and Who Knew About It?" *Health Education Research* 5: 87–97.

Novelli, W. D. (1990). "Applying Social Marketing to Health Promotion and Disease Prevention," in *Health Behavior and Health Education: Theory, Research, and Practice*, K. Glanz, F. M. Lewis, and B. K. Rimer, eds. (San Francisco, CA: Jossey-Bass).

Nursing Development Conference Group (1973). *Concept Formalization in Nursing: Process and Product* (Boston: Little, Brown).

Nutbeam, D. (1985). *Health Promotion Glossary* (Copenhagen: World Health Organization Regional Office for Europe, July).

Nutbeam, D. and J. Catford (1987). "The Welsh Heart Programme Evaluation Strategy: Progress, Plans, and Possibilities," *Health Promotion* 2: 5–18.

Nutbeam, D., C. Smith, and J. Catford (1990). "Evaluation in Health Education: A Review of Possibilities and Problems," *Journal of Epidemiology and Community Health* 44: 83–89.

Nutting, P. A. (1986). "Health Promotion in Primary Medical Care: Problems and Potential," *Preventive Medicine* 15: 537–48.

Nutting, P. A., ed. (1987). *Community-Oriented Primary Care: From Principle to Practice.* (Washington, DC: U.S. Department of Health and Human Services, Health Resources and Services Administration, HRS-A-PE 86-1).

Nutting, P. A. (1990). "Community-Oriented Primary Care: A Critical Area of Research for Primary Care," *Primary Care Research: An Agenda for the 90s* (Washington, DC: U.S. Department of Health and Human Services, Agency for Health Care Policy and Research).

Nyswander, D. (1942). *Solving School Health Problems* (New York: Oxford University Press).

Nyswander, D. (1956). "Education for Health: Some Principles and Their Application," *California's Health* 14: 65–70.

O'Connell, J. K., J. H. Price, S. M. Roberts et al. (1985). "Utilizing the Health Belief Model to Predict Dieting and Exercising Behavior of Obese and Nonobese Adolescents," *Health Education Quarterly* 12: 343–51.

O'Donnell, M. (1985). "Research on Drinking Locations of Alcohol-Impaired Drivers: Implication for Prevention Policies," *Journal of Public Health Policy* 6: 510–25.

O'Donnell, M. P. (1986). "Definition of Health Promotion," *American Journal of Health Promotion* 1: 4–5.

O'Donnell, M. P. (1989). "Definition of Health Promotion: Part III: Expanding the Definition," *American Journal of Health Promotion* 3: 5.

O'Donnell, M. P. and T. Ainsworth, eds. (1984). *Health Promotion in the Workplace* (New York: Wiley).

Office of Disease Prevention and Health Promotion (1981). *Toward a Healthy Community: Organizing Events for Community Health Promotion* (Washington, DC: U.S. Department of Health and Human Services, Pub. No. PHS 80-50113).

Office of Health and Medical Affairs, Department of Management and Budget and Center for Health Promotion, Michigan Department of Health (1987). *Health Promotion Can Produce Economic Savings* (Lansing, MI: Center for Health Promotion, Michigan Department of Public Health).

Office on Smoking and Health (1987). *Health Consequence of Smoking: Cardiovascular Disease* (Washington, DC: U.S. Government Printing Office).

Okafor, F. C. (1985). "Basic Needs in Nigeria," *Social Indicators Research*, 17: 115–25.

Oldridge, N. (1982). "Compliance and Exercise in Primary and Secondary Prevention of Coronary Heart Disease: A Review," *Preventive Medicine* 11: 56–70.

Oldridge, N. B. (1984). "Adherence to Adult Exercise Fitness Programs," in *Behavioral Health*, J. D. Matarazzo, S. M. Weiss, J. A. Herd et al., eds. (New York: Wiley), pp. 467–87.

Oliver, R. and P. Berger (1979). "A Path Analysis of Preventive Health Care Decision Models," *Journal of Consumer Research* 6: 113–22.

Orem, D. E. (1971). *Nursing: Concepts of Practice* (New York: McGraw-Hill, 1971).

Orlandi, M. A. (1986). "Community-Based Substance Abuse Prevention: A Multicultural Perspective," *Journal of School Health* 56: 394–401.

Orlandi, M. A. (1987). "Promoting Health and Preventing Disease in Health Care Settings: An Analysis of Barriers," *Preventive Medicine* 16: 119–30.

Orleans, C. and R. Shipley (1982). "Worksite Smoking Cessation Initiatives: Review and Recommendations," *Addictive Behaviors* 7: 1–16.

Orleans, C. T., L. K. George, J. L. Houpt, and K. H. Brodie (1985). "Health Promotion in Primary Care: A Survey of U.S. Family Practitioners," *Preventive Medicine* 14: 636–647.

O'Rourke, T. W. and D. M. Macrina (1989). "Beyond Victim Blaming: Examining the Micro-Macro Issue in Health Promotion," *Wellness Perspectives: Research, Theory, and Practice* 6: 7–17.

Orthoefer, J., D. Bain, R. Empereur, and T. Nesbit (1988). "Consortium Building Among Local Health Departments in Northwest Illinois," *Public Health Reports* 103: 500–07.

Osgood, G. E., G. J. Cuci, and P. H. Tannenbaum (1961). *The Measurement of Meaning* (Urbana: University of Illinois Press).

Ostrow, D. G. (1989). "AIDS Prevention Through Effective Education," *Daedalus: Journal of the American Academy of Arts and Sciences* 118: 229–254.

Ottoson, J. M. and L. W. Green (1987). "Reconciling Concept and Context: Theory of Implementation," in *Advances in Health Education and Promotion*, vol. 2, W. B. Ward and M. H. Becker, eds. (Greenwich, CT: JAI Press), pp. 353–82.

Paehlke, R. C. (1989). *Environmentalism and the Future of Progressive Politics* (New Haven: Yale University Press).

Page, R. M. and R. S. Gold (1983). "Assessing Gender Differences in College Cigarette Smoking: Intenders and Non-Intenders," *Journal of School Health* 53: 531–35.

Parcel, G. S. (1976). "Skills Approach to Health Education: A Framework for Integrating Cognitive and Affective Learning," *Journal of School Health* 66: 403–06.

Parcel, G. S. (1984). "Theoretical Models for Application in School Health Education Research," *Journal of School Health* 54: 39–49.

Parcel, G. S. and Baranowski, T. (1981). "Social Learning Theory and Health Education," *Health Education* 12(3): 14–18.

Parcel, G. S., J. G. Bruhn, and J. L. Murray (1983). "Preschool Health Education Program (PHEP): Analysis of Education and Behavioral Outcomes," *Health Education Quarterly* 10: 149–72.

Parcel, G. S., M. P. Eriksen, C. Y. Lovato et al. (1989). "The Diffusion of School-Based Tobacco-Use Prevention Programs: Project Description and Baseline Data," *Health Education Research* 4: 111–24.

Parcel, G. S., L. W. Green, and B. Bettes (1989). "School-Based Programs to Prevent or Reduce Obesity," in *Childhood Obesity: A Biobehavioral Perspective*, N. A. Krasnagor, G. D. Grave, and N. Kretchmer, eds. (Caldwell, NJ: Telford Press), pp. 143–57.

Parcel, G. S., L. D. Muraskin, and C. M. Endert (1988). "Community Education: Study Group Report" [of Society for Adolescent Medicine], *Journal of Adolescent Health Care* 9: 41S–45S.

Parcel, G. S., B. G. Simons-Morton, and L. J. Kolbe (1988). "Health Promotion: Integrating Organizational Change and Student Learning Strategies," *Health Education Quarterly* 15: 435–50.

Parcel, G. S., B. G. Simons-Morton, N. M. O'Hara et al. (1989). "School Promotion of Healthful Diet and Physical Activity: Impact on Learning Outcomes and Self-Reported Behavior," *Health Education Quarterly* 16: 181–99.

Parcel, G. S., D. G. Simons-Morton, S. G. Brink et al. (1987). *Smoking Control Among Women: A CDC Community Intervention Handbook* (Atlanta: Centers for Disease Control).

Parkinson, R. S. and Associates, eds. (1982). *Managing Health Promotion in the Workplace: Guidelines for Implementation and Evaluation* (Palo Alto., CA: Mayfield).

Parlette, N., E. Glogow, and C. N. D'Onofrio (1981). "Public Health Administration and Health Education Training Need More Integration," *Health Education Quarterly* 8: 123–46.

Parsons, T. (1964). "The Superego and the Theory of Social Systems," in *The Family: Its Structure and Functions*, R. L. Coser, ed. (New York: St. Martin's Press), pp. 433–449.

PATCH: Planned Approach to Community Health (Atlanta: Centers for Disease Control, 1985).

Pate, R. R. (1983). "A New Definition of Fitness," *The Physician and Sports Medicine* 11: 77–82.

Patient Information and Prescription Drugs: Parallel Surveys of Physicians and Pharmacists (1983). (New York: Louis Harris and Associates).

Patrick, D. and P. Erickson (1987). *Assessing Health-Related Quality of Life in General Population Surveys: Issues and Recommendations* (Washington, DC: National Center for Health Statistics).

Patton, C. (1985). *Sex and Germs: The Politics of AIDS* (Boston: South End Press).

Patton, M. Q. (1978). *Utilization-Focused Evaluation* (Beverly Hills: Sage).

Patton, M. Q. (1980). *Qualitative Evaluation Methods* (Beverly Hills: Sage).

Patton, R. D. and W. B. Cissell, eds. (1989). *Community Organization: Traditional Principles and Modern Application* (Johnson City, TN: Latchpins Press).

Pechacek, T. F., B. H. Fox, D. M. Murray, and R. V. Luepker (1984). "Review of Techniques for Measurement of Smoking Behaviors," in *Behavioral Health: A Handbook of Health Enhancement and Disease Prevention*, J. Matarazzo, S. M. Weiss, J. A. Herd et al., eds. (New York: Wiley).

Pederson, L. L. and J. C. Baskerville (1983). "Multivariate Prediction of Smoking Cessation Following Physician Advice to Quit Smoking: A Validation Study," *Preventive Medicine* 12: 430–36.

Pederson, L., J. Wanklin, and J. Baskerville (1984). "The Role of Health Beliefs in Compliance with Physician Advice to Quit Smoking," *Social Science and Medicine* 19: 573–80.

Pelletier, K. R., N. L. Klehr, and S. J. McPhee (1988). "Town and Gown: A Lesson in Collaboration," *Business and Health* (Feb): 34–39.

Pelletier, K. R. and R. Lutz (1988). "Healthy People – Healthy Business: A Critical Review of Stress Management Programs in the Workplace," *American Journal of Health Promotion* 2(3): 5–12.

Pels, R. J., D. H. Bor, and R. S. Lawrence (1989). "Decision Making for Introducing Clinical Preventive Services," *Annual Review of Public Health* 10: 363–83.

Pennington, J. T., L. A. Wisniowski, and G. B. Logan (1988). "In-Store Nutrition Information Programs," *Journal of Nutrition Education* 20: 5–10.

Pentz, M. A. (1986). "Community Organization and School Liaisons: How to Get Programs Started," *Journal of School Health* 56: 382–88.

Pentz, M. A., J. H. Dwyer, D. P. MacKinnon et al. (1989). "A Multicommunity Trial for Primary Prevention of Drug Abuse," *Journal of the American Medical Association* 261: 3259–66.

Pentz, M. A., D. P. Mackinnon, J. H. Dwyer et al. (1989). "Longitudinal Effects of the Midwestern Prevention Project on Regular and Experimental Smoking in Adolescents," *Preventive Medicine* 18: 304–21.

Perera, D. R., J. P. LoGerfo, E. Shulenberger et al. (1983). "Teaching Sigmoidoscopy to Primary Care Physicians: A Controlled Study of Continuing Medical Education." *Journal of Family Practice* 16: 785–99.

Permut, S. (1986). "Corporate Liability for Occupational Medicine Programs," in *Occupational Stress: Health and Performance at Work*, S. Wolf and A. Finestone, eds. (Littleton, MA: PSG Publishing), pp. 136–52.

Perry, C. L., ed. (1986). "Special Issue on Community Programs for Drug Abuse Prevention," *Journal of School Health* 56(9): 357–418.

Perry, C. L., R. V. Luepker, D. M. Murray et al. (1988). "Parent Involvement with Children's Health Promotion: The Minnesota Home Team," *American Journal of Public Health* 78: 1156–60.

Perspectives on Health Promotion and Disease Prevention in the United States (Washington, DC: Institute of Medicine, National Academy of Sciences, 1978).

Pertschuk, M. and A. Erikson (1987). *Smoke Fighting: A Smoking Control Movement Building Guide* (New York: American Cancer Society).

Pertschuk, M. and Schaetzel, W. (1989). *The People Rising: The Campaign Against the Bork Nomination* (New York: Thunder's Mouth Press).

Pesznecher, B. L. and J. McNeil (1975). "Relationship Among Health Habits, Social Psychologic Well-Being, Life Change, and Alterations in Health Status," *Nursing Research* 24: 442–47.

Peters, T. J. and R. H. Waterman, Jr. (1984). *In Search of Excellence: Lessons from America's Best Run Companies* (New York: Warner Books).

Peterson, C. and A. J. Stunkard (1989). "Personal Control and Health Promotion," *Social Science and Medicine* 28: 819–28.

Pierce, J. P., P. Macaskill, and D. Hill (1990). "Long-Term Effectiveness of Mass Media Led Antismoking Campaigns in Australia," *American Journal of Public Health* 80: 565–69.

Pigg, R. M. (1989). "The Contribution of School Health Programs to the Broader Goals of Public Health: The American Experience," *Journal of School Health* 59: 25–30.

Pilisuk, M., S. Parks, J. Kelly, and E. Turner (1982). "The Helping Network Approach: Community Promotion of Mental Health." *Journal of Primary Prevention* 3: 116–32.

Pokorny, A., P. Putnam, and J. E. Fryer (1980). "Drug Abuse and Alcoholism Teaching in U.S. Medical and Osteopathic Schools, 1975–77," in *Alcohol and Drug Abuse in Medical Education*, M. Galanter, ed. (Washington, DC: U.S. Government Printing Office, DHEW Pub. No. (ADM)79-81).

Polissar, L., D. Sim, and A. Francis (1981). "Survival of Colorectal Cancer Patients in Relation to Duration of Symptoms and Other Prognostic Factors," *Diseases of the Colon and Rectum* 24: 364–69.

Pollock, M. (1987). *Planning and Implementing Health Education in Schools* (Palo Alto, CA: Mayfield).

Pollock, M. and K. Middleton (1989). *Elementary School Health Instruction*, 2nd ed. (St. Louis: Times Mirror/Mosby).

Popkin, B., P. Haines, K. Reidy (1989). "Food Consumption Trends of U.S. Women: Patterns and Determinants Between 1977 and 1985," *American Journal of Clinical Nutrition* 49: 1307–19.

Porras, J. and S. Hoffer (1986). "Common Behavior Changes in Successful Organization Development Efforts," *Journal of Applied Behavioral Science* 22: 477–94.

Posavac, E. J. (1980). "Evaluations of Patient Education Programs: A Meta-Analysis," *Evaluation and the Health Professions* 3: 47–62.

Povar, G. J., M. Mantell, and L. A. Morris (1984). "Patients' Therapeutic Preferences in an Ambulatory Care Setting," *American Journal of Public Health* 74: 1395–97.

Powell, K. E., C. J. Caspersen, J. P. Koplan, and E. S. Ford (1989). "Physical Activity and Chronic Diseases," *American Journal of Clinical Nutrition* 49: 999–1006.

Powell, K. E., G. M. Christensen, and M. W. Kreuter (1984). "Objectives for the Nation: Assessing the Role Physical Education Must Play," *Journal of Physical Education, Recreation and Dance* 55: 18–20.

Powell, K. E., P. D. Thompson, C. J. Caspersen et al. (1987). "Physical Activity and the Incidence of Coronary Heart Disease," *Annual Review of Public Health* 8: 253–87.

Preparation and Practice of Community, Patient, and School Health Educators: Proceedings on Commonalities and Differences (1978). (Bethesda, MD: Bureau of Health Manpower, U.S. Department of Health, Education, and Welfare, HRA 78-71).

Prescription Drug Information for Patients and Direct-to-Consumer Advertising (1984). (Boston: Medicine in the Public Interest, Inc.).

Pressman, J. and A. Wildavsky (1973). *Implementation*, 2nd ed. (Berkeley: University of California Press).

Preston, M. A., T. Baranowski, and J. C. Higginbotham (1988–89). "Orchestrating the Points of Community Intervention," *International Quarterly of Health Education* 9: 11–34.

Prochaska, J. O. (1989). "What Causes People to Change from Unhealthy to Health Enhancing Behavior?" paper presented at the American Cancer Society meeting on Behavioral Research in Cancer, Bloomington, Indiana, 9-10 Aug.

Prochaska, J. O. and C. DiClemente (1983). "Stages and Processes of Self-Change in Smoking: Toward an Integrative Model of Change," *Journal of Consulting and Clinical Psychology* 5: 390-95.

Puska, P., A. McAlister, J. Pekkola, and K. Koskela (1981). "Television in Health Promotion: Evaluation of a National Programme in Finland," *International Journal of Health Education* 24: 2-14.

Puska, P., A. Nissinen, J. Tuomilehto et al. (1985). "The Community-Based Strategy to Prevent Coronary Heart Disease: Conclusions from the Ten Years of the North Karelia Project," *Annual Review of Public* 6: 147-93.

Radecki, S. E. and R. C. Mandenhall (1986). "Patient Counseling by Primary Care Physicians: Results of a Nationwide Survey," *Patient Education and Counseling* 8: 165-77.

Radius, S., M. Becker, I. Rosenstock et al. (1978). "Factors Influencing Mothers' Compliance with a Medical Regimen for Asthmatic Children," *Journal of Asthma Research* 15: 133-49.

Raeburn, J. M. and I. Rootman (1988). "Towards an Expanded Health Field Concept: Conceptual and Research Issues in a New Era of Health Promotion," *Health Promotion: An International Journal* 3: 383-92.

Ramirez, A. G. and A. L. McAlister (1989). "Mass Media Campaign—*A Su Salud*," *Preventive Medicine* 17: 608-21.

Ratcliff, J. and L. Wallack (1986). "Primary Prevention in Public Health: An Analysis of Basic Assumptions," *International Quarterly of Community Health Education* 6: 215-37.

Rayant G. and A. Sheiham (1980). "An Analysis of Factors Affecting Compliance with Tooth-Cleaning Recommendations," *Journal of Clinical Periodontology* 7: 289-99.

Redman, S., E. A. Spencer, and R. W. Sanson-Fisher (1990). "The Role of Mass Media in Changing Health-Related Behaviour: A Critical Appraisal of Two Models," *Health Promotion International* 5: 85-102.

Rein, M. and F. Rabinovitz (1977). "Implementation: A Theoretical Perspective," (Cambridge: Joint Center for Urban Studies of MIT and Harvard University, Working Paper No. 43).

Remington, P. L., M. Y. Smith, D. F. Williamson et al. (1988). "Design, Characteristics, and Usefulness of State-Based Behavioral Risk Factor Surveillance: 1981-87," *Public Health Reports* 103: 366-75.

Report of the Presidential Commission on the Human Immunodeficiency Virus Epidemic (1988). (Washington, DC: The White House, 24 June).

Report of the President's Committee on Health Education (New York: Public Affairs Institute, 1973).

Resnick, L. B. (1987). *Education and Learning to Think* (Washington, DC: National Academy Press).

Rezmovic, E. L. (1982). "Program Implementation and Evaluation Results: A Reexamination of Type III Error in a Field Experiment," *Evaluation and Program Planning* 5: 111-18.

Richie, N. D. (1976). "Some Guidelines for Conducting a Health Fair," *Public Health Reports* 91: 261-64.

Riger, S. and P. J. Lavrakas (1981). "Community Ties: Patterns of Attachment and Social Interaction in Urban Neighborhoods," *American Journal of Community Psychology* 9: 55-66.

Riggs, R. and M. Noland (1983). "Awareness, Knowledge, and Perceived Risk for Toxic Shock Syndrome in Relation to Health Behavior," *Journal of School Health* 53: 303-07.

Rimer, B. K. (1990). "Perspectives on Intrapersonal Theories in Health Education and Health Behavior," in *Health Behavior and Health Education: Theory, Research, and Practice*, K. Glanz, F. M. Lewis, and B. K. Rimer, eds. (San Francisco: Jossey-Bass), pp. 140-57.

Rimer, B. K., S. W. Davis, P. F. Engstrom et al. (1988). "Some Reasons for Compliance and Noncompliance in a Health Maintenance Organization Breast Cancer Screening Program," *Journal of Compliance in Health Care* 3: 103–14.

Rimer, B. K., W. Jones, C. Wilson et al. (1983). "Planning a Cancer Control Program for Older Citizens," *Gerontologist* 23: 384–89.

Rimer, B. K., M. K. Keintz, and L. Fleisher (1986). "Process and Impact of a Health Communications Program," *Health Education Research* 1: 29–36.

Rimer, B. K., M. Keintz, B. Glassman, and J. Kinman (1986). "Health Education for Older Persons: Lessons from Research and Program Evaluations," in *Advances in Health Education and Promotion*, vol. 1, pt B, Z. Salisbury, J. G. Zapka, and S. B. Kar, eds. (Greenwich, CT: JAI Press), pp. 369–96.

Risser, L. W., H. M. Hoffman, B. G. Gordon, and L. W. Green (1985). "A Cost-Benefit Analysis of Preparticipation Sports Examinations of Adolescent Athletes," *Journal of School Health* 55: 270–73.

Rivara, F. P., P. J. Sweeney, and B. F. Henderson (1985). "A Study of Low Socioeconomic Status, Black Teenage Fathers, and Their Nonfather Peers," *Pediatrics* 107: 648–56.

Roberts, M. C. (1987). "Public Health and Health Psychology: Two Cats of Kilkenny?" *Professional Psychology: Research and Practice* 18: 145–49.

Roccella, E. J. and G. W. Ward (1984). "The National High Blood Pressure Campaign: A Description of Its Utility as a Generic Program Model," *Health Education Quarterly* 11: 225–42.

Roesner, J. B. (1977). "Citizen Participation: Tying Strategy to Function," in *Citizen Participation Certification Community Development*, P. Marshall, ed. (Washington, DC: National Association of Housing and Redevelopment Officials).

Rogers, E. M. (1983). *Diffusion of Innovations*, 3rd ed. (New York: Free Press).

Rokeach, M. (1970). *Beliefs, Attitudes, and Values* (San Francisco: Jossey-Bass).

Romm, R. J., S. W. Fletcher, and B. S. Hulka (1981). "The Periodic Health Examination: Comparison of Recommendations and Internists' Performance," *Southern Medical Journal* 74: 265–71.

Roos, N. P. (1975). "Evaluating Health Programs: Where Do We Find the Data," *Journal of Community Health* 1: 39–51.

Rootman, I. (1988). "Canada's Health Promotion Survey," in *Canada's Health Promotion Survey: Technical Report*, I. Rootman, R. Warren, T. Stephens, and L. Peters, eds. (Ottawa: Minister of Supply and Services).

Rose, G., P. J. Hamilton, L. Colwell et al. (1982). "A Randomized Controlled Trial of Anti-Smoking Advice: 10 Year Results," *Journal of Epidemiology and Community Health* 36: 102–08.

Rosen, G. (1958). *A History of Public Health* (New York: MD Publications).

Rosenblatt, D. and L. Kabasakalian (1966). "Evaluation of Venereal Disease Information Campaign for Adolescents," *American Journal of Public Health* 56: 1104–13.

Rosenstock, I. M., M. Derryberry, and B. Carriger (1959). "Why People Fail to Seek Poliomyelitis Vaccination," *Public Health Reports* 74: 98–103.

Ross, H. S. and P. R. Mico (1980). *Theory and Practice in Health Education* (Palo Alto, CA: Mayfield).

Ross, J. G. and G. G. Gilbert (1985). "The National Children and Youth Fitness Study," *Journal of Health, Physical Education, Recreation and Dance* 56(1): 45–50.

Ross, M. (1955). *Community Organization: Theory and Principles* (New York: Harper & Row).

Ross, M. (1967). *Community Organization: Theory, Principles, and Practice* (New York: Harper & Row).

Rosser, W. W. (1987). "Benzodiapezine Use in a Family Medicine Center," *Drug Protocol* 2(10): 9–15.

Roter, D. L. (1977). "Patient Participation in the Patient-Provider Interaction: The Effects of Patient Question-Asking on the Quality of Interaction, Satisfaction, and Compliance," *Health Education Monographs* 5: 281–315.

Roter, D. L., J. A. Hall, and N. R. Katz (1988). "Patient-Physician Communication: A Descriptive Summary of the Literature," *Patient Education and Counseling* 12: 99–119.

Rothman, J. and E. R. Brown (1989). "Indicators of Societal Action to Promote Social Health," in *Health Promotion Indicators and Actions*, S. B. Kar, ed. (New York: Springer), pp. 202–220.

Rothman, J. and J. E. Tropman (1987). "Models of Community Organization and Macro Practice: Their Mixing and Phasing," in *Strategies of Community Organization*, 4th ed., F. M. Cox, J. Erlich, J. L. Rothman, and J. E. Tropman, eds. (Itasca, IL: F. E. Peacock), pp. 3–26.

Rubinson, L. and L. Baillie (1981). "Planning School-Based Sexuality Programs Using the PRECEDE Model," *Journal of School Health* 51: 282–87.

Ruchlin, H. S. and M. H. Alderman (1980). "Cost of Hypertension Control at the Workplace," *Journal of Occupational Medicine* 22: 795–800.

Rundall, T. G. and K. A. Phillips (1990). "Informing and Educating the Electorate About AIDS," *Medical Care Review* 47: 3–13.

Rundall, T. G. and J. R. C. Wheeler (1979). "The Effect of Income on Use of Preventive Care: An Evaluation of Alternative Explanations," *Journal of Health and Social Behavior* 20: 397–406.

Rundall, T. G. and J. R. C. Wheeler (1979). "Factors Associated with Utilization of the Swine Flu Vaccination Program Among Senior Citizens in Tompkins County," *Medical Care* 17: 191–200.

Russell, E. M. and E. L. Iljonforeman (1985). "Self-Care in Illness—A Review," *Family Practice* 2: 108–21.

Russell, L. B. (1986). *Is Prevention Better Than Cure?* (Washington, DC: Brookings Institution).

Sackett, D. L. and J. C. Snow (1979). "The Magnitude of Compliance and Noncompliance," in *Compliance in Health Care*, R. B. Haynes, D. W. Taylor, and D. L. Sackett, eds. (Baltimore: Johns Hopkins University Press).

Sallis, J. F., W. L. Haskell, S. P. Fortmann et al. (1986). "Predictors of Adoption and Maintenance of Physical Activity in a Community Sample," *Preventive Medicine* 15: 331–41.

Sallis, J. F., M. F. Hovell, C. R. Hoffstetter et al. (1990). "Distance Between Homes and Exercise Facilities Related to Frequency of Exercise Among San Diego Residents," *Public Health Reports* 105: 179–85.

Sallis, J. F., R. B. Pinski, R. M. Grossman et al. (1988). "The Development of Self-Efficacy Scales for Health-Related Diet and Exercise Behaviors," *Health Education Research* 3: 283–92.

Salloway, J., W. Pletcher, and J. Collins (1978). "Sociological and Social-Psychological Models of Compliance with Prescribed Regimens: In Search of Synthesis," *Sociological Symposium* 23: 100–21.

Saltz, R. (1987). "The Role of Bars and Restaurants in Preventing Alcohol-Impaired Driving: An Evaluation of Server Intervention," *Evaluation and Health Professions* 10: 5–27.

Samuels, S. E. (1990). "Project LEAN: A National Campaign to Reduce Dietary Fat Consumption," *American Journal of Health Promotion* 4: 435–40.

Sanders, I. T. (1950). *Preparing a Community Profile: The Methodology of a Social Reconnaissance* (Lexington, KY: Kentucky Community Series No. 7, Bureau of Community Services, University of Kentucky).

Sauer, W. J. and R. Warland (1982). "Morale and Life Satisfaction," in *Research Instruments in Social Gerontology*, vol. 1, D. J. Mangen and W. A. Peterson, eds. (Minneapolis: University of Minnesota Press), pp. 123–41.

Sayegh, J. and L. W. Green (1976). "Family Planning Education: Program Design, Training Component, and Cost-Effectiveness of a Post-Partum Program in Beirut," *International Journal of Health Education* 19(Suppl): 1–20.

Schaeffer, M. (1985). *Designing and Implementing Procedures for Health and Human Services* (Beverly Hills: Sage).

Schellstede, W. P. and R. L. Ciszewski (1984). "Social Marketing of Contraceptives in Bangladesh," *Studies in Family Planning* 15(1) (Jan/Feb): 30–39.

Schiller, P. L. and L. S. Levin (1983). "Is Self-Care a Social Movement?" *Social Science and Medicine* 17: 1343–52.

Schiller, P., A. Steckler, L. Dawson, and F. Patton (1987). *Participatory Planning in Community Health Education: A Guide Based on the McDowell County, West Virginia Experience* (Oakland, CA: Third Party Publishing).

Schilling, R. F., L. D. Gilchrist, and S. P. Schinke (1985). "Smoking in the Workplace: Review of Critical Issues," *Public Health Reports* 100: 473–79.

Schinke, S. P. (1982). "A School-Based Model for Teenage Pregnancy Prevention," *Social Work in Education* 4: 34–42.

Schlesinger, M. (1988). "The Perfectibility of Public Programs: Real Lessons from the Large-Scale Demonstration Projects (Editorial)," *American Journal of Public Health* 78: 899–902.

Schmidt, D. and I. E. Leppik, eds. (1988). *Compliance in Epilepsy* (Amsterdam: Elsevier Science Publishers B.V.).

"The School Health Education Evaluation Study" (1985). *Journal of School Health* 55(Oct): whole issue no. 6.

Schorr, L. (1988). *Within Our Reach: Breaking the Cycle of Disadvantage* (New York: Doubleday/Anchor).

Schott, F. W. (1985). "WELCOM: The Wellness Council of the Midlands," in *A Decade of Survival: Past, Present, Future. Proceedings of the 20th Annual Meeting* (Washington, DC: Society of Prospective Medicine).

Schunk, D. H. and J. P. Carbonari (1984). "Self-Efficacy Models," in *Behavioral Health: A Handbook of Health Enhancement and Disease Prevention*, J. D. Matarazzo, S. M. Weiss, J. A. Herd et al., eds. (New York: Wiley), pp. 230–47.

Schuurman, J. and W. de Haes (1980). "Sexually Transmitted Diseases: Health Education by Telephone," *International Journal of Health Education* 23: 94–106.

Schwartz, J. L., ed. (1978). *Progress in Smoking Cessation* (New York: American Cancer Society).

Schwartz, J. L. (1987). *Review and Evaluation of Smoking Cessation Methods: The United States and Canada 1978–1985* (Washington, DC: Department of Health and Human Services, National Institutes of Health, NIH 87–2940).

Scriven, M. (1972). "Pros and Cons About Goal-Free Evaluation," *Evaluation Comment* 3(4): 1–5.

Secretary's Task Force on Black and Minority Health (1985). *Report of the Secretary's Task Force on Black and Minority Health* (Washington, DC: U.S. Department of Health and Human Services).

Sederburg, W., R. Ortwein, and W. Durr (1985). *Michigan's Health Initiative* (Lansing, MI: Michigan State Legislature, no date).

Segall, M. E. and C. A. Wynd (1990). "Health Conception, Health Locus of Control, and Power as Predictors of Smoking Behavior Change," *American Journal of Health Promotion* 4: 338–44.

Shamian, J. and L. Edgar (1987). "Nurses as Agents for Change in Teaching Breast Self-Examination," *Public Health Nursing* 4: 29–34.

Shannon, B. M., H. Smickiklas-Wright, B. W. Davis, and C. A. Lewis (1983). "Peer Educator Approach to Nutrition for the Elderly," *The Gerontologist* 23: 123–26.

Shaw, G. B. (1930). *The Apple Cart: A Political Extravaganza* (London: Constable and Co.), pp. xiv–xv.

Shea, S. and C. E. Basch (1990). "A Review of Five Major Community-Based Cardiovascular Disease Prevention Programs. Part I: Rationale, Design, and Theoretical Framework," *American Journal of Health Promotion* 4: 203–13.

Shephard, R. J., P. Corey, P. Renzland et al. (1982). "The Influence of an Employee Fitness and Lifestyle Modification Program Upon Medical Care Costs," *Canadian Journal of Public Health* 73: 259–63.

Shimkin, D. (1986–87). "Improving Rural Health: The Lessons of Mississippi and Tanzania," *International Quarterly of Community Health Education* 7: 149–65.

Shine, M. S., M. C. Silva, and F. S. Weed (1983). "Integrating Health Education into Baccalaureate Nursing Education," *Journal of Nursing Education* 22: 22–27.

Shipley, R. (1987). "Smoking Reduction Programs Help Business Snuff Out Health Problems," *Occupational Health and Safety* 56: 73–77.

Shoemaker, J. and H. L. Nix (1972). "A Study of Reputational Leaders Using the Concepts of Exchange and Coordinative Positions," *The Sociological Quarterly* 13: 516–24.

Shor, I. and P. Freire (1987). *A Pedagogy for Liberation* (Boston: Bergin and Garvey Publishers).

Shumaker, S. A., S. Parker, and J. Wolle, eds. (1990). *The Handbook of Health Behavior Change* (New York: Springer).

Sigerist, H. E. (1946). *The University at the Crossroads: Addresses and Essays* (New York: Henry Schuman).

Silvers, I. J., M. F. Hovell, M. H. Weisman, and M. R. Mueller (1985). "Assessing Physician-Patient Perceptions in Rheumatoid Arthritis—A Vital Component in Patient Education," *Arthritis and Rheumatism* 28: 300–07.

Simmons, J., ed. (1975). "Making Health Education Work," *American Journal of Public Health* 65(Oct 1975, Suppl): 1–49.

Simon, K. J. and J. Das (1984). "An Application of the Health Belief Model Toward Educational Diagnosis for VD Education," *Health Education Quarterly* 11: 403–18.

Simons-Morton, B. G., S. G. Brink, G. S. Parcel et al. (1989). *Preventing Alcohol Misuse Among Adolescents and Young Adults: A CDC Community Intervention Handbook* (Atlanta: Centers for Disease Control).

Simons-Morton, B. G., S. G. Brink, G. S. Parcel et al. (1989). *Preventing Alcohol-Related Health Problems Among Adolescents and Young Adults: A CDC Intervention Handbook* (Atlanta: Centers for Disease Control).

Simons-Morton, B. G., S. G. Brink, D. G. Simons-Morton et al. (1989). "An Ecological Approach to the Prevention of Injuries Due to Drinking and Driving," *Health Education Quarterly* 16: 397–411.

Simons-Morton, B. G., G. S. Parcel, N. M. O'Hara et al. (1988). "Health-Related Physical Fitness in Childhood: Status and Recommendations," *Annual Review of Public Health* 9: 403–25.

Simons-Morton, B. G., G. S. Parcel, and N. M. O'Hara (1988). "Implementing Organizational Changes to Promote Healthful Diet and Physical Activity at School," *Health Education Quarterly* 15: 115–30.

Simons-Morton, D. G., G. S. Parcel, S. G. Brink et al. (1988). *Promoting Physical Activity Among Adults: A CDC Community Intervention Handbook* (Atlanta: Centers for Disease Control).

Simons-Morton, D. G., B. G. Simons-Morton, G. S. Parcel, and J. G. Bunker (1988). "Influencing Personal and Environmental Conditions for Community Health: A Multilevel Intervention Model," *Family and Community Health* 11: 25–35.

Simpson, G. W. and B. E. Pruitt (1989). "The Development of Health Promotion Teams as Related to Wellness Programs in Texas Schools," *Health Education* 20(1): 26–28.

Skiff, A. W. (1974). "Experiences with Methods for Patient Teaching from a Public Health Service Hospital," *Health Education Monographs* 2(1): 48–53.

Sleet, D. A. (1987). "Health Education Approaches to Motor Vehicle Injury Prevention," *Public Health Reports* 102: 606–08.

Slenker, S., J. Price, S. Roberts, and S. Jurs (1984). "Joggers Versus Nonexercisers: An Analysis of Knowledge, Attitudes, Beliefs About Jogging," *Research Quarterly for Exercise and Sport* 55: 371–78.

Sloan, R. P., J. C. Gruman, and J. P. Allegrante (1987). *Investing in Employee Health: A Guide to Effective Health Promotion in the Workplace* (San Francisco: Jossey-Bass).

Slovic, P. (1986). "Informing and Educating the Public About Risk," *Risk Analysis* 6: 403–15.

Smith, C., J. L. Roberts, and L. L. Pendleton (1988). "Booze on the Box – The Portrayal of Alcohol on British Television: A Content Analysis," *Health Education Research* 3: 267–72.

Smith, G. S. and J. F. Kraus (1988). "Alcohol and Residential, Recreational, and Occupational Injuries: A Review of the Epidemiologic Evidence," *Annual Review of Public Health* 9: 99–122.

Smith, H. (1988). *The Power Game, How Washington Works* (New York: Random House).

Smith, J. A. and D. L. Scammon (1987). "A Market Segment Analysis of Adult Physical Activity: Exercise Beliefs, Attitudes, Intentions, and Behaviors," *Advances in Nonprofit Marketing*, vol. 2 (Greenwich, CT: JAI Press).

Smith, P. (1989). "National School Boards Association, and Center for Chronic Disease Prevention and Health Promotion, CDC, School Policies and Programs on Smoking and Health – United States, 1988," *Morbidity and Mortality Weekly Report* 38: 202–03; also in *Journal of the American Medical Association* 261(1989): 2488.

Smith, T. (1973). "Policy Roles: An Analysis of Policy Formulators and Policy Implementors," *Policy Sciences* 4: 297–307.

Sobal, J., C. M. Valente, H. L. Muncie, Jr. et al (1986). "Physicians' Beliefs About the Importance of 25 Health Promoting Behaviors," *American Journal of Public Health* 75: 1427–28.

Sobel, D. and F. Hornbacher (1973). *An Everyday Guide to Your Health* (New York: Grossman).

Society for Public Health Education (1977). "Guidelines for the Preparation and Practice of Professional Health Educators," *Health Education Monographs* 5: 75–89.

Soen, D. (1981). "Citizen and Community Participation in Urban Renewal and Rehabilitation – Comments on Theory and Practice," *Community Development Journal* 16: 105–17.

Sogaard, A. J. (1988). "The Effect of a Mass-Media Dental Health Education Campaign," *Health Education Research* 3: 243–55.

Solomon, M. Z. and W. DeJong (1986). "Recent Sexually Transmitted Disease Prevention Efforts and Their Implications for AIDS Health Education," *Health Education Quarterly* 13: 301–16.

Somers, A., ed. (1976). *Health Promotion and Consumer Health Education* (Greenbelt, MD: Aspen Systems).

Somers, A. and R. Somers (1987). "Four 'Orphan' Areas in Current Medical Education: What Hope for Adoption?" *Family Medicine* 19: 137–40.

Sorensen, A. A. and J. S. Sinacore (1979). "Developing a Regional Health Education Program," *Regional Health Education* 3(2): 79–84.

Source Book of Health Insurance Data (1989). (New York: Health Insurance Association of America).

Spain, C., E. Eastman, and K. Kizer (1989). "Model Standards Impact on Local Health Department Performance in California," *American Journal of Public Health* 79: 969–74.

Spiegel, C. V. and F. C. Lindaman (1977). "Children Can't Fly: A Program to Prevent Childhood Morbidity and Mortality from Window Falls," *American Journal of Public Health* 67: 1143–46.

Spretnak, C. and F. Capra (1984). *Green Politics* (New York: E.P. Dutton).

Squyres, W., ed. (1980). *Patient Education: An Inquiry into the State of the Art* (New York: Springer).

Squyres, W. and Associates (1985). *Patient Education and Health Promotion in Medical Care* (Palo Alto, CA: Mayfield).

Stainbrook, G. and L. W. Green (1982). "Behavior and Behaviorism in Health Education," *Health Education* 13: 14–19.

Starfield, B. (1982). "Family Income, Ill Health, and Medical Care of U.S. Children," *Journal of Public Health Policy* 3: 244–59.

Starfield, B. and P. Budetti (1985). "Child Health Risk Factors," *Health Services Research* 19(6, Pt 2): 817–86.

State School Health Education Project (1981). *Recommendations for School Health Education: A Handbook for State Policymakers* (Denver: Education Commission of the States).

Statistics Canada and Department of the Secretary of State of Canada (1986). *Report of the Canadian Health and Disability Survey* (Ottawa: Minister of Supply and Services Canada, Catalog No. 82-555).

Steckler, A. (1989). "The Use of Qualitative Evaluation Methods to Test Internal Validity: An Example in a Work Site Health Promotion Program," *Evaluation and the Health Professions* 12: 115–33.

Steckler, A. and L. Dawson (1978). "Determinants of Consumer Influence in a Health Systems Agency," *Health Education Monographs* 6: 377–93.

Steckler, A. and L. Dawson (1982). "The Role of Health Education in Public Policy Development," *Health Education Quarterly* 9: 275–92.

Steckler, A., L. Dawson, R. M. Goodman, and N. Epstein (1987). "Policy Advocacy: Three Emerging Roles for Health Education," in *Advances in Health Education and Promotion*, vol. 2, W. B. Ward, ed. (Greenwich, CT: JAI Press), pp. 5–27.

Steckler, A., L. Dawson, and A. Williams (1981). "Consumer Participation and Influence in a Health Systems Agency," *Journal of Community Health* 6: 181–93.

Steckler, A. and R. M. Goodman (1989). "How to Institutionalize Health Promotion Programs," *American Journal of Health Promotion* 3: 34–44.

Steckler, A. and R. M. Goodman (1989). "A Model for the Institutionalization of Health Promotion Programs," *Family and Community Health* 11: 63–78.

Steckler, A., K. Orville, E. Eng, and L. Dawson (1989). *PATCHing It Together: A Formative Evaluation of CDC's Planned Approach to Community Health (PATCH) Program* (Chapel Hill, NC: Department of Health Behavior and Health Education, School of Public Health, University of North Carolina).

Steinfeld, J., W. Griffiths, K. Ball, and R. M. Taylor, eds. (1977). *Smoking and Health: Health Consequences, Education, Cessation Activities, and Government Action*, vol. 2 (Washington, DC: Department of Health, Education and Welfare, NIH 77-1413).

Stephens, T. (1987). "Secular Trends in Adult Physical Activity: Exercise Boom or Bust," *Research Quarterly for Exercise and Sport* 58: 95.

Stephens, T., D. R. Jacobs, Jr., and C. C. White (1985). "A Descriptive Epidemiology of Leisure-Time Physical Activity," *Public Health Reports* 100: 147–58.

Stephens, T. and C. A. Schoenborn (1988). "Adult Health Practices in the United States and Canada," in National Center for Health Statistics, *Vital and Health Statistics* (Washington, DC: U.S. Government Printing Office, Series 5, No. 3, DHHS-PHS 88-1479).

Stockman, D. A. (1986). *The Triumph of Politics: How the Reagan Revolution Failed* (New York: Harper & Row).

Stone, E. J., C. L. Perry, and R. V. Luepker (1989). "Synthesis of Cardiovascular Behavioral Research for Youth Health Promotion," *Health Education Quarterly* 16: 155–69.

Strategies for Promoting Health in Special Populations (Washington, DC: Office of Disease Prevention and Health Promotion, 1981), reprinted in *Journal of Public Health Policy* 8(1987): 369–423.

Strecher, V. J., B. M. DeVellis, M. H. Becker, and I. M. Rosenstock (1986). "The Role of Self-Efficacy in Achieving Health Behavior Change," *Health Education Quarterly* 13: 73–92.

Strehlow, M. S. (1983). *Education for Health* (London: Harper & Row).

Stuart, G. W. (1969). "Planning and Evaluation in Health Education," *International Journal of Health Education* 12: 65–76.

Suchman, E. (1967). "Preventive Health Behavior: A Model for Research on Community Health Campaigns," *Journal of Health and Social Behavior* 8: 197–209.

Sutherland, M., C. Pittman-Sisco, T. Lacher, and N. Watkins (1987). "The Application of a Health Education Planning Model to a School-Based Risk Reduction Model," *Health Education* 18(3): 47–51.

Syme, L. W. (1986). "Strategies for Health Promotion," *Preventive Medicine* 15: 492–507.

Targets for Health for All (1986). (Copenhagen: World Health Organization Regional Office for Europe).

Tarlov, A. R., B. H. Kehrer, D. P. Hall et al. (1987). "Foundation Work: The Health Promotion Program of the Henry J. Kaiser Family Foundation," *American Journal of Health Promotion* 2: 74–80.

Tash, R., R. O'Shea, and L. Cohen (1969). "Testing a Preventive-Symptomatic Theory of Dental Health Behavior," *American Journal of Public Health* 59: 514–21.

Taylor, C. W. (1984). "Promoting Health and Strengthening Wellness Through Environmental Variables," in *Behavioral Health: A Handbook of Health Enhancement and Disease Prevention*, J. D. Matarazzo, S. M. Weiss, J. A. Herd et al., eds. (New York: Wiley), pp. 130–49.

Taylor, D. (1979). "A Test of the Health Belief Model in Hypertension," in *Compliance in Health Care*, R. B. Haynes, D. W. Taylor, and D. L. Sackett, eds. (Baltimore: Johns Hopkins University Press): 103–09.

Taylor, D. (1982). *Medicines, Health, and the Poor World* (London: Office of Health Economics).

Terris, M. (1975). "Approaches to an Epidemiology of Health," *American Journal of Public Health* 65: 1037–45.

Terris, M. (1976). "The Epidemiologic Revolution, National Health Insurance, and the Role of Health Departments," *American Journal of Public Health* 66: 1155–64.

Terris, M. (1978). "Public Health in the United States: The Next 100 Years," *Journal of Public Health Policy* 93: 602–08.

Terris, M. (1986). "What Is Health Promotion?" *Journal of Public Health Policy* 7: 147–51.

Terry, P. B., V. L. Wang, B. S. Flynn et al. (1981). "A Continuing Medical Education Program in Chronic Obstructive Pulmonary Diseases: Design and Outcome," *American Review of Respiratory Distress* 123: 41–46.

Thoits, P. (1982). "Conceptual, Methodological, and Theoretical Problems in Studying Social Support as a Buffer Against Life Stress," *Journal of Health and Social Behavior* 23: 145–59.

Thomas, S. B. (1990). "Community Health Advocacy for Racial and Ethnic Minorities in the United States: Issues and Challenges for Health Education," *Health Education Quarterly* 17: 13–19.

Thompson, R. S., S. Taplin, A. P. Carter et al. (1988). "A Risk-Based Breast Cancer Screening Program," *HMO Practice* 2: 177–91.

Thoresen, C. E. and K. Kirmil-Gray (1983). "Self-Management Psychology and the Treatment of Childhood Asthma," *Journal of Allergy and Clinical Immunology* 72(Nov, Suppl) 596–606.

Thornberry, O. T., R. W. Wilson, and P. M. Golden (1986). "Health Promotion Data for the 1990 Objectives. Estimates from the National Health Interview Survey of Health Promotion and Disease Prevention: United States, 1985," *Advance Data from Vital and Health Statistics* 126(Sept 19, 1986), DHHS No. (PHS) 86-1250.

Thornton, M. A. (1979). "Preventive Dentistry in the Veterans Administration," *Dental Hygiene* 53: 121–24.

Tirrell, B. and L. Hart (1980). "The Relationship of Health Beliefs and Knowledge to Exercise Compliance in Patients After Coronory Bypass," *Heart and Lung* 9: 487–93.

Titmus, R. (1972). *The Gift Relationship from Human Blood to Social Policy* (New York: Vintage Books).

Tjerandsen, C. (1980). *Education for Citizenship: A Foundation's Experience* (Santa Cruz, CA: Emil Schwarzhaupt Foundation).

Todaro, V., J. Denard, P. Clarke et al. (1987). "Survey of Worksite Smoking Policies," *Morbidity and Mortality Weekly Report* 36: 177–79.

Tones, B. K. (1979). "Past Achievement and Future Success," in *Health Education – Perspectives and Choices*, I. Sutherland, ed. (London: Allen & Unwin), chap. 12.

Tonin, M. O. (1980). "Concepts in Community Participation," *International Journal of Health Education* 23(Suppl): 1–13.

Toward a Healthy Community: Organizing Events for Community Health Promotion (Washington, DC: U.S. Department of Health and Human Services, Office of Disease Prevention and Health Promotion, PHS 80-50113, 1980).

Trends: Consumer Attitudes and the Supermarket (1989). (Washington, DC: Food Marketing Institute).

Tuckett, D. A., M. Boulton, and M. Olson (1985). "A New Approach to the Measurement of Patients' Understanding of What They Are Told in Medical Consultations," *Journal of Health and Social Behavior* 26: 27–38.

Udry, J., L. Clark, C. Chase et al. (1972). "Can Mass Media Advertising Increase Contraceptive Use?" *Family Planning Perspectives* 4: 37–44.

U.S. Bureau of the Census (1989). *Statistical Abstract of the United States: 1990*, 109th ed. (Washington, DC: U.S. Government Printing Office).

U.S. Department of Education, Office of Educational Research and Improvement (1988). *Youth Indicators 1988: Trends in the Well-Being of American Youth* (Washington, DC: U.S. Government Printing Office).

U.S. Department of Health, Education and Welfare (1979). *Healthy People: Surgeon General's Report on Health Promotion and Disease Prevention* (Washington, DC: Public Health Service, DHEW-PHS-79-55071).

U.S. Department of Health and Human Services (1981). *National Conference for Institutions Preparing Health Educators: Proceedings* (Washington, DC: U.S. Office of Health Information and Health Promotion, PHS 81-50171).

U.S. Department of Health and Human Services (1981). *Promoting Health in Special Populations* (Washington, DC: Office of Disease Prevention and Health Promotion), reprinted in *Journal of Public Health Policy* 8(1987): 369–423.

U.S. Department of Health and Human Services (1985). *Report of the Secretary's Task Force on Black and Minority Health* (Washington, DC: U.S. Government Printing Office).

U.S. Department of Health and Human Services (1986). *The 1990 Health Objectives for the Nation: A Midcourse Review* (Washington, DC: Office of Disease Prevention and Health Promotion).

U.S. Department of Health and Human Services (1988). *Surgeon General's Report on Nutrition and Health* (Washington, DC: Public Health Service, Publ. No. 88-50210).

U.S. Department of Health and Human Services (1990). *The Health Consequences of Smoking Cessation: A Report of the Surgeon General* (Washington, DC: PHS, Office on Smoking and Health).

U.S. Department of Health and Human Services (1990). *Promoting Health/Preventing Disease: Year 2000 Objectives for the Nation* (Washington, DC: Office of the Assistant Secretary for Health, Public Health Service, Draft).

U.S. Preventive Services Task Force (1989). *Guide to Clinical Preventive Services: An Assessment of the Effectiveness of 169 Interventions* (Baltimore: William & Wilkens).

Valente, C. M., J. Sobal, H. L. Muncie, Jr. et al. (1986). "Health Promotion: Physicians' Beliefs, Attitudes, and Practices," *American Journal of Preventive Medicine* 2: 82–88.

Van de Ven, A. H. and A. L. Delbecq (1972). "The Nominal Group as a Research Instrument for Exploratory Health Studies," *American Journal of Public Health* 62: 337–42.

Van Meter, D. and C. Van Horn (1975). "The Policy Implementation Process: A Conceptual Framework," *Administration and Society* 6: 445–88.

Vartiainen, E. and P. Puska (1987). "The North Karelia Youth Project 1978–80: Effects of Two Years of Educational Intervention on Cardiovascular Risk Factors and Health Behavior in Adolescence," in *Cardiovascular Risk Factors in Childhood: Epidemiology and Prevention*, B. Hetzel and G. S. Berenson, eds. (Dublin: Elsevier), pp. 183–202.

Vickers, Sir G. (1958). "What Sets the Goals of Public Health," *New England Journal of Medicine* 258: 12.

Vickery, D. M. and J. F. Fries (1981). "Effect of Self-Care Book," *Journal of the American Medical Association* 245(1981): 341–42.

Vickery, D. M., H. Kalmer, D. Lowry et al. (1983). "Effect of a Self-Care Education Program on Medical Visits," *Journal of the American Medical Association* 250: 2952–56.

Viet, C. T. and J. E. Ware, Jr. (1982). "Measuring Health and Health-Care Outcomes: Issues and Recommendations," in *Values and Long-Term Care*, R. L. Kane and R. A. Kane, eds. (Lexington, MA: Lexington Books).

Vincent, M. L., A. F. Clearie, C. G. Johnson and P. A. Sharpe (1988). *Reducing Unintended Adolescent Pregnancy Through School/Community Education Interventions: A South Carolina Case Study* (Columbia, SC: School of Public Health, University of South Carolina).

Vincent, M. L., A. F. Clearie, and M. D. Schluchter (1987). "Reducing Adolescent Pregnancy Through School and Community-Based Education," *Journal of the American Medical Association* 257: 3382–86.

Viseltear, A. (1976). "A Short History of P.L. 94-317," in *Preventive Medicine USA*, American College of Preventive Medicine and Fogerty Center, eds. (New York: Prodist).

Vojtecky, M. A. (1986). "Commentary: A Unified Approach to Health Promotion and Health Protection," *Journal of Community Health* 11: 219–21.

Wagner, E. H. and P. A. Guild (1989). "Primer on Evaluation Methods: Choosing an Evaluation Strategy," *American Journal of Health Promotion* 4: 134–39.

Waitzkin, H. (1985). "Information Giving in Medical Care," *Journal of Health and Social Behavior* 26: 81–101.

Wallack, L. M. (1980). "Assessing Effects of Mass Media Campaigns: An Alternative Perspective," *Alcohol, Health and Research World* 5: 17–29.

Wallack, L. M. (1981). "Mass Media Campaigns: The Odds Against Finding Behavior Change," *Health Education Quarterly* 8: 209–60.

Wallack, L. M. (1983). "Mass Media Campaigns in a Hostile Environment: Advertising as Anti-Health Education," *Journal of Drug Addiction* 28: 51–63.

Wallack, L. M. (1985). "Health Educators and the New Generation of Strategies," *Hygie* 4(2): 23–30.

Wallack, L. M. (1990). "Media Advocacy: Promoting Health Through Mass Communication," in *Health Behavior and Health Education: Theory, Research, and Practice*, K. Glanz, F. M. Lewis, and B. K. Rimer, eds. (San Francisco: Jossey-Bass), chap. 16.

Wallack, L. and N. Wallerstein (1986–87). "Health Education and Prevention: Designing Community Initiatives," *International Quarterly of Community Health Education* 7: 319–42.

Wallerstein, N. (1990). [Book review of] "P. Schiller, A. Steckler, L. Dawson, and F. Patton (1987). *Participatory Planning in Community Health Education: A Guide Based on the McDowell County, West Virginia Experience* (Oakland, CA: Third Party Publishing), in *Health Education Quarterly* 17: 119–21.

Wallerstein, N. and E. Bernstein (1988). "Empowerment Education: Freire's Ideas Adapted to Health Education," *Health Education Quarterly* 15: 379–94.

Wallston, B., S. Alagna, B. DeVellis, and R. DeVellis (1983). "Social Support and Physical Health," *Health Psychology* 2: 367–91.

Wallston, B. S. and K. A. Wallston (1978). "Locus of Control and Health: A Review of the Literature," *Health Education Monographs* 6: 107–17.

Walsh, D. C. (1984). "Corporate Smoking Policies: A Review and an Analysis," *Journal of Occupational Medicine* 26: 17–22.

Walsh, D. C. and V. McDougall (1988). "Current Policies Regarding Smoking in the Workplace," *American Journal of Industrial Medicine* 13: 181–90.

Walter, H. J. (1989). "Primary Prevention of Chronic Disease Among Children: The School-Based 'Know Your Body' Intervention Trials," *Health Education Quarterly* 16: 201–14.

Walter, H. J. and E. L. Wynder (1989). "The Development, Implementation, Evaluation, and Future Directions of a Chronic Disease Prevention Program for Children: The 'Know Your Body' Studies," *Preventive Medicine* 18: 59–71.

Wang, V. L., P. Ephross, and L. W. Green (1975). "The Point of Diminishing Returns in Nutrition Education Through Home Visits by Aides: An Evaluation of EFNEP," *Health Education Monographs* 3: 70–88; also in *The SOPHE Heritage Collection of Health Education Monographs*, vol. 3, J. Zapka, ed. (Oakland, CA: Third Party Publishing), pp. 155–73.

Wang, V. L., P. Terry, B. S. Flynn et al. (1979). "Multiple Indicators of Continuing Medical Education Priorities for Chronic Lung Diseases in Appalachia," *Journal of Medical Education* 54: 803–11.

Ward, G. H. (1978). "Changing Trends in Control of Hypertension," *Public Health Reports* 93: 31–34.

Ware, B. G. (1985). "Occupational Health Education: A Nontraditional Role for a Health Educator," in *Advancing Health Through Education: A Case Study Approach*, H. P. Cleary, J. M. Kichen, and P. G. Ensor, eds. (Palo Alto, CA: Mayfield), pp. 319–23.

Warnecke, R., S. Graham, S. Rosenthal, and C. Manfredi (1978). "Social and Psychological Correlates of Smoking Behavior Among Black Women," *Journal of Health and Social Behavior* 19: 397–410.

Warner, K. E. (1977). "The Effects of the Anti-Smoking Campaign on Cigarette Consumption," *American Journal of Public Health* 67: 645–50.

Warner, K. E. (1981). "Cigarette Smoking in the 1970's: The Impact of the Anti-Smoking Campaign on Consumption," *Science* 211(13): 729–31.

Warner, K. E. (1986). *Selling Smoke: Cigarette Advertising and Public Health* (Washington, DC: American Public Health Association).

Warner, K. E. (1987). "Selling Health Promotion to Corporate America: Uses and Abuses of the Economic Argument," *Health Education Quarterly* 14: 39–55.

Warner, K. E. (1989). "Effects of the Antismoking Campaign: An Update," *American Journal of Public Health* 79: 144–51.

Warner, K. E. and H. A. Murt (1983). "Premature Deaths Avoided by the Antismoking Campaign," *American Journal of Public Health* 73: 672–77.

Webb, G. R., R. W. Sanson-Fisher, and J. A. Bowman (1988). "Psychosocial Factors Related to Parental Restraint of Pre-School Children in Motor Vehicles," *Accident Analysis and Prevention* 20: 87–94.

Wechsler, H., S. Levine, R. K. Idelson et al. (1983). "The Physician's Role in Health Promotion: Survey of Primary Care Practitioners," *New England Journal of Medicine* 308: 97–100.

Weeks, M. F., R. A. Kulka, J. T. Lessler et al. (1983). "Personal Versus Telephone Surveys for Collecting Household Health Data at the Local Level," *American Journal of Public Health* 73: 1389–94.

Weinberg, M., S. A. Mazzuca, S. J. Cohen, and C. J. McDonald (1982). "Physicians' Ratings of Information Sources About Their Preventive Medicine Decisions," *Preventive Medicine* 11: 717–23.

Weinberger, M., J. Greene, J. Mamlin, and M. Jerin (1981). "Health Beliefs and Smoking Behavior," *American Journal of Public Health* 71: 1253–55.

Weiss, C. H. (1972). *Evaluation Research: Methods of Assessing Program Effectiveness* (Englewood Cliffs, NJ: Prentice-Hall).

Weiss, C. H. (1973). "Between the Cup and the Lip," *Evaluation*, 1(2): 54.

Weiss, S. M., J. A. Herd, and B. Fox, eds. (1981). *Perspectives on Behavioral Medicine* (New York: Academic Press).

Weitzel, M. H. and P. R. Waller (1990). "Predictive Factors for Health-Promotive Behaviors in White, Hispanic, and Black Blue-Collar Workers," *Family and Community Health* 13: 23–34.

Wells, B. L., J. D. DePue, T. M. Lasater, and R. A. Carleton (1988). "A Report on Church Site Weight Control," *Health Education Research* 3: 305–16.

Wells, K. B., C. E. Lewis, B. Leake et al. (1986). "The Practices of General and Subspecialty Internists in Counseling About Smoking and Exercise," *American Journal of Public Health* 76: 1009–13.

Wells, K. B., J. E. Ware, and C. E. Lewis (1984). "Physicians' Attitudes in Counseling Patients About Smoking," *Medical Care* 22: 360–65.

Werden, P. (1974). "Health Education for Indian Students," *Journal of School Health* 44: 319–23.

Werner, D. (1980). "Health Care and Human Dignity," in *Health: The Human Factor: Readings in Health, Development, and Community Participation*, S. B. Rifkin, ed. (Geneva: CMC, World Council of Churches, Special Series No. 3).

Westberg, J. (1986). "Gaining Physician Support for Effective Patient Education," *Patient Education and Counseling* 8: 407–14.

Wheeler, J. R. C. and T. G. Rundall (1980). "Secondary Preventive Health Behavior," *Health Education Quarterly* 7: 243–62.

Williams, A. F. and H. Wechsler (1972). "Interrelationship of Preventive Actions in Health and Other Areas," *Health Services Reports* 87: 969–76.

Williams, L. S. (1986). "AIDS Risk Reduction: A Community Health Education Intervention for Minority High Risk Group Members," *Health Education Quarterly* 13: 407–22.

Williams, R. M. (1990). "Rx: Social Reconnaissance," *Foundation News* 31(4): 24–29.

Williams, W. and R. Elmore, eds. (1976). *Social Program Implementation* (New York: Academic Press).

Williamson, J. and J. M. Chapin (1980). "Adverse Reactions to Prescribed Drugs in the Elderly: A Multicare Investigation," *Age and Aging* 9: 73–80.

Williamson, J. W., S. Aronovitch, L. Simonson et al. (1975). "Health Accounting: An Outcome-Based System of Quality Assurance—Illustrative Application to Hypertension," *Bulletin of the New York Academy of Medicine* 51: 727–38.

Williamson, N. B., M. J. Burton, W. B. Brown et al. (1988). "Changes in Mastitis Management Practices Associated with Client Education and the Effects of Adopting Recommended Mastitis Control Procedures on Herd Production," *Preventive Veterinary Medicine* 5: 213–23.

Wilson, R. (1981). "Do Health Indicators Indicate Health?" *American Journal of Public Health* 71: 461.

Wilson, R. W. and J. Elinson (1981). "National Survey of Personal Health Practices and Consequences: Background, Conceptual Issues, and Selected Findings," *Public Health Reports* 96: 218–25.

Wilson, R. W. and D. C. Iverson (1982). "Federal Data Bases for Health Education Research," *Health Education* 13(3): 30–34.

Wilson, W. J. (1987). *The Truly Disadvantaged: The Inner City, the Underclass, and Public Policy* (Chicago: The University of Chicago Press).

Winder, A. E. (1985). "The Mouse That Roared: A Case History of Community Organization for Health Practice," *Health Education Quarterly* 12: 353–63.

Windom, R., J. M. McGinnis, and J. E. Fielding (1987). "Examining Worksite Health Promotion Programs," *Business and Health* 4: 26–37.

Windsor, R. A. (1984). "Planning and Evaluation of Public Health Education Programs in Rural Settings: Theory into Practice," in *Advancing Health Through Education: A Case Study Approach*, H.P. Cleary, J. M. Kichen, P. G. Ensor, eds. (Palo Alto, CA: Mayfield), pp. 273–84.

Windsor, R. A., T. Baranowski, N. Clark, and G. Cutter (1984). *Evaluation of Health Promotion and Education Programs* (Palo Alto, CA: Mayfield).

Windsor, R. A., L. W. Green, and J. M. Roseman (1980). "Health Promotion and Maintenance for Patients with Chronic Obstructive Pulmonary Disease: A Review," *Journal of Chronic Disease* 33: 5–12.

Windsor, R. A. and C. T. Orleans (1986). "Guidelines and Methodological Standards for Smoking Cessation Intervention Research Among Pregnant Women: Improving the Science and Art," *Health Education Quarterly* 13(2): 131–61.

Winett, R. A., D. G. Altman, and A. C. King (1990). "Conceptual and Strategic Foundations for Effective Media Campaigns for Preventing the Spread of HIV Infection," *Evaluation and Program Planning* 13: 91–104.

Winickoff, R. N., K. L. Coltin, M. M. Morgan et al. (1984). "Improving Physician Performance Through Peer Companions," *Medical Care* 22: 527–34.

Winkleby, M. A., S. P. Fortmann, and D. C. Barrett (1990). "Social Class Disparities in Risk Factors for Disease: Eight-Year Prevalence Patterns by Level of Education," *Preventive Medicine* 19: 1–12.

Winslow, C. E. A. (1920). "The Untilled Fields of Public Health," *Science* 51: 23.

Wishner, W. J. and M. D. O'Brien (1978). "Diabetes and the Family," *Medical Clinics of North America* 62: 849–56.

Wojtowicz, G. G. (1990). "A Secondary Analysis of the School Health Education Evaluation Data Base," *Journal of School Health* 60: 56–59.

Wolinsky, F. D., R. M. Coe, D. K. Miller, and J. M. Prendergast (1985). "Correlate of the Elderly," *Journal of Community Health* 11: 93–107.

Woo, B., B. Woo, F. Cook et al. (1985). "Screening Procedures in the Asymptomatic Adult: Comparison of Physicians' Recommendations, Patients' Desires, Published Guidelines, and Actual Practice," *Journal of the American Medical Association* 254: 1480–84.

Woolhandler, S. and D. U. Himmelstein (1988). "Reverse Targeting of Preventive Care Due to Lack of Health Insurance," *Journal of the American Medical Association* 259: 2872–74.

Worden, J. K., B. S. Flynn, B. M. Geller et al. (1988). "Development of a Smoking Prevention Mass-Media Program Using Diagnostic and Formative Research," *Preventive Medicine* 17: 531–58.

Worden, J. K., L. J. Solomon, B. S. Flynn et al. (1990). "A Community-Wide Program in Breast Self-Examination Training and Maintenance," *Preventive Medicine* 19: 254–69.

World Bank (1983). *World Development Report, 1983* (New York: Oxford University Press).

World Health Assembly (1982). *New Policies for Health Education in Primary Health Care: Background Document for the Technical Discussions of the Thirty-Sixth World Health Assembly* (Geneva: World Health Organization, 661 TD/HED/82.1).

World Health Assembly (1985). *New Policies for Health Education in Primary Health Care: Technical Discussions of the Thirty-Sixth World Health Assembly* (Geneva: World Health Organization).

World Health Organization (1978). *Alma-Ata 1978: Primary Health Care* (Geneva: World Health Organization, "Health for All" Series No. 1).

World Health Organization (1979). *Report of the Task Force on Health Education in Family Health* (Geneva: WHO Technical Report Series 45).

World Health Organization (1981). *Health Program Evaluation: Guiding Principles* (Geneva, World Health Organization).

World Health Organization (1983). *Expert Committee on New Approaches to Health Education in Primary Health Care* (Geneva: World Health Organization Tech. Rep. Series 690).

World Health Organization (1984). *Health Promotion: A Discussion Document on the Concepts and Principles* (Copenhagen: WHO Regional Office for Europe, ICP/HSR 602).

World Health Organization (1986). *Targets for Health for All* (Copenhagen: WHO Regional Office for Europe).

World Health Organization and United Nations Children's Fund (1986). *Helping a Billion Children Learn About Health: Report of the WHO/UNICEF International Consultation on Health Education for School-Age Children, 1985* (Geneva: World Health Organization).

Wurtele, S., M. Roberts, and J. Leeper (1982). "Health Beliefs and Intentions: Predictors of Return Compliance in a Tuberculosis Detection Drive," *Journal of Applied Social Psychology* 53: 19–21.

Wyllie, A. and S. Casswell (1989). "The Response of New Zealand Boys to Corporate and Sponsorship Alcohol Advertising on Television," *British Journal of Addiction* 84: 639–46.

Xin-Zhi, W., H. Zhao-guang, and C. Dan-yang (1987). "Smoking Prevalence in Chinese Aged 15 and Above," *Chinese Medical Journal* 100: 686–92.

Young, K. E., C. M. Chambers, H. R. Kells et al. (1983). *Understanding Accreditation* (San Francisco: Jossey-Bass).

Zapka, J. G. (1985). "Management Functions of the Health Education Director: Examples of Data Management Activities," in *Advancing Health Through Education: A Case Study Approach*, H. P. Cleary, J. Kitchen, and P. Ensor, eds. (Palo Alto, CA: Mayfield).

Zapka, J. G. and S. Dorfman (1982). "Consumer Participation: Case Study of the College Health Setting," *Journal of American College Health* 30: 197–203.

Zapka, J. G. and J. A. Mamon (1982). "Integration of Theory, Practitioner Standards, Literature Findings, and Baseline Data: A Case Study in Planning Breast Self-Examination Education," *Health Education Quarterly* 9: 330–56.

Zapka, J. G. and J. A. Mamon (1986). "Breast Self-Examination in Young Women. II. Characteristics Associated with Proficiency," *American Journal of Preventive Medicine* 2: 70–78.

Zapka, J. G. and R. M. Mazur (1977). "Peer Sex Training and Evaluation," *American Journal of Public Health* 67: 450–54.

Zapka, J. G., A. Stoddard, and R. Barth et al. (1989). "Breast Cancer Screening Utilization by Latina Community Health Center Clients," *Health Education Research* 4: 461–68.

Zapka, J. G., A. M. Stoddard, M. E. Costanza, and H. L. Greene (1989). "Breast Cancer Screening by Mammography: Utilization and Associated Factors," *American Journal of Public Health* 79: 1499–502.

Zeldman, M. and Myrom, S. (1983). *How to Plan Projects and Keep Them on Schedule* (San Diego: Integrated Software Systems Corp.).

Zelnik, M. and Y. J. Kim (1982). "Sex Education and Its Association with Teenage Sexual Activity," *Family Planning Perspectives* 14: 117–26.

Zill, N. and C. C. Rogers (1988). "Recent Trends in the Well-Being of Children in the United States and Their Implications for Public Policy," in *Family Change and Public Policy*, A. Cherlin, ed. (Washington, DC: Urban Institute Press).

Index